Endocrinology and Metabolism: Clinical Research

Endocrinology and Metabolism: Clinical Research

Editor: Dante Banks

FOSTER
ACADEMICS
www.fosteracademics.com

www.fosteracademics.com

FOSTER ACADEMICS

Cataloging-in-Publication Data

Endocrinology and metabolism : clinical research / edited by Dante Banks.
p. cm.
Includes bibliographical references and index.
ISBN 978-1-63242-641-3
1. Endocrinology. 2. Metabolism. 3. Internal medicine. 4. Metabolism--Disorders. I. Banks, Dante.
RC648 .E53 2019
616.4--dc23

Foster Academics,
118-35 Queens Blvd., Suite 400,
Forest Hills, NY 11375, USA

ISBN 978-1-63242-641-3 (Hardback)

Printed and bound in China.

Contents

Preface

Endocrinology is a branch of medicine and biology that is concerned with the diseases and conditions of the endocrine system and the hormones associated with it. Metabolism refers to the life-sustaining chemical reactions occurring in the living organism. Since most organisms live under constantly changing environments, metabolic reactions should be finely regulated to maintain homeostasis. This metabolic regulation further allows organisms to interact actively with the environment and respond to signals. Metabolic regulation occurs extrinsically or intrinsically. In extrinsic control, cells respond to signals from other cells, transmitted in the form of hormones, growth factors and other soluble messengers. A good example of this is the endocrine hormone insulin that regulates glucose metabolism. Therefore, any hormonal imbalance in the endocrine system leads to metabolic syndromes. This book explores all the important aspects of endocrinology and metabolism. It provides significant information of these disciplines to help develop a good understanding of associated endocrine and metabolic disorders. Those in search of information to further their knowledge will be greatly assisted by this book.

Various studies have approached the subject by analyzing it with a single perspective, but the present book provides diverse methodologies and techniques to address this field. This book contains theories and applications needed for understanding the subject from different perspectives. The aim is to keep the readers informed about the progresses in the field; therefore, the contributions were carefully examined to compile novel researches by specialists from across the globe.

Indeed, the job of the editor is the most crucial and challenging in compiling all chapters into a single book. In the end, I would extend my sincere thanks to the chapter authors for their profound work. I am also thankful for the support provided by my family and colleagues during the compilation of this book.

Editor

1

Papillary thyroid microcarcinoma: characteristics at presentation, and evaluation of clinical and histological features associated with a worse prognosis in a Latin American cohort

José M. Domínguez[1], Flavia Nilo[1], María T. Martínez[1], José M. Massardo[1], Sueli Muñoz[1], Tania Contreras[1], Rocío Carmona[1], Joaquín Jerez[1], Hernán González[2], Nicolás Droppelmann[2], Augusto León[2]

[1] Department of Endocrinology, Faculty of Medicine, Pontificia Universidad Católica de Chile, Santiago, Región Metropolitana, Chile
[2] Department of Surgery, Faculty of Medicine, Pontificia Universidad Católica de Chile, Santiago, Región Metropolitana, Chile

Correspondence to:
José M. Domínguez
Diagonal Paraguay 362,
4th floor, Santiago,
Región Metropolitana, Chile
jdomingu@uc.cl

ABSTRACT

Objective: We aimed to describe the presentation of papillary microcarcinoma (PTMC) and identify the clinical and histological features associated with persistence/recurrence in a Latin American cohort. **Subjects and methods:** Retrospective study of PTMC patients who underwent total thyroidectomy, with or without radioactive iodine (RAI), and who were followed for at least 2 years. Risk of recurrence was estimated with ATA 2009 and 2015 classifications, and risk of mortality with 7th and 8th AJCC/TNM systems. Clinical data obtained during follow-up were used to detect structural and biochemical persistence/recurrence. **Results:** We included 209 patients, predominantly female (90%), 44.5 ± 12.6 years old, 183 (88%) received RAI (90.4 ± 44.2 mCi), followed-up for a median of 4.4 years (range 2.0–7.8). The 7th and 8th AJCC/TNM system classified 89% and 95.2% of the patients as stage I, respectively. ATA 2009 and ATA 2015 classified 70.8% and 78.5% of the patients as low risk, respectively. Fifteen (7%) patients had persistence/recurrence during follow-up. In multivariate analysis, only lymph node metastasis was associated with persistence/recurrence (coefficient beta 4.0, p = 0.016; 95% CI 1.3-12.9). There were no PTMC related deaths. **Conclusions:** Our series found no mortality and low rate of persistence/recurrence associated with PTMC. Lymph node metastasis was the only feature associated with recurrence in multivariate analysis. The updated ATA 2015 and 8th AJCC/TNM systems classified more PTMCs than previous classifications as low risk of recurrence and mortality, respectively. Arch Endocrinol Metab. 2018;62(1):6-13

Keywords
Thyroid cancer; head and neck; endocrine

INTRODUCTION

Papillary thyroid microcarcinoma (PTMC) is defined as a papillary thyroid cancer (PTC) whith a diameter 1 cm or less, and its incidence has increased during the last decades (1,2). PTMC comprises nearly 50% of PTC diagnosed worldwide and is associated with a favorable prognosis, which varies depending on the extension of the disease. Intrathyroidal incidental PTMC has the best prognosis, with recurrence and mortality rates as low as 0.5% and 0%, respectively (3-6). On the other hand, the 1-2.8% of patients with PTMC who have distant metastases at diagnosis have a worse prognosis, with high rates of persistence/recurrence (7). Previous studies have associated multifocality, bilateral disease, lymph node (LN) metastasis, tumor diameter of > 0.5 cm, a sum of multifocal tumor diameters greater than 2 cm, and minimal extra thyroidal extension (ETE) with a higher risk of recurrence (8-10).

Due to its good prognosis, some experts have proposed renaming PTMC as "micropapillary tumor" thus avoiding the word "cancer" and its implications regarding overtreatment and the deterioration of patient´s quality of life (11,12). Additionally, the favorable prognosis of PTMC has suggested the need for a less intense treatment with regard to surgery extension, radioactive iodine (RAI) ablation and TSH suppression, without increasing recurrence and mortality (13). Furthermore, active surveillance of selected PTMC patients has shown promising results, with a low risk of enlargement and LN metastases after 10 years of follow-up (14).

These less intense strategies for PTMC treatment are consistent with the updated versions of the 2015 American Thyroid Association (ATA) guidelines and the 8th AJCC/TNM system, which suggest changes in the stratification of the risks of recurrence and mortality, respectively (8,13,15). The most important changes include the following: i) the impact of LN metastases is now said to depend on both their number and size but not on their sole presence; ii) the role of minimal ETE has been reduced; and; iii) the age that determines a higher risk of mortality has been increased from 45 to 55 years (15,16).

Although PTMC represents nearly 50% of PTC patients, there is scarce information on this subject in relation to the Latin American population (5,17-19). Our aim was to describe the characteristics of PTMC at diagnosis and to identify the clinical and histological features associated with persistence/recurrence in a Latin American cohort. We hypothesized that our patients would have low rates of recurrence and mortality. We also expected that the updated ATA 2015 classification and the 8th AJCC/TNM system would induce significant changes in both recurrence and mortality risk stratification, respectively.

SUBJECTS AND METHODS

After receiving the approval of the Ethics Committee, we retrospectively reviewed the electronic medical records of 673 consecutive patients with PTC who were 18 years old or older, who had undergone total thyroidectomy between 2009 and 2013, and who had been followed-up for at least 2 years. We included every patient with PTMC. LN dissection was performed in patients whose preoperative ultrasound, fine needle aspiration biopsy, or intra-operative findings, suggested LN metastases. We used fixed RAI activities based on the extent of the initial disease, and the dose administered was decided by the attending physician, following ATA 2009 and institutional guidelines (8,20). A post-therapy whole body scan (WBS) was performed after RAI. Considering the results of preoperative ultrasound, intra-operative findings, pathology and WBS result, the patients were risk-stratified using the 7th and 8th edition of the AJCC/UICC staging system and the ATA 2009 and ATA 2015 risk of recurrence stratification systems (8,13). Of the 673 potentially eligible patients, a total of 209 patients satisfied the inclusion criteria.

After initial therapy, all patients received levothyroxine to keep TSH between 0.5 and 1.0 uUI/mL, and had at least two neck ultrasounds and two serum thyroglobulin (Tg) and anti-Tg antibodies (TgAb) determinations, either suppressed or stimulated by levothyroxine withdrawal.

Patients were routinely followed every 6 months during the first year, and at 6–12 month intervals thereafter at the discretion of the attending physician, based on the risk of the individual patient and the clinical course of the disease.

Structural neck persistent/recurrent PTC was defined as suspicious LN in neck ultrasound, accompanied by histocytological or Tg in an aspirate study that proved the presence of PTC. Extra-cervical structural persistent/recurrent PTC was defined as the presence of suspicious images on cross-sectional studies (computed tomography scan, or magnetic resonance imaging) or functional imaging (diagnostic WBS or ^{18}FDG PET-scan), requested according to the attending physician criteria. Biochemical persistent/recurrent PTC was defined as the presence of suppressed 1st generation Tg $\geq$ 0.9 ng/mL or stimulated Tg $\geq$ 2.0 ng/mL, without structural disease. At final follow-up, the absence of abnormal images in radiological studies accompanied by stimulated Tg < 2.0 ng/mL or suppressed 1st generation Tg < 0.9 ng/mL, were considered no clinical evidence of disease (NED).

Tg was measured using a chemiluminescent assay (Immulite 2000, Siemens, Los Angeles, CA, USA) with a functional sensitivity of 0.9 ng/mL, normalized to CRM 457. TgAb were measured using a chemiluminescent assay (Architect i1000, Laboratories, Abbott Park, IL, USA) (reference value of up to 4.11 IU/mL, analytical sensitivity 1.0 IU/mL). Since May 12th, 2014, second generation Tg was measured using a chemiluminescent assay (Elecsys II, Roche Diagnostics, Rotkreuz, Switzerland) with a functional sensitivity of 0.1 ng/mL, normalized to CRM 457.

Categorical variables are expressed as number and frequencies; continuous variables are expressed as mean ± SD, or median and ranges, as appropriate. Proportions were compared using a Fisher's exact chi2 test. Continuous variables were compared using parametric or non-parametric tests, as appropriate. Analysis was performed using SPSS software (version 15.0.0: SPSS, Inc., Chicago, IL). P-values < 0.05 were considered to be statistically significant.

RESULTS

Patients were predominantly female (90%) and 44.5 ± 12.6 years old: A total of 183 (88%) received RAI (90.4 ± 44.2 mCi) and were followed-up for a median of 4.4 years (range 2.0–7.8 years). Most patients (78%) had classical variant PTC, 61.2% had unifocal, 76.1% had unilateral disease, 17.9% had minimal ETE (microscopic or involving strap muscles), 16.7% had LN metastasis and none had distant metastases at diagnosis (Table 1).

According to the 7th AJCC/TNM system, 89%, 10% and 1% of the patients were classified as stage I, stage III and stage IVA disease, respectively. Using the updated 8th AJCC/TNM system, 95.2% and 4.8% of the patients were classified as stage I and stage II

Table 1. Characteristics of the patients at baseline

	Total Cohort (N = 209)	Persistence/Recurrence		P-value
		No (n = 194)	Yes (n = 15)	
Age at diagnosis (years)	44.5 ± 12.6	44.7 ± 12.8	40.8 ± 9.4	0.08
Female gender	188 (90%)	173 (89.1%)	15 (100%)	0,18
Histological subtype of PTC				0.6
Classical variant	163 (78%)	150 (77.3%)	13 (87.0%)	
Follicular variant	36 (17.2%)	34 (17.7%)	2 (13.0%)	
Other variants	10 (4.8%)	10 (5.130%)	0 (0%)	
Tumor diameter (cm)	0.62 ± 0.25	0,62 ± 0.26	0.65 ± 0.25	0.75
Sum of diameters (cm)	0.83 ± 0.54	0.83 ± 0.55	0.9 ± 0.48	0.9
Sum of all foci diameters > 2 cm	10 (4.8%)	10 (5.1%)	0 (0%)	0.36
Unifocal disease	128 (61.2%)	121 (62.4%)	7 (47.0%)	0.3.
Three or more foci	35 (16.7%)	30 (15.5%)	5 (33.3%)	0.07
Bilateral disease	50 (23.9%)	46 (23.7%)	4 (26.7%)	0.80
Minimal extra thyroidal extension	37 (17.7%)	31 (16.0%)	6 (40.0%)	0.019
Lymphocytic thyroiditis	88 (42.1%)	83 (42.8%)	5 (33.3%)	0.37
T				0.33
1a	172 (82.3%)	154 (82.8%)	8 (61.5%)	
3	37 (17.7%)	32 (17.2%)	5 (38.5%)	
N*				0.001
0	174 (83.3%)	166 (86.0%)	8 (53.3%)	
1	35 (16.7%)	28 (14.0%)	7 (46.7%)	
RAI ablation	183 (88.0%)	168 (86.6%)	15 (100%)	0.40
RAI dose (mCi)	90.4 ± 44.2	88.2 ± 44.2	116.7 ± 36.2	0.69
Length of follow-up (years)	4.4 (2.0-7.8)	4.4 (2.0 – 7.8)	4.2 (2.1 – 6.3)	0.37
AJCC 7th				
I	186 (89%)	173 (89.2%)	13 (86.6%)	0.06
III	21 (10%)	20 (10.3%)	1 (6.7%)	
IVA	2 (1.0%)	1 (0.5%)	1 (6.7%)	
AJCC 8th				0.34
I	199 (95.2%)	184 (95.0%)	15 (100%)	
II	10 (4.8%)	10 (5.0%)	0 (0%)	
ATA 2009				0.006
Low	148 (70.8%)	142 (73.2%)	6 (40%)	
Intermediate	61 (29.2%)	52 (26.8%)	9 (60%)	
ATA 2015				0.002
Low	164 (78.5%)	157 (81%)	7 (46.7%)	
Intermediate	45 (21.5%)	37 (19%)	8 (53.3%)	

* N0 includes patients subjected to lymph node dissection whose biopsy found no tumor, and in whom physical exam, preoperative ultrasound and intraoperative evaluation found no evidence of lymph node metastases.

disease, respectively, with no patients classified as stage III or stage IVA. Regarding risk of recurrence, ATA 2009 classified 70.8% and 29.2% of the patients as low and intermediate risk, respectively, while ATA 2015 categorized 78.5% and 21.5% of the patients as low and intermediate risk, respectively (Table 1).

Of the whole cohort, 194 (93%) patients had no persistence/recurrence, while 3 (1.5%) and 12 (5.5%) had biochemical and structural persistence/recurrence, respectively. There were no PTMC related deaths and the characteristics of patients who recurred are shown in Tables 1 and 2.

In univariate analysis, minimal ETE (OR 3.5 (95% CI 1.2-10.6)) and cervical LN metastasis (OR 5.2 (95% CI 1.7-15.4)) were associated with persistence/recurrence (Table 1). In multivariate analysis, only LN metastasis kept its significance (beta coefficient 4.0 ($p = 0.016$; 95% CI 1.3-12.9)).

The characteristics of the 15 patients who had persistence/recurrence are detailed in Table 2. Preoperative neck ultrasound was performed in only 5 (33%) of them. The median time between initial treatment and persistence/recurrence was 1.2 years (range 0.8-5.8) and 9 cases (60%) were diagnosed earlier than 1.5 years after initial treatment. Among the 12 patients with structural persistence/recurrence, 11 had cervical LN metastases: 5 underwent surgery and RAI, 3 underwent surgery alone, 1 received RAI alone and 2 underwent active surveillance: at the time of analysis, none of the patients showed progression of structural disease, while 7 accomplished a 2nd generation Tg ≤ 0.2 ng/dL, consistent with an excellent response to treatment.

The additional patient with structural disease was a 43-year old woman who had been treated initially with total thyroidectomy and RAI ablation (50 mCi) for a low risk PTMC. She achieved an excellent response (negative neck ultrasound and serum Tg of 0.1 ng/dL), but a 1.7 cm pulmonary metastasis was incidentally diagnosed on a chest X-ray 5.8 years after initial treatment. The lung metastasis was resected, an additional 100 mCi dose of RAI was given and the patient currently has NED.

Of the 3 patients with biochemical persistence/recurrence, all three underwent active surveillance. At the end of the follow-up, none had evidence of structural disease and 2 had achieved Tg ≤ 0.2 ng/dL, demonstrating an excellent response.

Of 194 patients with no persistence/recurrence, 2nd generation Tg was obtained in 146: 143 (98%) had Tg ≤ 0.2 ng/mL, while 3 patients had values between 0.3 and 0.9 ng/mL. None of them developed structural disease.

We found no significant differences for gender, histological subtypes, rate of multifocal disease, ETE, TNM/AJCC system, or risk of recurrence classifications among patients who had received and those who had not received RAI.

DISCUSSION

In this study, in which we evaluated a cohort of 209 Latin American patients, PTMC was associated with good prognosis: there were no PTMC related deaths, 7% of patients had persistence/recurrence, and 204 (98%) had NED at the end of the follow-up. These results are consistent with previously published series, which report mortality and recurrence rates of between 0-3.0% and 0.5-7.9%, respectively (9).

Previous reports have shown that non-incidental PTMC has higher risk of recurrence than incidental PTMC (6). The patients included in our series have a similar profile as those with non-incidental PTMC according to the previous series: predominantly female, 44.5 ± 12.6 years old, tumor diameter 0.62 ± 0.25 cm, multifocality (38.8%), bilaterality (23.9%), minimal ETE (17.7%), and LN metastasis (16.7%) (6). This similarity to non-incidental PTMC may explain why the recurrence rate was close to the highest reported.

Published data reported rates of LN metastases between 10-50%, with the highest rates found when prophylactic central LN dissection is performed (21). In our series, only 16.7% of PTMC had LN metastases, which is probably due to our policy of performing therapeutic neck dissection exclusively in patients with clinical evidence of N1 disease. This might also explain the impact of LN metastases in persistence/recurrence after multivariate analysis. It is currently known that the impact of LN metastases on recurrence depends on the number and size of the metastases, and on the presence of extra-nodal extension (8). Although it was controversial in the past, retrospective studies have not found lower rates of recurrence in PTC patients subjected to prophylactic central neck dissection, but may be associated with higher risks of complications (22,23).

Table 2. Characteristics of 15 patients with persistent or recurrent disease

Patient number	ATA 2015	Type of persistence/ recurrence	Time between initial treatment and to persistence/ recurrence (years)	Preoperative neck ultrasound done	Serum Tg (ng/mL)		Follow-up neck US	FNA	Therapy	2nd Gen Tg (ng/mL)	Length of follow-up (years)	Status at end of follow-up
					Suppressed	Stimulated						
1837	Low	Structural	0.8	No	< 0.9	NA	(+)	(+)	Sx	< 0.1	6.8	NED
1897	Low	Structural	2.2	No	3.6	NA	(+)	(+)	Sx + RAI	< 0.1	6.7	NED
2015	Intermediate	Structural	1.4	No	10.6	NA	(+)	NA	RAI	0.7	3.9	Biochemical disease
1952	Low	Structural	0.9	No	3.4	NA	(+)	(+)	Sx + RAI	< 0.1	6.1	NED
1997	Low	Structural	5.81	No	0.1	3.2	(-)	Chest CT and Dx scan compatible with 1.7 cm pulmonary metastasis	Sx + RAI	0.1	6.5	NED
1511	Low	Structural	1.2	No	5.5	NA	(+)	(+)	Sx + RAI	< 0.1	7.5	NED
1732	Intermediate	Structural	1.0	No	1.2	33	(+)	(+)	Sx + RAI	6.5	0.2	NED
2172	Intermediate	Structural	0.6	No	5.0	NA	(+)	(+)	Sx	4.8	<0.1	NED
2174	Intermediate	Structural	0.7	No	3.8	21	(+)	(+)	Sx	5.0	0.2	NED
2315	Low	Structural	1.96	Negative	< 0.9	NA	(+)	(+)	AS	0.2	4.5	Neck US non-specific nodule (granuloma) + negative chest CT
2232	Intermediate	Structural	4.0	No	< 0.9	NA	1 cm suspicious lateral cervical lymph node	Not done	AS	< 0.1	4.9	Stable neck US
2296	Intermediate	Structural	1.8	Cervical lymph nodes (+)	1.0	1.8	(+)	(+)	Sx + RAI	< 0.1	4.3	NED
1506	Low	Biochemical	0.9	Negative	2.4	27.1	(-)	(-)	AS	1.0	6.9	Biochemical disease (negative neck US and ^{18}FDG PET- CT)
1520	Intermediate	Biochemical	2.4	Cervical lymph nodes (+)	< 0.9	2.8	(-)	NA	AS	< 0.1	7.5	NED
2195	Intermediate	Biochemical	1.1	Negative	< 0.9	2.7	(-)	NA	AS	0.2	4.8	NED Neck US + Chest CT negative

Tg: thyroglobulin; NA: not applicable; Sx: surgery; RAI: radioactive iodine; NED: not evidence of disease; CT: computed tomography; Dx scan: ^{131}I diagnostic scan; AS: active surveillance; US: ultrasound.

In our series, minimal ETE had no impact on recurrence/persistence. Although it may be controversial and ATA 2015 guidelines still consider its presence to be criterion with which to classify patients as being at intermediate risk of recurrence, our findings are consistent with other studies that found no association with recurrence (10,24). Furthermore, the updated 8th TNM/AJCC system discouraged its role as a predictor of high risk of mortality in PTC, and recent data has shown poor agreement among expert pathologists in terms of defining its presence (15,25).

As patients were treated following older guidelines, 183 (93%) patients received RAI: they had similar characteristics at presentation to those who were not ablated, and RAI had no impact on recurrence/persistence, which is consistent with ATA 2015 recommendations and other series (13,26). We also recognize that currently a significant number of these patients would not undergo total thyroidectomy, as PTMC prognosis is similar in patients treated with partial thyroidectomy (13,27).

In our series, most patients with persistence/recurrence disease, 11 of 15, had structural regional disease. When analyzing their characteristics, only one third of them had preoperative neck ultrasound, and in two thirds persistence/recurrence was diagnosed within 1.5 years of initial treatment. These two facts suggest that the incomplete preoperative stratification is an explanation for the increased rate of structural persistent disease found early on in the follow-up. They also emphasize that the need for a comprehensive preoperative ultrasound staging in patients with PTMC is as important as it is in non-PTMC patients (28). From 2012 onwards, preoperative ultrasound staging was established as part of our routine protocol for every patient with diagnosis of thyroid cancer.

Of the 11 patients with cervical persistent/recurrence, 9 were actively treated with surgery, RAI, or a combination of both. The remaining 2 patients underwent active surveillance: one had NED and the other had stable findings at the end of the follow-up. This finding supports a less aggressive management of low volume cervical LN disease in properly selected patients, which has been previously associated with 5-10% risks of local progression, without or without very low risk of distant metastases (29,30).

Only one patient developed a distant metastasis during follow-up, which was incidentally discovered in a chest X-ray 5.81 years after initial treatment with total thyroidectomy and RAI. The patient had had a long period of excellent response, making recurrence very unlikely. After a lung metastasis resection and an additional RAI dose, the patient currently has NED.

An additional interesting finding is the impact of the updated risk of mortality and recurrence classifications. Regarding recurrence, in our series the rate of low risk patients rose from 70.8% to 78.5% according to ATA 2009 and 2015 classifications, respectively, which is consistent with the low rates of recurrence found in PTMC (8,13). Based on the recently published 8th AJCC/TNM system, the rate of stage I disease increased to 95%, and none of the patients were classified as stage III (8,13,15). These two changes are consistent with the very low risk of death related to PTMC in our and others series (6,16,31). These improvements in the stratification of PTMC patients should allow physicians to better adjust the intensity of therapy and avoid overtreatment in most patients with PTMC, which has been associated with side effects and deterioration of quality of life (9). Even more, in properly selected patients, active surveillance has shown to be feasible, with low risk of progression of disease and lower rates of side effects related to therapy (14,32).

A limitation of this study is the short time of follow-up, a median of 4.4 years (range 2.0-7.8). However, although PTC may recur a long time after initial treatment, nearly 50% and up to 80% of the recurrences occur during the first 3 and 5 years after initial treatment, respectively (33). In addition, it is important to note that among the 194 patients who did not have persistence/recurrence, 2nd generation Tg was available in 146: 143 had Tg $\leq$ 0.2 ng/mL, which is consistent with an excellent response to treatment and a very low risk of recurrence (13,34,35). The remaining 3 patients had negative imaging studies and stable serum Tg of between 0.3 and 0.9ng/mL, which is consistent with an indeterminate response, a category that still has good prognosis, with less than 1% risk of death and nearly 15% risk of structural progression (13).

In conclusion, we found a low rate of recurrence and no mortality associated with PTMC in Latin American patients. LN metastasis was the only feature associated with higher risk of recurrence, which emphasizes the importance of a comprehensive preoperative neck ultrasound evaluation. Updated ATA 2015 and 8th AJCC/TNM systems had a significant impact on patient stratification by increasing the rate of patients classified as at low risk of recurrence and mortality, respectively.

REFERENCES

1. Hedinger C, Williams ED, Sobin LH. The WHO histological classification of thyroid tumors: a commentary on the second edition. Cancer. 1989;63:908-11.
2. Davies L, Welch HG. Current thyroid cancer trends in the United States. JAMA Otolaryngol Head Neck Surg. 2014;140:317-22.
3. Lee YS, Lim H, Chang HS, Park CS. Papillary thyroid microcarcinomas are different from latent papillary thyroid carcinomas at autopsy. J Korean Med Sci. 2014;29:676-9.
4. Hughes DT, Haymart MR, Miller BS, Gauger PG, Doherty GM. The most commonly occurring papillary thyroid cancer in the United States is now a microcarcinoma in a patient older than 45 years. Thyroid. 2011;21:231-6.
5. Mosso L, Campusano C, González H, Domínguez JM, Salman P, Suazo V, et al. [From macro to micro thyroid carcinoma: records of a clinical hospital from 1991 to 2010]. Rev Med Chil. 2013;141:442-8.
6. Mehanna H, Al-Maqbili T, Carter B, Martin E, Campain N, Watkinson J, et al. Differences in the recurrence and mortality outcomes rates of incidental and nonincidental papillary thyroid microcarcinoma: a systematic review and meta-analysis of 21 329 person-years of follow-up. J Clin Endocrinol Metab. 2014;99:2834-43.
7. Bernet V. Approach to the patient with incidental papillary microcarcinoma. J Clin Endocrinol Metab. 2010;95:3586-92.
8. American Thyroid Association (ATA) Guidelines Taskforce on Thyroid Nodules and Differentiated Thyroid Cancer, Cooper DS, Doherty GM, Haugen BR, Kloos RT, Lee SL, Mandel SJ, et al. Revised American Thyroid Association management guidelines for patients with thyroid nodules and differentiated thyroid cancer. Thyroid. 2009;19:1167-214.
9. Leboulleux S, Tuttle RM, Pacini F, Schlumberger M. Papillary thyroid microcarcinoma: time to shift from surgery to active surveillance? Lancet Diabetes Endocrinol. 2016;4:933-42.
10. Kluijfhout WP, Pasternak JD, Kwon JS, Lim J, Shen WT, Gosnell JE, et al. Microscopic Positive Tumor Margin Does Not Increase the Risk of Recurrence in Patients with T1-T2 Well-Differentiated Thyroid Cancer. Ann Surg Oncol. 2016;23:1446-51.
11. Rosai J, LiVolsi VA, Sobrinho-Simoes M, Williams ED. Renaming papillary microcarcinoma of the thyroid gland: the Porto proposal. Int J Surg Pathol. 2003;11:249-51.
12. Rosario PW. Papillary microtumor or papillary microcarcinoma of the thyroid? A prospective analysis of the Porto Proposal. Int J Surg Pathol. 2013;21:639-40.
13. Haugen BR, Alexander EK, Bible KC, Doherty GM, Mandel SJ, Nikiforov YE, et al. 2015 American Thyroid Association Management Guidelines for Adult Patients with Thyroid Nodules and Differentiated Thyroid Cancer: The American Thyroid Association Guidelines Task Force on Thyroid Nodules and Differentiated Thyroid Cancer. Thyroid. 2016;26:1-133.
14. Ito Y, Miyauchi A, Kihara M, Higashiyama T, Kobayashi K, Miya A. Patient age is significantly related to the progression of papillary microcarcinoma of the thyroid under observation. Thyroid. 2014;24:27-34.
15. Tarasova VD, Tuttle RM. Current Management of Low Risk Differentiated Thyroid Cancer and Papillary Microcarcinoma. Clin Oncol (R Coll Radiol). 2017;29:290-7.
16. Nixon IJ, Wang LY, Migliacci JC, Eskander A, Campbell MJ, Aniss A, et al. An International Multi-Institutional Validation of Age 55 Years as a Cutoff for Risk Stratification in the AJCC/UICC Staging System for Well-Differentiated Thyroid Cancer. Thyroid 2016;26:373-80.
17. Monteros Alvi M, Gonorazky S, Virgili E, Soler G, Fernández M, van Cauwlaert L. [Non-incidental papillary microcarcinomas of the thyroid]. Medicina (B Aires). 2008;68:139-43.
18. Cordioli MI, Canalli MH, Coral MH. Increase incidence of thyroid cancer in Florianopolis, Brazil: comparative study of diagnosed cases in 2000 and 2005. Arq Bras Endocrinol Metabol. 2009;53:453-60.
19. Frigugliettí CU, Dutenhefner SE, Brandao LG, Kulcsar MA. Classification of papillary thyroid microcarcinoma according to size and fine-needle aspiration cytology: Behavior and therapeutic implications. Head Neck. 2011;33:696-701.
20. Pitoia F, Ward L, Wohllk N, Friguglietti C, Tomimori E, Gauna A, et al. Recommendations of the Latin American Thyroid Society on diagnosis and management of differentiated thyroid cancer. Arq Bras Endocrinol Metabol. 2009;53:884-7.
21. Qu N, Zhang L, Ji QH, Chen JY, Zhu YX, Cao YM, et al. Risk Factors for Central Compartment Lymph Node Metastasis in Papillary Thyroid Microcarcinoma: A Meta-Analysis. World J Surg. 2015;39:2459-70.
22. Moreno MA, Edeiken-Monroe BS, Siegel ER, Sherman SI, Clayman GL. In papillary thyroid cancer, preoperative central neck ultrasound detects only macroscopic surgical disease, but negative findings predict excellent long-term regional control and survival. Thyroid. 2012;22:347-55.
23. Wada N, Duh QY, Sugino K, Iwasaki H, Kameyama K, Mimura T, et al. Lymph node metastasis from 259 papillary thyroid microcarcinomas: frequency, pattern of occurrence and recurrence, and optimal strategy for neck dissection. Ann Surg. 2003;237:399-407.
24. Hay ID, Johnson TR, Thompson GB, Sebo TJ, Reinalda MS. Minimal extrathyroid extension in papillary thyroid carcinoma does not result in increased rates of either cause-specific mortality or postoperative tumor recurrence. Surgery 2016;159:11-9.
25. Su HK, Wenig BM, Haser GC, Rowe ME, Asa SL, Baloch Z, et al. Inter-Observer Variation in the Pathologic Identification of Minimal Extrathyroidal Extension in Papillary Thyroid Carcinoma. Thyroid. 2016;26:512-7.
26. Kwon H, Jeon MJ, Kim WG, Park S, Kim M, Kim TY, et al. Lack of Efficacy of Radioiodine Remnant Ablation for Papillary Thyroid Microcarcinoma: Verification Using Inverse Probability of Treatment Weighting. Ann Surg Oncol. 2017;24:2596-602.
27. Donatini G, Castagnet M, Desurmont T, Rudolph N, Othman D, Kraimps JL. Partial Thyroidectomy for Papillary Thyroid Microcarcinoma: Is Completion Total Thyroidectomy Indicated? World J Surg. 2016;40:510-5.
28. Ito Y, Tomoda C, Uruno T, Takamura Y, Miya A, Kobayashi K, et al. Preoperative ultrasonographic examination for lymph node metastasis: usefulness when designing lymph node dissection for papillary microcarcinoma of the thyroid. World J Surg. 2004;28:498-501.
29. Tomoda C, Sugino K, Matsuzu K, Uruno T, Ohkuwa K, Kitagawa W, et al. Cervical Lymph Node Metastases After Thyroidectomy for Papillary Thyroid Carcinoma Usually Remain Stable for Years. Thyroid; 2016;26:1706-11.
30. Robenshtok E, Fish S, Bach A, Domínguez JM, Shaha A, Tuttle RM. Suspicious cervical lymph nodes detected after thyroidectomy for papillary thyroid cancer usually remain stable over years in properly selected patients. J Clin Endocrinol Metab. 2012;97:2706-13.
31. Hay ID, Hutchinson ME, Gonzalez-Losada T, McIver B, Reinalda ME, Grant CS, et al. Papillary thyroid microcarcinoma: a study of 900 cases observed in a 60-year period. Surgery. 2008;144:980-987; discussion 987-8.

32. Brito JP, Ito Y, Miyauchi A, Tuttle RM. A Clinical Framework to Facilitate Risk Stratification When Considering an Active Surveillance Alternative to Immediate Biopsy and Surgery in Papillary Microcarcinoma. Thyroid. 2016;26:144-9.
33. Durante C, Montesano T, Torlontano M, Attard M, Monzani F, Tumino S, et al. Papillary thyroid cancer: time course of recurrences during postsurgery surveillance. J Clin Endocrinol Metab. 2013;98:636-42.
34. Giovanella L, Treglia G, Sadeghi R, Trimboli P, Ceriani L, Verburg FA. Unstimulated highly sensitive thyroglobulin in follow-up of differentiated thyroid cancer patients: a meta-analysis. J Clin Endocrinol Metab. 2014;99:440-7.
35. Malandrino P, Latina A, Marescalco S, Spadaro A, Regalbuto C, Fulco RA, et al. Risk-adapted management of differentiated thyroid cancer assessed by a sensitive measurement of basal serum thyroglobulin. J Clin Endocrinol Metab. 2011;96:1703-9.

Long term maintenance of glucose and lipid concentrations after Roux-en-Y gastric bypass

Fernanda Cristina Carvalho Mattos Magno[1], Priscila Alves Medeiros de Sousa[1], Marcelo Paiva Rodrigues[2], Lícia Lopes Pio Pereira[2], José Egídio Paulo de Oliveira[1], Eliane Lopes Rosado[1], João Régis Ivar Carneiro[1]

[1] Universidade Federal do Rio de Janeiro (UFRJ), Rio de Janeiro, RJ, Brasil
[2] Instituto Fernando Luiz Barroso, Rio de Janeiro, RJ, Brasil

Correspondence to:
alves_priscila@hotmail.com

ABSTRACT

Objective: Roux-en-Y gastric bypass (RYGB) reduces body weight and the comorbidities associated with obesity. The aim of this study was to evaluate whether glucose and lipid profiles were maintained during a 5-year follow-up period after RYGB. Subjects and methods: Anthropometric and laboratory data from 323 patients who had undergone this operation were analyzed. Differences in laboratory variables between the baseline and 12, 24, 36, 48 and 60 months postoperatively (PO) were assessed using a one-way ANOVA test to compare the three groups. Delta significance using one-way ANOVA was performed to assess anthropometric variable in the postoperative period ($p < 0.05$). Results: 77 patients (24%) were included in Group 1 (G1), 101 (32%) in Group 2 (G2), and 141 (44%) in Group 3 (G3). The majority of patients, 71.7% in G1, 82.8% in G2, and 70% in G3, showed high triglycerides (TG) before surgery. A decrease in weight loss was observed in all groups followed by an increase in body weight in G2 and G3 at 36, 48 and 60 months. Laboratory results for G1, G2 and G3 showed no significant differences between groups at baseline and during the post-operative period. Conclusion: Our results suggest that weight regain after RYGB has no significant impact on the long-term evolution of the lipid profile and glycemia. Arch Endocrinol Metab. 2018;62(3):346-51

Keywords
Bariatric surgery; weight regain; lipemia; glycemia

INTRODUCTION

Obesity is considered a risk factor for the development of various comorbidities, including impaired glucose homeostasis and cardiovascular disease (1). Roux-en-Y gastric bypass (RYGB) is the most commonly performed surgical treatment for obesity; however, although it is well documented that RYGB results in weight loss and metabolic improvements, some degree of weight regain has been observed 2–3 years after surgery (2), supporting the hypothesis that obesity is a chronic, incurable and progressive disease (3).

RYGB includes the anatomical diversion of the upper gastrointestinal tract. These changes in intestinal anatomy are thought to alter the function of the nutrient-driven enteroendocrine system, causing beneficial effects on glucose homeostasis that are independent of weight loss itself (4). In addition, weight loss elicits metabolic and cardiovascular benefits after RYGB, but evidence suggests that surgery might also activate weight-independent lipid amelioration mechanisms (1). Garcia-Marirrodriga and cols. (5) reported significant associations between lipid subfractions and excess weight loss after RYGB. However, a recent study conducted by Bradley and cols. (6) does not support the notion of clinically meaningful, weight loss-independent effects of RYGB surgery on β cell function and insulin sensitivity in non diabetic obese subjects after they have experienced considerable weight loss.

Weight loss results in improvements in glycemia and lipemia, and this is most evident in patients who have undergone RYGB (7). However, an elegant review by Shah and cols. (8) showed that the initial improvements seen following surgery decreased over a long-term follow-up period, possibly because of weight regain or unsatisfactory weight loss. Since weight gain can be considered a risk factor for dyslipidemia and changes in glucose levels, the aim of this study was to evaluate whether glucose and lipid profiles were maintained during a 5-year follow-up period after RYGB.

SUBJECTS AND METHODS

Subjects

This retrospective study was conducted by examining the medical records of 323 patients who underwent RYGB in a private clinic in Rio de Janeiro from 2000 to 2007 and maintained regular postoperative follow-up visits for at least 24 months after surgery. Personal, anthropometric and laboratory data were obtained from the medical records. This study was approved by the Research and Ethics Committee of the Clementino Fraga Filho University Hospital (176/09).

Three groups were classified according to the rate of inclination of each individual weight over time using linear regression slope for subjects with at least 36 months follow-up. The slope was obtained from the first 24 months after surgery, when patients' body weight is expected to stabilize. Negative slopes were considered G1 (patients without weight regain). Positive slopes (variation between 0 and 2 kg) were considered G2 (patients who might or might not regain weight). Positive slopes (over to 2 kg) were considered G3 (patients with weight regain).

Anthropometric and laboratory assessment

Anthropometric variables which were assessed included height and weight measured during the preoperative period and at 12, 24, 36, 48 and 60 months PO. Body mass index (BMI) was calculated by dividing the body weight in kilograms (kg) by the square of the height in meters (m^2) (9). Total body mass and stature were measured following Gibson, using a mechanical anthropometric balance (Welmy®) with a maximum capacity of 300 kg, divided by 100 g, and the stadiometer from the anthropometric balance with a scale of 0.1 cm (10). The patients were barefoot and wore minimal clothing when weighed.

Laboratory parameters assessed included total cholesterol (TC), low-density lipoprotein cholesterol (LDLc), high-density lipoprotein cholesterol (HDLc), triglycerides (TG) and glucose. These were measured during the preoperative period and at 12, 24, 36, 48 and 60 months PO. TC, HDLc, TG and glucose were determined by the enzymatic-colorimetric method (11). Concentrations of LDLc were calculated based on Friedwald's equation (12). Concentrations of serum lipids that were considered normal were those provided in the guidelines of the National Cholesterol Education Program – Adult Treatment Panel III (NCEP/ATPIII): CT < 200 mg/dL, TG < 150 mg/dL, HDLc > 40 mg/dL e LDL-c < 130 mg/dL (13). A concentration of ≤ 100 mg/dL was considered normal for fasting blood glucose (14).

Statistical analysis

Means and standard deviations (SD) were determined for quantitative data. All data were assessed for normality using the Kolmogorov-Smirnov test. The Chi-square test was used for the comparison of proportions of abnormal values in TC, LDLc, HDLc, TG and glucose to baseline. Differences in laboratory variables between the baseline and at 12, 24, 36, 48 and 60 months PO were assessed using a one-way ANOVA test to compare the groups. Delta significance using one-way ANOVA was used to assess anthropometric variables PO. Statistical significance was defined as two-tailed $p < 0.05$. Statistical analysis was performed using SPSS (Statistical Package for the Social Sciences) software, version 21.0 for Windows.

RESULTS

Of the 323 patients included in this study, 77 were included in G1 (24%), 101 in G2 (32%), and 141 in G3 (44%). Demographic data and the proportion of patients with abnormal laboratory values at baseline are shown in Table 1.

Table 2 showed no difference in the proportion of groups with abnormal values for the lipid subtractions and glucose concentration at baseline. Most patients from the 3 groups showed high TG before surgery.

Figure 1 shows weight loss for G1, G2 and G3 during the postoperative period. Comparing these groups, a decrease in weight loss was observed in all groups followed by an increase in body weight for G2 and G3 at 36, 48, and 60 months ($p < 0.01$).

Table 1. Baseline characteristics of the patients who received RYGB over 5 years of follow-up

	Number of patients (n = 323)
Female	72% (233/323)
Male	29% (90/323)
Age (years)	38 ± 10
Height (m)	1,65 ± 0,86
Baseline Weight (kg)	123,91 ± 21,9
Baseline BMI (Kg/m^2)	45,4 ± 6,1
TC > 200 mg/dL	40% (86/217)
LDLc > 130 mg/dL	31% (64/206)

BMI: body mass index, TC: total cholesterol; LDLc: Low-density lipoprotein cholesterol; HDLc: high density lipoprotein cholesterol; TG: triglycerides.

Table 2. Laboratorial profile with abnormal levels at baseline

Laboratorial data	G1		G2		G3		p value
	n	Percentage	N	Percentage	n	Percentage	
TC > 200 mg/dL	19	36.5%	28	43.1%	39	39%	0.76
LDLc > 130 mg/dL	16	32%	20	32.8%	64	31.1%	0.90
HDLc < 40 mg/dL	16	32%	22	34.4%	30	30.9%	0.90
TG> 100 mg/dL	38	71.7%	53	82.8%	70	70%	0.17
Glucose> 100 mg/dL	15	28.8%	34	48.6%	43	41.7%	0.08

TC: total cholesterol; LDLc: low-density lipoprotein cholesterol; HDLc: high-density lipoprotein cholesterol; TG: triglycerides.

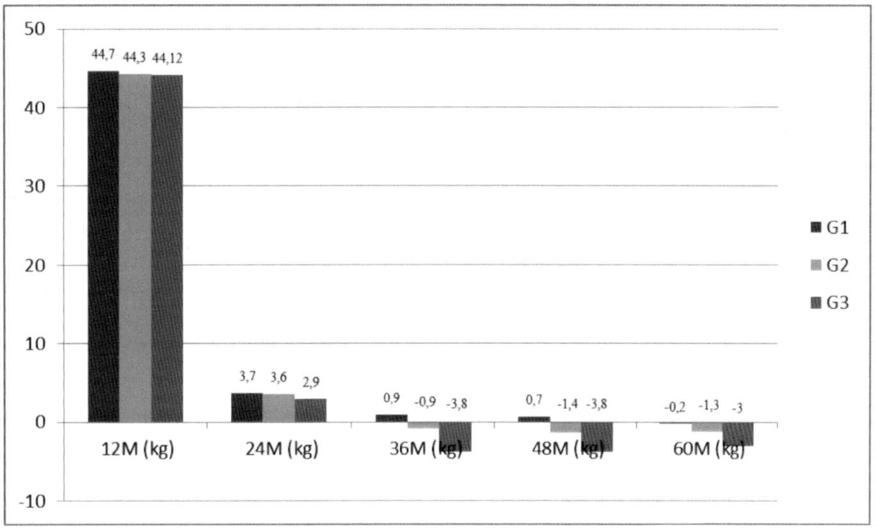

Figure 1. Weight loss (mean) in kilograms per year in patients who underwent RYGB.
M: months; kg: kilograms; G1: group 1; G2: group 2; G3: group 3.

Laboratory results for G1, G2 and G3 are shown in Table 3. No differences between groups at baseline and during the post-operative period were found.

DISCUSSION

This study examines the impact of weight regain on plasma glucose concentrations and lipid profiles in obese subjects during a 5-year follow-up period after marked RYGB-induced weight loss. The three groups of patients were comparable in terms of age, gender, anthropometric characteristics and laboratory results at baseline.

After the second or third year PO, long-term studies have shown a tendency for a weight increase in gastric bypass patients (15-20). In this study, weight loss did not differ significantly over the first 24 months after surgery.

Weight reduction can improve the lipid profile, alter carbohydrate metabolism, reduce morbidity and mortality, and generally enhance the quality of life of morbidly obese patients (21). Upper gastrointestinal tract diversion results in weight loss, but also may have weight loss-independent metabolic effects. Studies have reported contradictory findings regarding weight-loss dependent and independent effects of gastric bypass on glucose homeostasis and lipid profiles (1,8).

The RYGB technique may itself improve total cholesterol and LDLc levels (22). An observational study in obese patients confirmed that BMI is correlated with levels of TG and HDLc, but not with LDLc levels (23). In our study, glucose and lipid profiles were lower in all groups after surgery and this was not related to weight. Further studies analyzing laboratory parameters and weight dynamics after RYGB might contribute to clarifying whether the metabolic improvements seen after RYGB rely on weight loss or are an effect of the surgical technique itself.

The proportion of patients with abnormal total cholesterol concentrations prior to surgery was high in all groups but decreased during the long-term outcomes. Brolin and cols. (24) found that the greatest

Table 3. Lipid profiles and glucose concentrations (means and standard deviation) of patients who underwent RYGB

Variable	Groups	Baseline		12 mPO		24 mPO		36 mPO		48 mPO		60 mPO	
		N	Mean/SD	n	Mean/SD	N	Mean/SD	N	Mean/SD	N	Mean/SD	n	Mean/SD
TC	G1	52	196±43	65	164 ± 33	56	170 ± 30	48	169 ± 43	20	164 ± 31	17	171 ± 32
	G2	65	200 ± 46	87	162 ± 28	77	170 ± 32	65	170 ± 34	44	170 ± 35	25	179 ± 32
	G3	100	200 ± 47	127	170 ± 34	107	170 ± 32	83	176 ± 36	71	180 ± 34	39	174 ± 41
	p value	--	0.85	--	0.18	--	0.99	--	0,48	--	0.12	--	0.77
LDL	G1	50	120 ± 35	64	93 ± 24	54	93 ± 22	48	84 ± 27	21	89 ± 28	17	89 ± 17
	G2	61	124 ± 43	86	90 ± 23	78	90 ± 27	65	90 ± 23	44	91 ± 27	38	89 ± 22
	G3	95	119 ± 36	125	95 ± 28	105	93 ± 24	81	95 ± 28	70	97 ± 30		88 ± 24
	p value	--	0.70	--	0.45	--	0.66	--	0.07	--	0.38	--	0.98
HDL	G1	50	46 ± 10	62	56 ± 17	54	57 ± 14	48	65 ± 20	22	64 ± 15	19	67 ± 17
	G2	64	47 ± 15	86	56 ± 12	78	63 ± 17	64	64 ± 16	43	64 ± 16	25	68 ± 23
	G3	97	46 ± 11	123	55 ± 11	106	62 ± 15	80	67 ± 18	71	65 ± 20	41	61 ± 25
	p value	--	0.90	--	0.94	--	0.06	--	0.68	--	0.85	--	0.35
TG	G1	53	147 ± 70	62	87 ± 34	56	85 ± 37	46	83 ± 46	21	84 ± 35	17	89 ± 46
	G2	64	160 ± 93	86	78 ± 31	77	77 ± 29	63	78 ± 35	43	83 ± 41	25	84 ± 34
	G3	100	143 ± 63	125	86 ± 35	109	78 ± 32	82	78 ± 29	71	82 ± 34	37	86 ± 24
	p value	--	0.38	--	0.18	--	0.29	--	0.70	--	0.95	--	0.89
Glucose	G1	52	99 ± 20	63	83 ± 12	51	85 ± 8	44	83 ± 8	19	85 ± 8	14	89 ± 13
	G2	70	110 ± 36	87	85 ± 9	77	84 ± 8	58	87 ± 12	41	87 ± 12	21	89 ± 10
	G3	103	104 ± 29	127	83 ± 12	106	84 ± 6	78	89 ± 30	68	90 ± 32	35	86 ± 8
	p value	--	0.12	--	0.56	--	0.51	--	0.43	--	0.65	--	0.35

TC: total cholesterol; LDLc: low-density lipoprotein cholesterol; HDLc: high-density lipoprotein cholesterol; TG: triglycerides; 12 mPO: 12 months post-operative; 24 mPO: 24 months post-operative; 36 mPO: 36 months post-operative; 48 mPO: 48 months post-operative; 60 mPO: 60 months post-operative.

postoperative reductions in cholesterol and triglycerides generally occur in patients with the highest preoperative elevations, which is in accordance with our results for TG. Previous studies have shown a decline in total cholesterol and TG concentrations, and an elevation in HDLc concentrations, during the PO period. These changes were sustained over a long period of time in those patients who kept lost weight off as well as in those who experienced weight regain over time. Jamal and cols. (25) reported that the amelioration of the overall lipid profile was sustained over a 6-year PO follow-up.

Laguna and cols also showed that TG and LDL-C levels decreased 30% with respect to preoperative levels, while HDL-C increased 97% over initial values. Both TC:HDL-C and TG:HDL-C ratios normalized after RYGB and values were sustained over the weight regain period until the end of the study (26).

Bradley and cols. (6) support the idea that weight loss itself is primarily responsible for the clinical effects of RYGB on insulin sensitivity, β cell function, and oral glucose tolerance in non diabetic obese adults. On the other hand, Reed and cols. (27) showed improved fasting insulin and glucose levels a week after RYGB, despite persistent insulin resistance. Peterli and cols. (28) also reported early and augmented insulin responses as early as a week PO, potentially mediating improved early glycemic control. In our study, improved blood glucose levels were maintained throughout the postoperative period, regardless of weight regain. This may be associated with the enteroendocrine effects of RYGB, and suggests that glucose homeostasis after RYGB is weight-independent. Postoperative reduction in the levels of gastric inhibitory protein (GIP), and enhanced production of the antidiabetic hormone glucagon-like peptide (GLP-1), may underlie the changes in glucose seen after surgery (29). In addition, patients who participated in a prospective human study of gastric bypass had increased intestinal peptide YY (PYY) and GLP-1 responses, which were sustained even more than a year PO (30).

Numerous other factors have been implicated as potential contributors to the metabolic improvement observed after bariatric surgery, including other intestinal gut hormones (GLP-2, PYY), ghrelin (an anorexic hormone secreted by the gastric fundus), adipokines, the increased energy expenditure following surgery, changes in the gut microbiome, and bile acid metabolism (31).

Weight regain after gastric bypass has been attributed to multiple factors, including dilation of the gastric reservoir and gastrojejunostomy site, increased calorie intake of high glycemic index carbohydrates and fats, intolerance to red meat, hormonal alterations resulting from the adaptive process, binge eating, alcohol and drug consumption (32,33), difficulty promoting behavior changes, and lack of physical exercise. However, low adherence to follow-up with the multidisciplinary team PO is notoriously prevalent and problematic following bariatric surgery (34). Wardé-Kamar and cols. (35) suggest that such low adherence may occur due to underestimation of, or misinformation about, the surgery's consequences after long periods of time. Patients who regain weight may also feel embarrassed to seek help from the care service center where they had the operation. Reasons such as loss or change of health insurance, job loss, moving to another city or simply choosing not to continue the treatment after surgery may also reduce follow-up participation.

The limitations of our study include the retrospective nature of the analysis, incomplete follow-up, reduced sample size at the end of the study, and difficulty contacting patients who did not attend their scheduled follow-up appointments. These limitations are commonly reported in the literature for this kind of study. As laboratory results might change with further increases in body weight, a follow-up period of longer than 5 years would be necessary to establish whether they eventually return to preoperative levels (impairing the surgery's success and the patient's health). However, in spite of these limitations, long-term studies are crucial to determine long-term patient outcomes after bariatric surgery.

In conclusion, our results suggest that weight regain has no significant impact in the long-term evolution of the lipid profile and glycemia after RYGB. This study highlights the need for closer follow-up of RYGB patients, and for the implementation of actions aimed at improving adherence to the treatment protocols established by multidisciplinary teams. Additional long-term studies are required to establish whether a weight regain threshold might affect laboratory results, and to elucidate the exact mechanisms leading to these effects and their clinical consequences for the patient's health.

Acknowledgements: we thank Fernando Luiz Barroso.

REFERENCES

1. Stefater M, Kohli R, Inge T. Advances in the surgical treatment of morbid obesity. Mol Aspects Med. 2013;34(1):84-94.
2. Christou N, Look D, Maclean L. Weight gain after short- and long-limb gastric bypass in patients followed for longer than 10 years. Ann Surg. 2006;244(5):734-40.
3. Malinowski S. Nutritional and metabolic complications of bariatric surgery. Am J Med Sci. 2006;331(4):219-25.
4. Buchwald H, Estok R, Fahrbach K, Banel D, Jensen MD, Pories WJ, et al. Weight and type 2 diabetes after bariatric surgery: systematic review and meta-analysis. Am J Med. 2009;122(3):248-256.e5.
5. Garcia-Marirrodriga I, Amaya-Romero C, Ruiz-Diaz GP, Férnandez S, Ballesta-López C, Pou JM, et al. Evolution of lipid profiles after bariatric surgery. Obes Surg. 2012;22(4):609-16.
6. Bradley D, Conte C, Mittendorfer B, Eagon JC, Varela JE, Fabbrini E, et al. Gastric bypass and banding equally improve insulin sensitivity and β cell function. J Clin Invest. 2012;122(12):4667-74.
7. Schauer PR, Burguera B, Ikramuddin S, Cottam D, Gourash W, Hamad G, et al. Effect of laparoscopic Roux-en Y gastric bypass on type 2 diabetes mellitus. Ann Surg. 2003 Oct;238(4):467-84.
8. Shah M1, Simha V, Garg A. Review: Review: long-term impact of bariatric surgery on body weight, comorbidities, and nutritional status. J Clin Endocrinol Metab. 2006;91(11):4223-31.
9. World Health Organization: Physical Status: the use and interpretation of anthropometry: Technical report series 854. Geneva; 1998. p. 1-452.
10. Gibson S. Principles of nutritional dymatic. New York: Oxford; 1990. p. 691.
11. McGowan MW, Artiss JD, Strandbergh DR, Zak B. A peroxidase-coupled method for the colorimetric determination of serum triglycerides. Clin Chem. 1983;29(3):538-42.
12. Friedwald W, Levy R, Fredrickson D. Estimation of the concentration of low-density lipoprotein cholesterol in plasma, without use of the preparative ultracentrifuge. Clin Chem. 1972;18(6):499-502.
13. Expert Panel on Detection, Evaluation, and Treatment of High Blood Cholesterol in Adults. Executive Summary of The Third Report of The National Cholesterol Education Program (NCEP) Expert Panel on Detection, Evaluation, And Treatment of High Blood Cholesterol In Adults (Adult Treatment Panel III). JAMA. 2001;285(19):2486-97.
14. American Diabetes Association. Standards of medical care in diabetes--2012. Diabetes Care. 2012;35:11-63.
15. Dalcanale L, Oliveira CP, Faintuch J, Nogueira MA, Rondó P, Lima VM, et al. Long-term nutritional outcome after gastric bypass. Obes Surg. 2010;20(2):181-7.
16. Faria SL, de Oliveira Kelly E, Lins RD, Faria OP. Nutritional management of weight regain after bariatric surgery. Obes Surg. 2010;20(2):135-9.
17. Meguid MM, Glade MJ, Middleton FA. Weight regain after Roux-en-Y: a significant 20% complication related to PYY. Nutrition. 2008;24(9):832-42.
18. Pories WJ. Bariatric surgery: risks and rewards. J Clin Endocrinol Metab. 2008 Nov;93(11 Suppl 1):S89-96.

19. Lopez P, Patel N, Koche L. Outpatient complications encountered following Roux-en-Y gastric bypass. Med Clin North Am. 2007;91(3):471-83, xii.
20. Christou N, Look D, Maclean L. Weight gain after short- and long-limb gastric bypass in patients followed for longer than 10 years. Ann Surg. 2006;244(5):734-40.
21. Francischi R, Pereira L, Freitas C, Klopfer M, Santos RC, Vieira P, et al. Obesidade: atualização sobre sua etiologia, morbidade e tratamento. Rev Nutr. 2000;13(1):17-28.
22. Benaiges D, Goday A, Ramon JM, Hernandez E, Pera M, Cano JF; Obemar Group. Laparoscopic sleeve gastrectomy and laparoscopic gastric bypass are equally effective for reduction of cardiovascular risk in severely obese patients at one year of follow-up. Surg Obes Relat Dis. 2011;7(5):575-80.
23. Sundquist J, Winkleby M, Pudaric S. Cardiovascular disease risk factors among older black, Mexican-American, and white women and men: an analysis of NHANES III, 1988-1994. Third National Health and Nutrition Examination Survey. Third National Health and Nutrition Examination Survey. J Am Geriatr Soc. 2001;49(2):109-16.
24. Brolin RE, Bradley LJ, Wilson AC, Cody RP. Lipid risk profile and weight stability after gastric restrictive operations for morbid obesity. J Gastrointest Surg. 2000;4(5):464-9.
25. Jamal M, Wegner R, Heitshusen D, Liao J, Samuel I. Resolution of hyperlipidemia follows surgical weight loss in patients undergoing Roux-en-Y gastric bypass surgery: a 6-year analysis of data. Surg Obes Relat Dis. 2011;7(4):473-9.
26. Laguna S, Andrada P, Silva C, Rotellar F, Valenti V, Gil MJ, et al. Body weight-independent variations in HDL-cholesterol following gastric bypass. In: Anales del Sistema Sanitario De Navarra. Navas Tolosa 21, Pamplona, 31002, Spain: Gobierno de Navarra, 2016. p. 23-33.
27. Reed MA, Pories WJ, Chapman W, Pender J, Bowden R, Barakat H, et al. Roux-en-Y gastric bypass corrects hyperinsulinemia implications for the remission of type 2 diabetes. J Clin Endocrinol Metab. 2011;96(8):2525-31.
28. Peterli R, Wölnerhanssen B, Peters T, Devaux N, Kern B, Christoffel-Courtin C, et al. Improvement in glucose metabolism after bariatric surgery: comparison of laparoscopic Roux-en-Y gastric bypass and laparoscopic sleeve gastrectomy: a prospective randomized trial. Ann Surg. 2009;250(2):234-41.
29. Korner J, Bessler M, Inabnet W, Taveras C, Holst JJ. Exaggerated glucagon-like peptide-1 and blunted glucose-dependent insulinotropic peptide secretion are associated with Roux-en-Y gastric bypass but not adjustable gastric banding. Surg. Surg Obes Relat Dis. 2007;3(6):597-601.
30. Pournaras DJ, Osborne A, Hawkins SC, Mahon D, Ghatei MA, Bloom SR, et al. The gut hormone response following Roux-en-Y gastric bypass: cross-sectional and prospective study. Obes Surg. 2010;20(1):56-60.
31. Corcelles R, Daigle CR, Schauer PR. Management of endocrine disease: metabolic effects of bariatric surgery. Eur J Endocrinol. 2016;174(1):R19-28.
32. Barhouch AS, Zardo M, Padoin AV, Colossi FG, Casagrande DS, Chatkin R, et al. Excess weight loss variation in late postoperative period of gastric bypass. Obes Surg. 2010;20(11):1479-83.
33. Odom J, Zalesin KC, Washington TL, Miller WW, Hakmeh B, Zaremba DL, et al. Behavioral predictors of weight regain after bariatric surgery. Obes Surg. 2010;20(3):349-56.
34. Silver HJ, Torquati A, Jensen GL, Richards WO. Weight, dietary and physical activity behaviors two years after gastric bypass. Obes Surg. 2006;16(7):859-64.
35. Wardé-Kamar J, Rogers M, Flancbaum L, Laferrère B. Calorie intake and meal patterns up to 4 years after Roux-en-Y gastric bypass surgery. Obes Surg. 2004;14(8):1070-9.

Influence of maternal weight gain on birth weight: a gestational diabetes cohort

Livia S. Mastella[1], Letícia S. Weinert[1], Vanessa Gnielka[1], Vânia N. Hirakata[2], Maria Lúcia R. Oppermann[3], Sandra P. Silveiro[1,4], Angela J. Reichelt[4]

[1] Programa de Pós-Graduação em Ciências Médicas: Endocrinologia, Universidade Federal do Rio Grande do Sul (UFRGS), Porto Alegre, RS, Brasil
[2] Unidade de Bioestatística, Hospital de Clínicas de Porto Alegre (HCPA), Porto Alegre, RS, Brasil
[3] Serviço de Obstetrícia e Ginecologia, Hospital de Clínicas de Porto Alegre (HCPA), Porto Alegre, RS, Brasil
[4] Serviço de Endocrinologia, Hospital de Clínicas de Porto Alegre (HCPA), Porto Alegre, RS, Brasil

Previous presentation: preliminary results presented as abstract/ poster during the Scientific IADPSG Meeting 2016, held in Buenos Aires, Argentina, March 21-23, 2016.

Correspondence to:
Livia S. Mastella
Rua Ramiro Barcelos, 2350, Prédio 12, 4º andar
90035-003 – Porto Alegre, RS, Brasil
livia_mastella@yahoo.com.br

ABSTRACT

Objective: Our objective was to evaluate gestational weight gain (GWG) patterns and their relation to birth weight. Subjects and methods: We prospectively enrolled 474 women with gestational diabetes mellitus (GDM) at a university hospital (Porto Alegre, Brazil, November 2009-May 2015). GWG was categorized according to the 2009 Institute of Medicine guidelines; birth weight was classified as large (LGA) or small (SGA) for gestational age. Adjusted relative risks (aRRs) and 95% confidence intervals (95% CIs) were determined. Results: Adequate GWG occurred in 121 women [25.5%, 95% CI: 22, 30%]; excessive, in 180 [38.0%, 95% CI: 34, 43%]; and insufficient, in 173 [36.5%, 95% CI: 32, 41%]. In women with normal body mass index (BMI), the prevalence of SGA was higher in those with insufficient compared to adequate GWG (30% vs. 0%, $p < 0.001$). In women with BMI ≥ 25 kg/m^2, excessive GWG increased the prevalence of LGA [aRR 2.58, 95% CI: 1.06, 6.29] and protected from SGA [aRR 0.25, 95% CI: 0.10, 0.64]. Insufficient vs. adequate GWG did not influence the prevalence of SGA [aRR 0.61, 95% CI: 0.31, 1.22]; insufficient vs. excessive GWG protected from LGA [aRR 0.46, 95% CI: 0.23, 0.91]. Conclusions: One quarter of this cohort achieved adequate GWG, indicating that specific ranges have to be tailored for GDM. To prevent inadequate birth weight, excessive GWG in women with higher BMI and less than recommended GWG in normal BMI women should be avoided; less than recommended GWG may be suitable for overweight and obese women. Arch Endocrinol Metab. 2018;62(1):48-56

Keywords

Gestational diabetes mellitus; weight gain; birth weight

INTRODUCTION

Gestational diabetes mellitus (GDM) is typically diagnosed approximately 24-28 weeks using an oral glucose tolerance test (1). Adverse outcomes associated with GDM include increased risk of maternal hypertensive disorders and cesarean section as well as perinatal risks of macrosomia, shoulder dystocia and hypoglycemia (2).

Maternal obesity contributes to GDM and, in an independent fashion, to many other adverse maternal pregnancy outcomes, including pregnancy hypertensive disorders, cesarean section, weight retention, and postpartum diabetes. Adverse outcomes for offspring, including congenital anomalies, macrosomia and indicated preterm delivery, are also increased (3). Excessive weight gain *per se* contributes to an increased prevalence of large for gestational age (LGA) and macrosomia (4).

In 2009, the American Institute of Medicine (IOM) updated their recommendations on weight gain in pregnancy without a specific recommendation for GDM (4). Weight gain has been evaluated in several GDM cohort studies, with variable frequencies of adequate, insufficient or excessive weight gain being reported (5-8).

The objectives of this study were to evaluate how the 2009 IOM recommendations on gestational weight gain (GWG) applied to a contemporary cohort of GDM pregnancies and how the patterns of GWG in GDM impacted birth weight.

SUBJECTS AND METHODS

We studied a cohort of 508 women with GDM with singleton pregnancies, with at least one prenatal appointment, who delivered at Hospital de Clínicas de Porto Alegre (HCPA), a university hospital. HCPA is located in the Southern state of Brazil, Rio Grande do Sul (population ~11 million inhabitants) and provides medical care through the *Sistema Único de Saúde* (SUS), the national health system. In 2015, more than 600,000 general consultations were performed; approximately 4,000 babies were delivered; and the cesarean rate was 32.8% (9). From November 2009 to May 2015, all eligible women referred from primary care units were consecutively included; a multidisciplinary team provided prenatal care. Women gave their consent after being fully informed, and the authors signed the confidentiality document for data use. The hospital ethics committee approved the study protocol (number 2010-0364). We followed the STROBE statement for the study report (10).

Thirty-four women were excluded: one due to an abortion, one for having congenital achondroplasia and 32 due to missing data on maternal weight or infant birth weight. GDM was diagnosed with a 75-g oral glucose tolerance test (OGTT) using the criteria of fasting plasma glucose ≥110 mg/dL or 2-h plasma glucose ≥140 mg/dL in 232 women (49%) (11). After 2010, the International Association of Diabetes and Pregnancy Study Groups (IADPSG) recommendation was adopted; 242 (51%) of the women met these criteria (12).

Pregestational weight was self-reported, and pre-pregnancy BMI was classified according to the World Health Organization criteria (13). Weight and height were measured with light clothes and no shoes. All women were prescribed a normocaloric diet, emphasizing the intake of low glycemic index carbohydrates and fiber-rich food. Capillary glucose targets were ≤95 mg/dL for pre-meal and ≤120 mg/dL for 2-h postprandial measures (14). If goals were not met after 2 weeks of nutritional therapy, pharmacological treatment was initiated. Data on pregnancy evolution, delivery, and maternal and newborn outcomes were obtained from hospital registries.

Ethnicity was self-reported. Schooling was categorized as ≤ 11 years or > 11 years. Total weight gain was the weight measured at admission to delivery minus the pre-pregnancy weight; weight gains until diagnosis and from diagnosis to delivery were calculated. The 2009 IOM guidance on GWG by BMI was used, including the following ranges: underweight women, 12.5 to 18 kg; normal weight, 11.5 to 16 kg; overweight, 7 to 11 kg and obese, 5 to 9 kg (4). An A1C test was measured at booking (initial A1C test) and during the 3rd trimester (3rd trimester A1C test). Pregnancy-related hypertension disorders included any diagnosis of gestational hypertension or preeclampsia/eclampsia (15), and the composite of maternal risk factors included hypertensive disorders of pregnancy plus smoking.

Newborns were classified as small for gestational age (SGA) or as LGA according to the Alexander birth weight chart (16), which is routinely used at our hospital. Macrosomia was defined as a term birth weight ≥ 4,000 g, and preterm birth was defined as a delivery before the completion of 37 gestational weeks (17).

Plasma glucose was measured by the enzymatic method and an A1C test using HPLC (Variant II Turbo HbA1C, BioRad Laboratories, Hercules, CA, USA, aligned to DCCT recommendations).

Statistical analysis

We described the prevalence of adequate gestational weight gain as n (%) and evaluated the 95% confidence intervals [95% CIs]. Student's t test, χ^2 test, ANOVA, and Pearson correlation were applied as appropriate.

Relative risks (RR) and 95% CIs for SGA and LGA were determined according to maternal weight gain within normal or elevated BMI ranges (≥ 25 kg/m^2). Skin color, living with a partner, schooling, gravidity, weight gain grouped by IOM category, fasting glucose at the time of the diagnostic test, use of pharmacologic treatment, 3rd trimester A1C test, and the composite of maternal risk factors were explored in univariable and multivariable models for SGA. For LGA analysis, we added family history of diabetes to the models. Poisson regression with robust estimation was employed in multivariable analyses. Variables were included if a p value of at least < 0.10 was obtained in univariable analysis or if considered clinically important (gravidity and maternal risk factor).

We used SPSS software version 18.8 for statistical analyses. Statistical significance was set at 0.05, two-sided.

RESULTS

There were some slight differences in baseline clinical characteristics between women classified by the two

GDM diagnostic criteria (Table 1). We analyzed them as a single group because we assumed that dissimilarities were related to distinct profiles captured by each criterion. The main differences were observed for a family history of diabetes (54.3% vs. 42.6%, $p = 0.011$), pregestational BMI (29.4 ± 6.5 vs. 30.7 ± 7.0 kg/m^2, $p = 0.046$); the 2-hour glucose in the diagnostic OGTT (170.7 ± 29.1 vs. 148.5 ± 37.1 mg/dL, $p < 0.001$); the baseline A1C value (5.7% ± 0.8% vs. 5.4% ± 0.6%, $p < 0.001$), the latter measurement being within the range of laboratory references (6.0%); and weight at delivery (84.0 ± 17.3 vs. 89.1 ± 18.5 kg, $p = 0.002$). No differences were found regarding key maternal and perinatal outcomes.

Among the 474 women, only one had a BMI < 18.5 kg/m^2, and this case was analyzed in the normal BMI group; 119 had normal BMIs (n = 120, 25%, 95% CI: 21, 29%); and 354 (75%, 95% CI: 71, 79%) had BMIs ≥ 25 kg/m^2. Adequate weight gain occurred in 121 women [25.5%, 95% CI: 22, 30%], excessive in 180

Table 1. Comparison of women with gestational diabetes according to two diagnostic criteria

Characteristic/outcome	Brazilian criteria N = 232	IADPSG criteria N = 242	p
	Mean ± SD or %	Mean ± SD or %	
Maternal			
Age (years)	31.4 ± 6.2	31.2 ± 6.7	0.755
White ethnicity	75.4	78.9	0.365
Education (> 11 years)	49.6	47.5	0.656
With partner	63.4	45.5	< 0.001
Pregnancies (n)	2.7 ± 1.6	2.8 ± 1.7	0.789
Current smoker	0.9	3.3	0.064
Family history of diabetes	54.3	42.6	0.011
Previous GDM	13.4	13.2	0.964
Pre-pregnancy BMI (kg/m^2)	29.4 ± 6.5	30.7 ± 7.0	0.046
Systolic BP (mmHg)*	115.8 ± 11.9	117.0 ± 12.3	0.287
Diastolic BP (mmHg)*	72.5 ± 10.2	73.0 ± 9.8	0.591
Glycemia in the OGTT (mg/dL)**			
Fasting	100.0 ± 27	97.2 ± 16.4	0.177
1 hour (n = 180)	–	178.4 ± 35.8	–
2 hour	170.7 ± 29.1 n = 226	148.5 ± 37.1 n = 200	< 0.001
2nd trimester A1C test (%)***	5.7 ± 0.8	5.4 ± 0.6	< 0.001
3rd trimester weight gain (kg)	2.0 ± 4.0	2.7 ± 4.2	0.066
Weight at delivery (kg)	84.0 ± 17.3	89.1 ± 18.5	0.002
Total gestational weight gain (kg)	10.5 ± 7.5	10.1 ± 7.9	0.598
Hypertensive disorders of pregnancy	13.8	12.0	0.556
Cesarean section	58.6	52.1	0.151
Offspring			
Birth weight (g)	3,221.6 ± 578.7	3,246.6 ± 602.8	0.645
Birth weight category			0.681
SGA	9.9	12.0	
AGA	78.9	75.6	
LGA	11.2	12.4	
Macrosomia	7.3	8.3	0.704

IADPSG: International Association of Diabetes in Pregnancy Study Groups; GDM: gestational diabetes mellitus; BMI: body mass index; BP: blood pressure; OGTT: oral glucose tolerance test; SGA: small for gestational age; AGA: adequate for gestational age; LGA: large for gestational age.

* n = 230 for the Brazilian criteria and 241 for the IADPSG criteria; ** n = 226 for the Brazilian criteria and 200 for the IADPSG criteria; *** n = 206 for the Brazilian criteria and 207 for the IADPSG criteria.

[38%, 95% CI: 34, 43%] and insufficient in 173 [36.5%, 95% CI: 32, 41%]. Pre-pregnancy hypertension was present in 12.4% of the women, and preeclampsia/gestational hypertension was present in 9.5% of the women. The average gestational age at delivery was 38 ± 1.5 weeks (range: 30-41 weeks), and the rate of cesarean section was 55.3%. The baseline characteristics of the 474 women according to gestational weight gain categories are presented in Table 2.

When demographic and social characteristics across GWG categories (insufficient vs. adequate vs. excessive) were analyzed, maternal age was higher in women with insufficient GWG compared to those with excessive gain (Table 2). Fasting plasma glucose (mg/dL) in the OGTT was available for all women (98 ± 18 vs. 98 ± 26 vs. 100 ± 23, $p = 0.455$), 1 h glucose was available for 180 women (182 ± 35 vs. 185 ± 38 vs. 171 ± 34, $p = 0.104$) and 2 h glucose was available for 426 women (162 ± 31 vs. 162 ± 40 vs. 158 ± 35, $p = 0.558$). The initial A1C level was measured in 413 women at a mean gestational age of 31 ± 5.8 weeks and was similar across groups (5.6% ± 0.7% vs. 5.5% ± 0.8% vs. 5.7% ± 0.8%, $p = 0.070$).

Women who gained insufficient weight were more likely to be receiving pharmacological treatment (insulin or oral agents) compared to those with adequate gain (58% vs. 40%, $p = 0.009$). Metformin treatment was less frequent in those with adequate weight gain (31%) compared to those with insufficient weight gain (47%, $p = 0.023$), but in the excessive weight gain group (42%), the rates were not different compared to the two other groups. Insulin use was similar across all three groups (19.0% vs. 13.2% vs. 16.1%, $p = 0.407$).

The primary data on maternal weight gain by IOM category for the two BMI groups (normal and overweight/obese) are displayed in Table 3. Total weight gain increased significantly across the groups. Weight at delivery increased significantly across the three IOM categories in normal BMI women (63.3 ± 6.4 vs. 69.9 ± 6.7 vs. 80.7 ± 7.3 kg, $p = 0.001$). In women with BMI ≥ 25 kg/m^2, the average weight gain was almost 10 kg higher in the excessive weight gain group.

Table 3 depicts offspring outcomes according to GWG categories. The mean ± SD birth weight was 3.234 ± 591 g; 242 (51%) newborns were male; 52 (11%) were SGA and 56 (12%) LGA; and 37 (7.8%) were macrosomic. The preterm birth rate was 16.5% and was similar across groups (insufficient, 20%, adequate, 13% and excessive, 16%, $p = 0.315$).

The Pearson correlation (r) between GWG and birth weight in normal BMI women was weak, 0.47 ($p < 0.001$), with a coefficient of determination (r^2) of 0.22; in the group with overweight/obesity, r was lower, 0.24 ($p < 0.001$), and r^2 was 0.06. The overall r coefficient was 0.26 ($p < 0.001$), and r^2 was 0.07.

We could not run univariable analyses in the normal BMI group due to the lack of SGA babies and the presence of only one LGA baby in the adequate gain category (Table 3). Pharmacological treatment,

Table 2. Baseline characteristics of 474 women with gestational diabetes according to the 2009 Institute of Medicine weight gain categories

Characteristic	Weight gain category				p value
	Total n = 474	Insufficient n = 173 (36.5)	Adequate n = 121 (25.5)	Excessive n = 180 (38)	
Age (years)[&]	31 ± 6.4	33 ± 6.0	31 ± 6.6	30 ± 6.5	0.001
White ethnicity	366 (77)	138 (80)	99 (82)	129 (72)	0.073
Education, > 11 years	230 (49)	84 (49)	57 (47)	89 (49)	0.924
With partner	257 (54)	101 (58)	67 (55)	89 (49)	0.232
Pregnancies (n)	2.7 ± 1.7	2.8 ± 1.6	2.9 ± 1.6	2.6 ± 1.7	0.347
Current smoker	10 (2)	4 (2.3)	2 (1.7)	4 (2.2)	0.920
Family history of diabetes	229 (48)	74 (43)	63 (52)	92 (51)	0.185
Previous GDM	63 (13)	26 (15)	15 (12)	22 (12)	0.699
Pre-pregnancy BMI (kg/m^2)	30.1 ± 6.8	30.7 ± 7.8	29.2 ± 6.5	29.9 ± 5.8	0.194
Systolic BP (mmHg), n = 471	116 ± 12	115 ± 13	116 ± 12	118 ± 12	0.120
Diastolic BP (mmHg), n = 471	73 ± 10	73 ± 10	71 ± 9	74 ± 11	0.163

GDM: gestational diabetes mellitus; BMI: body mass index; BP: blood pressure.

Data represent the mean ± standard deviation (SD) or n (%). ANOVA and Tukey's test for multiple comparisons χ^2 test and Z test for proportion with Bonferroni adjustment.

[&] Insufficient and excessive groups are significantly different.

excessive total GWG and excessive gain in the 3rd trimester were all statistically significant in the BMI ≥ 25 kg/m² group and were included in the multivariable model, as were gravidity and 3rd trimester A1C. A maternal risk factor composite was added to SGA model, and the fasting plasma glucose at the OGTT was added to the LGA model.

Analyses were run including the total GWG and 3rd trimester gain separately, with adequate weight gain as the reference category. Comparisons of the effect of insufficient GWG on LGA risk were also performed, with excessive GWG as reference. Overall, we analyzed 328 pregnancies with 34 SGA and 42 LGA infants in multivariable models.

As observed in Table 4, the SGA risk decreased 75% with excessive total GWG and 23% with each kilogram gained during the third trimester but was not enhanced by insufficient weight gain. The LGA risk increased independently with total GWG; each kilogram gained in the 3rd trimester increased the risk by 10%. In

Table 3. Pregnancy outcomes according to pre-pregnancy body mass index and 2009 Institute of Medicine weight gain categories in 474 women with gestational diabetes

Outcome according to BMI	Weight gain category			p value
	Insufficient	Adequate	Excessive	
BMI < 25 kg/m² (n = 120)	**n = 54**	**n = 34**	**n = 32**	
Maternal				
3rd trimester weight gain#	-0.7 ± 4.6	2.4 ± 2.3	4.1 ± 5.3	< 0.001
Weight at delivery (kg)¶	63.3 ± 6.4	69.9 ± 6.7	80.7 ± 7.3	< 0.001
Total weight gain (kg)¶	6.8 ± 3.0	13.3 ± 1.3	22.6 ± 5.0	< 0.001
Hypertensive disorders of pregnancy	7 (13)	2 (6)	2 (6)	0.427
Cesarean section	24 (44)	18 (53)	16 (50)	0.722
Maternal risk factors	12 (22)	2 (6)	4 (13)	0.101
Offspring				
Birth weight (g)#	2868 ± 478	3284 ± 368	3413 ± 454	< 0.001
Birth weight category				< 0.001
SGA#	16 (30)	0 (0)	1 (3)	
AGA£	37 (69)	33 (97)	25 (78)	
LGA&	1 (2)	1 (3)	6 (19)	
BMI ≥ 25 kg/m² (n = 354)	**n = 119**	**n = 87**	**n = 148**	
Maternal				
3rd trimester weight gain¶	0.7 ± 2.8	2.2 ± 3.4	4.1 ± 4.3	< 0.001
Weight at delivery (kg)†	88.0 ± 18.0	88 ± 16.0	98 ± 14	< 0.001
Total weight gain (kg) ¶	1.8 ± 3.1	8.2 ± 1.8	16.4 ± 5.8	< 0.001
Hypertensive disorders of pregnancy	11 (9)	12 (14)	27 (18)	0.110
Cesarean section	66 (56)	49 (56)	89 (60)	0.715
Maternal risk factors*	35 (29)	23 (26)	43 (29)	0.882
Offspring				
Birth weight (g)†	3157 ± 642	3157 ± 569	3425 ± 586	< 0.001
Birth weight category				< 0.001
SGA§	12 (10)	17 (20)	6 (4)	
AGA	94 (79)	64 (74)	113 (76)	
LGA§	13 (11)	6 (7)	29 (20)	

* Maternal risk factors include: hypertensive disorders of pregnancy plus smoking.

BMI: body mass index; n: number; SGA: small for gestational age; AGA: adequate for gestational age; LGA: large for gestational age. Data represent the mean ± standard deviation (SD) or n (%).

ANOVA and Tukey's test for multiple comparisons χ^2 test and Z test for proportion with Bonferroni adjustment.

insufficient group is significantly different from the adequate or excessive groups; £ insufficient and adequate groups were different; & insufficient and excessive groups were different; † insufficient and adequate groups were different from the excessive group; ¶ all groups were different; § adequate and excessive groups were different.

addition to weight gain, pharmacological treatment increased the LGA risk in the model with total GWG (RR 2.60, 95% CI: 1.11, 5.81). In the model with 3rd trimester weight gain, the risks were also independently increased with pharmacological treatment (RR 2.38; 95% CI: 1.10, 5.28) and 3rd trimester A1C (RR 1.72; 95% CI: 1.28, 2.31). Both adequate and insufficient weight gain had a protective effect upon LGA risk when compared to excessive weight gain.

Table 4. Risk for small and large for gestational age babies in women with gestational diabetes with BMI ≥ 25 kg/m² according to gestational weight gain

Risk factor	Multivariable analysis*	
	aRR [95% CI]	p value
	Small for gestational age	
Total GWG (adequate as reference)		
Excessive	0.25 [0.10,0.64]	0.004[a]
Insufficient	0.61 [0.31,1.22]	0.161
3rd trimester weight gain (kg)	0.87 [0.81,0.95]	0.001[a]
	Large for gestational age	
Total GWG (adequate as reference)		
Excessive	2.58 [1.06,6.29]	0.037[b]
Insufficient	1.17 [0.42,3.29]	0.768
3rd trimester weight gain (kg)	1.11 [1.05,1.17]	< 0.001[b]
Total GWG (excessive as reference)		
Adequate	0.39 [0.16,0.95]	0.037[b]
Insufficient	0.46 [0.23,0.91]	0.026

aRR [95% CI]: adjusted relative risk (95% confidence interval); GWG: gestational weight gain.
* Poisson regression with robust estimation.
[a] Adjusted for gravidity, pharmacological treatment, maternal risk factors, and 3rd trimester A1C.
[b] Adjusted for gravidity, fasting plasma glucose in the oral glucose tolerance test, pharmacological treatment, and 3rd trimester A1C.

COMMENTS

In this GDM cohort, adequate weight gain was attained by only one quarter of women. Those with normal BMI had increased SGA rates with insufficient weight gain. In women with overweight or obesity, excessive GWG increased the LGA risk and protected from SGA, while there was a trend towards a decreased risk of LGA when GWG was insufficient.

Overweight and obesity were frequent in our cohort (75%), with a rate quite similar to that described for type 2 diabetes pregnancies, 80% (18), reflecting the pattern described in 49.1% of non-pregnant Brazilian women in a recent survey (19). Variable rates of obesity, 17 to 71%, have been reported in GDM cohorts; different study populations and diagnostic criteria may explain this wide range (5-7,20,21). Maternal and offspring outcomes can be worsened if women enter pregnancy in the overweight or obese categories; deleterious effects are further magnified by excessive weight gain (22). The high frequency of excessive GWG found (38%) was expected, since up to 65% women were reported gaining more weight than recommended in several cohort studies in GDM (5,7,8,22). This is not exclusive to GDM pregnancies; a similar rate (32.9%) was observed in women in a large Brazilian cohort (n=2,244) (23). Less than recommended GWG was 33.4% in the latter cohort, close to our rate (36.5%) and to those described in GDM (up to 40% of women) (7,8). The influence of GWG on GDM outcomes may therefore be uncertain, leading to the conclusion by a National Institutes of Health committee that evidence was insufficient "because of inconsistency across studies and imprecise effect estimates" (24).

We observed higher weight gain until GDM diagnosis followed by lower gain thereafter, as described in other studies (25,26); this reinforces the idea that more than intervention *per se*, being labeled GDM may increase treatment compliance (27). Moreover, we suppose that excessive weight might be perceived as deleterious by GDM mothers, since overweight and obese women gained approximately 5 kg less than their normal BMI counterparts along pregnancy. Women with insufficient weight gain in our cohort frequently needed pharmacological treatment; this association was also found in the Atlantic-DIP cohort, where insulin use was common in women with lower weight gain (5), in contrast to what was previously described (25). A possible explanation could be the presence of a more severe degree of metabolic disorder. We could not further explore this possibility because we did not measure insulin or C-peptide. We can speculate that this may in part also explain the interesting finding that women gaining insufficient weight were older than those with excessive weight gain. Another explanation for this latter finding could be ascribed to the presence of some degree of placental insufficiency in the oldest group or to compliance being greater due to their previous life experiences.

Although excessive and insufficient weight gain were frequent, maternal outcomes seemed unaffected in our study, opposing findings described by other authors: a higher weight gain in GDM pregnancies increased risks of cesarean section (7,22) and pregnancy-related hypertension by almost two-fold in Irish women with excessive weight gain (5).

Regarding offspring outcomes, we found that only 7% of birth weight could be explained by maternal GWG. Despite this, normal BMI women who gained less than the recommended GWG delivered more SGA babies, while in overweight/obese women we did not observe this association. Furthermore, the SGA rate was close to that of the LGA rate for the whole group, an unexpected finding. We could speculate that close surveillance of diet and weight gain could eventually be an explanation for both an increased rate of SGA in normal BMI women and a decreased rate of LGA in women with adequate or insufficient weight gain, while in women with excessive GWG, high rates of LGA remained. In non-diabetic pregnancies, delivery of SGA or low birth weight babies (< 2,500 g) is associated with multiple factors, such as hypertension, smoking and insufficient weight gain (27). No difference in hypertension or smoking rates across the weight gain groups was found. High rates of SGA were not expected, as it is well established that GDM treatment *per se* does not increase this risk (28). However, 22% of birth weight was ascribed to GWG in normal BMI women in our study, which could partially explain our findings. Weight gain below recommendations was not related to increased rates of SGA in other GDM cohorts (8,25) nor was it in a type 2 diabetes cohort (18); of note, the results were not adjusted by pre-pregnancy BMI categories. Weight loss in GDM women with BMI ≥25 kg/m^2 resulted in increased SGA in a large American cohort, despite protecting against LGA and macrosomia, although in the study, the last weight measurement was taken around a mean gestational age of 34.8 weeks (29). The linkage between SGA and poor maternal weight gain, which is stronger in underweight women, is not well established yet for other BMI categories in non-GDM pregnancies and not even in GDM, though it is described in large cohort studies and remains positive when adjusted for confounders such as smoking and hypertension (4). It is tempting to speculate that other factors such as vitamin D deficiency might play a role. Maternal vitamin D deficiency and an increased rate of SGA births have been previously described in our cohort (30).

Excessive birth weight is conditioned by maternal obesity and hyperglycemia as well as by excessive weight gain (21,31,32). The association of birth weight with maternal weight gain has been described in women with type 2 diabetes (18), in obese-only women (31), and in obese GDM women (33), reflecting the independent role of those factors. Gestational diabetes leads to excessive birth weight irrespective of diagnostic criteria (2), while proper treatment has been associated with decreased risk (28). In our cohort, as in others, higher rates of LGA were associated with excessive weight gain mainly in overweight and obese women (7,8,25). In the Atlantic-DIP cohort, adjusted risks of similar magnitude to ours were reported for LGA (5), while in another cohort, LGA was increased in obese, but not in overweight, women (6). It is worthy of consideration that those studies calculated GWG from the time of booking. The independent effects of hyperglycemia and weight gain on birth weight were recently quantified: an A1C test < 5.0% avoided 47% of LGA, while adequate GWG avoided 52% of LGA (32). Finally, total GWG was not the only important factor in our study; weight gain in the third trimester also independently influenced LGA risk. A trend towards LGA risk was previously reported in women with excessive GWG after GDM diagnosis (34).

Insufficient GWG and its influence on LGA have been less commonly evaluated. A tendency toward a decreased LGA risk was previously reported in obese GDM women, as well as in overweight women (aRR 1.05, 95% CI: 0.68, 4.19), with a risk magnitude similar to ours (aRR 1.17 (95% CI: 0.42, 3.29) (6). The protective effect of lower GWG on LGA risk compared to excessive gaining was expected, as we compared two extremes, but it is worth saying that women with insufficient GWG had a trend toward delivering more LGA babies than those gaining adequate weight. We believe that the independent effects of hyperglycemia and increased BMI could prevail over that of GWG because their additive effects, which are mediated through maternal hyperlipidemia and relative insulin insufficiency, further stimulate insulin secretion by the fetal pancreas, promoting intrauterine overgrowth (21). Appropriate treatment strategies, including reduced weight gain, potentially counteract these metabolic effects (35).

The main strength of our study is the possibility to evaluate the 2009 IOM recommendation on GWG in a mixed ethnic cohort with a typical GDM profile of excessive BMI at the beginning of pregnancy. In addition to the well-known effects of excessive GWG, we demonstrated that less than recommended GWG might not be deleterious in GDM pregnancies.

A study limitation, the influence of treatment on pregnancy outcomes, is inherent to the study design and is mitigated by the similar antenatal care offered throughout the time period.

In conclusion, only one quarter of this cohort achieved weight gain within the 2009 IOM guidance, perhaps indicating that specific ranges should be tailored for GDM pregnancies. Less than currently recommended GWG should be avoided in normal BMI women, although it may be suitable for overweight and obese women because it prevents excessive birth weight. Excessive GWG should be prevented in overweight and obese women to reduce the risk of large for gestational age babies.

Author's contributions: LSM, SPS and AJR designed research; LSM, LSW and VG conducted research; VNH and AJR performed statistical analysis; MLRO, SPS and AJR contributed to discussion, wrote the manuscript and are responsible for the final content. All authors revised the manuscript.

Acknowledgments: the authors acknowledge Professors Maria Inês Schmidt, Michele Drehmer and Themis Zelmanovitz, from Universidade Federal do Rio Grande do Sul (UFRGS), Porto Alegre, Brazil, for useful suggestions; Natália Jaeger for helping with language review and Scientific Linguagem Ltda. for manuscript preparation.

Financial disclosure: fund for Research and Event Promotion, Hospital de Clínicas de Porto Alegre (FIPE-HCPA).

REFERENCES

1. World Health Organization. WHO Guidelines Approved by the Guidelines Review Committee. Diagnostic criteria and classification of hyperglycemia first detected in pregnancy. Geneva: World Health Organization Copyright; 2013.
2. Wendland EM, Torloni MR, Falavigna M, Trujillo J, Dode MA, Campos MA, et al. Gestational diabetes and pregnancy outcomes – A systematic review of the World Health Organization (WHO) and the International Association of Diabetes in Pregnancy Study Groups (IADPSG) diagnostic criteria. BMC Pregnancy Childbirth. 2012 Mar 31;12:23.
3. Yogev Y, Catalano PM. Pregnancy and obesity. Obstet Gynecol Clin North Am. 2009;36(2):285-300, viii.
4. Institute of Medicine and National Research Council Committee to Reexamine (IOMPWG). The National Academies Collection: Reports funded by National Institutes of Health. Washington: National Academies Press; 2009.
5. Egan AM, Dennedy MC, Al-Ramli W, Heerey A, Avalos G, Dunne F. ATLANTIC-DIP: excessive gestational weight gain and pregnancy outcomes in women with gestational or pregestational diabetes mellitus. J Clin Endocrinol Metabol. 2014;99(1):212-9.
6. Berggren EK, Stuebe AM, Boggess KA. Excess Maternal Weight Gain and Large for Gestational Age Risk among Women with Gestational Diabetes. Am J Perinatol. 2015;32(3):251-6.
7. Horosz E, Bomba-Opon DA, Szymanska M, Wielgos M. Maternal weight gain in women with gestational diabetes mellitus. J Perinat Med. 2013;41(5):523-8.
8. Wong VW, Russell H. Weight gain during pregnancy in women with gestational diabetes: How little is too little? Diabetes Res Clin Pract. 2013;102(2):e32-4.
9. Hospital de Clínicas de Porto Alegre. Relatório de Gestão do Exercício de 2015-2016 [2016 Nov 01]. Available from: http://https://www.hcpa.edu.br/downloads/ccom/inst_gestao_publicacoes/relatorio_de_2015.pdf.
10. von Elm E, Altman DG, Egger M, Pocock SJ, Gotzsche PC, Vandenbroucke JP, et al. The Strengthening the Reporting of Observational Studies in Epidemiology (STROBE) statement: guidelines for reporting observational studies. Lancet. 2007;370(9596):1453-7.
11. Reichelt AAJ, Oppermann MLR, Schmidt MI. [Guidelines of the 2nd Meeting of the diabetes and pregnancy task force]. Arq Bras Endocrinol Metab. 2002;46(5):574-81.
12. International Association of D, Pregnancy Study Groups Consensus P, Metzger BE, Gabbe SG, Persson B, Buchanan TA, Catalano PA, Damm P, et al. International association of diabetes and pregnancy study groups recommendations on the diagnosis and classification of hyperglycemia in pregnancy. Diabetes Care. 2010;33(3):676-82.
13. World Health Organization. Physical status: the use and interpretation of anthropometry. Report of a WHO Expert Committee. 1995;854:435-45.
14. Weinert LS, Silveiro SP, Oppermann ML, Salazar CC, Simionato BM, Siebeneichler A, et al. [Gestational diabetes management: a multidisciplinary treatment algorithm]. Arq Bras Endocrinol Metab. 2011;55(7):435-45.
15. Tranquilli AL, Dekker G, Magee L, Roberts J, Sibai BM, Steyn W, et al. The classification, diagnosis and management of the hypertensive disorders of pregnancy: a revised statement from the ISSHP. Pregnancy Hypertens. 2014;4(2):97-104.
16. Alexander GR, Himes JH, Kaufman RB, Mor J, Kogan M. A United States national reference for fetal growth. Obstet Gynecol. 1996;87(2):163-8.
17. International Association of Diabetes in Pregnancy Study Group Working Group on Outcome D, Feig DS, Corcoy R, Jensen DM, Kautzky-Willer A, Nolan CJ, Oats JJ, et al. Diabetes in pregnancy outcomes: a systematic review and proposed codification of definitions. Diabetes Metab Res Rev. 2015;31(7):680-90.
18. Parellada CB, Asbjornsdottir B, Ringholm L, Damm P, Mathiesen ER. Fetal growth in relation to gestational weight gain in women with type 2 diabetes: an observational study. Diabet Med. 2014;31(12):1681-9.
19. Brasil. Ministério da Saúde. Vigitel: Vigilância de fatores de risco e proteção para doenças crônicas por inquérito telefônico 2014. Brasília; 2014. Available from: http://portalsaude.saude.gov.br/images/pdf/2015/abril/15/PPT-Vigitel-2014-.pdf.
20. Kase BA, Cormier CM, Costantine MM, Hutchinson M, Ramin SM, Saade GR, et al. Excessive gestational weight gain in women with gestational and pregestational diabetes. Am J Perinatol. 2011;28(10):761-6.
21. Catalano PM, McIntyre HD, Cruickshank JK, McCance DR, Dyer AR, Metzger BE, et al. The hyperglycemia and adverse pregnancy outcome study: associations of GDM and obesity with pregnancy outcomes. Diabetes Care. 2012;35(4):780-6.
22. Ouzounian JG, Hernandez GD, Korst LM, Montoro MM, Battista LR, Walden CL, et al. Pre-pregnancy weight and excess weight gain are risk factors for macrosomia in women with gestational diabetes. J Perinatol. 2011;31(11):717-21.

23. Drehmer M, Duncan BB, Kac G, Schmidt MI. Association of second and third trimester weight gain in pregnancy with maternal and fetal outcomes. PloS One. 2013;8(1):e54704.
24. Hartling L, Dryden DM, Guthrie A, Muise M, Vandermeer B, Donovan L. Benefits and harms of treating gestational diabetes mellitus: a systematic review and meta-analysis for the U.S. Preventive Services Task Force and the National Institutes of Health Office of Medical Applications of Research. Ann Intern Med. 2013;159(2):123-9.
25. Park JE, Park S, Daily JW, Kim SH. Low gestational weight gain improves infant and maternal pregnancy outcomes in overweight and obese Korean women with gestational diabetes mellitus. Gynecol Endocrinol. 2011;27(10):775-81.
26. Stewart ZA, Wallace EM, Allan CA. Patterns of weight gain in pregnant women with and without gestational diabetes mellitus: an observational study. Aust N Z J Obstet Gynaecol. 2012;52(5):433-9.
27. Han Z, Lutsiv O, Mulla S, Rosen A, Beyene J, McDonald SD, et al. Low gestational weight gain and the risk of preterm birth and low birthweight: a systematic review and meta-analyses. Acta Obstet Gynecol Scand. 2011;90(9):935-54.
28. Falavigna M, Schmidt MI, Trujillo J, Alves LF, Wendland ER, Torloni MR, et al. Effectiveness of gestational diabetes treatment: a systematic review with quality of evidence assessment. Diabetes Res Clin Pract. 2012;98(3):396-405.
29. Yee LM, Cheng YW, Inturrisi M, Caughey AB. Gestational weight loss and perinatal outcomes in overweight and obese women subsequent to diagnosis of gestational diabetes mellitus. Obesity. 2013;21(12):E770-4.
30. Weinert LS, Silveiro SP. Maternal-fetal impact of vitamin D deficiency: a critical review. Matern Child Health J. 2015;19(1):94-101.
31. Gavard JA, Artal R. The association of gestational weight gain with birth weight in obese pregnant women by obesity class and diabetic status: a population-based historical cohort study. Matern Child Health J. 2014;18(4):1038-47.
32. Barquiel B, Herranz L, Hillman N, Burgos MA, Grande C, Tukia KM, et al. HbA1c and Gestational Weight Gain Are Factors that Influence Neonatal Outcome in Mothers with Gestational Diabetes. J Womens Health. 2016;25(6):579-85.
33. Gante I, Amaral N, Dores J, Almeida MC. Impact of gestational weight gain on obstetric and neonatal outcomes in obese diabetic women. BMC Pregnancy Childbirth. 2015;15:249.
34. Harper LM, Tita A, Biggio JR. The institute of medicine guidelines for gestational weight gain after a diagnosis of gestational diabetes and pregnancy outcomes. Am J Perinatol. 2015;32(3):239-46.
35. Friedman JE. Obesity and Gestational Diabetes Mellitus Pathways for Programming in Mouse, Monkey, and Man—Where Do We Go Next? The 2014 Norbert Freinkel Award Lecture. Diabetes Care. 2015;38(8):1402-11.

4

An update of genetic basis of PCOS pathogenesis

Raiane P. Crespo[1], Tania A. S. S. Bachega[1], Berenice B. Mendonça[1], Larissa G. Gomes[1]

[1] Divisão de Endocrinologia e Laboratório de Hormônios e Genética Molecular (LIM-42), Hospital das Clínicas da Faculdade de Medicina da Universidade de São Paulo (HCFMUSP), São Paulo, SP, Brasil

Correspondence to:
Larissa Garcia Gomes
Av. Dr. Enéas de Carvalho Aguiar, 155, 2° andar, Bloco 6
05403-000 – São Paulo, SP, Brasil
larissag.gomes@gmail.com

ABSTRACT

Polycystic ovary syndrome (PCOS) is a common and complex endocrine disorder that affects 5-20% of reproductive age women. PCOS clinical symptoms include hirsutism, menstrual dysfunction, infertility, obesity and metabolic syndrome. There is a wide heterogeneity in clinical manifestations and metabolic complications. The pathogenesis of PCOS is not fully elucidated, but four aspects seem to contribute to the syndrome to different degrees: increased ovarian and/or adrenal androgen secretion, partial folliculogenesis arrest, insulin resistance and neuroendocrine axis dysfunction. A definitive etiology remains to be elucidated, but PCOS has a strong heritable component indicated by familial clustering and twin studies. Genome Wide Association Studies (GWAS) have identified several new risk loci and candidate genes for PCOS. Despite these findings, the association studies have explained less than 10% of heritability. Therefore, we could speculate that different phenotypes and subphenotypes are caused by rare private genetic variants. Modern genetic studies, such as whole exome and genome sequencing, will help to clarify the contribution of these rare genetic variants on different PCOS phenotypes. Arch Endocrinol Metab. 2018;62(3):352-61

Keywords

Polycystic ovary syndrome; PCOS; genetics; pathogenesis; complex genetic trait

INTRODUCTION

Polycystic ovary syndrome (PCOS) is a common and complex endocrine disorder that affects 5 to 20% of reproductive age women, and it is a major cause of hirsutism and anovulatory infertility (1). However, PCOS is more than a reproductive disease; it is associated with a wide range of metabolic disorders, such as glucose intolerance, diabetes, dyslipidemia, hypertension, hepatic steatosis, and increased cardiovascular surrogate markers. An increased prevalence of cardiovascular outcomes and mortality has not yet been demonstrated in this population (2).

PCOS diagnosis is currently based on a combination of the following signs and symptoms: hyperandrogenism and/or hyperandrogenemia, ovulatory dysfunction and polycystic ovarian morphology (PCOM). In the first attempt to define diagnostic criteria, the National Institutes of Health (NIH) Conference proposed in 1990 that the presence of both hyperandrogenism and chronic anovulation were mandatory for diagnosis (3) (Table 1). In 2003, the Rotterdam Consensus included PCOM finding as a criterion, and defined that the presence of at least two out of the three main characteristics were necessary to confirm the diagnosis (Table 1) (4). Therefore, the Rotterdam Consensus expanded the possibilities of combinations of the three classic manifestations, allowing the characterization of four main phenotypes (Table 2). In 2006, the Androgen Excess Society proposed a modification, in which hyperandrogenism would be an essential condition for diagnosis, reducing the number of phenotypic possibilities (5). More recently, a Consensus by NIH tried to unify the recommendations, suggesting the use of the Rotterdam Consensus for PCOS diagnosis in order to include the four phenotypes possibilities, and thus expanding the population with PCOS to its largest number (6).

CLINICAL ASPECTS: WIDE HETEROGENEITY

There is wide clinical heterogeneity, in terms of not only the main components of the syndrome, but also of the metabolic aspects. Cross-sectional studies have shown that metabolic abnormalities are more common in the classic and NIH phenotypes, often classified together with the denomination of classic (also adopted in this current review), compared to the other Rotterdam phenotypes, namely, ovulatory and normoandrogenic (Table 2). Moghetti and cols. found that the prevalence of each phenotype is about 70% for classic, 15% for ovulatory and 15% for normoandrogenic phenotypes (7). Other epidemiological studies in unselected populations reported the prevalence of 40–45% for classic phenotype, ~35% for ovulatory phenotype and ~20% for normoandrogenic phenotype (8). The prevalence of insulin resistance in PCOS patients is around 70%; however, insulin resistance differs among phenotypes: 80% in the classic, 65% in the ovulatory and only 38% in the normoandrogenic phenotype (7). The presence of metabolic syndrome also differs among these groups. Çelik and cols. compared 183 normoandrogenic PCOS patients with 504 classic/ovulatory PCOS patients and found a significantly higher prevalence of metabolic syndrome (OR 2.95) in the classic/ovulatory group (9). This clinical and metabolic heterogeneity could be explained by distinct pathogenic causes.

Table 1. Diagnostic criteria for PCOS

NIH 1990	Rotterdam 2003	AE-PCOS Society 2006
• Chronic anovulation • Clinical and/or biochemical signs of hyperandrogenism *(Both criteria needed)*	• Oligo- and/or anovulation • Clinical and/or biochemical signs of hyperandrogenism • Polycystic ovaries *(Two of three criteria needed)*	• Clinical and/or biochemical signs of hyperandrogenism • Ovarian dysfunction (Oligo-anovulation and/or polycystic ovarian morphology) *(Both criteria needed)*

Table 2. PCOS phenotypes according to each diagnostic criteria

Phenotypes	1	2	3	4
	Classic	NIH	Ovulatory	Normoandrogenic
Hyperandrogenism	Yes	Yes	Yes	No
Chronic anovulation	Yes	Yes	No	Yes
Polycystic ovaries	Yes	No	Yes	Yes
NIH 1990	X	X		
Rotterdam 2003	X	X	X	X
AE-PCOS Society 2006	X	X	X	

PCOS PATHOGENESIS ASPECTS

Ovarian and adrenal hyperandrogenism

There are considerable evidences, an that PCOS is an intrinsic disorder of the ovaries and that the primary defect resides in the increased androgen biosynthesis. Normally, ovarian theca cells produce androgens in response to LH. The theca cells express the *CYP17A1* gene, which encodes the P450c17 enzyme, catalyzing both 17α-hydroxylase and 17,20-lyase activity, the rate-limiting step in sex steroid synthesis. Androgen production is cyclical and modulated by intra-ovarian and extra-ovarian mechanisms. As LH rises, a downregulation of LH receptors and a decrease in CYP17A1 expression occur, minimizing the androgenic production. Estrogen and androgen inhibit 17α-hydroxylase and 17,20-lyase activity in a paracrine and autocrine negative feedback loop. In contrast, insulin and IGFs stimulate the P450c17 enzyme and up-regulate LH receptor sites (10) (Figure 1).

PCOS ovaries are typically hypersensitive to LH, which is caused by partial escape from LH receptor downregulation. The imbalance of the intra-ovarian regulatory system seems to play a role in this increased sensitivity to LH. Exogenous factors, such as insulin resistance and hyperinsulinemia, are examples of extra-ovarian modulators that disrupt normal intra-ovarian regulatory mechanisms (10) (Figure 1).

In vitro studies have demonstrated that isolated theca cells or tissues from PCOS women secrete more androgen than cells from normal controls. The increased androgen synthesis in PCOS theca cells results from increased expression of 17α-hydroxylase/17,20-lyase and the cholesterol side-chain cleavage enzyme, suggesting an intrinsic theca cell defect (11). Taken together, these data indicate that ovarian cells from PCOS patients have intrinsic and stable characteristics that contribute to their phenotype, even after exclusion of gonadotrophin, hyperinsulinemia and hyperandrogenism stimulus.

Although the ovaries are considered the main source of androgens in PCOS, increased adrenal androgens, mainly DHEA and DHEAS, are present in around 20–30% of PCOS women (12). Normal adrenal *zona reticularis* steroidogenic enzymes resemble theca cell enzymes, favoring the formation of DHEA, which is rapidly sulfated to DHEAS by sulfotransferase 2A1 (SULT2A1). DHEAS is the most abundant adrenal precursor, but it is an inert terminal product. However, DHEAS can be converted to DHEA, which can be metabolized into more potent androgens. Genetic variants in *SULT2A1* have been shown to alter the DHEAS/DHEA ratio in PCOS (13).

Increased adrenal P450c17 activity is also suggested in PCOS women with adrenal hyperandrogenism. This adrenal hyperandrogenism does not seem to depend on an increased hypothalamic–pituitary-adrenal drive, but it reflects a generalized adrenal hyper-responsiveness for androgenic biosynthesis (12).

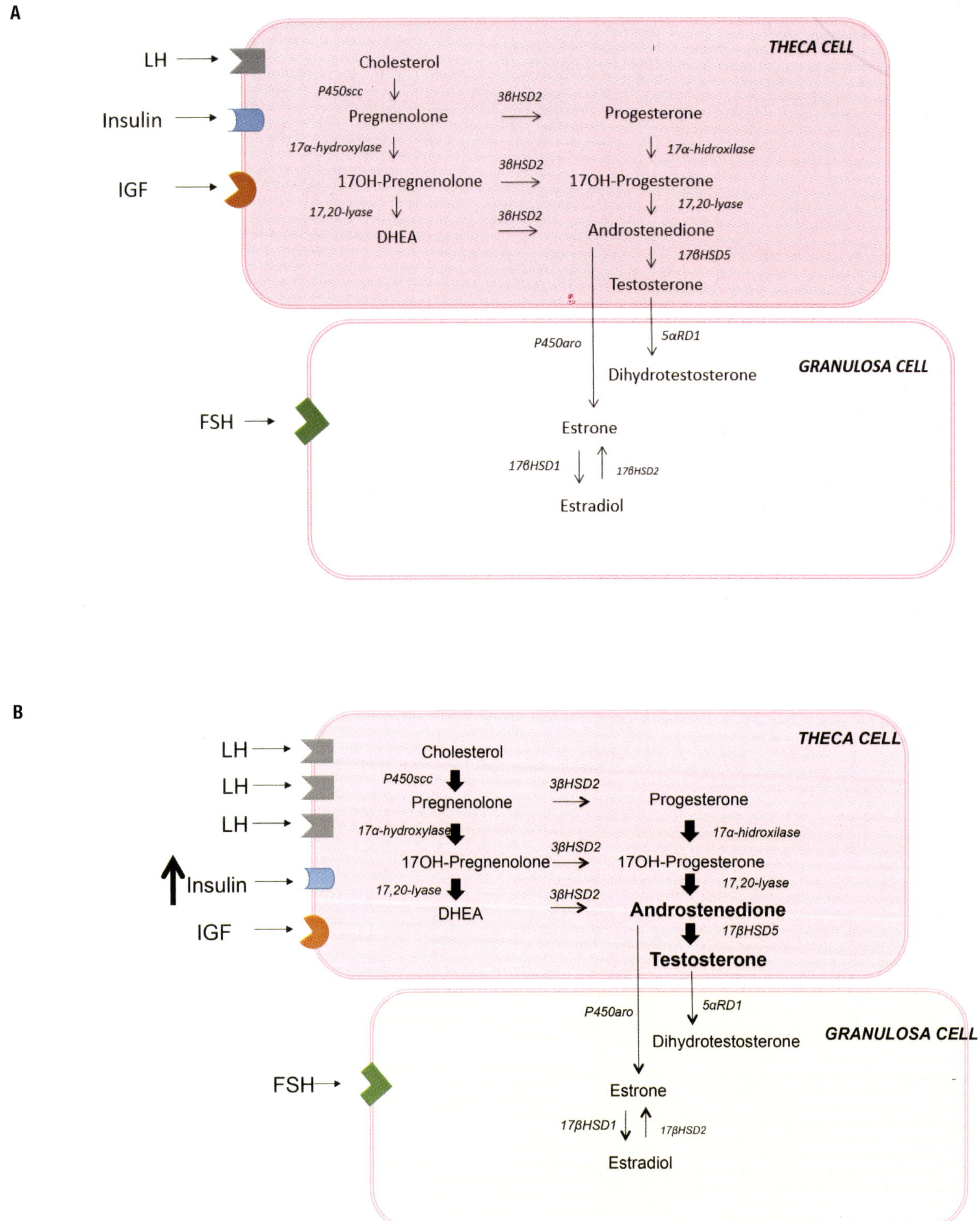

Figure 1. Ovarian steroidogenesis. (**A**) Normal ovarian steroid synthesis. (**B**) PCOS ovarian steroid synthesis. In comparison to normal theca cells, PCOS theca cells show increased expression of LH receptor and increased expression of CYP17A1 gene, leading to enhance of 17α-hydroxylase and 17,20-lyase activity, and amplifying androgen synthesis. Exogenous factors, such as hyperinsulinemia and IGFs are modulatory hormones that can disrupt normal intra-ovarian regulatation of steroidogenesis.

Genetic and epigenetic factors are probably implicated in the theca cell and adrenal steroidogenesis dysfunction. An example of a genetic cause of adrenal PCOS is cortisone reductase deficiency. The original study described mutations in 11β-hydroxysteroid dehydrogenase (11βHSD) type I and hexose-6-phosphate dehydrogenase in a digenic triallelic mode of inheritance. In11β-HSD type I deficiency, cortisone is not convert into cortisol, with a consequent elevation of ACTH, which stimulates androgen production, leading to the PCOS phenotype (14).

Ovarian folliculogenesis

The beginning of follicular recruitment is an intrinsic ovarian process, independent of gonadotropins. The primordial follicles are maintained in the quiescence state by epithelial-mesenchymal interactions, inhibitory transcription factors (LKB1/STK11/ BMP4) and pro-apoptotic factors (FOX) secreted by oocytes. A set of local follicular factors regulates follicular recruitment (GDF9, BMP6 and BMP9) (10), follicle growth and development. For example, BMP15 acts synergistically with GDF9 proliferating the granulosa cells (10).

Another important modulator of folliculogenesis is AMH, a member of the GFR-beta superfamily that is produced by the granulosa cells of small growing follicles. The highest expression of AMH is detected in preantral and small antral follicles of ≤ 4 mm. Once the follicles reach > 8 mm, AMH expression is reduced, and these follicles become more sensitive to FSH action, culminating with increased follicle growth and estrogen production, selection of the dominant follicle and subsequent ovulation in the normal ovary (15). AMH acts to prevent the initial FSH-independent recruitment of primary follicles from the primordial follicle pools, inhibits FSH-dependent follicular maturation and the selection of the dominant follicle (1) (Figure 2).

Several studies have shown that serum AMH levels are significantly higher in patients with PCOS (15-17), and this finding is compatible with the large number of follicles in the preantral and antral stages, both of which are stages of maximum AMH production. Pellatt and cols. demonstrated that the production of AMH per cell is 75 times greater in the granulosa cells of anovulatory PCOS patients (16). This finding suggests that high serum AMH levels are not only a consequence of the increased granulosa cell mass in anovulatory patients, but are also a potential causal factor for anovulation in PCOS (15,16). However, the cause for the increased production of AMH per granulosa cell remains unknown. Several other signals produced by granulosa cells and oocytes modulate (positively and negatively) the ovarian environment for oocyte maturation. These factors include inhibin B, TGF-beta superfamily members (ex. BMPs), cytokines (ex. TNF-alpha), and microRNAs (10).

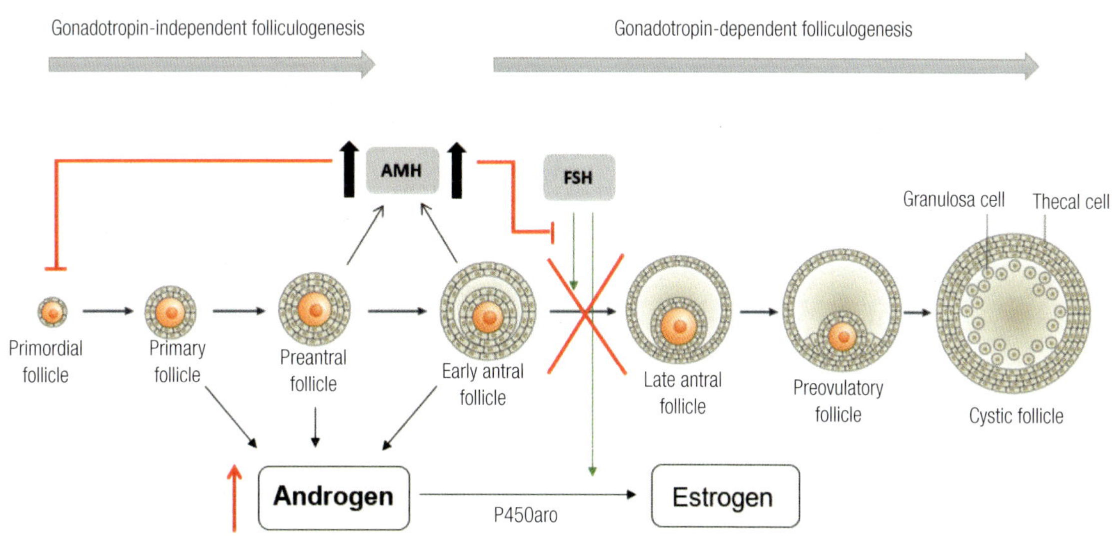

Figure 2. Role of AMH in folliculogenesis. AMH has an inibitory effect on initial recruitment of primary follicles, on FSH-dependent follicular maturation and selection of dominant follicle, and on FSH-induced aromatase expression on granulosa cells, reducing the conversion of testosterone into estradiol. Higher AMH levels in PCOS patients turns the follicles more resistant to FSH action, culminating in inhibition of follicular maturarion and ovulation, and in inhibiton of aromatase expression, and consequently, leading to hyperandrogenism. Adapted from Azziz and cols. 2016 (1).

Regulatory folliculogenesis factors, such as GDF9 and BMP15, have already been studied as possible causes of PCOS, but there is still no evidence that these molecules are responsible for abnormal folliculogenesis (18). Mutations of *BMP15* have been implicated in early ovarian failure caused by ovarian dysgenesis (19).

FOX transcription factors have also demonstrated a potential role in PCOS pathogenesis. Mikaeili and cols. correlated FOX03 expression and activation in granulosa cells with apoptosis rates, and found a positive correlation between them, making this transcription factor a potential candidate target (20).

Insulin resistance

In 1970, rare forms of severe insulin resistance (IR), *acanthosis nigricans* and hyperandrogenism, were described (Insulin Resistance type A, Rabson-Mendenhall Syndrome and Leprechaunism) (21). The molecular mechanism of insulin resistance in these diseases was explained by a reduction in the binding of insulin to its receptor and by a defect in insulin receptor autophosphorylation (22,23). Family forms of lipodystrophy with severe IR were also associated with hyperandrogenism at the same time (24). Remarkable hyperinsulinemia, as a common feature of these syndromes, suggested for the first time that insulin could directly stimulate androgen production (24).

In 1980, Burghen and cols. reported that women with PCOS had increased insulin levels in response to the oral glucose tolerance test that were not justified only by obesity (25). In addition, women with classical PCOS had acanthosis nigricans, which gave them a phenotypic picture similar to the rare IR syndromes described previously (25).

Observational studies suggest that in obese PCOS women, metabolic abnormalities related to IR and obesity have a greater impact on anovulation mechanisms than excess androgens (26). However, IR in PCOS patients is not necessarily associated with obesity. Some lean patients with PCOS present with IR, and even obese women have IR disproportionate to the degree of adiposity (27). Therefore, insulin resistance in PCOS is an intrinsic characteristic aggravated by obesity and not simply a consequence of obesity.

In PCOS syndrome, IR is not generalized in all tissues. Defects in metabolic actions of insulin occur in muscle and adipose tissues, but mitogenic and steroidogenic actions of insulin in ovaries are preserved (28). By acting on the ovarian insulin receptor, insulin amplifies the response of theca cells to LH and increases the expression of P450c17 and 3β-HSD2, leading to increased androgen production (29). This pathway is well illustrated by studies in rats presenting IR induced by an obesogenic diet; in these studies, the knock-out of insulin receptors improved hyperandrogenism and anovulation (30). Reaffirmation of the role of insulin in steroidogenesis is observed in the treatment of PCOS. All treatments that reduce serum insulin levels, whether weight loss due to lifestyle changes, bariatric surgery, metformin or thiazolidinedione, significantly diminish anovulation and hyperandrogenemia (31,32).

Neuroendocrine axis

Since ovarian steroidogenesis is directly related to the gonadotropic stimulus, alterations of LH are indicated as one of the factors involved in the development of PCOS.

Progesterone is the primary regulator of GnRH pulsatility. It is known that PCOS patients present a GnRH-generating pulse resistance to negative feedback by progesterone, which results in a higher LH pulses frequency and/or amplitude (33). This phenomenon has already been attributed to hyperandrogenemia in several studies, in which treatment with flutamide for 4 weeks restored hypothalamic sensitivity to ovarian steroids (34). At this point, alterations of the gonadotropic axis appear to be secondary to hyperandrogenemia. Moreover, LH excess is an inconstant feature of PCOS, thus, it is difficult to attribute a primary role to LH excess in the pathogenesis of all PCOS patients. However, in patients with congenital virilization, changes in LH pulsatility appear to be determinant for the PCOS phenotype (10).

Therefore, ovarian and adrenal hyperandrogenism, altered folliculogenesis, increased insulin resistance and neuroendocrine axis dysfunction could have a greater or lesser role in PCOS pathogenesis (Figure 3). The classification of specific clinical patterns in patients with PCOS could improve the search for genetic determinants and potentially the development of specific treatment regimens.

PCOS GENETIC HERITABILITY

Since 1968, studies have suggested an important genetic role contributing to the etiology of PCOS (35). First-degree relatives of PCOS patients have a higher

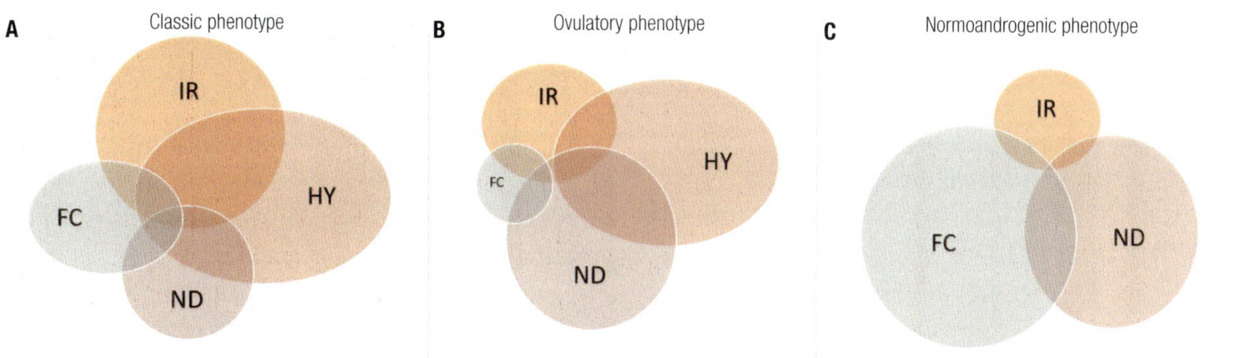

Figure 3. Schematic components of PCOS pathogenesis. Four main physiologic mechanisms contribute to PCOS pathogenesis: hyperandrogenism (HY), insulin resistance (IR), folliculogenesis dysfunction (FC), and neuroendocrine axis dysfunction (ND). These mechanisms contribute to each phenotype in different degrees. The classical phenotype shows alterations in all four mechanism, being HY and IR the main ones (**A**). In the ovulatory phenotype, HY and ND predominate and folliculogenesis seems not compromised (**B**). In contrast, in the normoandrogenic phenotype, FC seems to play the most important role in the pathogenesis, while HY is not present (**C**).

risk of being affected by the syndrome compared to the general population. Kahsar-Miller and cols. studied first-degree relatives of 93 PCOS patients and found that 35% of non-menopausal mothers and 40% of sisters were also affected (36).

Examining a large twin cohort of 1332 monozygotic and 1873 dizygotic twin sisters, Vink and cols. found a higher correlation for PCOS in monozygotic compared to dizygotic twins. This study concluded that the genetic component contributes to over 70% of PCOS pathogenesis (37). Therefore, PCOS is a complex genetic disease with high inheritance rates and heterogeneous phenotypes.

Studies based on candidate genes for PCOS have not been successful. Studies involving more than 100 candidate genes, especially those related to reproductive axis, insulin resistance and chronic inflammation have not shown reproducible results (38,39). The lack of consistency across studies may stem from the small sample size, phenotypic heterogeneity among patients, an inadequate control group, the lack of comorbidity matching (obesity, insulin resistance), or the limitation to only one or two variants genotyped in each gene of interest instead of the whole gene (40).

The genome-wide association study (GWAS) is a more recent genomic approach to understanding the genetics of complex diseases. This method searches the genome for single nucleotide variants that occur more frequently in people with a particular disease than in people without the disease. The goal is to identify genetic risk factors for common diseases. Two GWAS conducted in Han Chinese women identified 11 loci, accounting for 17 SNPs, with a strong association risk for PCOS (41,42) (Table 3). These data were validated in Caucasians, confirming the presence of 12 out of the 17 variants with the same risk effect, indicating a similar genetic risk profile in different populations (43-48). However, the frequency of risk alleles differs significantly among populations (43).

Table 3. PCOSGWAS susceptibility gene markers

Han Chinese: 2011 (41), 2012 (42)	European 1 2015 (47)	European 2 2015 (48)
LHCGR	*GATA4/NEIL2*	*ERBB4*
FSHR	*FSHB*	*FSHB*
C9orf3	*C9orf3*	*RAD50*
THADA		*THADA*
DENND1A		*KRR1*
YAP1		*YAP1*
RAB5B5		
HMGA2		
TOX3		
INSR		

GWAS results have provided new insights into the biological pathways that may be involved in PCOS pathogenesis. The *DENND1A* (Differentially Expressed in Normal and Neoplastic Development isoform A1) gene was identified as a potential risk marker. *DENND1A* encodes a protein (connecdenn 1) associated with clathrin-coated pits where cell-surface receptors reside. The DENND1A protein is located in the cytoplasm and in the nuclei of theca cells (10). This gene has two major transcripts: DENND1A variant 1 (DENND1A.V1), which encodes a 1,009-aa protein with a C-terminal proline-rich domain, and

DENND1A variant 2 (DENND1A.V2), which encodes a truncated 559-aa protein that contains the DENN domain and a clathrin-binding domain; however, the protein lacks the proline-rich domain and includes a C-terminal 33-aa sequence that is not found in the larger connecdenn variant 1 (49). McAllister's group showed that DENND1A.V2 protein is more expressed in PCOS theca cells compared to normal theca cells. They also forced overexpression of DENND1A.V2 in normal theca cells, resulting in increased CYP17A1 and CYP11A1 expression and increased androgen biosynthes, compatible with PCOS theca cells profile. Additionally, knock-out of DENND1A.V2 in PCOS theca cells reduced CYP17A1 and CYP11A1 expression and androgen biosynthesis (10,49). Recently, DENND1A expression in the adrenal *zona reticularis* was shown (50). Taking all these data into consideration, the DENND1A variant 2 is potentially one of the mechanisms involved with the intrinsic abnormality in ovarian theca cells steroidogenesis in PCOS.

Some other genes (*LHCGR, FSHR, INRS, THADA, HMGA2, RAB5B, SUOX, YAP, ZNF217*) located in susceptibility loci indicated by GWAS studies were related to the gonadotropic regulatory axis, glucose and lipid metabolism, and cell cycle regulation.

- The *LHCGR* (luteinizing hormone/ choriogonadotropin receptor) gene is a G protein-coupled receptor, which is expressed in granulosa cells, mainly in the preovulatory follicles. Increased LHCGR expression in granulosa cells in preovulatory follicles allows these follicles to respond to the LH peak in the middle of the cycle, resulting in ovulation. Inactivating mutations of this gene result in increased LH levels, amenorrhea or oligomenorrhea and infertility (51,52). In contrast, activating mutations of this gene are associated with hyperandrogenism (53).
- The *FSHR* (follicle stimulating hormone receptor) gene is related to the ovarian response to FSH and appears to be a highly plausible candidate gene for PCOS. Inactivating mutations of FSHR lead to hypergonadotropic hypogonadism and follicles stagnation in the preantral stage (50). Polymorphic variations of this gene in patients with PCOS have been associated with increased FSH concentrations (44) and resistance to exogenous ovarian stimulation with gonadotrophins and clomiphene (54).
- The *INRS* gene is the most prominent gene associated with insulin resistance indicated by GWAS. Mutations in the tyrosine kinase domain of the insulin receptor are known causes of insulin resistance and severe hyperinsulinemia (55). Polymorphic variants in different exons have been reported as risk factors for PCOS, but the results were generally not consistent in subsequent studies (50).
- *THADA* and *HMGA2* genes have also been described in the GWAS studies involving patients with DM2 (56). *RAB5B* and *SUOX* genes are located at the susceptibility locus for DM1 (57). *YAP* and *ZNF217* genes do not have a known ovarian function but they are related to cell proliferation and apoptosis (58).

The wide genetic possibilities indicated by GWAS could be related to the phenotypic heterogeneity. However, these loci identified in GWAS so far explain less than 10% of PCOS heritability. The rationale for GWAS large-scale sequencing studies is "common disease is associated with common variants", postulating that common diseases are related to allelic variants present in more than 1-5% of the population. From this principle, GWAS studies allow the identification of an enormous number of genetic variants associated with complex diseases; however, most of the variants individually or in combination confer small increments in risk (1.1-1.5 fold). Variants with lower frequency and larger effect size that are not captured by GWAS may account for the deficit in heritability found using this method (59).

Moreover, the associations of the PCOS risk variants and some PCOS features, such as testosterone levels, hyperinsulinemia, and ovarian morphology could not be clearly established. The next step in genomics era is understanding how these variants contribute to disease's pathogenesis as discussed by Jones and Goodarzi (60).

GENETIC APPROACH IN PCOS POS-GWAS DISCOVERIES

Currently, GWAS have provided insights into the genetics of PCOS, pointing to some susceptible *loci*, usually in a non-coding region associated with the disease, but at the same time, these studies have shown that this complex disease cannot be explained by a limited number of variants with a low effect on phenotype. Much of the speculation about missing heritability from PCOS GWAS studies has focused on the role of rare genetic variants with substantial effect on phenotype.

It is in this context that massive parallel sequencing, which can process millions of sequences in parallel, provides a mechanism to screen the whole exome or to sequence the whole genome for rare variants. Whole exome sequencing (WES) has been able to advance the understanding of complex diseases via two approaches: searching for lower frequency coding variants that may only be present in subsets of the population and sequencing individuals with a severe phenotype. Rare variants with large effects in a specific gene may be found in extreme phenotypes, which can provide insights into the underlying pathophysiology of the common disorder (61).

Recently, Gorsic and cols. identified 18 rare variants in PCOS patients using WES, and 17 of 18 (94%) of the variants were associated with reduced AMH signaling. They hypothesize that these AMH mutations lead to the PCOS phenotype by disrupting AMH's transcriptional inhibition of *CYP17A1*, leading to increased androgen biosynthesis (62). As demonstrated, WES seems promising in identifying rare genetic variants that contribute to PCOS pathogenesis and in mapping genetic variants that contribute to different aspects of each phenotype of the syndrome.

In conclusion, major advances in the genetics knowledge, combining with functional data and epigenetic studies in PCOS might increase our understanding of the etiology of this disease, with possible translational implications. The determination of genetic markers may improve the diagnosis of the syndrome and its phenotypes, allowing early intervention in associated co-morbidities and adequating treatment in a more individualized way.

REFERENCES

1. Azziz R, Carmina E, Chen Z, Dunaif A, Laven JS, Legro RS, et al. Polycystic ovary syndrome. Nat Rev Dis Primers. 2016;2:16057.
2. Gunning MN, Fauser BCJM. Are women with polycystic ovary syndrome at increased cardiovascular disease risk later in life? Climacteric. 2017;20(3):222-7.
3. JK Z. Diagnostic criteria of polycystic ovary syndrome; towards a rational approach. In: Dunaif A, editor. Polycystic Ovary Syndrome ed. Boston, MA: Blackwell Scientific; 1992.
4. Group REA-SPCW. Revised 2003 consensus on diagnostic criteria and long-term health risks related to polycystic ovary syndrome. Fertil Steril. 2004;81(1):19-25.
5. Azziz R, Carmina E, Dewailly D, Diamanti-Kandarakis E, Escobar-Morreale HF, Futterweit W, et al. Positions statement: criteria for defining polycystic ovary syndrome as a predominantly hyperandrogenic syndrome: an Androgen Excess Society guideline. J Clin Endocrinol Metab. 2006;91(11):4237-45.
6. Legro RS, Arslanian SA, Ehrmann DA, Hoeger KM, Murad MH, Pasquali R, et al. Diagnosis and treatment of polycystic ovary syndrome: an Endocrine Society clinical practice guideline. J Clin Endocrinol Metab. 2013;98(12):4565-92.
7. Moghetti P, Tosi F, Bonin C, Di Sarra D, Fiers T, Kaufman JM, et al. Divergences in insulin resistance between the different phenotypes of the polycystic ovary syndrome. J Clin Endocrinol Metab. 2013;98(4):E628-37.
8. Lizneva D, Suturina L, Walker W, Brakta S, Gavrilova-Jordan L, Azziz R. Criteria, prevalence, and phenotypes of polycystic ovary syndrome. Fertil Steril. 2016;106(1):6-15.
9. Çelik E, Türkçüoğlu I, Ata B, Karaer A, Kırıcı P, Eraslan S, et al. Metabolic and carbohydrate characteristics of different phenotypes of polycystic ovary syndrome. J Turk Ger Gynecol Assoc. 2016;17(4):201-8.
10. Rosenfield RL, Ehrmann DA. The Pathogenesis of Polycystic Ovary Syndrome (PCOS): The Hypothesis of PCOS as Functional Ovarian Hyperandrogenism Revisited. Endocr Rev. 2016;37(5):467-520.
11. Nelson VL, Legro RS, Strauss JF, McAllister JM. Augmented androgen production is a stable steroidogenic phenotype of propagated theca cells from polycystic ovaries. Mol Endocrinol. 1999;13(6):946-57.
12. Goodarzi MO, Carmina E, Azziz R. DHEA, DHEAS and PCOS. J Steroid Biochem Mol Biol. 2015;145:213-25.
13. Louwers YV, de Jong FH, van Herwaarden NA, Stolk L, Fauser BC, Uitterlinden AG, et al. Variants in SULT2A1 affect the DHEA sulphate to DHEA ratio in patients with polycystic ovary syndrome but not the hyperandrogenic phenotype. J Clin Endocrinol Metab. 2013;98(9):3848-55.
14. Draper N, Walker EA, Bujalska IJ, Tomlinson JW, Chalder SM, Arlt W, et al. Mutations in the genes encoding 11beta-hydroxysteroid dehydrogenase type 1 and hexose-6-phosphate dehydrogenase interact to cause cortisone reductase deficiency. Nat Genet. 2003;34(4):434-9.
15. Garg D, Tal R. The role of AMH in the pathophysiology of polycystic ovarian syndrome. Reprod Biomed Online. 2016;33(1):15-28.
16. Pellatt L, Hanna L, Brincat M, Galea R, Brain H, Whitehead S, et al. Granulosa cell production of anti-Müllerian hormone is increased in polycystic ovaries. J Clin Endocrinol Metab. 2007;92(1):240-5.
17. Fallat ME, Siow Y, Marra M, Cook C, Carrillo A. Müllerian-inhibiting substance in follicular fluid and serum: a comparison of patients with tubal factor infertility, polycystic ovary syndrome, and endometriosis. Fertil Steril. 1997;67(5):962-5.
18. Wei LN, Huang R, Li LL, Fang C, Li Y, Liang XY. Reduced and delayed expression of GDF9 and BMP15 in ovarian tissues from women with polycystic ovary syndrome. J Assist Reprod Genet. 2014;31(11):1483-90.
19. Dixit H, Rao LK, Padmalatha VV, Kanakavalli M, Deenadayal M, Gupta N, et al. Missense mutations in the BMP15 gene are associated with ovarian failure. Hum Genet. 2006;119(4):408-15.
20. Mikaeili S, Rashidi BH, Safa M, Najafi A, Sobhani A, Asadi E, et al. Altered FoxO3 expression and apoptosis in granulosa cells of women with polycystic ovary syndrome. Arch Gynecol Obstet. 2016;294(1):185-92.
21. Kahn CR, Flier JS, Bar RS, Archer JA, Gorden P, Martin MM, et al. The syndromes of insulin resistance and acanthosis nigricans. Insulin-receptor disorders in man. N Engl J Med. 1976;294(14):739-45.

22. Musso C, Cochran E, Moran SA, Skarulis MC, Oral EA, Taylor S, et al. Clinical course of genetic diseases of the insulin receptor (type A and Rabson-Mendenhall syndromes): a 30-year prospective. Medicine (Baltimore). 2004;83(4):209-22.
23. Taylor SI, Cama A, Accili D, Barbetti F, Quon MJ, de la Luz Sierra M, et al. Mutations in the insulin receptor gene. Endocr Rev. 1992;13(3):566-95.
24. Garg A, Peshock RM, Fleckenstein JL. Adipose tissue distribution pattern in patients with familial partial lipodystrophy (Dunnigan variety). J Clin Endocrinol Metab. 1999;84(1):170-4.
25. Burghen GA, Givens JR, Kitabchi AE. Correlation of hyperandrogenism with hyperinsulinism in polycystic ovarian disease. J Clin Endocrinol Metab. 1980;50(1):113-6.
26. Robinson S, Kiddy D, Gelding SV, Willis D, Niththyananthan R, Bush A, et al. The relationship of insulin insensitivity to menstrual pattern in women with hyperandrogenism and polycystic ovaries. Clin Endocrinol (Oxf). 1993;39(3):351-5.
27. Dunaif A, Segal KR, Futterweit W, Dobrjansky A. Profound peripheral insulin resistance, independent of obesity, in polycystic ovary syndrome. Diabetes. 1989;38(9):1165-74.
28. Diamanti-Kandarakis E, Dunaif A. Insulin resistance and the polycystic ovary syndrome revisited: an update on mechanisms and implications. Endocr Rev. 2012;33(6):981-1030.
29. Miller WL, Tee MK. The post-translational regulation of 17,20 lyase activity. Mol Cell Endocrinol. 2015;408:99-106.
30. Wu S, Divall S, Nwaopara A, Radovick S, Wondisford F, Ko C, et al. Obesity-induced infertility and hyperandrogenism are corrected by deletion of the insulin receptor in the ovarian theca cell. Diabetes. 2014;63(4):1270-82.
31. Nestler JE, Jakubowicz DJ. Decreases in ovarian cytochrome P450c17 alpha activity and serum free testosterone after reduction of insulin secretion in polycystic ovary syndrome. N Engl J Med. 1996;335(9):617-23.
32. Eid GM, Cottam DR, Velcu LM, Mattar SG, Korytkowski MT, Gosman G, et al. Effective treatment of polycystic ovarian syndrome with Roux-en-Y gastric bypass. Surg Obes Relat Dis. 2005;1(2):77-80.
33. Pastor CL, Griffin-Korf ML, Aloi JA, Evans WS, Marshall JC. Polycystic ovary syndrome: evidence for reduced sensitivity of the gonadotropin-releasing hormone pulse generator to inhibition by estradiol and progesterone. J Clin Endocrinol Metab. 1998;83(2):582-90.
34. Eagleson CA, Gingrich MB, Pastor CL, Arora TK, Burt CM, Evans WS, et al. Polycystic ovarian syndrome: evidence that flutamide restores sensitivity of the gonadotropin-releasing hormone pulse generator to inhibition by estradiol and progesterone. J Clin Endocrinol Metab. 2000;85(11):4047-52.
35. Cooper HE, Spellacy WN, Prem KA, Cohen WD. Hereditary factors in the Stein-Leventhal syndrome. Am J Obstet Gynecol. 1968;100(3):371-87.
36. Kahsar-Miller MD, Nixon C, Boots LR, Go RC, Azziz R. Prevalence of polycystic ovary syndrome (PCOS) in first-degree relatives of patients with PCOS. Fertil Steril. 2001;75(1):53-8.
37. Vink JM, Sadrzadeh S, Lambalk CB, Boomsma DI. Heritability of polycystic ovary syndrome in a Dutch twin-family study. J Clin Endocrinol Metab. 2006;91(6):2100-4.
38. Urbanek M, Legro RS, Driscoll DA, Azziz R, Ehrmann DA, Norman RJ, et al. Thirty-seven candidate genes for polycystic ovary syndrome: strongest evidence for linkage is with follistatin. Proc Natl Acad Sci U S A. 1999;96(15):8573-8.
39. Talbot JA, Bicknell EJ, Rajkhowa M, Krook A, O'Rahilly S, Clayton RN. Molecular scanning of the insulin receptor gene in women with polycystic ovarian syndrome. J Clin Endocrinol Metab. 1996;81(5):1979-83.
40. Mykhalchenko K, Lizneva D, Trofimova T, Walker W, Suturina L, Diamond MP, et al. Genetics of polycystic ovary syndrome. Expert Rev Mol Diagn. 2017;17(7):723-33.
41. Chen ZJ, Zhao H, He L, Shi Y, Qin Y, Li Z, et al. Genome-wide association study identifies susceptibility loci for polycystic ovary syndrome on chromosome 2p16.3, 2p21 and 9q33.3. Nat Genet. 2011;43(1):55-9.
42. Shi Y, Zhao H, Cao Y, Yang D, Li Z, Zhang B, et al. Genome-wide association study identifies eight new risk loci for polycystic ovary syndrome. Nat Genet. 2012;44(9):1020-5.
43. Louwers YV, Stolk L, Uitterlinden AG, Laven JS. Cross-ethnic meta-analysis of genetic variants for polycystic ovary syndrome. J Clin Endocrinol Metab. 2013;98(12):E2006-12.
44. Mutharasan P, Galdones E, Peñalver Bernabé B, Garcia OA, Jafari N, Shea LD, et al. Evidence for chromosome 2p16.3 polycystic ovary syndrome susceptibility locus in affected women of European ancestry. J Clin Endocrinol Metab. 2013;98(1):E185-90.
45. Goodarzi MO, Jones MR, Li X, Chua AK, Garcia OA, Chen YD, et al. Replication of association of DENND1A and THADA variants with polycystic ovary syndrome in European cohorts. J Med Genet. 2012;49(2):90-5.
46. Welt CK, Styrkarsdottir U, Ehrmann DA, Thorleifsson G, Arason G, Gudmundsson JA, et al. Variants in DENND1A are associated with polycystic ovary syndrome in women of European ancestry. J Clin Endocrinol Metab. 2012;97(7):E1342-7.
47. Hayes MG, Urbanek M, Ehrmann DA, Armstrong LL, Lee JY, Sisk R, et al. Genome-wide association of polycystic ovary syndrome implicates alterations in gonadotropin secretion in European ancestry populations. Nat Commun. 2015;6:7502.
48. Day FR, Hinds DA, Tung JY, Stolk L, Styrkarsdottir U, Saxena R, et al. Causal mechanisms and balancing selection inferred from genetic associations with polycystic ovary syndrome. Nat Commun. 2015;6:8464.
49. McAllister JM, Modi B, Miller BA, Biegler J, Bruggeman R, Legro RS, et al. Overexpression of a DENND1A isoform produces a polycystic ovary syndrome theca phenotype. Proc Natl Acad Sci U S A. 2014;111(15):E1519-27.
50. McAllister JM, Legro RS, Modi BP, Strauss JF. Functional genomics of PCOS: from GWAS to molecular mechanisms. Trends Endocrinol Metab. 2015;26(3):118-24.
51. Toledo SP, Brunner HG, Kraaij R, Post M, Dahia PL, Hayashida CY, et al. An inactivating mutation of the luteinizing hormone receptor causes amenorrhea in a 46,XX female. J Clin Endocrinol Metab. 1996;81(11):3850-4.
52. Latronico AC, Chai Y, Arnhold IJ, Liu X, Mendonca BB, Segaloff DL. A homozygous microdeletion in helix 7 of the luteinizing hormone receptor associated with familial testicular and ovarian resistance is due to both decreased cell surface expression and impaired effector activation by the cell surface receptor. Mol Endocrinol. 1998;12(3):442-50.
53. Latronico AC, Lins TS, Brito VN, Arnhold IJ, Mendonca BB. The effect of distinct activating mutations of the luteinizing hormone receptor gene on the pituitary-gonadal axis in both sexes. Clin Endocrinol (Oxf). 2000;53(5):609-13.
54. Overbeek A, Kuijper EA, Hendriks ML, Blankenstein MA, Ketel IJ, Twisk JW, et al. Clomiphene citrate resistance in relation to follicle-stimulating hormone receptor Ser680Ser-polymorphism in polycystic ovary syndrome. Hum Reprod. 2009;24(8):2007-13.
55. Moller DE, Yokota A, White MF, Pazianos AG, Flier JS. A naturally occurring mutation of insulin receptor alanine 1134 impairs tyrosine kinase function and is associated with dominantly inherited insulin resistance. J Biol Chem. 1990;265(25):14979-85.
56. Voight BF, Scott LJ, Steinthorsdottir V, Morris AP, Dina C, Welch RP, et al. Twelve type 2 diabetes susceptibility loci identified through large-scale association analysis. Nat Genet. 2010;42(7):579-89.

57. Barrett JC, Clayton DG, Concannon P, Akolkar B, Cooper JD, Erlich HA, et al. Genome-wide association study and meta-analysis find that over 40 loci affect risk of type 1 diabetes. Nat Genet. 2009;41(6):703-7.
58. Li T, Zhao H, Zhao X, Zhang B, Cui L, Shi Y, et al. Identification of YAP1 as a novel susceptibility gene for polycystic ovary syndrome. J Med Genet. 2012;49(4):254-7.
59. Manolio TA, Collins FS, Cox NJ, Goldstein DB, Hindorff LA, Hunter DJ, et al. Finding the missing heritability of complex diseases. Nature. 2009;461(7265):747-53.
60. Jones MR, Goodarzi MO. Genetic determinants of polycystic ovary syndrome: progress and future directions. Fertil Steril. 2016;106(1):25-32.
61. de Bruin C, Dauber A. Insights from exome sequencing for endocrine disorders. Nat Rev Endocrinol. 2015;11(8):455-64.
62. Gorsic LK, Kosova G, Werstein B, Sisk R, Legro RS, Hayes MG, et al. Pathogenic Anti-Müllerian Hormone Variants in Polycystic Ovary Syndrome. J Clin Endocrinol Metab. 2017;102(8):2862-72.

Short-term insulin intensive therapy decreases MCP-1 and NF-κB expression of peripheral blood monocyte and the serum MCP-1 concentration in newly-diagnosed type 2 diabetics

Yang Lin[1,2], Shandong Ye[1,3], Yuanyuan He[3], Sumei Li[3], Yan Chen[4], Zhimin Zhai[5]

[1] School of Medicine, Shandong University, Jinan, Shandong 250100, China
[2] Department of Pediatrics, Anhui Provincial Hospital, Hefei, Anhui 230001, China
[3] Department of Endocrinology, Anhui Provincial Hospital, Hefei, Anhui 230001, China
[4] Endocrinological Laboratory, Anhui Provincial Hospital, Hefei, Anhui 230001, China
[5] Department of Central lab, Anhui Provincial Hospital, Hefei, Anhui 230001, China

Correspondence to:
Shandong YE,
Shandong University,
Jinan, 250100, China
ysd196406@163.com

ABSTRACT

Objective: To observe the effect of short-term insulin intensive treatment on the monocyte chemoattractant protein-1 (MCP-1) as well as on the nuclear factor-kappa B (NF-κB) expression of peripheral blood monocyte. This is also in addition to observing the serum MCP-1 level in newly-diagnosed type 2 diabetic patients and probing its anti-inflammation effects. Subjects and methods: Twenty newly-diagnosed type 2 diabetic patients were treated with an insulin intensive treatment for 2 weeks. MCP-1 and NF-κB expression on the monocyte surface were measured with flow cytometry, the serum MCP-1 level was measured by enzyme linked immunosorbent assay (ELISA) during pre-treatment and post-treatment. Results: After 2 weeks of the treatment, MCP-1 and NF-κB protein expression of peripheral blood monocyte and serum MCP-1 levels decreased significantly compared with those of pre-treatment, which were (0.50 ± 0.18)% vs (0.89 ± 0.26)% (12.22 ± 2.80)% vs (15.53 ± 2.49)% and (44.53 ± 3.97) pg/mL vs (49.53 ± 3.47) pg/mL, respectively ($P < 0.01$). The MCP-1 expression on monocyte surface had a significant positive relationship with serum MCP-1 levels ($r = 0.47$, $P < 0.01$). Conclusions: Short-term insulin intensive therapy plays a role in alleviating the increased inflammation reaction in type 2 diabetics. Arch Endocrinol Metab. 2018;62(2):212-20

Keywords
Type 2 diabetes; insulin intensive therapy; MCP-1; NF-κB

INTRODUCTION

The world has seen a rapid increase in the incidence of diabetes generally, and type 2 diabetes mellitus (T2DM) has become the most common metabolic disease globally (1). Experimental data have shown that hyperglycemia may induce a chronic inflammatory state in the vessel wall, thus accelerating the development of diabetic chronic complications (2). T2DM and obesity are insulin-resistant (IR) disorders characterized by chronic inflammation (3).

NF-κB is a family of transcription factors that controls the production of pro-inflammatory proteins. The NF-κB pathway unites the inflammatory and metabolic responses, and, as a well-studied mediator of inflammation, represents an entry point for an improved understanding of metabolic diseases. MCP-1 is a member of chemotactic cytokines (CC) sub-family chemokines, which plays a pivotal role in the development of inflammatory reactions. MCP-1 accelerates the development and progress of diabetic nephropathy (DN) and macrovascular complications through inducing inflammatory cells from the circulation to artery endothelium and kidney. It also contributes to the proliferation of arterial smooth muscle cells, which constitute the key cellular components of atherosclerotic plaques (4).

Insulin has been shown to suppress inflammatory changes through the down-regulation of pro-inflammatory cytokines, reactive oxygen species (ROS) (5) and acute phase proteins (6), and the up-regulation of anti-inflammatory cytokines (7). In this report, we aim to demonstrate an anti-inflammatory effect of short insulin intensive therapy through comparing changes in MCP-1 expression on the monocyte surface, NF-κB expression in the monocyte, and serum MCP-1 level in newly-diagnosed T2DM patients pre-short-term insulin intensive treatment with those of post-treatment.

SUBJECTS AND METHODS

The subjects are 20 newly-diagnosed T2DM patients (HbA1c 9.02 ± 0.17%, women, n = 6; men, n = 14; mean age, 51.25 ± 5.71 years) admitted to department of endocrinology, Anhui provincial hospital, which is consistent with the diabetes diagnostic criteria of the World Health Organization (WHO) in 1999. To reduce the possibility of confounding, patients were selected according to the following exclusion criteria: pregnancy, concomitant diseases, smoking, and alcohol intake of more than 10 g/d. Patients with allergic diathesis regarding both type 1 e type 2 immune responses and/or reporting respiratory, gastrointestinal, or genitourinary tracts infections during the last three months were also screened out. The acute complications and severe chronic complications of diabetes have not appeared in type 2 diabetics recently, and the urinary albumin relative to the urinary creatinine was below 300 mg/gCr. None of the patients were receiving statins, aldosterone receptor antagonists, angiotensin-converting enzyme inhibitors, or angiotensin receptor antagonists, antibiotics, non-steroidal anti-inflammatory drugs, corticosteroids, or cytotoxic drugs at the time of the study. The other 20 healthy volunteers (women, n = 9; men, n = 11; mean age, 54.30 ± 7.39 years) were chosen from the Health Medical Examination Center of Anhui Provincial Hospital, serving as control subjects.

Research design

Blood samples were obtained from all participants after a 12-hour fast to measure the blood glucose, insulin, glycosylated haemoglobin A1c (HbA1c), white blood cell count (WBC), the neutrocyte percents (N%), cholesterol (TC), triglyceride (TG), low density lipoprotein cholesterol (LDL-C), MCP-1 expression on the monocyte surface, serum MCP-1 level and NF-κB expression in monocyte. Random spot urine samples were collected for the examination of urinary Albumin and creatinine levels. To eliminate the effect of urine volume, we expressed the level of urinary albumin (UALB) relative to the urinary creatinine (UCr) excretion, which was abbreviated as UACR (UALB/UCr ratio). Clearance of Creatinine Rate (Ccr) was calculated to stand for the glomerular filtration rate (GFR), using the formula raised by Cockcroft and Gault in 1976 (8). The patients in the observation group then received insulin intensive treatment consisting of regular pre-meal and bedtime neutral protamine hagedorn (NPH) insulin injections for two weeks. The indexes mentioned above were measured again at the study's conclusion. All laboratory tests were performed in the Biochemical Laboratory and Endocrinology Laboratory of Anhui Provincial Hospital.

The 20 newly-diagnosed T2DM patients, with an average HbA1c (9.02%), indicated that they had poor blood-glucose control, so the insulin treatment was necessary. Fasting blood glucose (FBG) and postprandial 2h blood glucose (P2hBG) were measured daily, and daily insulin doses (in units) were approximately 1 unit per kilogram; the dosage of insulin was adjusted according to blood glucose levels, FBG were controlled among 3.9~8.3 mmol/L while P2hBG were controlled < 10 mmol/L, and 3-5 days were limited to reach the determined blood glucose levels.

METHODS

Measurement of Serum MCP-1 Level (by ELISA)

Fasting serum samples were collected to measure serum MCP-1 level. For purposes of analysis, samples were thawed and vortexed vigorously, and MCP-1 level (pg/mL) was measured in duplicate according to the manufacturer's instructions with a commercially available ELISA (Biosource Inc).

Measurement of MCP-1 expression on the monocyte surface (by flow cytometry)

Five mL peripheral vein blood were drawn with the heparin supplemented tube. The measurement tube was supplemented with mouse monoclonal antibody to the human CD14 antigen stained with PE-Cy5 (Caltag Laboratories) 2.5 ul and mouse monoclonal antibody to the human MCP-1 antigen stained with PE (eBioscience) 1.25 ul. Mouse monoclonal antibody was added in the control tube to the human CD14 antigen stained with PE-Cy5 2.5 ul and Armenian hamster IgG isotype control stained with PE (eBioscience) 1.25 ul, then both the measurement tube and the control tube were injected with 100 ul blood followed by shaking in order to misce bene. Subsequently, both tubes were protected from light for 20 min at room temperature, and then each tube was added with hemolytic agent 2 mL. 10 min later, the two tubes were centrifugated at 1500 r/min for 5 min, abandoned the supernatant and supplemented with 2 mL PBS, repeated 1500 r/min centrifugalization for 5 min. Each tube was then washed three times with PBS, abandoned the supernatant, and then both the two tubes were supplemented with normal sodium to 500 ul, shaken to misce bene before measured by flow cytometry.

Measurement of NF-κB expression in the monocyte (by flow cytometry)

One milligram peripheral vein blood were drawn with heparin supplemented tube. The measurement tube and the control tube were supplemented with mouse monoclonal antibody to the human CD14 antigen stained with PE-Cy5 (Caltag Laboratories) 2.5 ul, then were added with 100 ul blood followed by shaking in order to misce bene. Subsequently, both tubes were protected from light for 20 min at room temperature, and then the tubes were added with 100 ul Fixation Medium A to fix. The tubes were then protected from light for 15 min at room temperature, then supplemented with 2 mL PBS, followed by 1500 r/min centrifugalization for 5 min, abandoned the supernatant and supplemented with 100 ul permeabilization medium B to rupture the membrane of monocyte. The measurement tube was added with mouse monoclonal antibody to the human NF-κB P65 antigen that stained with PE (eBioscience) 5 ul while the control tube had Armenian hamster IgG isotype control stained with PE added (eBioscience) 5 ul, followed by shaking in order to misce bene. Following this, both tubes were protected from light for 20 min at room temperature, supplemented with 2 mL PBS, repeated 1500 r/min centrifugalization for 5 min, and abandoned the supernatant. After this, both tubes were supplemented with normal sodium to 500 ul, shaked to misce bene before measured by flow cytometry.

Statistical analysis

Data were presented as means ± SD and analyzed using the Statistical Package for the Social Sciences 13.0. After testing data for normality, we used Student's paired *t* test to compare values before and after two weeks of insulin intensive treatment. The relationship between MCP-1 expression on monocyte surface and serum MCP-1 level, the relationships between MCP-1, NF-κB, and the change of FBG and P2hBG were performed by linear correlation. In all cases, a *P* value ≤ 0.05 was considered statistically significant.

RESULTS

The comparisons of data between diabetic patients and control group

The FBG, P2hBG, HbA1C, TC, TG, LDL-C, UACR, the expression of MCP-1 on monocyte and NF-κB in monocyte and serum MCP-1 level in diabetic patients were higher significantly than those in the control group, which were (11.18 ± 1.73) mmol/L vs (4.52 ± 0.15) mmol/L (17.92 ± 2.08) mmol/L vs (5.26 ± 0.34) mmol/L (9.02 ± 0.17)% vs (5.37 ± 0.08)% (5.45 ± 0.65) mmol/L vs (4.51 ± 0.53) mmol/L (2.02 ± 0.35) mmol/L vs (1.40 ± 0.30) mmol/L (3.85 ± 0.59) mmol/L vs (2.32 ± 0.69) mmol/L (71.98 ± 31.62) mg/gCr vs (12.88 ± 1.35) mg/gCr (0.89 ± 0.26)% vs (0.28 ± 0.09)% (Figures 1 and 2), (15.53 ± 2.49)% vs (3.67 ± 1.68)% (Figures 4 and 5) (49.53 ± 3.47) pg/mL vs (39.14 ± 7.43) pg/mL, respectively, $P < 0.05$. But there were no significant differences in age, BMI, GFR, SBP and DBP between the diabetic patients and the control group, which were (51.25 ± 5.71)y vs (54.30 ± 7.39)y, (23.26 ± 0.40) kg/m^2 vs (22.15 ± 0.62)kg/m^2, (99.35 ± 10.30) mL/min vs (105.10 ± 8.74) mL/min, (128.63 ± 2.41) mmHg vs (125.28 ± 5.31) mmHg, (75.21 ± 2.12) mmHg vs (70.31±2.48) mmHg, respectively, $P > 0.05$ (Table 1).

Table 1. The comparisons of paremeters between diabetic patients and control group

	NC	DM
AGE (y)	54.30 ± 7.39	51.25 ± 5.71
BMI (kg/m^2)	22.15 ± 0.62	23.26 ± 0.40
SBP (mmHg)	125.28 ± 5.31	128.63 ± 2.41
DBP (mmHg)	70.31 ± 2.48	75.21 ± 2.12
TC (mmol/L)	4.51 ± 0.53	5.45 ± 0.65*
TG (mmol/L)	1.40 ± 0.30	2.02 ± 0.35*
LDL-C (mmol/L)	2.32 ± 0.69	3.85 ± 0.59*
GFR (mL/min)	105.10 ± 8.74	99.35 ± 10.30
UACR (mg/gCr)	12.88 ± 1.35	71.98 ± 31.62*
FBG (mmol/L)	4.52 ± 0.15	11.18 ± 1.73*
P2hBG (mmol/L)	5.26 ± 0.34	17.92 ± 2.08*
HbA1c (%)	5.37 ± 0.08	9.02 ± 0.17*
serum MCP-1 (pg/mL)	39.14 ± 7.43	49.53 ± 3.47*
MCP-1 expression (%)	0.28 ± 0.09	0.89 ± 0.26*
NF-κB expression in monocyte (%)	3.67 ± 1.68	15.53 ± 2.49*

vs normal control group, * $P < 0.05$.

The changes of the MCP-1 and NF-κB expression before and after insulin intensive therapy in diabetic group are as follows:

After 2 weeks of the insulin intensive treatment, the MCP-1 expression on monocyte surface and serum MCP-1 level decreased significantly compared with those of pre-treatment, which were (0.50 ± 0.18)% vs (0.89 ± 0.26)%, (44.53 ± 3.97) pg/mL vs (49.53 ± 3.47) pg/mL, respectively, (P < 0.01) (Table 2, Figures 2 and 3); NF-κB expression in monocyte also decreased significantly compared that of pre-treatment, which were (12.22 ± 2.80)% vs (15.53 ± 2.49)% (P < 0.01) (Table 2, Figures 5 and 6).

The changes of FBG, P2hBG, Homa-IR (log), WBC and N% before and after insulin intensive therapy in diabetic group are as follows:

The FBG, P2hBG, Homa-IR(log), WBC and N% all significantly decreased after two weeks of insulin intensive treatment compared with those of pre-treatment, which were (6.37 ± 1.07) mmol/L vs (11.18 ± 1.73) mmol/L, (8.27 ± 2.12) mmol/L vs (17.92 ± 2.08) mmol/L, (0.71 ± 0.04) vs (0.78 ± 0.03), (5.52 ± 1.12) × 10^9/L vs (7.39 ± 1.56) × 10^9/L, (56.23 ± 4.71)% vs (64.61 ± 5.45)% (Table 2).

Relationship analysis

The MCP-1 expression on monocyte surface had a significant and positive relationship with serum MCP-1 level ($r = 0.47$, $P < 0.01$).

The expression of NF-κB in monocyte had a positive relationship with the MCP-1 expression on monocyte surface ($r = 0.51$, $P < 0.01$) and serum MCP-1 level ($r = 0.49$, $P < 0.01$).

The changes of FBG had no significant relationship with the changes of MCP-1 expression on monocyte surface ($r = 0.31$ $P > 0.05$), serum MCP-1 ($r = 0.33$, $P > 0.05$) and expression of NF-κB in monocyte ($r = 0.28$, $P > 0.05$).

The changes of P2hBG had no significant relationship with the changes of MCP-1 expression on monocyte surface ($r = 0.32$, $P > 0.05$), serum MCP-1 ($r = 0.28$, $P > 0.05$) and expression of NF-κB in monocyte ($r = 0.31$, $P > 0.05$).

The incidence of hypoglycemia

Hypoglycemia was recorded as blood glucose < 3.9 mmol/L with symptoms such as hunger, shakiness, nervousness, sweating, or dizziness. Twenty-six percent of patients were recorded to have had a hypoglycemic attack at least once in the T2DM patients. No hypoglycemia occurred in the control group.

DISCUSSION

T2DM is characterized by two major defects: a dysregulation of pancreatic hormone secretion (quantitative and qualitative – early phase, pulsatility – decrease of insulin secretion, increase in glucagon secretion), and a decrease of insulin action on target tissues (IR) (9). Now, T2DM is also recognized as a disease of chronic inflammation, which may play an important role in the development of IR, impairment of islet function, and

Table 2. The changes of indexes in diabetic group before and after insulin intensive therapy

	N	pre-treatment	post-treatment	t	p
FBG (mmol/L)	20	11.18 ± 1.73	6.37 ± 1.07	11.77	< 0.01
P2hBG (mmol/L)	20	17.92 ± 2.08	8.27 ± 2.12	19.14	< 0.01
Homa-IR(log)	20	0.78 ± 0.03	0.71 ± 0.04	6.43	< 0.01
WBC × 109/L	20	7.39 ± 1.56	5.52 ± 1.12	5.54	< 0.01
N%	20	64.61 ± 5.45	56.23 ± 4.71	5.72	< 0.01
BMI (kg/m^2)	20	23.26 ± 0.40	22.43 ± 0.52	1.856	> 0.05
TC (mmol/L)	20	5.45 ± 0.65	5.32 ± 0.51	2.77	< 0.05
TG (mmol/L)	20	2.02 ± 0.35	1.82 ± 0.31	8.91	< 0.01
LDL-C (mmol/L)	20	3.85 ± 0.59	3.55 ± 0.53	6.88	< 0.01
GFR (mL/min)	20	99.35 ± 10.30	101.20 ± 8.84	1.78	> 0.05
UACR (mg/gCr)	20	71.98 ± 31.62	53.52 ± 24.99	6.50	< 0.01
serum MCP-1 level (pg/mL)	20	49.53 ± 3.47	44.53 ± 3.97	4.21	< 0.01
MCP-1 expression (%)	20	0.89 ± 0.26	0.50 ± 0.18	8.48	< 0.01
NF-κB expression in monocyte (%)	20	15.53 ± 2.49	12.22 ± 2.80	3.96	< 0.01

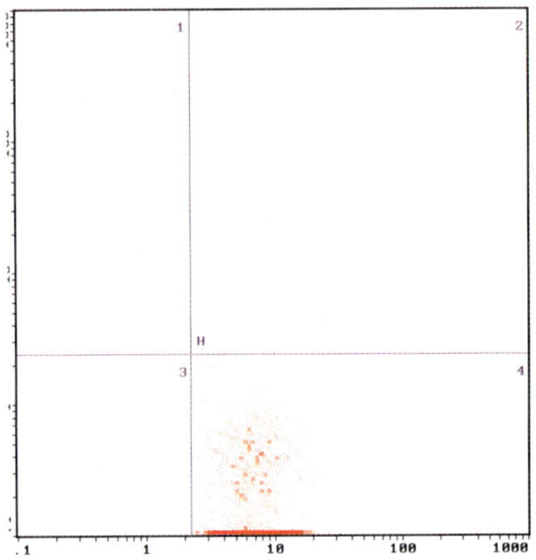

Figure 1. The MCP-1 expression on monocyte surface measured by flow cytometry in normal control group.

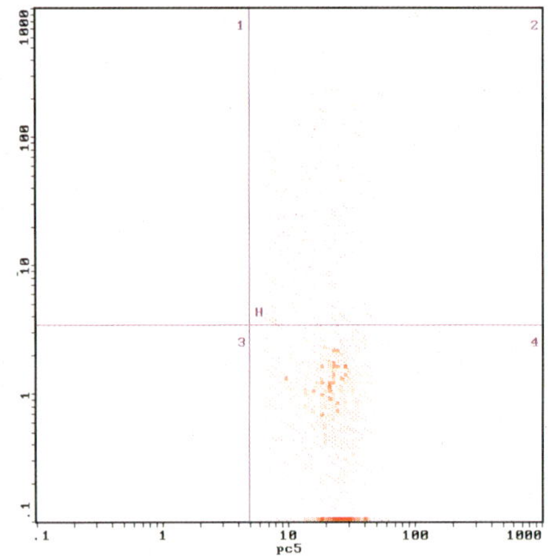

Figure 2. The MCP-1 expression on monocyte surface measured by flow cytometry before the treatment

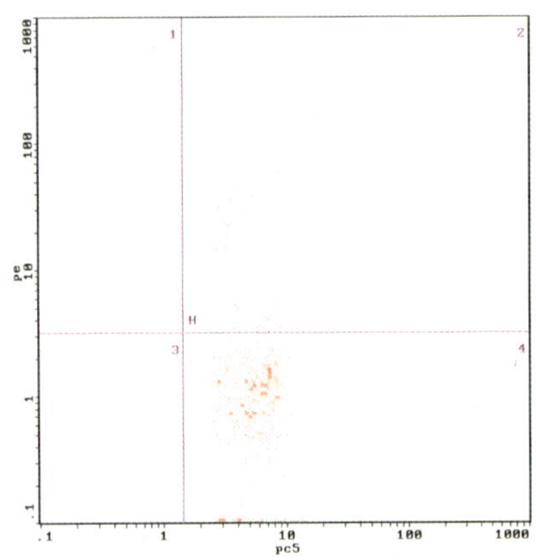

Figure 3. The MCP-1 expression on monocyte surface measured by flow cytomery after the treatment.

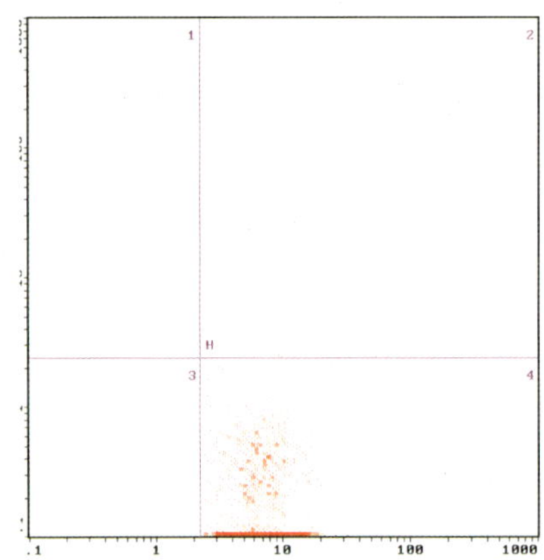

Figure 4. The expression of monocyte NF-κB measured by flow cytometry in normal control group.

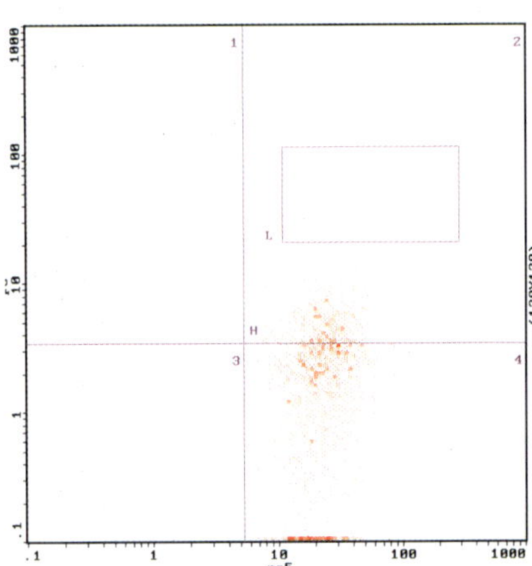

Figure 5. The expression of monocyte NF-κB measured by flow cytometry before the treatment.

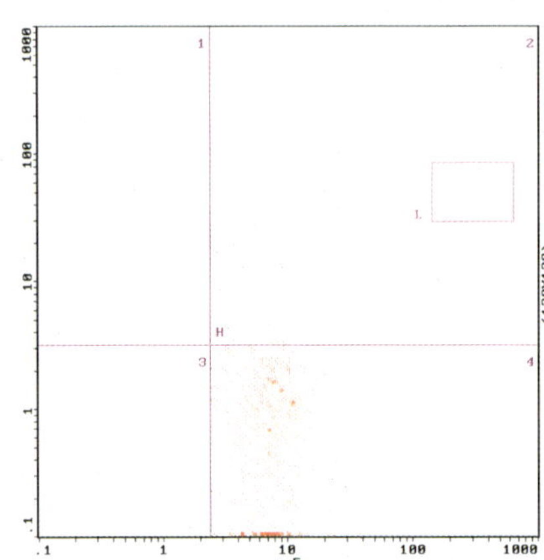

Figure 6. The expression of monocyte NF-κB measured by flow cytometry after the treatment

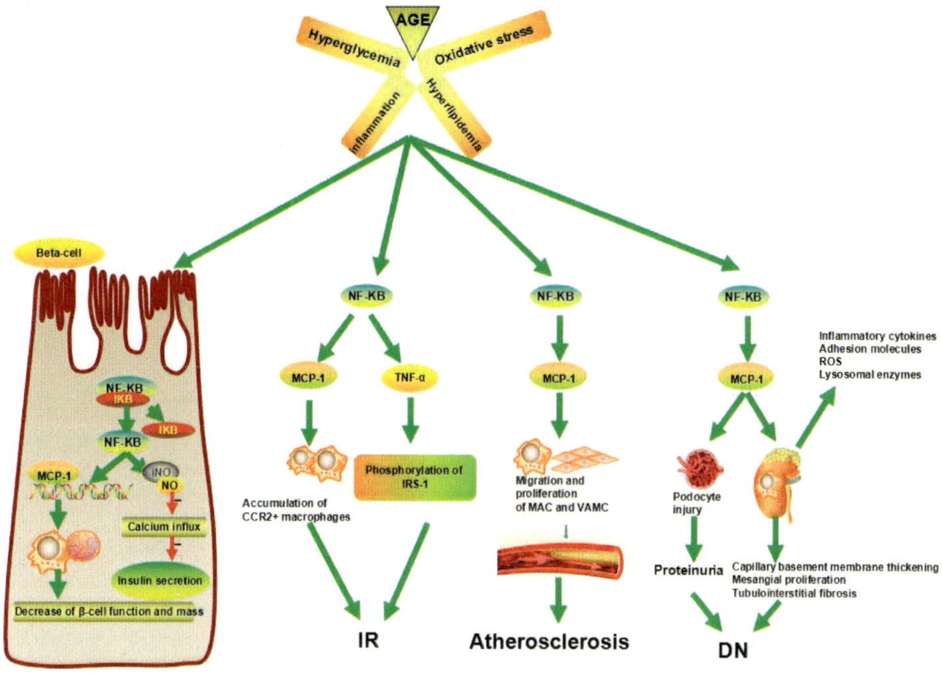

Figure 7. The pathophysiology of NF-κB and MCP-1 in T2DM.

diabetic chronic complications (10). Hyperglycemia, a main metabolic disorder in T2DM patients, activates the body's inflammatory defense mechanism, causing the waterfall release of numerous inflammatory mediators and cytokines, and eventually leading to organ damage (11). The dyslipidemia of T2DM also results in an increase in circulation concentrations of inflammatory cytokines (12). Previous studies have shown that many inflammatory factors, such as NF-κB, MCP-1, TNF-α, C reactive protein (CRP), IL-6, etc., not only take part in the dys-regulation of pancreatic hormone secretion and IR, but also in the development of the chronic complications of diabetes, such as its microvascular and macrovascular complications (12). In this study, the result also showed that the expressions of MCP-1 on monocyte and NF-κB in monocyte and serum MCP-1 level increased significantly in newly-diagnosed diabetic patients, which further indicates that increased chronic inflammation is present in T2DM patients.

Data accumulated in recent years suggest that activated NF-κB signaling pathway may be involved in the pathogenesis of IR, stress response, and inflammation by controlling gene network expression (13-15). NF-κB is present in the cytoplasm complexed to its inhibitory protein known as inhibitory κB (Iκ-B). Following activation, the phosphorylation of IκB molecules promotes their degradation and the release of NF-κB, which then translocates to the nucleus to promote the transcription of target genes (16). The NF-κB signaling pathway controls the expression of genes including inflammatory cytokines, chemokines, and adhesion molecules (17), such as MCP-1, IL-6, TNF-α, etc., which in turn initiate local inflammation and leukocyte accumulation (18).

MCP-1 is expressed by a variety of cell types, including monocyte, macrophage, endothelial cell (EC), vascular smooth muscle cell (VSMC), podocyte, adipocyte and fibroblast, etc. The expression of MCP-1 in all kinds of cells listed above is low under normal physiological conditions, once given the stimulations such as increased blood glucose, advanced glycation end products (AGEs), hyper-lipemia, angiotensin II (Ang II), oxidative stress, interleukin-1 (IL-1), TNF-α, et al., the expression of MCP-1 is obviously up-regulated (19,20). Increased serum MCP-1 level in humans correlates with markers of metabolic disorder including obesity, IR, and T2DM (21-23). MCP-1 accelerates the onset of atherosclerosis, as it attracts monocytes to the inflammatory sites of vascular subendothelial space, initiating the migration of monocytes into the arterial wall to form excessive macrophage-derived foam cells (24). It also participates in the early renal injury through activation of lysosomal enzymes and proteolytic enzymes in mononuclear macrophages and overproduction of ROS (25). Chow and cols. (26) reported that the MCP-1 genetic knockout mouse displayed amelioration of diabetic albuminuria, reduction in renal fibrosis, preservation of kidney clearance function, and decreased accumulation of macrophages.

Increasing evidence shows that short-term insulin intensive therapy can alleviate glucose toxicity, lipotoxicity and IR, and improve islet β cell function in newly diagnosed type 2 diabetics, but the study about its effect in inhibiting the MCP-1 and NF-κB expression in diabetic patients in vivo has not been reported. Two large, prospective, randomized controlled studies showed that intensive insulin therapy in hyperglycemic patients in a surgical intensive care unit (ICU) resulted in a 50% reduction in mortality, along with several other benefits, including a reduction in the incidence of renal failure, septicemia and ICU neuropathy. Insulin infusion also lowered circulating levels of MCP-1, intracellular adhesion molecule-1 (ICAM-1) and E-selectin in patients with prolonged critical illness (27,28). Aljada and cols. (29) reported that insulin could inhibit NF-κB and MCP-1 expression in human aortic endothelial cells. Treatment of Akita mice with insulin implants for 20 weeks normalized hyperglycemia and decreased urinary albumin excretion (30). This study showed that two weeks of intensive insulin therapy reduced MCP-1 expression on the monocyte surface, serum MCP-1 level, NF-κB expression in monocyte, peripheral blood WBC and N%, which further demonstrated the anti-inflammatory effect of insulin therapy. So an earlier initiation of insulin intensive treatment may be more effective in providing long-term efficacy against the complications of T2DM.

The mechanisms underlying the anti-inflammatory effect of insulin therapy are, however, unclear, but it can be proved as follows: 1) Insulin can activate some signaling pathways, including PI3K, protein kinase B/Akt, and mitogen-activated protein kinases (MAPK) such as p38, p42/p44, and JNK (31), activation of those signaling pathway is known to limit pro-inflammatory gene expression (28,32-34). 2) Insulin therapy has been reported to increase the production and release of anti-inflammatory cytokines such as IL-2 and IL-4 IL-10, and anti-inflammatory signal transcription factor mRNA expression of SOCS-3 and RANTES (35). 3) Long-term hyperglycemia has been proven to activate NF-κB and upregulate the expression of MCP-1 gene, insulin intensive treatment can control hyperglycemia more quickly (36). 4) Hyperglycemia can induce intracellular oxidative stress which results in the expression of pro-inflammatory cytokines gene. Dandona and cols. (37) showed that insulin therapy could decrease the production of ROS. Recent research also confirms that insulin played a significant role in the regulation of the cellular redox balance via Nrf-2 dependent pathway (38-40). 5) Insulin therapy can attenuate the IR, which is related to the inflammatory reaction in vivo. In this trial, we also found that short-term insulin intensive therapy improved IR in newly-diagnosed T2DM patients. 6) The dyslipidemia of T2DM also results in an increase in circulation concentrations of inflammatory cytokines (41). Hayashi (42) demonstrates that intensive insulin therapy reduced serum small dense LDL particles and TG levels in type 2 diabetics. In the present study, we also found that serum TC, TG, LDL-C levels in diabetic patients were higher than those in the control group, and, furthermore, their levels decreased after two weeks of intensive insulin therapy, which indicated that insulin may exert an anti-inflammatory effect partly through its hypolipidemic effects.

In this study, we observed that the UACR was also reduced in type 2 diabetics after two weeks of treatment, which indicates that insulin intensive treatment could ameliorate micro-albuminuria, which may be partially related to the reduction of the expression of MCP-1 and NF-κB.

In summary, our primary study shows that insulin therapy can reduce the MCP-1 expression on the monocyte surface, serum MCP-1 level and NF-κB expression in monocyte, which indicates that short-term insulin intensive treatment can alleviate the increased micro-inflammatory state in T2DM patients. But the mechanisms of insulin therapy in anti-inflammation must be further evaluated. We also discovered that reduced expression of MCP-1 and NF-κB were not related to the changes of FBG and P2hBG, which requires more cases and long-term studies to research whether or not the anti-inflammatory effect of insulin therapy is independent of its hypoglycemic effects.

Acknowledgments: the research presented in this paper was supported by the Natural Science Foundation (no. 11040606 M159) and the Natural Science Research Project (no. 1508085SMH227) of China's Anhui Province. Great help was offered by the Department of Endocrinology and Central Laboratory of Anhui Provincial Hospital.

REFERENCES

1. Chen S, Jiang H, Wu X, Fang J. Therapeutic Effects of Quercetin on Inflammation, Obesity, and Type 2 Diabetes. Mediators Inflamm. 2016 (2016):9340637.
2. Schmidt AM, Hofmann M, Taguchi A, Yan SD, Stern DM. RAGE: a multiligand receptor contributing to the cellular response in diabetic vasculopathy and inflammation. Semin Thromb Hemost. 2000;26(5):485-93.
3. Dubé JJ, Amati F, Stefanovic-Racic M, Toledo FG, Sauers SE, Goodpaster BH. Exercise-induced alterations in intramyocellular lipids and insulin resistance: the athlete's paradox revisited. Am J Physiol Endocrinol Metab. 2008;294(5):E882-8.
4. Han KH, Ryu J, Hong KH, Ko J, Pak YK, Kim JB, et al. HMG-CoA reductase inhibition reduces monocyte CC chemokine receptor 2 expression and monocyte chemoattractant protein-1-mediated monocyte recruitment in vivo. Circulation. 2005;111(11):1439-47.
5. Dandona P, Aljada A, Mohanty P, Ghanim H, Hamouda W, Assian E, et al. Insulin inhibits intranuclear nuclear factor kappaB and stimulates IkappaB in mononuclear cells in obese subjects: evidence for an anti-inflammatory effect? J Clin Endocrinol Metab. 2001;86(7):3257-65.
6. Hansen TK, Thiel S, Wouters PJ, Christiansen JS, Van den Berghe G. Intensive insulin therapy exerts antiinflammatory effects in critically ill patients and counteracts the adverse effect of low mannose-binding lectin levels. J Clin Endocrinol Metab. 2003;88(3):1082-8.
7. Jeschke MG, Klein D, Herndon DN. Insulin treatment improves the systemic inflammatory reaction to severe trauma. Ann Surg. 2004;239(4):553-60.
8. Cockcroft DW, Gault MH. Prediction of creatinine clearance from serum creatinine. Nephron. 1976;16(1):31-41.
9. Girard J. Contribution of free fatty acids to impairment of insulin secretion and action. mechanism of beta-cell lipotoxicity. Med Sci (Paris). 2005;21 Spec No:19-25.
10. Guclu M, Oz Gul O, Cander S, Unal O, Ozkaya G, Sarandol E, et al. Effect of Rosiglitazone and Insulin Combination Therapy on Inflammation Parameters and Adipocytokine Levels in Patients with Type 1 DM. J Diabetes Res. 2015;2015:807891.
11. Sun Q, Li J, Gao F. New insights into insulin: The anti-inflammatory effect and its clinical relevance. World J Diabetes. 2014;5(2): 89-96.
12. Kanagasabapathy G, Kuppusamy UR, Abd Malek SN, Abdulla MA, Chua KH, Sabaratnam V. Glucan-rich polysaccharides from Pleurotus sajor-caju (Fr.) Singer prevents glucose intolerance, insulin resistance and inflammation in C57BL/6J mice fed a high-fat diet. BMC Complement Altern Med. 2012;12:261.
13. Arkan MC, Hevener AL, Greten FR, Maeda S, Li ZW, Long JM, et al. IKK-beta links inflammation to obesity-induced insulin resistance. Nat Med. 2005;11(2):191-8.
14. Austin RL, Rune A, Bouzakri K, Zierath JR, Krook A. siRNA-mediated reduction of inhibitor of nuclear factor-kappaB kinase prevents tumor necrosis factor-alpha-induced insulin resistance in human skeletal muscle. Diabetes. 2008;57(8):2066-73.
15. Shoelson SE, Lee J, Goldfine AB. Inflammation and insulin resistance. J Clin Invest. 2006;116(7):1793-801.
16. Zhao Y, Chen SJ, Wang JC, Niu HX, Jia QQ, Chen XW, et al. Sesquiterpene lactones inhibit advanced oxidation protein product-induced MCP-1 expression in podocytes via an IKK/NF-κB-Dependent mechanism. Oxid Med Cell Longev. 2015;2015:934058.
17. Kim JE, Lee MH, Nam DH, Song HK, Kang YS, Lee JE, et al. Celastrol, an NF-κB inhibitor, improves insulin resistance and attenuates renal injury in db/db mice. PLoS One. 2013;8(4):e62068.
18. Ma ZJ, Zhang XN, Li L, Yang W, Wang S-S, Guo X, et al. Tripterygium glycosides tablet ameliorates renal tubulointerstitial fibrosis via the Toll-Like receptor 4/Nuclear Factor Kappa B signaling pathway in High-Fat diet fed and streptozotocin-induced diabetic rats. J Diabetes Res. 2015 (2015):390428.
19. Ehlermann P, Eggers K, Bierhaus A, Most P, Weichenhan D, Greten J, et al. Increased proinflammatory endothelial response to S100A8/A9 after preactivation through advanced glycation end products. Cardiovasc Diabetol. 2006 Mar 30;5:6.
20. Zhan Y, Brown C, Maynard E, Anshelevich A, Ni W, Ho IC, et al. Ets-1 is a critical regulator of Ang-mediated vascular inflammation and remodeling. J Clin Invest. 2005;115(9):2508-16.
21. Patsouris D, Cao JJ, Vial G, Bravard A, Lefai E, Durand A, et al. Insulin Resistance is Associated with MCP1-Mediated Macrophage Accumulation in Skeletal Muscle in Mice and Humans. PLoS One. 2014;9(10):e110653.
22. Kamei N, Tobe K, Suzuki R, Ohsugi M, Watanabe T, Kubota N, et al. Overexpression of monocyte chemoattractant protein-1 in adipose tissues causes macrophage recruitment and insulin resistance. J Biol Chem. 2006;281(36):26602-14.
23. Uchida Y, Takeshita K, Yamamoto K, Kikuchi R, Nakayama T, Nomura M, et al. Stress augments insulin resistance and prothrombotic state:role of visceral adipose-derived monocyte chemoattractant protein-1. Diabetes. 2012;61(6):1552-61.
24. Panee J. Monocyte Chemoattractant Protein-1(MCP-1) in Obesity and Diabetes. Cytokine. 2012;60(1):1-12.
25. Gu J, Ye S, Wang S, Sun W, Hu Y. Metformin inhibits nuclear factor-κB activation and inflammatory cytokines expression induced by high glucose via adenosine monophosphate-activated protein kinase activation in rat glomerular mesangial cells in vitro. Chin Med J (Engl). 2014;127(9):1755-60.
26. Chow FY, Nikolic-Paterson DJ, Ozols E, Atkins RC, Rollin BJ, Tesch GH. Monocyte chemoattractant protein-1 promotes the development of diabetic renal injury in streptozotocin-treated mice. Kidney Int. 2006;69(1):73-80.
27. Dandona P, Mohanty P, Chaudhuri A, Garg R, Aljada A. Insulin infusion in acute illness. J Clin Invest. 2005;115(8):2069-72.
28. Langouche L, Vanhorebeek I, Vlasselaers D, Vander Perre S, Wouters PJ, Skogstrand K, et al. Intensive insulin therapy protects the endothelium of critically ill patients. J Clin Invest. 2005;115(8):2277-86.
29. Aljada A, Ghanim H, Saadeh R, Dandona P. Insulin inhibits NF-kappaB and MCP-1 expression in human aortic endothelial cells. J Clin Endocrinol Metab. 2001;86(1):450-3.
30. Salem ES, Grobe N, Elased KM. Insulin treatment attenuates renal ADAM17 and ACE2 shedding in diabetic Akita mice. Am J Physiol Renal Physiol. 2014;306(6):F629-39.
31. Harbrecht BG, Nweze I, Smith JW, Zhang B. Insulin inhibits hepatocyte iNOS expression induced by cytokines by an Akt-dependent mechanism. Am J Physiol Gastrointest Liver Physiol. 2012;302(1):G116-22.
32. Fan W, Nakazawa K, Abe S, Inoue M, Kitagawa M, Nagahara N, et al. Inhaled aerosolized insulin ameliorates hyperglycemia-induced inflammatory responses in the lungs in an experimental model of acute lung injury. Crit Care. 2013;17(2):R83.
33. Ge D, Dauchy RT, Liu S, Zhang Q, Mao L, Dauchy EM, et al. Insulin and IGF1 enhance IL-17-induced chemokine expression through a GSK3B-dependent mechanism: a new target for melatonin's anti-inflammatory action. J Pineal Res. 2013;55(4):377-87.
34. Guenzl PM, Raim R, Kral J, Brunner J, Sahin E, Schabbauer G. Insulin Hypersensitivity Induced by Hepatic PTEN Gene Ablation Protects from Murine Endotoxemia. PLoS One. 2013 Jun 25;8(6):e67013.
35. Jeschke MG, Einspanier R, Klein D, Jauch KW. Insulin attenuates the systemic inflammatory response to thermal trauma. Mol Med. 2002;8(8):443-50.

36. Garvey WT, Olefsky JM, Griffin J, Hamman RF, Kolterman OG. The effect of insulin treatment on insulin secretion and insulin action in type II diabetes mellitus. Diabetes. 1985;34(3):222-34.

37. Dandona P, Aljada A, Mohanty P, Ghanim H, Hamouda W, Assian E, et al. Insulin inhibits intranuclear nuclear factor kappaB and stimulates IkappaB in mononuclear cells in obese subjects: evidence for an anti-inflammatory effect? J Clin Endocrinol Metab. 2001;86(7):3257-65.

38. Wang X, Tao L, Hai CX. Redox-regulating role of insulin: the essence of insulin effect. Mol Cell Endocrinol. 2012;349(2):111-27.

39. Wang X, Wu H, Chen H, Liu R, Liu J, Zhang T, et al. Does insulin bolster antioxidant defenses via the extracellular signal-regulated kinases-protein kinase B-nuclear factor erythroid 2 p45-related factor 2 pathway? Antioxid Redox Signal. 2012;16(10):1061-70.

40. Niture SK, Kaspar JW, Shen J, Jaiswal AK. Nrf2 signaling and cell survival. Toxicol Appl Pharmacol. 2010;244(1):37-42.

41. Bouchi R, Nakano Y, Fukuda T, Takeuchi T, Murakami M, Minami I, et al. Reduction of visceral fat by liraglutide is associated with ameliorations of hepatic steatosis, albuminuria, and micro-inflammation in type 2 diabetic patients with insulin treatment: a randomized contral trial. Endocr J. 2017;64(3):269-81.

42. Hayashi T, Hirano T, Yamamoto T, Ito Y, Adachi M. Intensive insulin therapy reduces small dense low-density lipoprotein particles in patients with type 2 diabetes mellitus: relationship to triglyceride-rich lipoprotein subspecies. Metabolism. 2006;55(7):879-84.

Association of different biomarkers of renal function with D-dimer levels in patients with type 1 diabetes mellitus (renal biomarkers and D-dimer in diabetes)

Caroline Pereira Domingueti[1], Rodrigo Bastos Fóscolo[2], Luci Maria S Dusse[3], Janice Sepúlveda Reis[4], Maria das Graças Carvalho[3], Karina Braga Gomes[3], Ana Paula Fernandes[3]

[1] Campus Centro Oeste Dona Lindu, Universidade Federal de São João del-Rei (UFSJ), Divinópolis, MG, Brasil
[2] Departamento de Clínica Médica, Faculdade de Medicina, Universidade Federal de Minas Gerais (UFMG), Belo Horizonte, MG, Brasil
[3] Departamento de Análises Clínicas e Toxicológicas, Faculdade de Farmácia, Universidade Federal de Minas Gerais (UFMG), Belo Horizonte, MG, Brasil
[4] Departamento de Endocrinologia e Metabologia, Instituto de Ensino e Pesquisa da Santa Casa de Belo Horizonte, Belo Horizonte, MG, Brasil

Correspondence to:
Caroline Pereira Domingueti
Universidade Federal de São João del-Rei,
Campus Centro Oeste Dona Lindu
Rua Sebastião Gonçalves Coelho, 400, Chanadour
35501-296 – Divinópolis, MG, Brasil
caroldomingueti@ufsj.edu.br

ABSTRACT

Objective: This study aimed to evaluate the association between different renal biomarkers with D-Dimer levels in diabetes mellitus (DM1) patients group classified as: low D-Dimer levels (< 318 ng/mL), which included first and second D-Dimer tertiles, and high D-Dimer levels (≥ 318 ng/mL), which included third D-Dimer tertile. Materials and methods: D-Dimer and cystatin C were measured by ELISA. Creatinine and urea were determined by enzymatic method. Estimated glomerular filtration rate (eGFR) was calculated using CKD-EPI equation. Albuminuria was assessed by immunoturbidimetry. Presence of renal disease was evaluated using each renal biomarker: creatinine, urea, cystatin C, eGFR and albuminuria. Bivariate logistic regression analysis was performed to assess which renal biomarkers are associated with high D-Dimer levels and odds ratio was calculated. After, multivariate logistic regression analysis was performed to assess which renal biomarkers are associated with high D-Dimer levels (after adjusting for sex and age) and odds ratio was calculated. Results: Cystatin C presented a better association [OR of 9.8 (3.8–25.5)] with high D-Dimer levels than albuminuria, creatinine, eGFR and urea [OR of 5.3 (2.2–12.9), 8.4 (2.5–25.4), 9.1 (2.6–31.4) and 3.5 (1.4–8.4), respectively] after adjusting for sex and age. All biomarkers showed a good association with D-Dimer levels, and consequently, with hypercoagulability status, and cystatin C showed the best association among them. Conclusion: Therefore, cystatin C might be useful to detect patients with incipient diabetic kidney disease that present an increased risk of cardiovascular disease, contributing to an early adoption of reno and cardioprotective therapies. Arch Endocrinol Metab. 2018;62(1):80-6

Keywords
D-Dimer, type 1 diabetes mellitus, cystatin C, creatinine, albuminuria

INTRODUCTION

Diabetic kidney disease is defined as a progressive increase in urinary albumin excretion (UAE), leading to glomerular filtration declining and, eventually, renal failure (1). It is the most important cause of end-stage renal disease, is an independent risk factor for cardiovascular disease and is responsible for increased mortality. It is estimated that nearly 30% of patients with diabetes develop renal disease (2,3).

Several biomarkers can be used to evaluate renal function in patients with diabetes, such as creatinine, urea, glomerular filtration rate (GFR), UAE and cystatin C. Creatinine is derived from metabolism of creatine and phosphocreatine of muscle cells, while urea is the major nitrogenous metabolite derived from the degradation of proteins (4,5). However, various factors can influence their levels aside from renal disease; therefore, the estimative of GFR is more often used in clinical practice (4,5). UAE is an important biomarker of renal injury, which is used for the diagnosis and prognosis of diabetic kidney disease, since it enables early detection of renal parenchyma injury (4,6). Cystatin C is a low molecular weight protein synthesized by all nucleated cells, whose function is to regulate cysteine proteases. It has been shown to be very promising in detecting early stages of renal disease in diabetic patients (6,7).

D-Dimer is a specific degradation product of cross-linked fibrin clots. It is a classic hypercoagulability biomarker, useful in the diagnosis of thromboembolic events (8). There is an association between D-Dimer levels with the development of atherothrombosis and cardiovascular complications in patients with diabetes, indicating that D-Dimer can be useful in evaluating the risk of cardiovascular disease in these patients (8-10). D-Dimer levels also increase with the progression of renal disease in patients with diabetes, indicating that hypercoagulability could be a link between diabetic kidney disease and the increased risk of cardiovascular outcomes (11-14).

A biomarker that is capable of detecting early stages of renal function decline and, therefore, could be simultaneously associated with a higher hypercoagulability status could be of great value. This is because it could be useful for detecting patients with incipient diabetic kidney disease that present an increased risk of cardiovascular disease, contributing to an early adoption of reno and cardioprotective therapies and, consequently, to a reduction of mortality.

Therefore, this study aimed to evaluate the association between D-Dimer levels and different biomarkers to assess the relationship between hypercoagulability and renal disease in patients with type 1 diabetes mellitus (DM1).

MATERIALS AND METHODS

The study was performed in accordance with the 2000 Declaration of Helsinki. It was approved by the Research Ethics Committee of *Universidade Federal de Minas Gerais* (CAAE – 0392.0.203.000-11), and informed consent was obtained from all participants.

Clinical records of 240 consecutive DM1 patients being assisted at Endocrinology Ambulatories of the Hospital das Clínicas and Santa Casa de Misericórdia of Belo Horizonte, Brazil, from November 2011 to September 2012, were analyzed. After the application of exclusion criteria, 125 patients with clinical and laboratorial diagnosis of DM1 (15), 18 to 60 years of age, were selected for this study. Criteria of exclusion consisted of hepatic disease, alcoholism, coagulation or hemostatic abnormalities, malignant diseases, acute infectious, history of kidney transplantation, pregnancy and hemodialysis. Data regarding age, sex, weight, height, time of diagnosis of DM1, use of antihypertensive, statin and acetylsalicylic acid were obtained from medical records.

Serum creatinine and urea were determined using an enzymatic method, serum albumin was assessed using a colorimetric method and HbA1c was determined through an immunoturbidimetric method, using dry chemistry technology. Cystatin C and D-Dimer were measured by ELISA. UAE was determined in urine samples collected after at least 4 hours of urinary retention, and urinary albumin was normalized by urinary creatinine. Urinary albumin was evaluated using an immunoturbidimetric method and urinary creatinine was assessed using an enzymatic method, using dry chemistry technology. UAE ≥ 30 mg/g of creatinine was confirmed in two out of three occasions during a period between three and six months, and the median was calculated (6). The estimated glomerular filtration rate (eGFR) was calculated using the CKD-EPI equation (16).

Statistical analysis was performed using SPSS software v. 20.0. Patients were divided into tertiles based on D-Dimer levels and were classified into two groups: low D-Dimer levels (< 318 ng/mL), which included first and second D-Dimer tertiles, and high D-Dimer levels (≥ 318 ng/mL), which included third D-Dimer tertile (17). The Shapiro-Wilk test was used to test the normality of the variables. Data normally distributed were expressed as mean ± SD and were compared using ANOVA and a t-est. Data not normally distributed were expressed as median (percentiles 25%-75%) and were compared using the Kruskal-Wallis H test and Mann-Whitney U test. Categorical variables were expressed as frequencies and compared using a chi-square test (χ^2). The presence of renal disease was evaluated using each renal biomarker; these were dichotomized using cutoff of ≥ 1.3 mg/dL, ≥ 40 mg/dL, ≥ 0.92 mg/L and ≥ 30 mg/g, for creatinine, urea, cystatin C and UAE, respectively (18-20). Bivariate logistic regression analysis was performed to assess which dichotomized renal biomarkers are associated with high D-Dimer levels and an odds ratio was calculated. Multivariate logistic regression analysis was performed to assess which dichotomized renal biomarkers are associated with high D-Dimer tertiles after adjusting for sex and age, and an odds ratio was calculated. The correlation between non-categorized renal biomarkers and D-Dimer levels were evaluated using the Spearman Correlation. Differences were considered significant when $p \leq 0.05$.

RESULTS

The characteristics and clinical variables of the DM1 patients included in this cross-sectional study are presented in Table 1.

Patients with high D-Dimer levels were older ($p = 0.003$) and presented an increased frequency of antihypertensive use than those with low D-Dimer levels ($p = 0.001$). The frequency of males was decreased in the high D-Dimer group compared to the low D-Dimer group ($p = 0.003$). There were no significant differences among groups regarding BMI, time of diagnosis, HbA1c levels, use of statin and use of AAS. Reduced serum albumin was observed in patients of the high D-Dimer group when compared to the low D-Dimer group ($p = 0.006$). Patients with high D-Dimer levels presented more increased levels of creatinine, eGFR, urea, cystatin C and UAE than patients with low D-Dimer levels ($p = 0.001$, $p < 0.001$, $p < 0.001$, $p < 0.001$ and $p = 0.004$, respectively).

Bivariate logistic regression analysis has demonstrated that patients with cystatin C ≥ 0.92 mg/L showed a better association with high D-Dimer levels [OR of 9.0 (3.8–21.1)], than patients with UAE ≥ 30 mg/g, creatinine ≥ 1.3 mg/dL, eGFR < 60 mL/min/1.73 m^2 and urea ≥ 40 mg/dL [OR of 5.0 (2.2–11.4), 5.3 (2.1–13.3), 6.0 (2.3–15.7) and 3.3 (1.5–7.3), respectively] (Table 2). A multivariate logistic regression analysis has shown that the association between all renal biomarkers and high D-Dimer levels remained, even after adjusting for sex and age (Table 2). After the adjustment for sex and age, patients with cystatin C ≥ 0.92 mg/L remained, presenting a better association with high D-Dimer levels [OR of 9.8 (3.8–25.5)] than patients with UAE ≥ 30 mg/g, creatinine ≥ 1.3 mg/dL, eGFR < 60 mL/min/1.73 m^2 and urea ≥ 40 mg/dL [OR of 5.3 (2.2–12.9), 8.4 (2.5–25.4), 9.1 (2.6–31.4) and 3.5 (1.4–8.4), respectively].

Cystatin C levels correlated better with D-Dimer levels ($r = 0.476$, $p < 0.001$) than other renal biomarkers ($r = 0.174$, $p = 0.070$ for creatinine; $r = 0.238$, $p = 0.012$ for urea; $r = -0416$, $p < 0.001$ for eGFR; $r = 0.314$, $p = 0.005$ for albuminuria) (Figure 1).

Table 1. Characteristics of patients with diabetes classified according to D-Dimer levels

	Low D-Dimer Group	High D-Dimer Group	p
Number of individuals (n)	82	43	
Age (years)	32 (24 – 37)	35 (30 – 45)*	0.003
Sex/male (n, %)	37 (45.1)	8 (18.6)*	0.003
BMI (kg/m^2)	24 ± 3	23 ± 3	NS
Time of diagnosis (years)	18 ± 8	20 ± 6	NS
Use of antihypertensive (n, %)	44 (53.7)	36 (83.7)*	0.001
Use of statin (n, %)	22 (26.8)	18 (41.9)	NS
Use of AAS (n, %)	10 (12.2)	11 (25.6)	NS
HbA1c (%)	8.5 (7.5 – 9.8)	8.4 (7.6 – 8.4)	NS
Creatinine (mg/dL)	0.81 (0.66 – 0.92)	1.02 (0.71 – 1.45)*	0.001
eGFR (mL/min/1.73 m^2)	112 (91 – 123)	76 (43 – 104)*	< 0.001
Urea (mg/dL)	31 ± 7	42 ± 17*	< 0.001
Albumin (g/dL)	4.1 ± 0.4	3.8 ± 0.4*	0.006
Cystatin C (mg/L)	0.74 (0.64 – 0.85)	1.11 (0.86 – 1.97)*	< 0.001
UAE (mg/g of creatinine)	8 (4 – 18)	44 (6 – 157)*	0.004
D-Dimer (ng/mL)	191 (134 – 233)	484 (381 – 639)*	< 0.001

Normally-distributed data were expressed as mean ± SD and compared by ANOVA and T test. Not normally distributed data were expressed as median (percentiles 25% – 75%) and compared by the Kruskal-Wallis H test and Mann-Whitney U test, followed by Bonferroni correction. Categorical variables were expressed as frequencies n (%) and compared using the chi-square test ($\chi 2$).

* $p < 0.05$ for high D-Dimer group compared to low D-Dimer group.

NS: not significant. BMI: body mass index. UAE: urinary albumin excretion. AAS: acetylsalicylic acid.

Table 2. Association between renal biomarkers and high D-Dimer levels

Variable	Odds ratio (95% confidence interval) unadjusted	p*	Odds ratio (95% confidence interval) adjusted for sex and age	p*
Creatinine ≥ 1.3 mg/dL	5.303 (2.106 – 13.357)	< 0.001	8.374 (2.464 – 28.459)	< 0.001
eGFR < 60 mL/min/1.73 m^2	6.048 (2.335 – 15.666)	< 0.001	9.110 (2.643 – 31.408)	< 0.001
Urea ≥ 40 mg/dL	3.340 (1.535 – 7.271)	< 0.001	3.480 (1.433 – 8.453)	0.008
Cystatin C ≥ 0.92 mg/L	9.018 (3.853 – 21.109)	< 0.001	9.844 (3.796 – 25.527)	< 0.001
UAE ≥ 30 mg/g	5.042 (2.222 – 11.440)	< 0.001	5.285 (2.160 – 12.926)	< 0.001

Data was evaluated by bivariate and multivariate logistic regression analysis and are presented as odds ratio (95% confidence interval). NS = not significant.
* $p < 0.05$ for high D-Dimer group compared to low D-Dimer group.

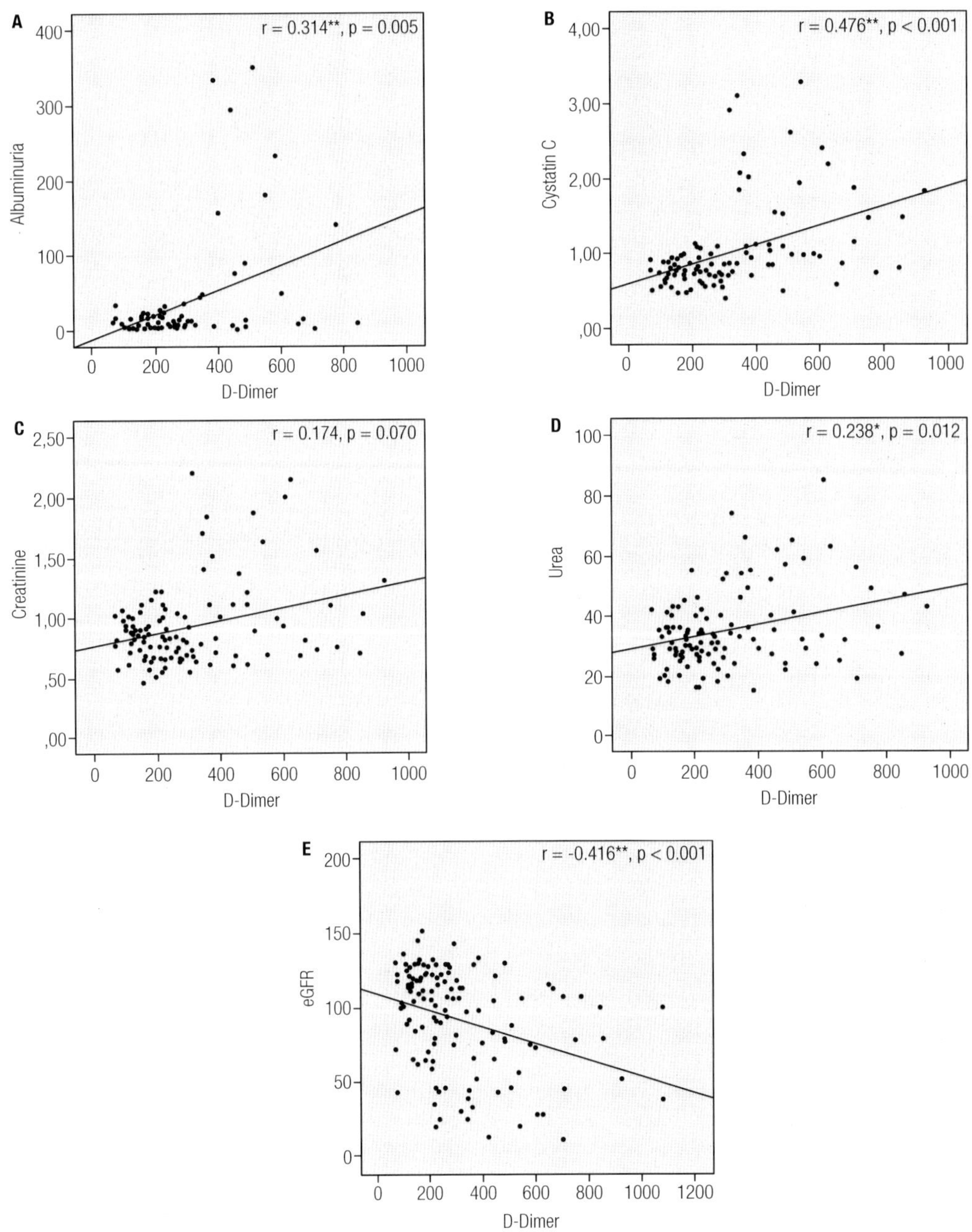

Figure 1. Spearman correlation of albuminuria (**A**), cystatin C (**B**), creatinine (**C**), urea (**D**) and (**E**) eGFR with D-Dimer levels.
* Correlation is significant at the 0.05 level. ** Correlation is significant at the 0.01 level.

DISCUSSION

Diabetic kidney disease is associated with an increased mortality, mainly due to cardiovascular outcomes (6). It has been demonstrated that the risk of cardiovascular death gradually increases with progressing stages of kidney disease (21,22). Therefore, simultaneous evaluation of early stages of renal function and hypercoagulability status using a unique biomarker would be of great value. Here, we have evaluated the association between different biomarkers of renal function with hypercoagulability status as assessed by D-Dimer levels in DM1 patients.

Some studies have found an association between increased D-Dimer levels and the presence of increased UAE levels and reduced eGFR in patients with diabetes (12-14,23). In this study, increased levels of different renal biomarkers, such as creatinine, urea, cystatin C, eGFR and UAE, were observed in patients with high D-Dimer levels. The association between renal dysfunction and increased levels of D-Dimer in DM1 patients may be explained by the increased synthesis of D-Dimer, but not by the reduced loss of D-Dimer in urine, since it has been shown that patients with diabetic kidney disease show higher urinary levels of D-Dimer than healthy individuals due to proteinuria (24). Proteinuria should also be responsible for the loss of important natural anticoagulant proteins, such as antithrombin, protein C and protein S, intensifying the hypercoagulability status and the production of D-Dimer (25).

It was verified that the decline of GFR also results in endothelial dysfunction and the release of the von Willebrand factor, which promotes platelet adhesion and aggregation and, consequently, microthrombi formation and increased D-Dimer levels (26). Endothelial dysfunction also impairs the activation of protein C, which depends on the endothelial protein C receptor and thrombomodulin, whose expression is reduced in damaged microvasculature, enhancing hypercoagulability status (27).

Haase and cols. (28) has demonstrated that D-Dimer plasma levels are higher in older adults and in females, which was also found in this study. These findings could be explained by the development of age-related changes in microcirculation and blood coagulation, which contribute to generate a hypercoagulability status and a gradual increase of D-Dimer levels with aging, as well as by the use of hormonal contraceptives in most of women. Such contraceptives can promote clotting mechanisms and increase D-Dimer levels (29,30). Increased frequency of antihypertensive use was observed in patients with high D-Dimer levels, which was expected, since these patients also showed an increased frequency of renal disease. Antihypertensive is commonly prescribed to patients with diabetes who have kidney disease to protect renal function (31). These patients also showed reduced serum albumin, which is in accordance to the increased UAE.

The relationship between increased UAE levels with a higher risk of cardiovascular disease in DM1 patients has been demonstrated by several authors (21,32,33). After the onset of proteinuria, median survival is only about seven years, and this increased mortality is mainly due to cardiovascular death rather than renal failure (34). High levels of serum creatinine and reduced eGFR have also been demonstrated to be indicative of progressive cardiovascular disease among diabetic patients (35,36), and increased levels of cystatin C have been associated with the development of cardiovascular events (37-40). Some authors have even shown that cystatin C is a stronger predictor of cardiovascular outcomes in patients with diabetes and elderly adults than creatinine and eGFR (39,40).

In agreement in this study, cystatin C presented a better association – when assessed by odds ratio analysis – with higher D-Dimer levels than urea, creatinine, eGFR and UAE, after adjusting for sex and age, which are variables that can influence D-Dimer levels (28). Cystatin C levels also presented a better correlation with D-Dimer levels than other renal biomarkers. These results suggest that cystatin C presents a better association with hypercoagulability status than other renal biomarkers and that it might be able to detect hemostatic changes that are not completely captured by measurements of urea, creatinine, eGFR and UAE. Cystatin C has been demonstrated to be a better biomarker to detect early stages of chronic kidney disease than creatinine and eGFR (41,42). This could partially explain the better association of this renal biomarker with higher D-Dimer levels, since cystatin C could detect a decline of renal function, and consequently a hypercoagulability state, that is not detected by other biomarkers. However, further longitudinal studies that directly assess the development of cardiovascular disease are still necessary to confirm the superiority of cystatin C to predict this risk in comparison to other renal biomarkers.

Some studies have reported that arteries with atherosclerosis contain more cysteine proteases than normal arteries, which may contribute to the degradation of atherosclerotic plaque (43,44). Cystatin C is a protein responsible for inhibit cysteine proteases and is a biomarker able to detect early stages of chronic kidney disease (41,42). Therefore, patients with renal disease present high levels of cystatin C, which may inhibit proteases that promote the degradation of atherosclerotic plaque. This contributes to the development of atherosclerosis and cardiovascular disease and explains why cystatin C is the renal biomarker that presents a better association with hypercoagulability status. However, this hypothesis should be further evaluated.

In conclusion, all renal biomarkers showed a good association with D-Dimer levels and, consequently, with hypercoagulability status. However, cystatin C showed the best association among them. These findings suggest that cystatin C might present an important utility to simultaneously evaluate renal function decline and the hypercoagulability status in DM1 patients.

Acknowledgments: the authors thank *Fundação de Amparo à Pesquisa do Estado de Minas Gerais* (Fapemig), *Coordenação de Aperfeiçoamento de Pessoal de Nível Superior* (CAPES) and *Conselho Nacional de Desenvolvimento Científico e Tecnológico* (CNPq).

REFERENCES

1. American Diabetes Association. Microvascular Complications and Foot Care. In: Standards of Medical Care in Diabetes – 2016. Diabetes Care. 2016;39:S72-S80.
2. Karnib HH, Ziyadeh FN. The cardiorenal syndrome in diabetes mellitus. Diabetes Res Clin Pract. 2010;89:201-8.
3. Gross JL, Silveiro SP, Canani LH, Friedman R, Leitão CB, Azevedo MJ. Nefropatia diabética e doença cardíaca. Arq Bras Endocrinol Metab. 2007;51:244-56.
4. Cirillo M. Evaluation of glomerular filtration rate and of albuminuria/proteinuria. J Nephrol. 2010;23:125-32.
5. Stevens LA, Levey AS. Measurement of kidney function. Med Clin North Am. 2005;89:457-73.
6. Murussi M, Murussi N, Campagnolo N, Silveiro SP. Detecção precoce da nefropatia diabética. Arq Bras Endocrinol Metabol. 2008;52:442-51.
7. Massey D. Commentary: clinical diagnostic use of cystatin C. J Clin Lab Anal. 2004;18:55-60.
8. Nwose EU, Richards RS, Jelinek HF, Kerr PG. D-Dimer identifies stages in the progression of diabetes mellitus from family history of diabetes to cardiovascular complications. Pathology. 2007;39:252-7.
9. Soares AL, Rosário PW, Borges MA, Sousa MO, Fernandes AP, Carvalho Md. PAI-1 and D-Dimer in type 2 diabetic women with asymptomatic macrovascular disease assessed by carotid Doppler. Clin Appl Thromb Hemost. 2010;16:204-8.
10. Krupinski J, Turu MM, Font MA, Ahmed N, Sullivan M, Rubio F, et al. Increased tissue factor, MMP-8, and D-dimer expression in diabetic patients with unstable advanced carotid atherosclerosis. Vasc Health Risk Manag. 2007;3:405-12.
11. Wakabayashi I, Masuda H. Association of D-Dimer with microalbuminuria in patients with type 2 diabetes mellitus. J Thromb Thrombolysis. 2009;27:29-35.
12. El Asrar MA, Adly AA, El Hadidy ES, Abdelwahab MA. D-dimer levels in type 1 and type 2 diabetic children and adolescents; Relation to microvascular complications and dyslipidemia "own data and review". Pediatr Endocrinol Rev. 2012;9:657-68.
13. Long ZF, Qu GY, Xu M. Relationship between the level of plasma D-dimer and diabetic microangiopathy. Hunan Yi Ke Da Xue Xue Bao. 2001;26:434-6.
14. Domingueti CP, Dusse LM, Fóscolo RB, Reis JS, Annichino-Bizzacchi JM, Orsi FL, et al. Von Willebrand factor, ADAMTS13 and D-Dimer are correlated with different levels of nephropathy in type 1 diabetes mellitus. PLoS One. 2015;10:e0132784.
15. American Diabetes Association. Diagnosis and classification of diabetes mellitus. Diabetes Care. 2013;36:dc13-S067.
16. Levey AS, Stevens LA, Schmid CH, Zhang YL, Castro AF 3rd, Feldman HI, et al. A new equation to estimate glomerular filtration rate. Ann Intern Med. 2009;150:604-12.
17. Akgul O, Uyarel H, Pusuroglu H, Gul M, Isiksacan N, Turen S, et al. Predictive value of elevated D-dimer in patients undergoing primary angioplasty for ST elevation myocardial infarction. Blood Coagul Fibrinolysis. 2013;24:704-10.
18. Kidney Disease: Improving Global Outcomes (KDIGO) CKD Work Group. KDIGO clinical practice guideline for the evaluation and management of chronic kidney disease. Kidney Int Suppl. 2013;3:1-150.
19. Finney H, Newman DJ, Price CP. Adult reference ranges for serum cystatin C, creatinine and predicted creatinine clearance. Ann Clin Biochem. 2000;37:49-59.
20. Bastos MG. Biomarcadores de Função Renal na DRC. In: Abensur H. Biomarcadores na Nefrologia. Soc Bras Nefrol e-Book. 2011;8-18.
21. Adler AI, Stevens RJ, Manley SE, Bilous RW, Cull CA, Holman RR; UKPDS GROUP. Development and progression of nephropathy in type 2 diabetes: the United Kingdom Prospective Diabetes Study (UKPDS 64). Kidney Int. 2003;63:225-32.
22. Lim CC, Teo BW, Ong PG, Cheung CY, Lim SC, Chow KY, et al. Chronic kidney disease, cardiovascular disease and mortality: A prospective cohort study in a multi-ethnic Asian population. Eur J Prev Cardiol. 2015;22:1018-26.
23. Wakabayashi I, Masuda H. Association of D-dimer with microalbuminuria in patients with type 2 diabetes mellitus. J Thromb Thrombolysis. 2009;27:29-35.
24. Shibata T, Magari Y, Mizunaga S, Okabe E, Sumie A, Ishii T, et al. Significance of urinary fibrin/fibrinogen degradation product (FDP) D-dimer measured by highly sensitive ELISA method with a new monoclonal antibody (D-D E72) in various renal diseases. Nihon Jinzo Gakkai Shi. 1994;36:805-12.
25. Kato S, Chernyavsky S, Tokita JE, Shimada YJ, Homel P, Rosen H, et al. Relationship between proteinuria and venous thromboembolism. J Thromb Thrombolysis. 2010;30:281-5.
26. Jenkins PV, O'Donnell JS. ABO blood group determines plasma von Willebrand factor levels: a biologic function after all? Transfusion. 2006;46:1836-44.
27. Scaldaferri F, Sans M, Vetrano S, Graziani C, De Cristofaro R, Gerlitz B, et al. Crucial role of the protein C pathway in governing microvascular inflammation in inflammatory bowel disease. J Clin Invest. 2007;117:1951-60.
28. Haase C, Joergensen M, Ellervik C, Joergensen MK, Bathum L. Age- and sex-dependent reference intervals for D-Dimer: evidence for a marked increase by age. Thromb Res. 2013;132:676-80.

29. Lippi G, Favaloro EJ, Cervellin G. A review of the value of D-dimer testing for prediction of recurrent venous thromboembolism with increasing age. Semin Thromb Hemost. 2014;40:634-9.
30. Fazio G, Ferrara F, Barbaro G, Alessandro G, Ferro G, Novo G, et al. Prothrombotic effects of contraceptives. Curr Pharm Des. 2010;16:3490-6.
31. Gross JL, de Azevedo MJ, Silveiro SP, Canani LH, Caramoni ML, Zelmanovitz T. Diabetic nephropathy: diagnosis, prevention, and treatment. Diabetes Care. 2005;28:164-76.
32. Deckert T, Yokoyama H, Mathiesen E, Ronn B, Jensen T, Feldt-Rasmussen B, et al. Cohort study of predictive value of urinary albumin excretion for atherosclerotic vascular disease in patients with insulin dependent diabetes. BMJ. 1996;312:871-4.
33. Kim WY, Astrup AS, Stuber M, Tarnow L, Falk E, Botnar RM, et al. Subclinical coronary and aortic atherosclerosis detected by magnetic resonance imaging in type 1 diabetes with and without diabetic nephropathy. Circulation. 2007;115:228-35.
34. Naidoo DP. The link between microalbuminuria, endothelial dysfunction and cardiovascular disease in diabetes. Cardiovasc J S Afr. 2002;13:194-9.
35. Karar T, Elfaki EM, Qureshi S. Determination of the serum levels of troponin I and creatinine among Sudanese type 2 diabetes mellitus patients. J Nat Sci Biol Med. 2015;6:S80-4.
36. Afkarian M, Katz R, Bansal N, Correa A, Kestenbaum B, Himmelfarb J, et al. Diabetes, kidney disease and cardiovascular outcomes in the Jackson Heart Study. Clin J Am Soc Nephrol. 2016;11:1384-91.
37. Ix JH, Shlipak MG, Chertow GM, Whooley MA. Association of cystatin C with mortality, cardiovascular events, and incident heart failure among persons with coronary heart disease: data from the Heart and Soul Study. Circulation. 2007;115:173-9.
38. Jernberg T, Lindahl B, James S, Larsson A, Hansson LO, Wallentin L. Cystatin C: a novel predictor of outcome in suspected or confirmed no n-ST-elevation acute coronary syndrome. Circulation. 2004;110:2342-8.
39. Schottker B, Herder C, Muller H, Brenner H, Rothenbacher D. Clinical utility of creatinine- and cystatin C-based definition of renal function for risk prediction of primary cardiovascular events in patients with diabetes. Diabetes Care. 2012;35:879-86.
40. Shlipak MG, Sarnak MJ, Katz R, Fried LF, Seliger SL, Newman AB, et al. Cystatin C and the risk of death and cardiovascular events among elderly persons. N Engl J Med. 2005;352:2049-60.
41. Pucci L, Triscornia S, Lucchesi D, Fotino C, Pellegrini G, Pardini E, et al. Cystatin C and estimatives of renal function: searching a better measure of kidney function in diabetic patients. Clin Chem. 2007;53:480-8.
42. Premaratne E, MacIsaac RJ, Finch S, Panagiotopoulos S, Ekinci E, Jerums G. Serial measurements of cystatin C are more accurate than creatinine-based methods in detecting declining renal function in type 1 diabetes. Diabetes Care. 2008;31:971-3.
43. Liu J, Sukhova GK, Sun JS, Xu WH, Libby P, Shi GP. Lysosomal cysteine proteases in atherosclerosis. Arterioscler Thromb Vasc Biol. 2004;24:1359-66.
44. Eriksson P, Jones KG, Brown LC, Greenhalgh RM, Hamsten A, Powell JT. Genetic approach to the role of cysteine proteases in the expansion of abdominal aortic aneurysms. Br J Surg. 2004;91:86-9.

Lifestyle intervention using the psychoeducational approach is associated with greater cardiometabolic benefits and retention of individuals with worse health status

Adriana Cezaretto[1], Camila Risso de Barros[1], Bianca de Almeida-Pititto[1], Antonela Siqueira-Catania[1], Milena Monfort-Pires[1], Luciana Gavilan Dias Folchetti[1], Sandra Roberta Gouvea Ferreira[1]

[1] Departamento de Epidemiologia, Faculdade de Saúde Pública, Universidade de São Paulo (FSP-USP), São Paulo, SP, Brasil

Correspondence to:
Sandra Roberta Gouvea Ferreira
Departamento de Epidemiologia,
Faculdade de Saúde Pública,
Universidade de São Paulo
Av. Dr. Arnaldo, 715
01246-904 – São Paulo, SP, Brasil
sandrafv@usp.br

ABSTRACT

Objective: This study aimed to compare the effects of two lifestyle intervention programs for type 2 diabetes mellitus (T2DM) prevention – traditional or interdisciplinary psychoeducation-based intervention – in daily habits and cardiometabolic risk factors and investigate the role of the psychoeducational approach for the retention of individuals in the program. **Subjects and methods:** Between 2008 and 2010, in a public health service, 183 pre-diabetic individuals were allocated to two 18-month interventions involving diet and physical activity. Physical activity, diet, quality of life (QOL) and depression and biochemical measurements were obtained. Linear mixed-effect models were used to assess the effect of the interventions. A student *t* test was used to compare dropouts versus non-dropouts. **Results:** Improvements in energy intake and physical activity were greater in the interdisciplinary than the traditional intervention. A decrease in fat mass and blood pressure was more pronounced with interdisciplinary intervention. Dropouts from the traditional intervention only had higher BMI and lower fiber intake and QOL than non-dropouts. **Conclusion:** The interdisciplinary psychoeducation-based intervention revealed useful for reducing cardiometabolic risk and retaining individuals with worse health profiles. This approach represents a feasible strategy for motivating high-risk individuals to adopt a long-term healthy lifestyle. Arch Endocrinol Metab. 2017;61(1):36-44

Keywords
Diabetes prevention; depression; lifestyle; psychoeducation; retention

INTRODUCTION

The modern lifestyle of populations, characterized by high consumption of energy-dense foods and physical inactivity, predisposes to weight gain and favors a growth in obesity-related diseases. In particular, abdominal obesity increases the risk of cardiometabolic disturbances, which in turn decrease the quality of life (QOL) and increase mortality (1-3).

Lifestyle interventions have yielded satisfactory results in preventing type 2 diabetes mellitus (T2DM) (4-6). In the Diabetes Prevention Program (5), modifications in dietary habits and physical activity were not only able to prevent T2DM but also induce greater improvement in QOL than the pharmacological arm, especially in individuals with considerable weight loss (7,8). However, long-term adherence to healthy behaviors remains a challenge for health professionals in real-life settings. This difficulty arises in part from the association of unhealthy habits with psychological problems. Among the latter, depression is highly prevalent and considered the number one cause of disability worldwide. This combination of unhealthy habits, excessive adiposity and mental disorders triggers a state of chronic low-grade inflammation and insulin resistance (9,10), which are underlying mechanisms of cardiometabolic diseases. Therefore, the management of psychological problems could facilitate achieving intervention goals and enhance QOL.

Psychoeducation is a therapeutic approach based on cognitive-behavioral theory, which involves the patients in solving their problems through communication and self-assertiveness training (11). Its effectiveness has been tested in prevention programs at the primary care level in developed countries (12,13) and was shown to be particularly effective when applied in interdisciplinary group sessions (14). Psychoeducational intervention was found to maintain benefits of psychiatric disease management with fewer relapses and higher levels of functioning (15-17) as well as improve the retention of alcohol-addicted individuals in a detoxification program (17). In clinical practice, the most disturbed patients and/or chronically ill, such as those with T2DM, are those who often fail to maintain treatment in healthcare systems.

In pre-diabetic conditions, psychoeducation was rarely applied in group sessions to promote a healthy lifestyle, being unclear whether this approach could improve retention of individuals at higher risk for T2DM.

Our group has reported benefits in QOL from lifestyle interventions in individuals at cardiometabolic risk treated under the Brazilian public health system (18). Psychoeducational techniques were applied in the interdisciplinary group sessions, whose participants showed greater improvement in QOL domains than those submitted to the traditional doctor-based intervention. A proportion of individuals interrupted participation in the interventions, which is worrisome since they are at risk for T2DM.

We hypothesized that an interdisciplinary psychoeducation-based intervention could be associated with greater clinical and psychological benefits and retention of individuals with a worse metabolic profile compared with a traditional intervention. Therefore, this study aimed to compare the effects of two lifestyle intervention programs for T2DM prevention – traditional or interdisciplinary psychoeducation-based intervention – in daily habits and cardiometabolic risk factors and investigate the role of the psychoeducational approach for the retention of individuals in the program.

SUBJECTS AND METHODS

Sample

A total of 438 individuals treated under the public health system in Sao Paulo, Brazil were screened for T2DM using a locally developed questionnaire (19) combined with a capillary to screen at-risk individuals. Those with values of random capillary glycemia > 140 mg/dL were invited to undergo clinical examination and laboratory tests. The inclusion criteria included the age range from 21 to 79 years and the presence of pre-diabetic conditions (impaired fasting glycemia and/or impaired glucose tolerance). Hypertensive participants had their blood pressure stabilized before starting the protocol, and anti-hypertensive schemes should be maintained during the intervention periods. The exclusion criteria included a medical history of neurological or psychiatric disturbances and liver, renal or infectious diseases. The institutional ethics committee approved the study and written consent was obtained from all participants. Those who developed diabetes were referred to medical treatment and pharmacological therapy. This trial was registered (RBR #65N292) on the ReBEC (ww.ensaiosclinicos.gov.br), the Brazilian registry center of the WHO International Clinical Trials Registry Platform.

Of the 230 eligible, 183 individuals agreed to participate in the interventions (www.fsp.usp.br/prevsm). Those who refused to participate were predominantly men, whereas non-participants did not differ from participants in terms of baseline socio-demographic, anthropometric and metabolic variables. Of these 183 individuals, 129 completed the study (Figure 1). The reasons for refusals were distance and time constraints to attend the intervention during business hours.

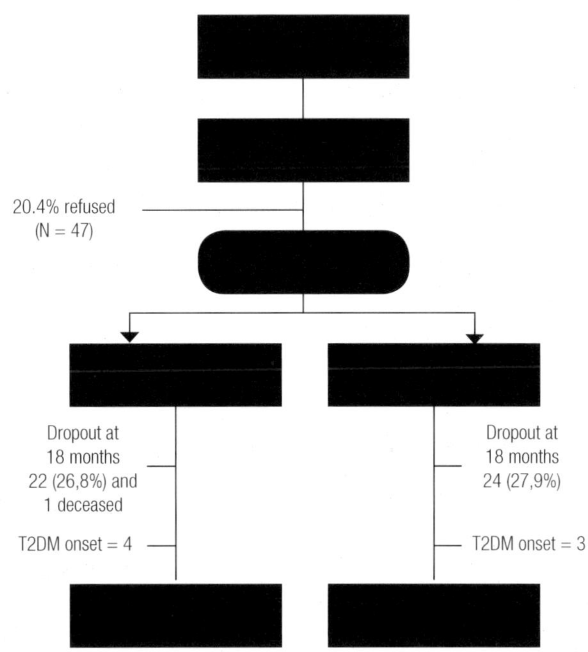

Figure 1. Flowchart of individuals in each stage of the study.

Protocol

In this 18-month interventional study, individuals were randomly assigned to one of two programs of modifications in dietary habits, physical activity and stress management. They were examined at baseline and again after 9 and 18 months of follow-up.

The traditional intervention consisted of quarterly medical visits with an endocrinologist, in which participants received usual written guidelines for changing diet and physical activity advocated by the Brazilian public health system. In addition to the medical visits, the interdisciplinary intervention with the psychoeducational approach included an individual appointment with a nutritionist and 16 group sessions conducted by a multiprofessional team (endocrinologist, psychologist, nutritionist and physical educator). Four two-hour group sessions were provided in the first month, two sessions in the second, followed by seven monthly sessions until the ninth month and three quarterly sessions up to the 18th month of the intervention (endpoint). Participants undergoing the interdisciplinary intervention also received printed materials to reinforce a healthy lifestyle. Group sessions dealt with issues related to daily routine, focusing on diet, physical activities and stressful situations and defining short-term targets. To enhance retention of the participants in the interventions, visits were arranged according to their convenience, and public transportation tickets were provided. Only for the interdisciplinary intervention, phone calls were made between sessions aimed at motivating and strengthening the participant-professional link.

Compliance was defined as 70% attendance to the interdisciplinary group sessions. Intervention goals were weight loss ≥ 5%, dietary fiber intake ≥ 20 grams/day, saturated fat ≤ 10% of total energy and moderate physical activity ≥ 150 minutes/week. The outcomes were the improvement in the risk profile, including blood pressure (BP) levels and glucose and lipid parameters.

Measures and variables

Measures were obtained by trained professionals. The physical activity level was assessed by the long version of the International Physical Activity Questionnaire (20,21) and dietary habits by three 24-hour recalls (two weekdays and one weekend day). Dietary data were analyzed using the Nutrition Data System for Research software (22). The Beck Depression Inventory (BDI) was applied to detect depression symptoms; its scores ranged from 0 to 63, and a value > 11 is indicative of the presence of depression (23). QOL was assessed using the Medical Outcome Study 36-Item Short-Form Health Survey (SF-36). This questionnaire includes 8 QOL domains (physical function, physical role, bodily pain, general health, vitality, social functioning, emotional role and mental health). Combined scores allowed calculation of the SF-36 physical and mental component summary health scales (24). BDI and SF-36 were previously translated and validated for the Brazilian population, taking into account the degree of literacy (25,26).

Height was taken using a fixed stadiometer and weight with individuals wearing light clothes and no shoes on a Filizola digital scale. Body mass index (BMI) was calculated as weight divided by height in meters squared. Waist circumference was measured at the midpoint between the bottom of the rib cage and above the top of the iliac crest during minimal respiration. Fat mass was measured by bioelectrical impedance analysis using a Quantum II – BIA Analyzer (RJL Systems, Inc., Clinton Township, Michigan, USA). BP was measured in a sitting position, three times with a 5-minute interval using an automatic blood pressure device (Omron HEM-712C, Omron Health Care, USA). The average of the last two measurements was used in analyses.

Participants were submitted to a 75-gram oral glucose tolerance test. Plasma glucose and lipid profiles were immediately determined in the local laboratory using enzymatic methods. Aliquots were frozen at -80 °C for further determinations. Insulin was determined by immunometric assay using a quantitative chemiluminescent kit (AutoDelfia, Perkin Elmer Life Sciences Inc, Norton, OH, USA) and adiponectin by ELISA (Human Adiponectin ELISA Kit, Millipore Corporation, MA, USA). Homeostasis model assessment (HOMA-IR) was used to assess insulin resistance (27).

Statistical analysis

Physical activity, dietary intake, depression, QOL and clinical data were expressed as mean and standard error or deviation. A student *t* test (or the Mann-Whitney test when indicated) was used to compare baseline variables between genders and intervention groups as well as to compare individuals who dropped out from each intervention versus those who were retained. A chi-square test was employed to compare retention rates.

Generalized Linear Mixed Models (GLMMs) were used to examine the change differences of outcomes between the intervention groups, considering an unstructured covariance matrix, which has the advantage of analyzing repeated measures over time, even when incomplete. This method assumes the random effects following a normal distribution and that missing data are missing at random. Mixed-effect models were built for each dependent variable (lifestyle, anthropometric and biochemical variables and QOL), considering the interaction between time and interdisciplinary intervention at 9 or 18 months of follow-up. All models were adjusted for sex and age as well as for the interdisciplinary intervention in order to control for differences between interventions at baseline.

Statistical analyses were performed using SPSS version 17.0 for Windows (SPSS Inc., Chicago, Illinois, USA) and the R statistical package (R Foundation for Statistical Computing, Vienna, Austria). A p-value < 0.05 was considered significant.

RESULTS

In the sample of 183 participants, 65% were women and the mean age was 54.7 ± 12.3 years. At baseline, 86% had a BMI ≥ 25 kg/m^2 and 61% had pre-diabetes. Stratifying according to sex, women had significantly higher BMI (31.7 versus 29.1, $p = 0.011$), HDL-cholesterol (44.7 versus 37.4, $p < 0.001$), adiponectin concentrations (16.7 versus 10.8, $p < 0.001$) and depression scores (14.8 versus 6.5, $p < 0.001$) as well as lower QOL in both physical (47.0 versus 51.8, $p < 0.001$) and mental (41.9 versus 49.4, $p < 0.001$) components than men, respectively. Seven participants (three in the traditional and four in the interdisciplinary intervention) became diabetic during the period and were excluded from this analysis.

At baseline, participants allocated to the interdisciplinary intervention and had a worse clinical profile (higher mean values of anthropometric measurements and diastolic BP and lower adiponectin concentration) than those allocated to the traditional intervention (Table 1).

Interdisciplinary intervention induced lower energy intake along 18 months. Both groups exhibited similar

Table 1. Baseline data according to type of intervention. Data expressed as mean (standard deviations) or percentages

	Traditional N = 86	Interdisciplinary N = 97	p-value
Women (%)	65.1	67.0	0.876
Schooling ≤ 8 yrs (%)	53.0	51.5	0.844
Employed (%)	65.0	59.8	0.106
QOL mental summary	44.7 (13.0)	44.2 (12.3)	0.807
QOL physical summary	49.1 (9.1)	48.3 (8.8)	0.532
Depression score#	11.4 (9.9)	12.4 (10.0)	0.441
Total energy intake (kcal)	1,754 (655)	1,861 (766)	0.315
Saturated fat intake (% total energy)	9.5 (2.6)	10.1(2.9)	0.188
Total fiber intake (per 1000 kcal)	9.2 (3.9)	9.1 (4.3)	0.883
Leisure physical activity (min/week)#	44.6 (73.4)	31.6 (61.7)	0.440
Body mass index (kg/m^2)	29.9 (5.7)	31.7 (5.7)	0.041
Waist circumference (cm)	98.6 (13.4)	103.6 (11.9)	0.010
Fat mass (%)	32.9 (9.4)	35.6 (9.0)	0.053
Systolic blood pressure (mmHg)	134.3 (17.7)	137.6 (20.3)	0.240
Diastolic blood pressure (mmHg)	80.3 (10.0)	84.9 (11.2)	0.034
Fasting plasma glucose (mg/dL)	99.1 (10.9)	99.4 (12.1)	0.837
Post-load plasma glucose (mg/dL)	115.1 (26.9)	121.2 (27.6)	0.131
LDL-cholesterol (mg/dL)	124.3 (41.9)	127.6 (35.6)	0.561
HDL-cholesterol (mg/dL)	41.7 (11.7)	42.7 (11.8)	0.553
Triglycerides (mg/dL)	150.4 (71.5)	151.4 (66.5)	0.916
HOMA-IR#	2.4 (1.8)	2.6 (1.7)	0.460
Adiponectin (ng/mL)#	18.1 (17.6)	11.6 (7.2)	0.001

Mann-Whitney test used for comparisons. QOL: quality of life.

patterns of change concerning saturated fat intake and fiber intake during the follow-up. However, participants of the interdisciplinary intervention had greater increase in leisure physical activity levels than those of the traditional one at the end of the follow-up (Table 2).

Table 2. Adjusted models of changes after 9 and 18 months in each clinical and psychological measure (outcomes) considering interaction between time and interdisciplinary intervention, by linear mixed models*

	Coefficient (SE)	P-value
Total energy intake (kcal)		
Change at 9 months	-191.8 (56.7)	< 0.001
Change at 18 months	-131.1 (58.1)	0.025
Interaction time 9 mo X intervention	-137.6 (78.1)	0.079
Interaction time 18 mo X intervention	-268.4 (80.2)	< 0.001
Physical activity (min/week)		
Change at 9 months	28.1 (11.1)	0.012
Change at 18 months	-9.07 (11.7)	0.439
Interaction time 9 mo X intervention	1.69 (15.3)	0.912
Interaction time 18 mo X intervention	35.9 (16.1)	0.026
Fat mass (percentage)		
Change at 9 months	0.71 (0.50)	0.161
Change at 18 months	0.31 (0.55)	0.574
Interaction time 9 mo X intervention	-1.56 (0.69)	0.026
Interaction time 18 mo X intervention	-1.65 (0.74)	0.027
Systolic blood pressure (mmHg)		
Change at 9 months	0.48 (2.11)	0.819
Change at 18 months	-1.98 (2.17)	0.362
Interaction time 9 mo X intervention	-6.62 (2.92)	0.024
Interaction time 18 mo X intervention	-8.78 (3.01)	0.004
Diastolic blood pressure (mmHg)		
Change at 9 months	-0.46 (1.17)	0.691
Change at 18 months	-1.43 (1.21)	0.234
Interaction time 9 mo X intervention	-5.72 (1.62)	< 0.001
Interaction time 18 mo X intervention	-6.06 (1.67)	< 0.001
Fasting glicemia (mg/dL)		
Change at 9 months	-1.89 (1.66)	0.256
Change at 18 months	-5.72 (1.71)	< 0.001
Interaction time 9 mo X intervention	-2.11 (2.29)	0.357
Interaction time 18 mo X intervention	4.98 (2.35)	0.040
Adiponectin (ng/mL)		
Change at 9 months	0.18 (1.43)	0.899
Change at 18 months	2.71 (1.48)	0.067
Interaction time 9 mo X intervention	4.96 (1.98)	0.013
Interaction time 18 mo X intervention	2.11 (2.04)	0.301

* All models were adjusted for gender and age.

Considering psychosocial measures, both physical ($\beta = 3.91$, $p < 0.001$) and mental ($\beta = 5.69$, $p < 0.001$) QOL components increased, and depression scores ($\beta = -5.04$, $p < 0.001$) had decreased after 18 months, but no difference was found when analyzing the interaction between time and intervention.

Greater reductions in BMI ($\beta = -0.79$, $p < 0.001$) and waist circumference ($\beta = -1.66$, $p = 0.023$) were observed after 9 months of the interdisciplinary intervention, but the difference between interventions lost statistical significance after 18 months. A greater decrease in fat mass in the interdisciplinary intervention was maintained until the end of the follow-up. Systolic and diastolic blood pressure reduced significantly over time, and these reductions were consistently greater in the interdisciplinary intervention than in the traditional intervention when considering interaction between time and intervention (Table 2).

The interdisciplinary intervention induced greater decreases in fasting plasma glucose than the traditional one only after 9 months. LDL-cholesterol and triglyceride concentrations did not change over time while significant elevations in HDL-cholesterol were observed for both intervention groups. HOMA-IR values decreased after 18 months ($\beta = -0.88$, $p < 0.001$), but no difference was found between interventions. Only participants of the interdisciplinary intervention had adiponectin concentrations increased at the ninth month (Table 2).

The percentage of individuals retained at the end of the follow-up was similar between interventions (traditional 70.7% and interdisciplinary 71.1%, $p = 0.95$). However, comparing baseline profiles, individuals who dropped out of the traditional intervention had worse depression scores, QOL, anthropometric measurements and dietary habits (lower fiber intake) than non-dropouts (Figure 2). On the other hand, the lifestyle data and clinical profile of dropouts and non-dropouts from the interdisciplinary intervention did not differ.

DISCUSSION

Translating research evidence derived from lifestyle interventions into practice poses a challenge, particularly in populations of developing countries due to economic and social limitations. The strategies used to address the challenges identified in our intervention among Brazilians may facilitate the adoption of preventive programs

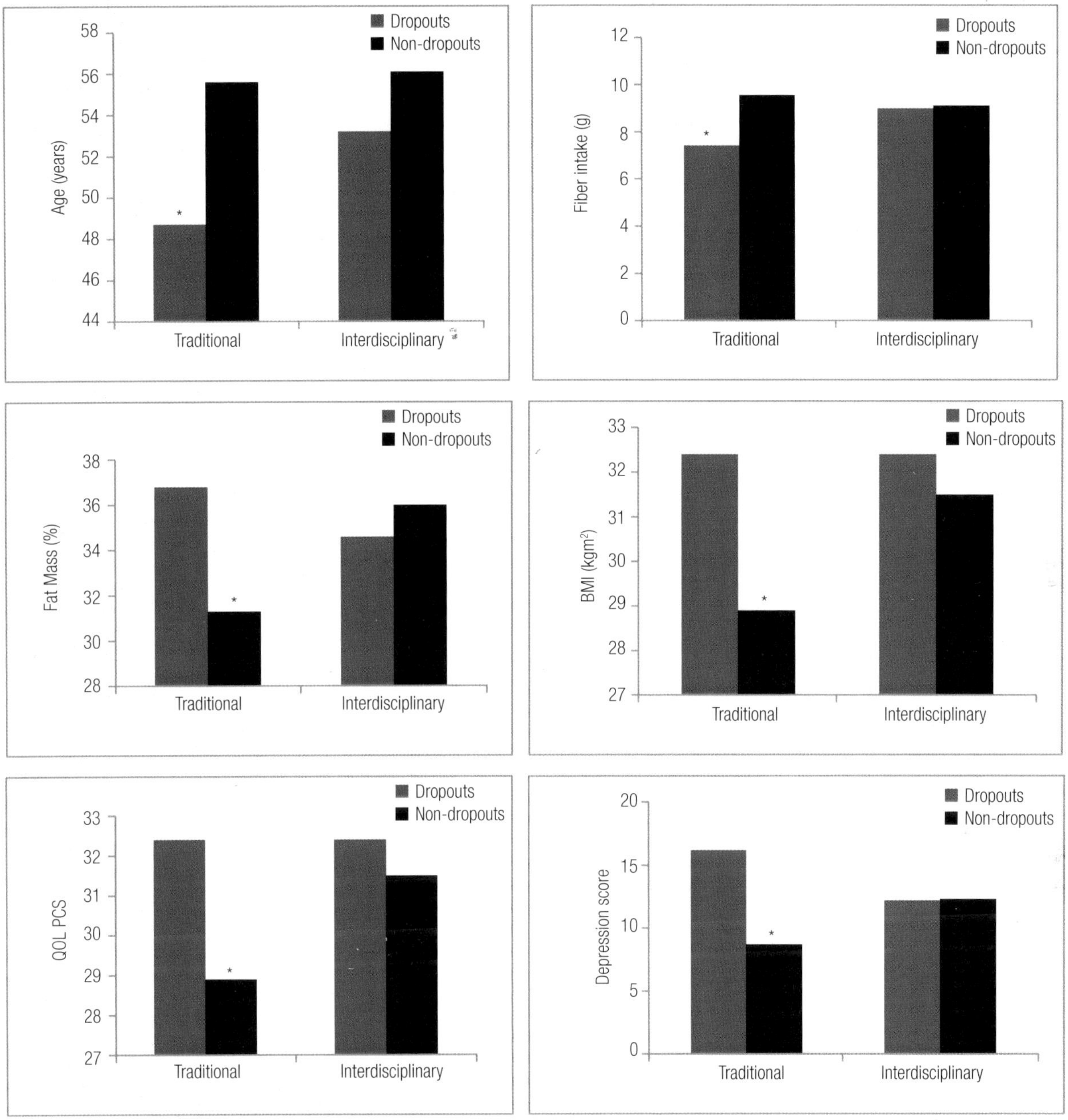

Student *t* test. * $p < 0.05$ versus non-dropouts.

BMI: body mass index; QOL: quality of life; PCS: physical component summary of SF-36.

Figure 2. Mean values of baseline data for dropouts and non-dropouts according to type of intervention.

in similar healthcare settings. The present study was able to demonstrate the superiority of an interdisciplinary intervention involving dietary and physical activity habits, which induced more pronounced benefits in body fatness, blood pressure levels and adiponectin concentrations than the traditional medical-centered intervention in individuals at cardiometabolic risk. Additionally, the psychoeducational approach retained individuals who most needed treatment, since this intervention was associated with greater retention of those exhibiting a worse metabolic profile at baseline.

By changing physical activity level and dietary habits, we sought to promote weight loss among the at-risk participants given the evidence of a protective effect against T2DM (4-6). In our study, the majority of the participants from the interdisciplinary intervention had increased time to do physical activity and decreased energy intake, suggesting that its approach could have encouraged this group to adopt healthier habits and resulting in favorable effects in body adiposity and blood pressure levels. During group sessions, participants had the opportunity to share problems and solutions by creating a forum for mutual help (28).

A beneficial effect of interdisciplinary intervention on anthropometric variables was seen at the ninth month; the rate of decline in fat mass but not in BMI was maintained until the end of the follow-up. The same pattern of changes, albeit to a smaller magnitude, was seen in the traditional intervention. This parallelism of the behaviors of both interventions could partially reflect a physiological defense against weight loss, mediated by a decrease in leptin levels (29). Although individuals from the interdisciplinary intervention started treatment with greater body adiposity than that of the participants from the traditional group, they showed more pronounced weight loss after follow-up. Previous studies have shown that motivational interviewing, such as psychoeducational groups, could be useful for achieving the goal of weight loss (30,31). The inclusion in our team of a professional who was aware of psychological concerns may have facilitated the maintenance of weight loss in the long term. This hypothesis is reinforced upon examining the clinical profile of individuals who completed each intervention.

The interdisciplinary intervention was able to retain a higher number of individuals with a worse clinical profile. By contrast, in the traditional intervention, individuals with lower fiber consumption, more severe obesity and worse QOL dropped out more frequently. These findings were interpreted as evidence that our psychoeducational approach improved motivation through life experience exchanges and mutual help. This probably helped participants manage their emotions, thereby facilitating behavioral changes. Healthier behavior and a better clinical profile were harder to be maintained by participants of the traditional group. Difficulties sustaining weight loss among obese individuals have been frequently reported, particularly in some specific populations such as low-income groups (32,33).

The benefits in cardiometabolic risk profile were achieved at the midpoint of our intervention but were attenuated by the end of the study. The same pattern has been described in other lifestyle interventions (34). Notably, we observed a sustained reduction in blood pressure for the interdisciplinary intervention only. This finding is in agreement with a 6-month trial adopting a similar approach to change lifestyle, in which significant blood pressure reduction was accompanied by weight loss (35). Such outcomes are relevant considering that even small decreases in these clinical parameters are able to lower the risk of chronic diseases such as T2DM, cardiovascular disease, osteoporosis and cancer (36).

Favorable effects in glucose and lipid metabolism were detected for both interventions. Plasma glucose and lipid concentrations decreased during the follow-up period, although no clear advantage of the interdisciplinary intervention was evident. Other behavioral population-based interventions have found clinical benefits, which were attributed to the mere fact that individuals had been followed up with (37). Unexpectedly, an increase in plasma glucose was detected after 18 months in the interdisciplinary group. Differences in the clinical characteristics of those retained in each intervention may have contributed to the more unfavorable outcomes of the participants in the interdisciplinary intervention. A relatively better metabolic profile of individuals from the traditional intervention at baseline might have also influenced the results. We speculate that this scenario may have attenuated the real benefits of the interdisciplinary intervention.

The limitations of our study include the small sample size and short duration of follow-up, precluding the evaluation of the incidence of concrete outcomes. Our reference group – the traditional intervention – is not representative of regular medical consultation under public healthcare systems since a specialist in endocrinology is not usually available in primary care units of developing countries. This could have reduced differences between the types of interventions, thus masking the real impact of the interdisciplinary intervention in its ability to change life habits. On the other hand, the results of the present study point to the importance of a traditional intervention having access to a diabetes specialist as an effective preventive strategy for high-risk individuals.

In conclusion, the interdisciplinary psychoeducation-based intervention proved useful for reducing cardiometabolic risk profile, most likely mediated by beneficial effects on daily habits. Moreover, this approach improves retention of at-risk individuals with worse health profiles. Interdisciplinary intervention, including group sessions, represents a feasible strategy for motivating individuals at a higher risk of adopting a long-term healthy lifestyle.

Acknowledgments: this study was supported by a grant from the São Paulo Foundation for Research Support – Fapesp, Sao Paulo, Brazil.

Sources of funding: funding was provided by the São Paulo Research Foundation (Fapesp process number: 11/06376-7) for a student (Adriana Cezaretto) and for a researcher (Sandra Roberta G. Ferreira; process number: 07/55120-0).

REFERENCES

1. Marks R, Allegrante JP, Lorig K. A review and synthesis of research evidence for self-efficacy-enhancing interventions for reducing chronic disability: implications for health education practice (part II). Health Promot Pract. 2005;6:148-56.
2. Slagter SN, van Vliet-Ostaptchouk JV, van Beek AP, Keers JC, Lutgers HL, van der Klauw MM, et al. Health-Related Quality of Life in Relation to Obesity Grade, Type 2 Diabetes, Metabolic Syndrome and Inflammation. PLoS One. 2015;16;10(10):e0140599.
3. Cameron AJ, Magliano DJ, Dunstan DW, Zimmet PZ, Hesketh K, Peeters A, et al. A bi-directional relationship between obesity and health-related quality of life: evidence from the longitudinal AusDiab study. Int J Obes. 2012;36(2):295-303.
4. Alberti KG, Zimmet P, Shaw J. Metabolic syndrome--a new world-wide definition. A Consensus Statement from the International Diabetes Federation. Diabet Med. 2006;23:469-80.
5. Knowler WC, Barrett-Connor E, Fowler SE, Hamman RF, Lachin JM, Walker EA, et al. Reduction in the incidence of type 2 diabetes with lifestyle intervention or metformin. N Engl J Med. 2002;346:393-403.
6. Tuomilehto J, Lindström J, Eriksson JG, Valle TT, Hämäläinen H, Ilanne-Parikka P, et al. Prevention of type 2 diabetes mellitus by changes in lifestyle among subjects with impaired glucose tolerance. N Engl J Med. 2001;344:1343-50.
7. Florez H, Pan Q, Ackermann RT, Marrero DG, Barrett-Connor E, Delahanty L, et al. Impact of lifestyle intervention and metformin on health-related quality of life: the diabetes prevention program randomized trial. J Gen Intern Med. 2012;27:1594-601.
8. Ackermann RT, Edelstein SL, Narayan KM, Zhang P, Engelgau MM, Herman WH, et al. Changes in health state utilities with changes in body mass in the Diabetes Prevention Program. Obesity (Silver Spring). 2009;17:2176-81.
9. Au B, Smith KJ, Gariépy G, Schmitz N. C-reactive protein, depressive symptoms, and risk of diabetes: results from the English Longitudinal Study of Ageing (ELSA). J Psychosom Res. 2014;77(3):180-6.
10. Young JJ, Bruno D, Pomara N. A review of the relationship between proinflammatory cytokines and major depressive disorder. J Affect Disord. 2014;169:15-20.
11. Anderson CM, Hogarty GE, Reiss DJ. Family treatment of adult schizophrenic patients: a psycho-educational approach. Schizophr Bull. 1980;6:490-505.
12. Cuijpers P, Munoz RF, Clarke GN, Lewinsohn PM. Psychoeducational treatment and prevention of depression: the "Coping with Depression" course thirty years later. Clin Psychol Rev. 2009;29:449-58.
13. Casañas R, Catalán R, Penadés R, Real J, Valero S, Muñoz MA, et al. Evaluation of the effectiveness of a psychoeducational intervention in treatment-naïve patients with antidepressant medication in primary care: a randomized controlled trial. Sci World J. 2015;2015:718607.
14. Pibernik-Okanović M, Hermanns N, Ajduković D, Kos J, Prašek M, Šekerija M, et al. Does treatment of subsyndromal depression improve depression-related and diabetes-related outcomes? A randomised controlled comparison of psychoeducation, physical exercise and enhanced treatment as usual. Trials. 2015;16:305.
15. Scott J, Colom F, Vieta E. A meta-analysis of relapse rates with adjunctive psychological therapies compared to usual psychiatric treatment for bipolar disorders. Int J Neuropsychopharmacol. 2007;10:123-9.
16. Sin J, Norman I. Psychoeducational interventions for family members of people with schizophrenia: a mixed-method systematic review. J Clin Psychiatry. 2013;74(12):e1145-62.
17. Odenwald M, Semrau P. Reducing dropout among traumatized alcohol patients in detoxification treatment: a pilot intervention study. Eur Addict Res. 2012;18:54-63.
18. Cezaretto A, Siqueira-Catania A, de Barros CR, Salvador EP, Ferreira SR. Benefits on quality of life concomitant to metabolic improvement in intervention program for prevention of diabetes mellitus. Qual Life Res. 2012;21:105-13.
19. de Barros CR, Cezaretto A, Curti ML, Pires MM, Folchetti LD, Siqueira-Catania A, et al. Realistic changes in monounsaturated fatty acids and soluble fibers are able to improve glucose metabolism. Diabetol Metab Syndr. 2014;7;6:136.
20. Craig CL, Marshall AL, Sjöström M, Bauman AE, Booth ML, Ainsworth BE, et al. International physical activity questionnaire: 12-country reliability and validity. Med Sci Sports Exerc. 2003;35:1381-95.
21. Florindo AA, Guimaraes VV, Cesar CL, Barros MB, Alves MC, Goldbaum M. Epidemiology of leisure, transportation, occupational, and household physical activity: prevalence and associated factors. J Phys Act Health. 2009;6:625-32.
22. Nutrition Coordinating Center (NCC) Nutrition data system for research-NDS-R. Minneapolis, University of Minnesota; 2005.
23. Beck AT, Steer RA, and Garbin MG. Psychometric properties of the Beck depression inventory: twenty-five years of evaluation. Clin Psychol Rev. 1988;8:77-100.
24. Ware JE Jr, Gandek B, Kosinski M, Aaronson NK, Apolone G, Brazier J, et al. The equivalence of SF-36 summary health scores estimated using standard and country-specific algorithms in 10 countries: results from the IQOLA Project. International Quality of Life Assessment. J Clin Epidemiol. 1998;51:1167-70.
25. Matthews DR, Hosker JP, Rudenski AS, Naylor BA, Treacher DF, Turner RC. Homeostasis model assessment: insulin resistance and beta-cell function from fasting plasma glucose and insulin concentrations in man. Diabetologia. 1985;28:412-9.
26. Bauml J, Frobose T, Kraemer S, Rentrop M, Pitschel-Walz G. Psychoeducation: a basic psychotherapeutic intervention for patients with schizophrenia and their families. Schizophr Bull. 2006;32 Suppl 1:S1-9.
27. Considine RV, Caro JF. Leptin and the regulation of body weight. Int J Biochem Cell Biol. 1997;29:1255-72.
28. Saffari M, Pakpour AH, Mohammadi-Zeidi I, Samadi M, Chen H. Long-term effect of motivational interviewing on dietary intake and weight loss in Iranian obese/overweight women. Health Promot Perspect. 2014;30;4(2):206-13.

29. Wadden TA, Butryn ML, Hong PS, Tsai AG. Behavioral treatment of obesity in patients encountered in primary care settings: a systematic review. JAMA. 2014;5;312(17):1779-91.
30. West DS, DiLillo V, Bursac Z, Gore SA, Greene PG. Motivational interviewing improves weight loss in women with type 2 diabetes. Diabetes Care. 2007;30:1081-7.
31. Ockene IS, Hayman LL, Pasternak RC, Schron E, Dunbar-Jacob J. Task force #4--adherence issues and behavior changes: achieving a long-term solution. 33rd Bethesda Conference. J Am Coll Cardiol. 2002;40:630-40.
32. Pekkarinen T, Kaukua J, Mustajoki P. Long-term weight maintenance after a 17-week weight loss intervention with or without a one-year maintenance program: a randomized controlled trial. J Obes. 2015;2015:651460.
33. den Boer AT, Herraets IJ, Stegen J, Roumen C, Corpeleijn E, Schaper NC, et al. Prevention of the metabolic syndrome in IGT subjects in a lifestyle intervention: Results from the SLIM study. Nutr Metab Cardiovasc Dis. 2013;23(11):1147-53.
34. Ilanne-Parikka P, Eriksson JG, Lindström J, Peltonen M, Aunola S, Hämäläinen H, et al. Effect of lifestyle intervention on the occurrence of metabolic syndrome and its components in the Finnish Diabetes Prevention Study. Diabetes Care. 2008;31:805-7.
35. Adami PE, Negro A, Lala N, Martelletti P. The role of physical activity in the prevention and treatment of chronic diseases. Clin Ter. 2010;161:537-41.
36. Reimers CD, Knapp G, Reimers AK. Does physical activity increase life expectancy? A review of the literature. J Aging Res. 2012;2012:243958.
37. Almeida-Pititto B, Hirai AT, Sartorelli DS, Harima HA, Gimeno SG, Ferreira SR. Predictive factors of non-deterioration of glucose tolerance following a 2-year behavioral intervention. Diabetol Metab Syndr. 2010;2:52.

The effect of metabolic surgery on type 1 diabetes: meta-analysis

Abdulzahra Hussain[1]

[1] Doncaster and Bassetlaw Teaching Hospitals, DN2 5LT, Doncaster, UK

Correspondence to:
azahrahussain@yahoo.com

ABSTRACT

Objective: Metabolic and bariatric surgery has a definite role in the management of obese patients with type 2 diabetes mellitus (T2DM). There is also evidence of such surgery improving the health of type 1 diabetic (T1DM) patients. The aim of this paper is to explore the effect of metabolic and bariatric surgery on T1DM. Materials and methods: A comprehensive search of PubMed and Google Scholar was performed to identify relevant papers reporting metabolic and bariatric surgery effects on T1DM. A statistical analysis is applied after data synthesis. A forest plot and Pearson correlation are then calculated. Results: Of the 567 papers that were identified, 558 articles did not fulfill the inclusion criteria and were therefore excluded. Nine studies involving 78 patients were selected for this meta-analysis. There was improvement in HBA1c (p value = 0.40), insulin dose (p value = 0.0001) and BMI (p value = 0.00001) after surgery. However, improvement in the HBA1c did not reach statistical significance. There was a weak correlation between postoperative insulin dose and BMI change after surgery (r = -0.177). There was a negligible correlation between HBA1c and BMI change after operations (r = -0.01). Conclusion: Current metabolic/bariatric surgery is improving T1DM in obese and morbidly obese patients. This is not exclusively related to excess weight loss (EWL) as previously thought. Therefore, there is a role for other factors, which are potential players to reproduce the same effect in nonobese T1DM patients. Arch Endocrinol Metab. 2018;62(2):172-8

Keywords

Bariatric surgery; metabolic surgery; type 1 diabetes mellitus; type 2 diabetes mellitus; HBA1c; insulin; body mass index

INTRODUCTION

Gastrointestinal surgery has excellent but variable outcomes on the glycemic control of diabetic patients depending on the type of surgery. The first report of gastrointestinal surgery ameliorating T2DM was reported by Friedman and cols. in 1955 (1), though its effect on T1DM was not recognized until recently when Czupryniak and cols. reported the first observation of T1DM improvement in a severely obese patient who underwent gastric bypass in 2004 (2). Hussain and cols. suggested the potential benefit of bariatric surgery for T1DM in 2009 (3), followed by Czupryniak and cols.'s case studies involving three patients in 2010 (4). Since then, several observational studies have reported changes in insulin requirement, HBA1c and BMI following different types of bariatric/metabolic surgery.

American Diabetic Association (ADA) and National Institute for Health and Care Excellence (NICE) guidelines have restricted the diagnosis of T1DM to situations in which the body does not produce insulin (5) or the destruction of insulin-producing beta cells in the pancreatic islets of Langerhans causes absolute insulin deficiency (6). This clear definition should avoid confusion in reporting insulin-dependent diabetic patients after bariatric/metabolic surgery, which could fall under either T1DM (when there is no insulin production) or T2DM (when insulin is produced but is not a sufficient amount for body requirements, or there is insulin resistance).

The metabolic effect of bariatric/metabolic surgery on T1DM has elicited significant interest because of the already-proven benefits on T2DM and the potential production of similar results for T1DM, which forms 10% of diabetic load (7-10). As there is no insulin production by pancreatic beta cells, the mechanisms of improving T1DM following metabolic/bariatric surgery are expected to be related to body mass index (BMI) change, reduction of insulin resistance, satiety/dietary change and possible neuroendocrine/hormonal or incretins influence. The aim of this paper is to explore current evidence regarding the effect of metabolic surgery on T1DM.

MATERIALS AND METHODS

The protocol of Preferred Reporting Items for Systematic Review and Meta-Analysis (PRISMA) is used

(Figure 1). Inclusion and exclusion criteria: All English literature reporting bariatric and metabolic surgery on T1DM patients (hyperglycemia, C-peptide negative and anti-glutamic acid carboxylase [GAC] antibodies positive) were included. The studies that reported less than three patients were excluded.

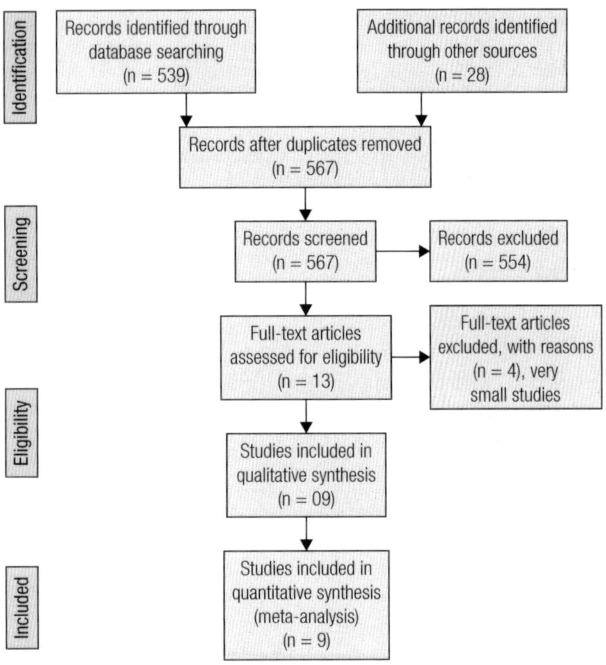

Source: Moher D, Liberati A, Tetzlaff J, Altman DG; The PRISMA Group (2009). Preferred Reporting Items for Systemic Reviews and Meta-Analyses: The PRISMA Statement. PLoS Med. 2009;6(7):e1000097.

Figure 1. Flow diagram.

Quality of the data

An assessment of the studies according to the Newcastle-Ottawa scoring system was performed (Table 1).

The data were reviewed and entered into the fields of Microsoft Excel. The data consisted of the following: sample size, authors, year of publication, HBA1c, insulin dose, BMI before and after the surgery and follow-up duration. All the studies were observational research, and no clinical trials were to have been performed for the studies to be included. Three of them were comparative protocols that included a T2DM arm. Only T1DM data were selected. Some of the studies lacked the calculation of standard deviation (SD), which is an important requirement for conducting the forest plot calculation. The SD of each study was calculated from the number of subjects, the largest and smallest value and the 95% confidence interval of 3.92. Some of the studies were lacking a mean of the specific data. Therefore, a calculation of the mean was performed. The patients' follow-ups varied, even within a single study. Some studies provided follow-up at 6 months, 1 year, 2 years, 3 years, 4 years or 5 years. The included data were taken from the longest follow-up to give more power to the results. Few studies reported insulin dose per kilogram (kg) of body weight/day, while the majority quoted total units/day. It was not possible to know the total units/day for these few studies (Table 2), so the reported unit/kg/day is used for analysis.

Table 1. Newcastle-Ottawa assessment of the quality of data

Studies	Selection	Comparability	Outcome
Blanco and cols. (2014)	****	*	**
Brethauer and cols. (2014)	***		**
Czupryniak and cols. (2010)	***		**
Maraka and cols. (2015)	****	*	**
Middelbeek and cols. (2015)	***		**
Raab and cols. (2013)	***		**
Robert and cols. (2015)	****	*	**
Lannoo and cols. (2014)	****		**
Mendez and cols. (2010)	***		**

Data synthesis

Data synthesis was completed and is shown in Table 2. Further calculation of change in the mean of three variables is depicted in Table 3. The forest plot was performed for HBA1c, Insulin dose and BMI changes after surgery (Figures 2, 3 and 4). Pearson correlation statistics were applied, and the results are shown in Table 4.

Statistical analysis

Review Manager software was used (Review Manager 5.3, version: 5.3.5). A 95% confidence interval (CI) and $p < 0.05$ limit was taken as significant. An odd ratio (OR), variance, standard errors and deviations were applied, and a forest plot for depicting the final results of each parameter was constructed. Different parameters such as age, insulin requirements, HBA1c, BMI and duration of diabetes were included in the final analysis. Further analysis was conducted to show the relations and degree of correlation between these 5 parameters. The correlation tests were performed using Excel (Microsoft 365, 2015) and also R software from the R Foundation for Statistical Computing (http://www.R-project.org). The test of normality was conducted for all data using Jarque-Bera and Anderson-Darling normality tests. The correlation coefficient (r) was calculated using the following equation: *R*

Calculation, $r = \Sigma((X - M_y)(Y - M_x)) / \sqrt{((SS_x)(SS_y))}$. Data synthesis was performed, and statistical analysis was conducted. The SD was lacking in some studies, and it was calculated using $SD = \sqrt{N}x\ (X\text{-}x)/3.92$ and a confidence interval of 95% (http://handbook.cochrane.org).

Table 2. Main data, the standard deviation is calculated using the formula $SD = \sqrt{n}\ x[X\text{-}x)^2/3.92$, n = number of subjects, X = upper limit value, x = lower limit, 3.92 = 95% confidence interval, CI. The values in the table represent the mean of the data plus SD when available. For insulin requirements, some data depicted as IU/kg/day rather than total unit/day

	Year	Age (mean) years	No of subjects	HBA1c before/after surgery	Insulin requirements before/after surgery IU/day (u/k/day)	BMI kg/m² before/ after surgery	Duration of T1DM in years	Follow up (month = m)
Czupryniak and cols.	2010	22 ± 6	3	10.13 ± 1.32/ 09.00 ± 0.73	94 ± 6.3/ 47.6 ± 6.42	42.2 ± 2.39/ 33.5 ± 2.65	11.60	5-8 years
Raab and cols.	2013	43	6	8.18 ± 2.17/ 6.95 ± 1.4	104.16 ± 11.59/ 36.75 ± 7.72	41.75 ± 5.89/ 27.82 ± 2.37	17.16	1 year
Robert and cols.	2015	39.2 ± 5.3	10	7.5 ± 1.9/ 7.1 ± 0.9	1.09 ± 0.7/ 0.44 ± 0.24	46.9 ± 6.3/ 30.34 ± 6.3	23.1 ± 11.8	4.5 years
Maraka and cols.	2015	50.6 ± 8.9	7	8.2 ±1.6/ 7.8 ±0.9	75.15 ± 6.4/ 55.45 ± 5.17	44.3 ± 8.0/ 31.2±9.9	20.6±11.4	2 years
Blanco and cols.	2014	38.2 ± 13.3	7	8.3 ± 1.2- 8.2 ± 0.9	0.61 ± 0.17/ 0.62 ± 0.12	39.4 ± 2.2/ 27.3 ± 2.2	27.3 ± 2.2	2 years
Middelbeek and cols.	2015	39.6 ± 8.4	10	8.1 ± 1.3/ 9.8 ± 1.9	53.0 ± 29.7/ 31.1 ± 22.8	43.5 ± 7.5/ 33.8 ± 7.5	24.6 ± 10.1	5 years
Brethauer and cols.	2014	45.6 ± 10.9	10	10 ± 1.6/ 8.9 ± 1.1	0.74 ± 0.32/ 0.40 ± 0	41.6 ± 3.9/ 30.5 ± 5.9	22	36.8 ± 32.3 (m)
Lannoo and cols.	2014	40.3 ± 8.5	22	8.4 ± 2.34/ 8.2 ± 2.11	92.5 ± 13.81/ 48.0 ± 11.36	39.7 ± 5.34/ 31.4 ± 2.86	25.3 ± 8.9	14.3 ± 10.1/ 37.8 ± 29.7
Mendez and cols.	2010	42.3	3	7.96 ± 0.67/ 8.03 ± 0.99	99.23 ± 9.36/ 42.9 ± 3.10	45.9 ± 3.11/ 29.4 ± 1.77	25	1 year

Table 3. Mean change in 3 variables BMI, HBA1c and insulin requirement, mean duration of T1DM (years) and age (years) are fixed

HBA1c	Insulin requirement	Duration of T1DM	BMI	AGE
1.13	46.40	11.60	08.70	22.0
1.23	67.41	17.16	13.95	43.0
0.40	00.65	23.10	16.56	39.2
0.40	19.70	20.60	13.10	50.6
0.10	00.01	27.30	12.10	38.2
-1.70	21.90	24.60	09.70	39.6
0.10	00.34	22.00	11.10	45.6
1.10	56.33	25.30	08.30	40.3
-0.07	44.50	25.00	16.50	42.3

Study or Subgroup	Post surgery Mean	Post surgery SD	Post surgery Total	Before surgery Mean	Before surgery SD	Before surgery Total	Weight	Std. Mean Difference IV, Random, 95% CI
Blanco et al 2014	8.2	0.9	7	8.3	1.2	7	9.9%	-0.09 [-1.14, 0.96]
Brethauer et al 2014	8.9	1.1	10	10	1.6	10	12.6%	-0.77 [-1.68, 0.15]
Czupryniak et al 2010	9	0.73	3	10.13	1.32	3	3.6%	-0.85 [-2.64, 0.95]
Lannoo et al 2014	8.2	2.11	22	8.4	2.34	22	26.0%	-0.09 [-0.68, 0.50]
Maraka et al 2015	7.8	0.9	7	8.2	1.6	7	9.8%	-0.29 [-1.34, 0.77]
Mendez et al 2010	8.03	0.99	3	7.96	0.67	3	4.5%	0.07 [-1.54, 1.67]
Middelbeek et al 2015	9.8	1.9	10	8.1	1.3	10	12.0%	1.00 [0.06, 1.94]
Raab et al 2013	6.95	1.4	6	8.18	2.17	6	8.1%	-0.62 [-1.79, 0.55]
Robert et al 2015	7.1	0.9	10	7.5	1.9	10	13.5%	-0.26 [-1.14, 0.62]
Total (95% CI)			**78**			**78**	**100.0%**	**-0.15 [-0.50, 0.20]**

Heterogeneity: $Tau^2 = 0.03$; $Chi^2 = 8.92$, df = 8 (P = 0.35); $I^2 = 10\%$
Test for overall effect: Z = 0.84 (P = 0.40)

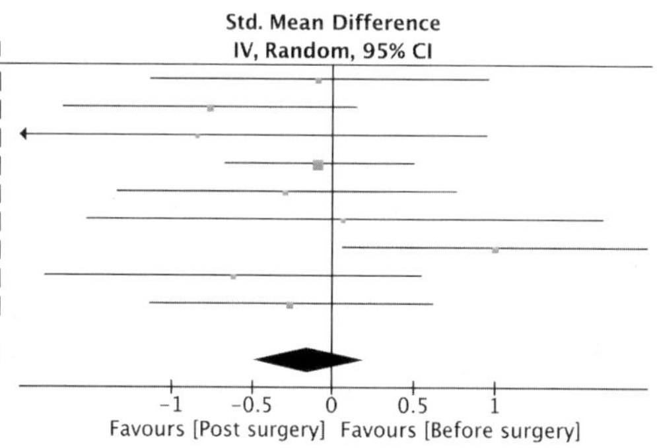

Figure 2. Forest plot, HBA1c.

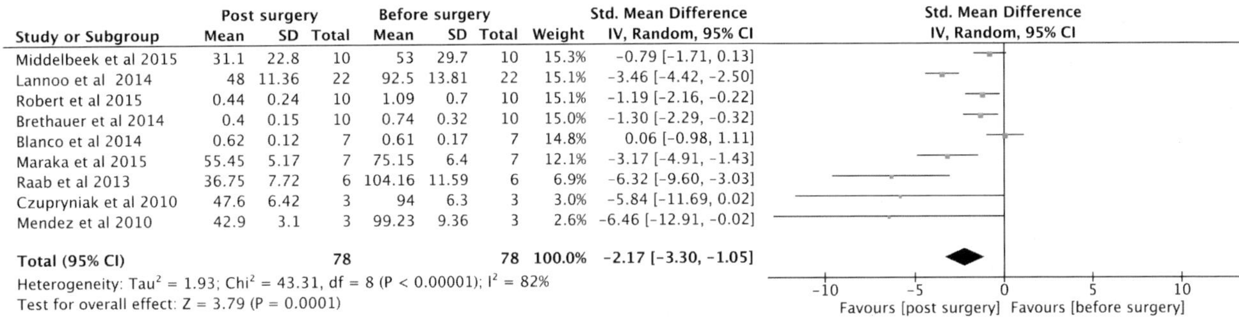

Figure 3. Forest plot, insulin.

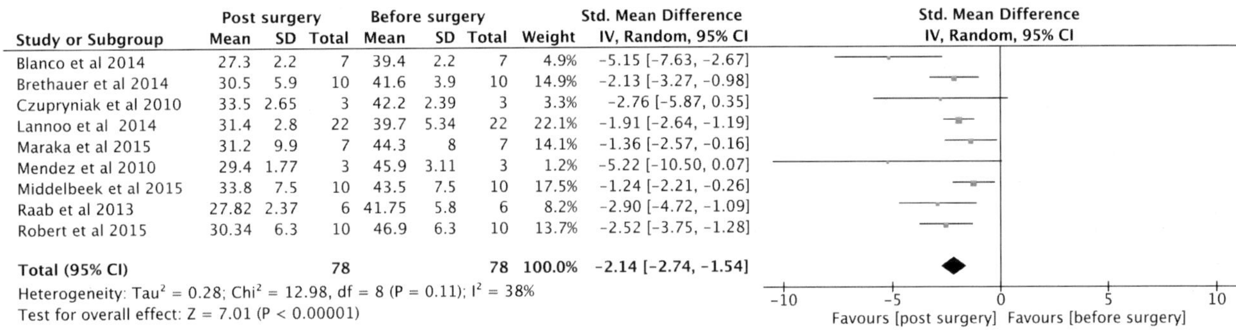

Figure 4. Forest plot, body mass index change after surgery.

Table 4. Pearson correlation for 2 constant (age and duration of T1DM) and 3 variable post operative parameters (insulin requirements, HBA1c change and BMI change) combination. Significant moderate correlation between any two parameters is depicted in grey color (0.-0.39 = weak, 0.4-0.59 moderate, 0.6-0.79 = strong, 0.8-1.0 = very strong, Evans guide 1996)

	Age	Duration of T1DM	Insulin requirement	HBA1c	BMI change after surgery
Age	-----	0.509	-0.208	-0.220	0.405
Duration of T1DM	0.509	------	-0.418	-0.513	0.204
Insulin requirement	-0.208	-0.418	------	0.475	-0.177
HBA1c	-0.210	-0.513	0.475	-----	-0.010
BMI	0.405	0.204	-0.177	-0.010	------

RESULTS

Type of bariatric/metabolic procedure

The included patients underwent laparoscopic adjustable gastric band (LAGB), 2 patients (2.5%); vertical sleeve gastrectomy (VSG), 11 patients (14%); laparoscopic Roux-en Y gastric bypass (LRYGB), 52 patients (67%); bilio-pancreatic diversion (BPD) 7 patients (9%); or bilio-pancreatic diversion plus duodenal switch (BPD-DS), 3 patients (3.8%). Except gastric bypass, all other operations included a small number of patients who fell short in terms of providing statistical power, and no subgroup analysis was conducted. Therefore, the outcomes were those of the 5 procedures.

HBA1c

HBA1c showed improvement after surgery; however, this improvement did not reach statistical significance, as the p value was 0.40 (Figure 2). HBA1c was moderately correlated with the duration of T1DM (r = -0.513) and insulin requirement (r = 0.475). HBA1c showed little or no correlation with BMI (r = 0.01) but a stronger correlation with age (r = -022).

Insulin requirement

Insulin requirement was significantly reduced after surgery, with p value = 0.00001 (Figure 3). It was moderately correlated with HBA1c, as expected (r = 0.475), and with duration of T1DM (r = -0.418). More importantly, it was weakly correlated with BMI change after surgery (r = -.0177) and also with age (r = -0.208) (Figures 2 and 4).

Duration of the diabetes

The mean duration of T1DM was 9.6 to 34.9 years, and it was correlated with age (r = 0.509). Duration of T1DM was moderately correlated with post-surgery insulin requirements and HBA1c and weakly correlated with BMI (r = -0.418, -0.513, 0.204, respectively) (Table 4).

Excess weight loss

All studies showed an acceptable amount of weight loss ranging from 8.3 to 16.56 kilograms/m^2. BMI change after surgery was weakly correlated with duration of diabetes, HBA1c and insulin requirement; however, it had significant correlation with age (r = 0.405) (Table 4).

Age group

The age group ranged from 16-65 years with mean of 40.16 years. There was a weak negative correlation with postoperative insulin dose and HBA1c (r = -0.205, -0.21, respectively). Age group was moderately correlated with duration of T1DM and BMI (r = 0.509, 0.405, respectively).

DISCUSSION

HBA1c and postoperative insulin dose are important parameters to assess glycemic control in T1DM patients following metabolic surgery. All but 2 studies (Middelbeek and cols. 2015 and Mendez and cols. 2010) showed a variable degree of improvement in HBA1c, although it did not reach statistical significance (4,11-18) (Figure 2). However, the insulin dose is significantly reduced following surgery, and it is moderately correlated with duration of T1DM and HBA1c level. This meta-analysis showed a weak correlation among postoperative HBA1c, insulin requirement and postoperative BMI loss. Therefore, the improvement in the HBA1c and insulin dose shortly after surgery is not entirely related to weight loss. The largest study of Lannoo and cols. (11) concluded that the insulin-sparing effect is probably related to insulin sensitivity following weight loss. However, according to this meta-analysis, the insulin-sparing effect is only weakly correlated with weight loss. We have to look beyond the anatomical configurations and physical effects of these procedures and explore the complex metabolic pathway of glucose homeostasis.

Incretins play a role in glucose regulation by reducing glucagon and food intake and increasing satiety (19). A recent review study highlighted the established roles of gut hormones in regard to diabetes (20). Metabolic and bariatric surgery may possibly produce insulin dose reduction and improve HBA1c through an incretins-related mechanism, but this does not exclude other potential factors that control glucose metabolism (21). The change in the nutrient flux could affect the balance of gut hormones (including hypothetical anti-incretins), and the change in hormone milieu might be responsible for changes in insulin sensitivity (22).

In their study, Kempf and cols. showed a rapid decrease of insulin requirement and an improvement in HBA1c in T2DM as a result of meal modification even before substantial weight loss occurred (23). Glycogenolysis, gluconeogenesis, carbohydrate intake and the modified response of the metabolism to post-metabolic/bariatric surgery in regard to anatomical, neuroendocrine and satiety changes are the primary cofactors for net glucose production. The interaction of these complex mechanisms produces the final blood glucose level, whether it is normal, hypoglycemic or hyperglycemic.

Following procedures such as gastric bypass, some T2DM patients develop hypoglycemia. The incidence of symptomatic hypoglycemia is less than 1% (24). However, asymptomatic post-bariatric/metabolic surgery hypoglycemia could reach 30% (25). In these patients, we possibly overdoing metabolic correction. On the other hand, in T1DM, the beta-cell influence on glucose homeostasis is absent, and therefore the entire set of regulatory mechanisms consists of the complex interactions among the gastrointestinal tract (GIT), liver, brain, adipose tissue, blood cells, muscles and kidneys. This results in the regulation of glucose entry into the circulation being influenced by additional factors such as hormones, the sympathetic nervous system and substrates (i.e., free fatty acid concentrations and availability of gluconeogenic precursors) (26).

The question regarding how to adjust the anatomical change of the gastrointestinal tract as a result of metabolic surgery and the inherent complex interactions among these systems to optimize the glucose level in T1DM is very difficult based on the current level of knowledge surrounding metabolic/bariatric surgery. Every single centimeter of the GIT is a complex unit, and any change caused by metabolic and bariatric surgery will result in a comparative impact to the glucose homeostasis. Such changes will never result in total glycemic control, and the patient will still need an insulin replacement, regardless of the preoperative insulin dose. Currently, we do not entirely know what each part of the GIT produces (except some factors such as incretins, PYY hormones and ghrelins), and we are still a far way from being in a position to perfect metabolic/bariatric surgery to produce the maximum benefit for T1DM patients. The interaction between diet and GIT has been a very important focus of interest. A very low calorie diet (VLCD) was found to produce similar effects to gastric bypass in terms of insulin sensitivity and beta-cell function improvement in T2DM (27). As diabetes is a spectrum of disease, the same effect could therefore be produced in T1DM. To date, no study has examined the potential effect of VLCD on T1DM. Bile acids are recognized effectors on the regulation of glucose and lipid metabolism through the FXR and TGR5 receptors (28). There is evidence that the alteration of bile acids following bariatric surgery improves insulin responsiveness and lowers fasting glucose in animal models (29). A similar effect may be reproduced in humans, and it may be a mechanism through which to explain the effect of metabolic surgery on diabetic patients.

There is no direct link between gut microbiota and improvement in glucose homeostasis following bariatric surgery. Gut microbiota does, however, have a direct effect on weight. An interesting study showed that transferring microbiota from an obese subject to a lean subject resulted in weight gain (30). The hepatocytes orchestrate the regulatory mechanisms of bile acids, microbiota and metabolome to affect glucose and lipid metabolism (31). Future research may prove the existence of a link between microbiota and beta-cell function.

Limitations of the study

This meta-analysis included 9 studies with some degree of heterogeneity that ranged from 10-82%. The studies are relatively small, with the largest reporting 22 patients. The patient follow-ups are different, as some studies reported 1 year, whereas others reported up to 5 years. The outcomes, especially HBA1c, may be creeping up with longer follow-up, as shown by Middelbeek and cols.'s 2015 study (12), and the current conclusion regarding HBA1c is represented by the mean follow-ups in these studies. Some studies included women only (like Middlbeek and cols. 2015), whereas others reported women as the majority. This would raise a question regarding the actual representation of the obese T1DM population; nevertheless, the studies are shedding a light on such patients who require extra help with glycemic control after having exhausted current nonsurgical methods.

CONCLUSION

Current metabolic/bariatric surgery is reducing postoperative insulin requirement and marginally improving HBA1c in obese and morbidly obese type 1 diabetic patients. This is not exclusively related to the EWL as previously thought. Therefore, there is a role for other factors, which are potential players to reproduce the same effect in nonobese T1DM patients. Further long-term studies are required to assess the real benefit of metabolic surgery for T1DM patients.

Acknowledgments: none.

REFERENCES

1. Friedman MN, Sancetta AJ, Magovern GJ. The amelioration of diabetes mellitus following subtotal gastrectomy. Surg Gynecol Obstet. 1955;100(2):201-4.
2. Czupryniak L, Strzelczyk J, Cypryk K, Pawlowski M, Szymanski D, Lewinski A, et al. Gastric bypass surgery in severely obese type 1 diabetic patients. Diabetes Care. 2004;27(10):2561-2.
3. Hussain A, Mahmood H, El-Hasani S. Can Roux-en-Y gastric bypass provide a lifelong solution for diabetes mellitus? Can J Surg. 2009;52(6):E269-75.
4. Czupryniak L, Wiszniewski M, Szymański D, Pawłowski M, Loba J, Strzelczyk J. Long-term results of gastric bypass surgery in morbidly obese type 1 diabetes patients. Obes Surg. 2010;20(4):506-8.
5. American Diabetic Association ADA. Available from: http://www.diabetes.org. Access on: Oct. 2, 2015.
6. National Institute for Health and Care Excellence (NICE). Available from: http://cks.nice.org.uk. Access on: Oct. 2, 2015.
7. Sieber P, Gass M2 Kern B, Peters T, Slawik M, Peterli R. Five-year results of laparoscopic sleeve gastrectomy. Surg Obes Relat Dis. 2014;10(2):243-9.
8. Brethauer SA, Aminian A, Romero-Talamás H, Batayyah E, Mackey J, Kennedy L, et al. Can diabetes be surgically cured? Long-term metabolic effects of bariatric surgery in obese patients with type 2 diabetes mellitus. Ann Surg. 2013 Oct;258(4):628-36.
9. Keating C, Neovius M, Sjöholm K, Peltonen M, Narbro K, Eriksson JK, et al. Health-care costs over 15 years after bariatric surgery for patients with different baseline glucose status: results from the Swedish Obese Subjects study. Lancet Diabetes Endocrinol. 2015;3(11):855-65

10. Sjöström L, Peltonen M, Jacobson P, Ahlin S, Andersson-Assarsson J, Anveden Å, et al. Association of bariatric surgery with long-term remission of type 2 diabetes and with microvascular and macrovascular complications. JAMA. 2014;311(22):2297-304.
11. Lannoo M, Dillemans B, Van Nieuwenhove Y, Fieuws S, Mathieu C, Gillard P, et al. Bariatric surgery induces weight loss but does not improve glycemic control in patients with type 1 diabetes. Diabetes Care. 2014;37(8):e173-4.
12. Middelbeek RJ, James-Todd T, Cavallerano JD, Schlossman DK, Patti ME, Brown FM. Gastric Bypass Surgery in Severely Obese Women With Type 1 Diabetes: Anthropometric and Cardiometabolic Effects at 1 and 5 Years Postsurgery. Diabetes Care. 2015;38(7):e104-5.
13. Mendez CE, Tanenberg RJ, Pories W.. Outcomes of Roux-en-Y gastric bypass surgery for severely obese patients with type 1 diabetes: a case series report. Diabetes Metab Syndr Obes. 2010;3:281-3.
14. Robert M, Belanger P, Hould FS, Marceau S, Tchernof A, Biertho L. Should metabolic surgery be offered in morbidly obese patients with type I diabetes? Surg Obes Relat Dis. 2015;11(4):798-805.
15. Raab H, Weiner RA, Frenken M, Rett K, Weiner S. Obesity and metabolic surgery in type 1 diabetes mellitus. Nutr Hosp. 2013 Mar;28 Suppl 2:31-4.
16. Maraka S, Kudva YC, Kellogg TA, Collazo-Clavell ML, Mundi MS. Bariatric surgery and diabetes: Implications of type 1 versus insulin-requiring type 2. Obesity (Silver Spring). 2015;23(3):552-7.
17. Blanco J, Jiménez A, Casamitjana R, Flores L, Lacy A, Conget I, et al. Relevance of beta-cell function for improved glycemic control after gastric bypass surgery. Surg Obes Relat Dis. 2014 ;10:9-13.
18. Brethauer SA, Aminian A, Rosenthal RJ, Kirwan JP, Kashyap SR, Schauer PR. Bariatric surgery improves the metabolic profile of morbidly obese patients with type 1 diabetes. Diabetes Care. 2014;37(3):e51-2.
19. Kim W, Egan JM. The role of incretins in glucose homeostasis and diabetes treatment. Pharmacol Rev. 2008;60(4):470-512.
20. Singh AK, Singh R, Kota SK. Bariatric surgery and diabetes remission: Who would have thought it? Indian J Endocrinol Metab. 2015;19(5):563-76.
21. Middelbeek RJ, James-Todd T, Patti ME, Brown FM. Short-term insulin requirements following gastric bypass surgery in severely obese women with type 1 diabetes. Obes Surg. 2014;24(9):1442-6.
22. Rubino F, R'bibo SL, del Genio F, Mazumdar M, McGraw TE. Metabolic surgery: the role of the gastrointestinal tract in diabetes mellitus. Nat Rev Endocrinol. 2010;6(2):102-9.
23. Kempf K, Schloot NC, Gärtner B, Keil R, Schadewaldt P, Martin S. Meal replacement reduces insulin requirement, HbA1c and weight long-term in type 2 diabetes patients with >100 U insulin per day. J Hum Nutr Diet. 2014;27 Suppl 2:21-7.
24. Foster-Schubert KE. Hypoglycemia complicating bariatric surgery: incidence and mechanisms. Curr Opin Endocrinol Diabetes Obes. 2011;18(2):129-33.
25. Goldfine AB, Mun EC, Devine E, Bernier R, Baz-Hecht M, Jones DB, et al. Patients with neuroglycopenia after gastric bypass surgery have exaggerated incretin and insulin secretory responses to a mixed meal. J Clin Endocrinol Metab. 2007;92(12):4678-85.
26. Shrayyef MZ, Gerich JE. Normal Glucose Homeostasis. Principles of Diabetes Mellitus. 2010; p. 19-35.
27. Jackness C, Karmally W, Febres G, Conwell IM, Ahmed L, Bessler M, et al. Very low-calorie diet mimics the early beneficial effect of Roux-en-Y gastric bypass on insulin sensitivity and □-cell Function in type 2 diabetic patients. Diabetes. 2013;62(9):3027-32.
28. Albaugh VL, Flynn CR, Tamboli RA, Abumrad NN. Recent advances in metabolic and bariatric surgery. F1000Res. 2016 May 24;5. pii: F1000 Faculty Rev-978.
29. Goncalves D, Barataud A, De Vadder F, Vinera J, Zitoun C, Duchampt A, et al. Bile Routing Modification Reproduces Key Features of Gastric Bypass in Rat. Ann Surg. 2015;262(6):1006-15.
30. Bäckhed F, Ding H, Wang T, Hooper LV, Koh GY, Nagy A, et al. The gut microbiota as an environmental factor that regulates fat storage. Proc Natl Acad Sci U S A. 2004;101(44):15718-23.
31. Duparc T, Plovier H, Marrachelli VG, Van Hul M, Essaghir A, Ståhlman M, et al. Hepatocyte MyD88 affects bile acids, gut microbiota and metabolome contributing to regulate glucose and lipid metabolism. Gut. 2017;66(4):620-32.

Is there an association between thyroid function abnormalities and breast cancer?

Anna Angelousi[1], Evanthia Diamanti-Kandarakis[2], Evangelia Zapanti[3], Afroditi Nonni[4], Eftuxios Ktenas[5], Aimilia Mantzou[6], Konstantinos Kontzoglou[7], Grigorios Kouraklis[8]

[1] Department of Internal Medicine, Laiko General Hospital, National and Kapodistrian University of Athens, Greece
[2] Department of Internal Medicine, Medical School, National and Kapodistrian University of Athens, Greece
[3] Department of Endocrinology and Diabetes, Alexandra Hospital, Athens, Greece
[4] Department of Pathology, Medical School, Laiko Hospital, National and Kapodistrian University of Athens, Greece
[5] National School of Public health, National and Kapodistrian University of Athens, Greece
[6] Endocrinology laboratory of Evgenidion hospital, Athens, Greece
[7] Department of Propaedeutic Surgery, Laiko General Hospital, University of Athens Medical School, Greece
[8] Department of Propaedeutic Surgery, Laiko General Hospital, University of Athens Medical School, Greece

Correspondence to:
Anna Angelousi
Andromachis 6 Street, 12135
Peristeri, Athens, Greece
a.angelousi@gmail.com

ABSTRACT

Objective: The aim of this study was to evaluate the association between thyroid function abnormalities and breast cancer and, in particular, the prognostic markers of breast cancer.. **Subjects and methods:** Baseline levels of thyrotropin, free triiodothyronine, free thyroxine and thyroid autoantibodies were measured in 97 women with primary breast cancer, 27 women with benign breast disease, and 4 women with atypical ductal hyperplasia. Their baseline levels were compared with those in 48 healthy women with a normal mammography in the last 2 years. **Results:** There were no significant associations between history of thyroid disease and breast cancer (p = 0.33). The mean baseline levels of triiodothyronine and thyrotropin did not differ significantly between the compared groups. The mean baseline levels of free thyroxine were found to be significantly higher in the breast cancer group, even after adjusting for thyroid replacement therapy. The presence of thyroid antibodies did not differ significantly between the compared groups. In a subgroup analysis, breast cancer cases with thyroid disease and particularly hypothyroidism had a significantly lower incidence of lymph node metastases compared with breast cancer cases without thyroid disease. **Conclusions:** Our data confirmed the proliferative effect of thyroid hormones on breast cells, which had previously been shown *in vitro*. Additionally, thyroid disease and particularly hypothyroid function appeared to be associated with a lower incidence of lymph node metastases. Further studies to determine the prognostic role of thyroid hormones in breast cancer are warranted. Arch Endocrinol Metab. 2017;61(1):54-61

Keywords
Breast cancer; hypothyroidism; hyperthyroidism; thyroid antibodies

INTRODUCTION

Thyroid hormones are involved in regulating mammalian development, cellular differentiation and metabolism (1). High affinity binding sites for 3-3-5 triiodothyronine (T3) have been identified in nuclei isolated from human tumors, including those in breast cancer (BC), suggesting that thyroid hormones may play a role in the development of BC at the cellular level (2).

Recent studies in human breast cancer cells lines (MCF-7 and MDA-MB-231) have shown proliferative effects of thyroid hormones on breast tissue through the same signal cascade utilized by estrogens involving phosphoinositol 3-kinase (PI3K) and the mitogen-activated protein kinase (MAPK) (3). In estrogen receptor positive (ER+) cell lines (MCF-7), T3 mimics estradiol via its binding to ER and induces the expression of progesterone receptor (PR) and growth factor-alpha (TGF-α) mRNAs (3). In other human cell lines, T3 has been shown to have a mitogenic effect by increasing the expression of the epithelial growth factor receptor (EGF-r) gene (4). In mammary cells, T3 can also activate the estrogen response element (ERE) (5), which is necessary for gene transcription and cell proliferation. Similarly, thyroxine (T4), much like estradiol, can activate the MAPK pathway and thus promote cell proliferation (6). Additionally, thyroid stimulating hormone (TSH) has been shown to have a direct effect on mammary cells. Recently, TSH receptors have been identified in BC tissue with the use of RT-PCR and were correlated to a lower grade of BC (7).

The potential correlation between thyroid disease and BC was based on the existence of common pathophysiological mechanisms in both glands. Thyroid hyperoxidase (TPO) and lactoperoxidase are immunologically similar enzymes that have been identified in both thyroid and breast tissue (8,9). Sodium-iodide symporter (NIS) (10) is an intrinsic plasma membrane glucoprotein of thyroid follicular cells that is also expressed physiologically in lactating breast tissue (11) as well as in BC in some cases (12,13). Despite this pre-clinical evidence, there is a lack of robust clinical evidence on the association between BC and thyroid function abnormalities. The aim of this single-center case control study was to evaluate the association between thyroid function abnormalities and BC and, in particular, the prognostic markers of BC.

SUBJECTS AND METHODS

Patient characteristics

One hundred thirty-three women with mammographic abnormalities were evaluated in the 2nd Surgical Department of the University of Athens (Greece) between June 2010 and March 2014; the women were evaluated before receiving any surgery or medical treatment (chemo and/or radiotherapy). All patients underwent fine needle aspiration of suspicious lesions followed by surgery. Three patients were excluded because of recurrence of known BC, and 2 patients were excluded because of a histological diagnosis of melanoma and sarcoma.

Our cohort consisted of 97 cases of primary BC, 27 cases of benign breast disease (BBD), primarily fibroadenomas and fibrocystic disease, and 4 cases of atypical ductal hyperplasia. Seventy-eight of the 97 cases with BC were diagnosed with ductal breast cancer; 75 cases (77.3%) were invasive ductal breast cancer, 3 (3.1%) were ductal *in situ* cancer (DCIS), and 19 (19.6%) were lobular infiltrating breast cancer. BC tumors were classified according to the Nottingham grading system and the American Joint Committee on Cancer stages. Fifty-nine (61%) of the 97 BC cases were grade I, 28 cases (29%) were grade II, and 10 cases (10%) were grade III. Three (3%) cases had stage 0 tumors (*in situ*), 44 (45.4%) had stage I, 29 (30%) had stage II, and 21 (21.6%) had stage III tumors. Seventy-five cases (77.6%) with primary BC showed positive ER and PR.

The control group consisted of 48 non-hospitalized healthy women who were recruited from the family members of the patients in the geriatric clinic of our hospital. All women were from the same geographical area as the cases, and they were required to have had a normal mammogram within the past 2 years.

Women (cases and controls) with a personal history of a previous cancer were excluded from the study. History of thyroid disease was retrieved from the patient's medical records and/or patient history.

Written informed consent was obtained for each patient and control. The protocol of the study was reviewed and approved by the scientific board of the institutional research committee (Laiko hospital, University of Athens) and was in accordance with the international ethical standards (Declaration of Helsinki).

Laboratory measurements

Thyroid function tests were performed before surgery or treatment for breast cancer. TSH (normal range: 0.3-4.0 mU/L) was measured with the double enzyme radioimmunoassay (RIA) 'sandwich' method (TSH-DiaSorin – CTK-3 Kit, Italy). Free thyroxine (fT4) (normal range: 10-25 pmol/L) and free triiodothyronine (fT3) (normal range: 2.3-5.3 pg/mL) were measured in serum using the double enzyme radioimmunoassay 'sandwich' method (ThermoScientific kit, USA). Autoantibodies against thyroglobulin (Tg-Abs) (positivity > 10 mU/L) and thyroid peroxidase (TPO-Abs) (positivity > 50 mU/L) were measured with RIA (ThermoScientific kit, USA). All TSH, fT3, fT4, TPO-Abs and Tg-Abs measurements were performed in the biochemical laboratory of the 'Laiko' hospital in Athens, Greece. The TSH receptor antibodies (TRAK) (positivity > 2 U/L) were measured with the receptor radioassay (RRA) method (Thermo Fisher-BRAHMS 101.5 kit, Germany) in the endocrinology laboratory of Evgenidion hospital in Athens, Greece.

Immunohistochemistry

ER and PR expression were immunohistochemically detected with the commercially available ER (clone EP1) and PR antibodies (clone PgR636) (DAKO), according to ASCO recommendations (14).

Statistical analysis

Continuous variables were initially evaluated with the Kolmogorov-Smirnov test. Variables with a normal distribution were evaluated using ANOVA. Variables without a normal distribution (values of fT3, fT4, TSH, TPO-Abs, Tg-Abs, and TRAK) were analyzed using the Kruskall-Wallis test. The categorical parameters were evaluated with Chi-Square test. The results were considered significant at $p < 0.05$ (95% CI). Cases with atypical ductal hyperplasia (n = 4) were excluded from the statistical analysis because of their small sample size. Statistical analyses were performed using SPSS software (version 20).

RESULTS

The clinical and epidemiological characteristics of the participants are summarized in Table 1. The 3 groups (controls, BC cases and BBD cases) differed significantly in mean age, age of menarche, menopausal status and alcohol use.

Table 1. Epidemiological characteristics of the studied population

Groups/Epidemiological data	Controls	BC	BBD	Atypical hyperplasia	Statistical significance (p)
Total number	48	97	27	4	
Age (mean ± SD)	54.27 ± 12.84	64.02 ± 14.11	52.07 ± 16.93	60.31 ± 13.86	p < 0.05[1]
BMI (kg/m²)	27.02 ± 7.53	28.00 ± 7.09	25.60 ± 5.30	27.42 ± 0.00	p = 0.226[1]
Age of menarche (mean ± SD)	13.43 ± 1.55	11.85 ± 3.07	12.26 ± 3.09	12.39 ± 2.75	p = 0.002[1]
Menopausal status					
Premenopausal (%)	17/48 (35%)	18/90 (20%)	13/24 (54%)	2/4	p = 0.044[1] (between pre and post-menopausal)
Postmenopausal (%)	30/48 (62.5%)	68/90 (76%)	10/24 (42%)	2/4	
Perimenopausal (%)	1/48 (2%)	4/90 (4%)	1/24 (4%)	0	
History of pregnancy					
Yes (%)	37/48 (78%)	80/91 (88%)	17/24 (71%)	¾	p = 0.44[1]
No (%)	11/48 (22%)	11/91 (12%)	7/24 (29%)	¼	
Parity					
1-2	34/37 (92%)	65/78 (83%)	10/17 (65%)		
> 3	3/37 (8%)	15/78 (17%)	4/17 (35%)		
Age of 1st birth					
< 20	6	8	4	0	
21-30	11	25	6	0	p = 0.46[1]
> 31	10	21	2	0	
Use of contraceptives					
Yes (%)	4/39 (10%)	8/79 (10%)	5/16 (31%)	0/2	p = 0.11[1]
No (%)	35/39 (90%)	71/79 (90%)	11/16 (69%)	2/2	
Smoking					
Yes (%)	12/48 (25%)	22/88 (25%)	6/25 (24%)	¼	p = 1.0[1]
No (%)	36/48 (75%)	66/88 (75%)	19/25 (76%)	¾	
Alcohol					
Yes (%)	1/48 (2%)	5/83 (6%)	5/24 (21%)	0/4	p = 0.025[1]
No (%)	47/48 (98%)	78/83 (94%)	19/24 (79%)	4/4	
1st degree family history of BC					
Yes	7/48 (15%)	14/93 (15%)	4/24 (16.6)	¼	p = 0.95[1]
No	41/48 (85%)	79/93 (85%)	20/24 (83.3)	¾	

[1] Statistical significance after comparison of controls, BC and BBD group (atypical hyperplasia group was excluding).

BC: breast cancer; BBD: breast benign disease; SD: standard deviation; BMI: body mass index.

Association between history of thyroid disease and histopathological parameters of breast tissue

The overall frequency of self-reported thyroid disease was 32 of 97 (33%) BC cases, 8 of 27 (29.6%) BBD cases, 3 of 4 (75%) patients in the atypical ductal hyperplasia group and 22 of 48 (45.8%) controls. History of thyroid disease did not significantly differ between the compared groups ($p = 0.33$) (Table 2). Autoimmune thyroid disease (Hashimoto's) and goiter were the most frequent thyroid diseases in the studied groups. Hashimoto's disease was more frequent in the controls than in the BC cases, whereas goiter was more frequent in BC cases than in controls; however, a statistical analysis was not possible because of the small sample size.

Twenty-one of the 97 patients in the BC group (22%), 7 of 27 in the BBD group (26%) and 7 of 47 (15%) in the control group reported levothyroxine treatment at the time of screening. The statistical analysis found no significant differences concerning levothyroxine treatment between the compared groups ($p = 0.79$). Three cases reported use of antithyroid drugs in the past, and one case reported treatment with iodide (I^{131}).

Association between thyroid function tests and histopathological parameters of breast tissue

The mean baseline values of TSH were 2.37 ± 2.3, 2.07 ± 1.04, 1.88 ± 1.07 and 2.05 ± 1.6 mU/L in the BC, BBD, atypical ductal hyperplasia and controls groups, respectively. Abnormally high levels of TSH (> 4.0 mU/L) were recorded in 15.3% of the BC cases and in 5% of the BBD cases. None of the controls had abnormally high levels of TSH. Abnormally low levels of TSH (< 0.3 mU/L) were recorded in 2.6% of the BC cases and in 2% of the controls. None of the BBD patients had abnormally low levels of TSH. No significant association was found between the mean levels of TSH ($p = 0.757$) of the compared groups, although BC cases showed slightly higher mean levels of TSH than the other groups (Table 3).

Table 2. Frequency of thyroid disorders and thyroid treatment in controls, BC and BBD cases

Groups/Frequency of thyroid disorder and treatment	Controls	BC	BBD	Atypical hyperplasia	Statistical significance (p)
History of thyroid disorders					
Yes (%)	22/48 (46%)	32/97 (33%)	8/27 (30%)	3/4	p = 0.33[1]
No (%)	26/48 (54%)	62/97 (64%)	17/27 (63%)	1/4	
No data	0	3/97 (3%)	2/27 (7%)	0	
Type of thyroid disorder					
Hashimoto (%)	7/22 (32%)	9/32 (28%)	3/8 (37.5%)	0	nd[2]
Primary hypothyroidism (other causes) (%)	0	4/32 (12.5%)	0	2	
Hyperthyroidism (%)	4/22 (18%)	4/32 (13%)	0	0	
Goiter (%)	2/22 (9%)	9/32 (28%)	5/8 (62.5%)	1	
Nodules (%)	9/22 (40%)	5/32 (16%)	0	0	
No data	0	1/32 (3%)	0	0	
Treatment					
Yes (substitution, antithyroid drugs)	7/47 (15%)*	21/97 (22%) 3/97 (3%)	7/27 (26%)	3/4	p = 0.79[1]
No	40/47 (85%)	73/97 (75%)	20/27 (74%)	1/4	

* One patient with hyperthyroidism at the past had received I^{131}. [1] Statistical analysis excluded the atypical hyperplasia group. [2] Statistical analysis not possible because of the small sample.
BC: breast cancer; BBD: breast benign disease; nd: no data.

Table 3. Mean baseline levels of thyroid hormones (fT3, fT4) and of TSH in controls, BC and BBD cases

Groups/Mean values ± SD, (n)	Controls	BC	BBD	Atypical hyperplasia	Statistical significance (p)
TSH (0,3-4,0 mU/L)	2.05 ± 1.57 (n = 42)	2.37 ± 2.30 (n = 78)	2.07 ± 1.03 (n = 20)	1.88 ± 1.90 (n = 4)	p = 0.757[1]
fT3 (2,3-5,3 pg/mL)	3.47 ± 1.93 (n = 41)	3.20 ± 0.74 (n = 69)	3.11 ± 0.83 (n = 16)	3.33 ± 0.37 (n = 3)	p = 0.622[1]
fT4 (10-25 pmol/L)	15.50 ± 3.76 (n = 41)	17.20 ± 3.30 (n = 67)	16.97 ± 3.29 (n = 16)	18.38 ± 2.80 (n = 4)	p = 0.035[1]

[1] Analysis was performed with the use of Kruskal-Wallis test. Cases with atypical hyperplasia were excluded from the analysis.
BC: breast cancer; BBD: breast benign disease; SD: standard deviation; TSH: thyroid stimulating hormone; fT3: free triiodothyronine; fT4: free thyroxine.

The mean baseline values of fT3 were 3.18 ± 0.74, 3.11 ± 0.83, 3.33 ± 0.37 and 3.47 ± 1.93 pg/mL in the BC, BBD, atypical ductal hyperplasia and controls groups, respectively. Abnormally low levels (< 2.3 pg/mL) of fT3 were recorded in 10% of the BC cases, 6% of the BBD cases and in 12% of the controls. Abnormally higher levels of fT3 (> 5.3 pg/mL) were recorded in only 2% of the controls. None of the cases (BC and BBD) had abnormally higher levels of fT3. No significant association was found between the compared groups' mean values of fT3 ($p = 0.622$) (Table 3).

The mean baseline values of fT4 were 17.2 ± 3.28, 16.9 ± 3.29, 18.38 ± 2.8 and 15.5 ± 3.76 pmol/L in the BC, BBD, atypical ductal hyperplasia and control groups, respectively. All BC cases and controls had normal levels of fT4. The mean values of fT4 were significantly higher in the BC group than in the other groups ($p = 0.035$). This statistical significance, although attenuated ($p = 0.055$), remained present when patients with levothyroxine treatment were excluded.

Association between thyroid autoantibodies and histopathological parameters of breast tissue

The frequency of positive TPO-Abs was 21.4% in the BC group, 33.3% in the BBD group, and 18% in controls. Positive Tg-Abs were found in 65% of the cases in the BC group, 55.5% in the BBD group and 16.6% in the control group. The levels of TPO-Abs and Tg-Abs did not significantly differ between the compared groups ($p = 0.43$ for TPO-Abs and $p = 1.00$ for Tg-Abs) (Table 4). The tests for TRAK antibodies were negative for the whole study population (cases and controls) (positivity > 2 U/L). The mean values of TRAK did not differ significantly ($p = 0.42$) between the groups.

Association between thyroid function and hormone dependent BC (ER and/or PR positivity)

Fifty-nine BC cases out of a total of 76 (77.6%) were found positive for estrogen and/or progesterone receptors through immunohistochemistry analysis (Table 5). Statistical analysis found no significant differences in the prevalence of history of thyroid disease between the hormone-dependent and hormone-independent BC cases ($p = 0.47$). Further analyses (not shown in Table 5) did not show any significant difference between hormone-dependent BC and positive thyroid autoantibodies (7 out of 25 hormone-dependent BC cases were positive for TPO-Abs, $p = 0.15$ and 6 of 11 hormone-dependent BC cases had positive Tg-Abs, $p = 1.00$) nor between the mean levels of thyroid hormones ($p = 0.486$ for TSH levels, $p = 0.229$ for fT3 levels and $p = 0.15$ for fT4 levels) and hormone-dependent BC.

Table 4. Frequency and mean baseline values of thyroid autoantibodies in the compared groups

Groups/Frequency and mean values ± SD, (n)	Controls	BC	BBD	Atypical hyperplasia	Statistical significance
TPO-Abs					
Mean values ± SD (n)	149.50 ± 495.54 (n = 39)	312 ± 810 (n = 42)	520 ± 1089 (n = 12)	20 ± 26.54 (n = 2)	p = 0.6[1]
Negative (< 50 mU/L)	32/39 (82%)	33/42 (78.5)	8/12 (66.6%)	2/2	p = 0.43[1]
Positive (> 50 mU/L)	7/39 (18%)	9/42 (21.4%)	4/12 (33.3%)	0/2	
Tg-Abs					
Mean values ± SD (n)	28.48 ± 64 (n = 12)	132 ± 238 (n = 17)	17.41 ± 14.65 (n = 9)	nd	p = 0.07[1]
Negative (< 10 mU/L)	10/12 (83%)	6/17 (35%)	4/9 (44.4%)	nd	p = 1.00
Positive (> 10 mU/L)	2/12 (16.6%)	11/17 (64.7%)	5/9 (55.5%)	nd	
TRAK					
Mean values ± SD (n)	0.71 ± 0.23 (n = 41)	0.64 ± 0.12 (n = 20)	0.66 ± 0.20 (n = 3)	nd	p = 0.42[1]
Negative (> 2 U/L)	41/41	20/20	3/3	nd	
Positive (< 2 U/L)	0	0	0	nd	

[1] Atypical hyperplasia was excluded from the statistical analysis. Analysis was performed with the use of Kruskal-Wallis test.

BC: breast cancer; BBD: breast benign disease; SD: standard deviation; nd: no data; TPO-Abs: thyroid hyperoxidase antibodies; TgAbs: thyroglobulin antibodies; TRAK: TSH receptors antibodies.

Table 5. Frequency of history of thyroid disease in the differenent T, N stages, the different grades (I, II, III) and the ER/PR positive BC

Thyroid disease/ Prognostic factors of BC	History of thyroid disease		Statistical significance (p)
	Yes	No	
TNM stage			
pT1	14 (14.4%)	27 (28%)	p = 0.805*
pT2	12 (12.4%)	24 (25%)	
pT3	4 (4%)	8 (8.2%)	
pT4	1 (1%)	2 (2%)	
pT+	8 (23.5%)	26 (76.5%)	p = 0.034
pT-	21 (46.6%)	24 (53.3%)	
Grade			
I	2 (25%)	6 (75%)	p = 0.83
II	17 (33%)	35 (66%)	
III	7 (22%)	18 (78%)	
Hormone-sensitivity			
ER +/PR +	20 (34%)	39 (66%)	p = 0.47
ER -/PR-	5 (33.5%)	10 (66.6%)	

* Cases with T4 tumors were excluded because of the small sample size.

BC: breast cancer; BBD: breast benign disease; ER: estrogen receptors; PR: progesterone receptors.

Association between thyroid disease and tumor size, nodal involvement or grading of BC

BC cases with a self-reported history of thyroid disease presented less frequently with lymph node infiltration (pN) than the BC cases without history of thyroid disease ($p = 0.035$) (Table 5). The frequency of primary hypothyroidism in BC cases with lymph node infiltration was 37.8% (2 patients with Hashimoto's and 1 with primary hypothyroidism out of 8 cases) and was 47.6% (7 patients with Hashimoto's and 3 with primary hypothyroidism out of 21 cases) in BC cases without lymph node infiltration.

BC cases with tumors with lymph node infiltration presented lower mean TSH levels and higher fT4 levels (mean value of TSH = 1.97 ± 1.4 mU/L, of fT3 = 3.37 ± 0.78 pg/mL and of fT4 = 17.68 ± 3.16 pmol/L) than the tumors without lymph node infiltration (mean value of TSH = 3.99 ± 1.0 mU/L, of fT3 = 3.09 ± 0.66 pg/mL and of fT4 = 16.33 ± 3.5 pmol/L), although there were no significant differences ($p = 0.148$ for TSH, $p = 0.26$ for fT3 and $p = 0.113$ for fT4). Due to the small sample of the T4 stage (n = 3), the corresponding statistical analyses were not performed.

The presence of positive thyroid autoantibodies was not significantly associated with the pT stage of BC ($p = 0.31$ for TPO-Ab and $p = 1.0$ for Tg-Ab), the pN stage of BC ($p = 0.87$ for TPO-Ab and $p = 0.76$ for Tg-Ab), nor the grade of BC ($p = 0.803$ for TPO-Ab and $p = 0.348$ for Tg-Ab (Table 5).

DISCUSSION

The present study showed that the mean baseline levels of fT4 were significantly higher in BC cases than in controls and patients with BBD. Additionally, history of thyroid disease was associated with a significantly lower frequency of lymph node metastases in BC cases. Recent data have shown that BC remains one of the most common cancers worldwide, with an estimated incidence of 464,000 new BC cases per 3.45 million new cases of cancer in Europe (15).

Previous studies are consistent with our results, showing no significant association between history of thyroid disease and histopathological characteristics of breast diseases (1,16-20). Nevertheless, other studies have demonstrated a higher (8,21,22) or a lower incidence of thyroid disease in BC cases (23). Hashimoto's disease, with or without positive thyroid antibodies (TPO-Abs and Tg-Abs), has been shown to be associated with an increased risk of BC (8,9,24-27) and, according to some studies, with a better prognosis and increased disease-free survival in BC cases (16,28). In our study, it seemed that Hashimoto's disease was not associated with BC; however, the small sample size precluded any definitive conclusions.

Our data showed that the mean baseline levels of fT4 were significantly higher in BC cases compared with the other groups, which is consistent with other studies in the literature (1,29). This correlation was sustained after exclusion of patients with levothyroxine treatment. Recently, it was found that fT4 levels in women without known thyroid disease and levothyroxine treatment were positively associated with risk of breast cancer, particularly in women with a BMI > 25 (28). However, hypothyroidism and low levels of fT4 (21) or only low levels of fT4 with normal TSH have also been shown to be related to an increased risk of BC risk in women (29).

As with fT4 levels, there have been reports suggesting an association of higher (1,30) or lower levels of fT3 with risk of BC (29,31,32). Surprisingly, we found no significant association between the mean baseline levels of fT3 and BC. One possible explanation for this result could be the short half-life of fT3 compared to fT4, which makes fT3 a less reliable marker of thyroid function. Another potential reason could be the circadian rhythm and periodicity concerning TSH and fT3 levels in particular. This circadian variation is not as evident in fT4 levels (33).

The mean baseline levels of TSH were not found to be significantly different between groups. Although there have been data associating low baseline levels of TSH (< 0.5 mU/l) in patients without known thyroid disease or treatment with a significantly increased risk of lung and prostate cancer, this association in BC has not been clearly demonstrated (34).

The association between positive thyroid autoantibodies and BC has been largely discussed in the literature (35,36). TPO-Abs are not thyroid-specific enzymes, and they can also be expressed in other tissues (24). In particular, TPO mRNA and protein have been found to be weakly but clearly expressed in BC tissues, peri-tumor tissues and in fat depots, and although they lack their functional activity, they maintain their antigenic role and can trigger B lymphocytes (37). Clinically, TPO-Abs have been associated with both an increased risk of BC (8,9,38) and a lower risk of BC; in some cases, TPO-Abs have even been associated with a lower frequency of distant metastases (39), a better outcome and better overall survival (27,38). Our data did not find an association between thyroid autoantibodies and risk of BC, which is consistent with a prospective study by Kuijpens and cols. (21).

Few data exist regarding the role of Tg-Abs and TRAB in BC. Tg-Abs have been associated with different oncological diseases and have been found to be more prevalent in patients with BC (23); however, they are not specific and may be influenced by different environmental factors (40). Extrathyroidal expression of TSH receptor has also been demonstrated in cardiac muscle and adrenal and kidney tissue (41) and was recently confirmed in BC tissue samples using RT-PCR (7). In clinical studies, TRAB levels have been found to be significantly higher in BC cases, particularly in low-grade BC cases (7), compared with healthy controls (40) and BBD cases (1).

The data in the literature associating thyroid function with prognostic markers of BC are scarce. In one study, BC cases with primary hypothyroidism showed a more indolent invasive breast cancer with less frequent lymph node metastases compared with euthyroid BC cases (23). According to other data, TPO-Ab levels (27) as well as the presence of nuclear TR-α receptors in breast cancer cells *in vitro* (2,41) were inversely correlated with lymph nodes metastases. Our findings showed that a history of thyroid disease was significantly correlated with a lower incidence of lymph nodes (pN stage) metastases in BC cases. The frequency of primary hypothyroidism (mainly Hashimoto's) was higher in BC cases with no lymph node involvement than in other thyroid diseases; however, the small sample size did not allow for a meaningful statistical analysis. We did not perform analyses for other prognostic markers such as Ki-67 and HER2 because of the limited data.

These data should be analyzed with caution because of the small size sample and because patients with known thyroid disease have more frequent access to hospital facilities and could thus be diagnosed with BC in earlier stages, which would explain the absence of lymph node metastases. Another limitation of this study was that patient's history of thyroid disease and treatment was based on medical interviews and files, and this could have led to misclassifications in the diagnosis of thyroid disease.

In conclusion, our findings showed that a history of thyroid disease was not associated with risk of BC. However, a history of thyroid disease was associated with a significantly lower frequency of lymph node metastases, suggesting the potential for a better prognosis in these BC cases. The significantly higher mean baseline levels of fT4 in the BC cases compared with the other two groups may suggest a thyroid hormone pattern that is distinct from that of low T3 syndrome. Further studies to determine the prognostic role of thyroid hormones in BC are warranted, as the small number of cases in the present study precludes definitive conclusions.

Acknowledgments: we thank Maggie Meitzler and Valsamo Anagnostou for their assistance in writing this manuscript.

REFERENCES

1. Ditsch N, Liebhardt S, Von Koch F, Lenhard M, Vogeser M, Spitzweg C, et al. Thyroid function in breast cancer patients. Anticancer Res. 2010; 30:1713-7.
2. Lemaire M, Baugnet-Mahieu L. Nuclear thyroid hormone receptors in human cancer tissues. Anticancer Res. 1986;6:695-700.
3. Nogueira CR, Brentani MM. Triiodothyronine mimics the effects of estrogen in breast cancer cell lines. J Steroid Biochem Mol Biol. 1996;59:271-9.
4. Humes HD, Cieslinski DA, Johnson LB, Sanchez IO. Triiodothyronine enhances renal tubule cell replication by stimulating EGF receptor gene expression. Am J Physiol. 1992;262:540-5.

5. Hall LC, Salazar EP, Kane SR, Liu N. Effects of thyroid hormones on human breast cancer cell proliferation. J Steroid Biochem Mol Biol. 2008;109:57-66.
6. Tang HY, Lin HY, Zhang S, Davis FB, Davis PJ. Thyroid hormone causes mitogen-activated protein kinase-dependent phosphorylation of the nuclear estrogen receptor. Endocrinology. 2004;145:3265-72.
7. Oh HJ, Chung JK, Kang JH, Kang WJ, Noh DY, Park IA, et al. The relationship between expression of the sodium/iodide symporter gene and the status of hormonal receptors in human breast cancer tissue. Cancer Res Treat. 2005;37:247-50.
8. Turken O, NarlnY, Demlrbas S, Onde ME, Sayan O, Kandemir EG, et al. Breast cancer in association with thyroid disorders. Breast Cancer Res. 2003;5:110-3.
9. Giani C, Fierabracci P, Bonacci R, Gigliotti A, Campani D, De Negri F, et al. Relationship between breast cancer and thyroid disease: relevance of autoimmune thyroid disorders in breast malignancy. J Clin Endocrinol Metab. 1996;81:990-94.
10. Dohán O, Carrasco N. Advances in Na(+)/I(-) symporter (NIS) research in the thyroid and beyond. Mol Cell Endocrinol. 2003;213:59-70.
11. Tazebay UH, Wapnir IL, Levy O, Dohan O, Zuckier LS, Zhao QH, et al. The mammary gland iodide transporter is expressed during lactation and in breast cancer. Nat Med. 2000;6:871-8.
12. Wapnir IL, van de Rijn M, Nowels K, Amenta PS, Walton K, Montgomery K, et al. Immunohistochemical profile of the sodium/iodide symporter in thyroid, breast, and other carcinomas using high density tissue microarrays and conventional sections. J Clin Endocrinol Metab. 2003;88:1880-8.
13. Rudnicka L, Sińczak A, Szybiński P, Huszno B, Stachura J. Expression of the Na(+)/I(-) symporter in invasive ductal breast cancer. Folia Histochem Cytobiol. 2003;41:37-40.
14. Pathologists' Guideline Recommendations for Immunohistochemical Testing of Estrogen and Progesterone Receptors in Breast Cancer. Breast Care. 2010;5:185-7.
15. Ferlay J, Steliarova-Foucher E, Lortet-Tieulent J, Rosso S, Coebergh JW, Comber H, et al. Cancer incidence and mortality patterns in Europe: estimates for 40 countries in 2012. Eur J Cancer. 2013;49:1374-403.
16. Michalaki V, Kondi-Pafiti A, Gennatas S, Antoniou A, Primetis H, Gennatas C. Breast cancer in association with thyroid disorders. J BUON. 2009;14:425-8.
17. Goldman MB, Monson RR, Maloof F. Cancer mortality in women with thyroid disease. Cancer Res. 1990;50:2283-9.
18. Kalache A, Vessey MP, McPherson K. Thyroid disease and breast cancer: findings in a large case-control study. Br J Surg. 1982;69:434-5.
19. Simon MS, Tang MT, Bernstein L, Norman SA, Weiss L, Burkman RT, et al. Do thyroid disorders increase the risk of breast cancer? Cancer Epidemiol Biomarkers Prev. 2002;11:1574-8.
20. Hoffman DA, McConahey WM, Brinton LA, Fraumeni JF Jr. Breast cancer in hypothyroid women using thyroid supplements. JAMA. 1984;251:616-19.
21. Kuijpens JL, Nyklíctek I, Louwman MW, Weetman TA, Pop VJ, Coebergh JW. Hypothyroidism might be related to breast cancer in post-menopausal women. Thyroid. 2005;15:1253-9.
22. Muller I, Pinchera A, Fiore E, Belardi V, Rosellini V, Giustarini E. High prevalence of breast cancer in patients with benign thyroid diseases. J Endocrinol Invest. 2011;34:349-52.
23. Cristofanilli M, Yamamura Y, Kau SW, Bevers T, Strom S, Patangan M, et al. Thyroid hormone and breast carcinoma. Primary hypothyroidism is associated with a reduced incidence of primary breast carcinoma. Cancer. 2005;103:1122-8.
24. Jiskra J, Barkmanova J, Limanova Z, Lánská V, Smutek D, Potlukova E, et al. Thyroid autoimmunity occurs more frequently in women with breast cancer compared to women with colorectal cancer and controls but it has no impact on relapse-free and overall survival. Oncol Rep. 2007;18:1603-11.
25. Giustarini E, Pinchera A, Fierabracci P, Roncella M, Fustaino L, Mammoli C, et al. Thyroid autoimmunity in patients with malignant and benign breast diseases before surgery. Eur J Endocrinol. 2006;154:645-9.
26. Hardefeldt PJ, Eslick GD, Edirimanne S. Benign thyroid disease is associated with breast cancer: a meta-analysis. Breast Cancer Res Treat. 2012;133:1169-77.
27. Smyth PP, Shering SG, Kilbane MT, Murray MJ, McDermott EW, Smith DF, et al. Serum thyroid peroxidase autoantibodies, thyroid volume, and outcome in breast carcinoma. J Clin Endocrinol Metab. 1998;83:2711-6.
28. Tosovic A, Becker C, Bondeson AG, Bondeson L, Ericsson UB, Malm J, et al. Prospectively measured thyroid hormones and thyroid peroxidase antibodies in relation to breast cancer risk. Int J Cancer. 2012;131:2126-33.
29. Takatani O, Okumoto T, Kosano H, Nishida M, Hiraide H, Tamakuma S. Relationship between the levels of serum thyroid hormones or estrogen status and the risk of breast cancer genesis in Japanese women. Cancer Res. 1989;49:3109-12.
30. Tosovic A, Bondeson AG, Bondeson L, Ericsson UB, Manjer J. Triiodothyronine levels in relation to mortality from breast cancer and all causes: a population-based prospective cohort study. Eur J Endocrinol. 2013;168:483-90.
31. Perry M, Goldie DJ, Self M. Thyroid function in patients with breast cancer. Ann R Coll Surg Engl. 1978;60:290-3.
32. Rose DP, Davis TE. Plasma thyronine levels in carcinoma of the breast and colon. Arch Intern Med. 1981;141:1161-4.
33. Russell W, Harrison RF, Smith N, Darzy K, Shalet S, Weetman AP, et al. Free triiodothyronine has a distinct circadian rhythm that is delayed but parallels thyrotropin levels. J Clin Endocrinol Metab. 2008;93:2300-6.
34. Hellevik AI, Asvold BO, Bjøro T, Romundstad PR, Nilsen TI, Vatten LJ. Thyroid function and cancer risk: a prospective population study. Cancer Epidemiol Biomarkers Prev. 2009;18:570-4.
35. Sandhu MK, Brezden-Masley C, Lipscombe LL, Zagorski B, Booth GL. Autoimmune hypothyroidism and breast cancer in the elderly. Breast Cancer Res Treat. 2009;115:635-41.
36. Brinton LA, Hoffman DA, Hoover R, Fraumeni JF Jr. Relationship of thyroid disease and use of thyroid supplements to breast cancer risk. J Chronic Dis. 1984;37:877-93.
37. Muller I, Giani C, Zhang L, Grennan-Jones FA, Fiore E, Belardi V, et al. Does thyroid peroxidase provide an antigenic link between thyroid autoimmunity and breast cancer? Int J Cancer. 2014;134:1706-14.
38. Fiore E, Giustarini E, Mammoli C, Fragomeni F, Campani D, Muller I, et al. Favorable predictive value of thyroid autoimmunity in high aggressive breast cancer. J Endocrinol Invest. 2007;30:734-8.
39. Szychta P, Szychta W, Gesing A, Lewiński A, Karbownik-Lewińska M. TSH receptor antibodies have predictive value for breast cancer – Retrospective analysis. Thyroid Res. 2013;6:8.
40. Dutton CM, Joba W, Spitzweg C, Heufelder AE, Bahn RS. Thyrotropin receptor expression in adrenal, kidney, and thymus. Thyroid. 1997;7:879-84.
41. Ditsch N, Toth B, Himsl I, Lenhard M, Ochsenkühn R, Friese K, et al. Thyroid hormone receptor (TR)alpha and TRbeta expression in breast cancer. Histol Histopathol. 2013;28:227-37.

A possible association between the -2518 A>G *MCP-1* polymorphism and insulin resistance in school children

Inés Matia-García[1], Lorenzo Salgado-Goytia[1], Luz Elena Ramos-Arellano[1], José Francisco Muñoz-Valle[2], Adakatia Armenta-Solís[3], Olga Lilia Garibay-Cerdenares[4], Mónica Ramírez[4], Isela Parra-Rojas[5]

[1] Facultad de Ciencias Químico Biológicas, Universidad Autónoma de Guerrero, Chilpancingo, Guerrero, México
[2] Instituto de Investigación en Ciencias Biomédicas, Departamento de Biología Molecular y Genómica, Centro Universitario de Ciencias de la Salud, Universidad de Guadalajara, Jalisco, México
[3] Facultad de Medicina, Universidad Autónoma de Guerrero, Acapulco, Guerrero, México
[4] Cátedra CONACyT, Facultad de Ciencias Químico Biológicas, Universidad Autónoma de Guerrero, Chilpancingo, Guerrero, México
[5] Laboratorio de Investigación en Obesidad y Diabetes, Facultad de Ciencias Químico Biológicas, Universidad Autónoma de Guerrero, Ciudad Universitaria, Guerrero, México

Correspondence to:
Isela Parra-Rojas Laboratorio de Investigación en Obesidad y Diabetes, Facultad de Ciencias Químico Biológicas, Universidad Autónoma de Guerrero, Ciudad Universitaria,Chilpancingo 39090, Guerrero, México
iprojas@yahoo.com

ABSTRACT

Objective: Monocyte chemoattractant protein 1 (MCP-1) has been suggested to be involved in the pathophysiology of insulin resistance (IR); therefore, variants in the *MCP-1* gene may contribute to the development of this disease. The aim of this study was to analyze the relationship of the -2518 A>G *MCP-1* (rs1024611) gene polymorphism with insulin resistance in Mexican children. Subjects and methods: A cross-sectional study was performed in 174 children, including 117 children without insulin resistance and 57 children with IR, with an age range of 6-11 years. Levels for serum insulin and high-sensitivity C-reactive protein were determined. The -2518 A>G *MCP-1* polymorphism was identified by the polymerase chain reaction-restriction fragment length polymorphism method. Insulin resistance was defined as a HOMA-IR in the upper 75th percentile, which was ≥ 2.4 for all children. Results: Genotype frequencies of the rs1024611 polymorphism for the insulin-sensitive group were 17% AA, 48% AG and 35% GG, and the frequency of G allele was 59%, whereas frequencies for the insulin-resistant group were 12% AA, 37% AG and 51% GG, and the frequency of G allele was 69%. The genotype and allele frequencies between groups did not show significant differences. However, the GG genotype was the most frequent in children with IR. The GG genotype was associated with insulin resistance (OR = 2.2, *P* = 0.03) in a genetic model. Conclusion: The -2518 A>G *MCP-1* gene polymorphism may be related to the development of insulin resistance in Mexican children. Arch Endocrinol Metab. 2018;62(1):72-9

Keywords
Insulin resistance; MCP-1; polymorphism; obesity; children

INTRODUCTION

The marked increase in pediatric obesity in the past decade has resulted in unprecedented increases in the incidence of type 2 diabetes mellitus among children and adolescents (1,2). There is substantial evidence that obesity is the main determinant of insulin resistance in children and that it increases the risk not only for the metabolic syndrome in adulthood but also for cardiovascular disease and type 2 diabetes later in life (3,4).

Obesity is associated with a chronic low-grade inflammatory state, characterized by enhanced production of multiple cytokines and chemokines. Monocyte chemoattractant protein-1 (MCP-1) is a chemokine produced by adipose tissue and other tissues. The production of MCP-1 in obesity is triggered when adipocytes are exposed to inflammatory cytokines and fatty acids. Other cells that produce MCP-1 in obesity include hepatocytes, skeletal muscle cells, monocytes, vascular smooth muscle and endothelial cells. MCP-1 production results in initiation and propagation of the inflammatory response in obesity (5,6). Some studies have found that plasma levels of MCP-1 are increased in obese adults (7) and in obese children (8) compared to lean controls. Furthermore, MCP-1 signaling has a direct role in the development of obesity. Younce and cols. reported that MCP-1-induced adipogenesis in 3T3-L1 cells is independent of PPAR gamma activation (9).

Mice with CCR2 deficiency had attenuated deposition of visceral fat and insulin resistance when challenged with a high fat diet (10). Moreover, *MCP-1* had an angiogenic effect on endothelial cells (11); therefore, it can contribute to the expansion and remodeling of adipose tissue (12).

In diabetic subjects, the high glucose-induced inflammatory process is characterized by the cooperation of a complex network of inflammatory molecules, such as cytokines, adhesion molecules, growth factors, and chemokines. The high glucose concentration induces an increase in the synthesis and release of MCP-1 by endothelial cells (EC) and smooth muscle cells (SMC) (13). MCP-1 is a potent chemotactic factor that regulates monocyte and macrophage migration and infiltration at sites of inflammation (14). The interaction of MCP-1 with its receptor CCR2 is considered pivotal in obesity-induced insulin resistance. Several groups have reported that mice with targeted deletions in the genes for *MCP-1/CCL2* and its receptor *CCR2* have reduced adipose tissue macrophage (ATM) content, decreased inflammation in fat and protection from high-fat (HF) diet-induced insulin resistance (15). Conversely, mice overexpressing MCP-1 in adipose tissue have an increased number of ATMs along with insulin resistance (16). Therefore, the MCP-1-CCR2 axis is of central importance for promoting ATM recruitment and insulin resistance in mice. Zineh and cols. reported that serum levels of MCP-1 increased in children with type 1 diabetes compared with the control group (17). In another study in adult subjects, serum concentrations of MCP-1 were higher in patients with type 2 diabetes than in normal subjects (18). The glucose and insulin appear to exert effects on MCP-1 secretion, and this interaction might be important for the development of insulin resistance in children (19).

A single nucleotide polymorphism characterized by a chance of A>G at position -2518 in the *MCP-1* distal promoter regulatory region affects MCP-1's transcription activity in response to IL-1β (20). This polymorphism has been associated with the development of chronic diseases such as obesity, hypertension, atherosclerosis, type 2 diabetes and insulin resistance (21-23). Briefly, in a German population, the *MCP-1* -2518G allele was associated with decreased prevalence of insulin resistance and type 2 diabetes (24). Another study carried out in a Japanese population found that in obese diabetics, -2518AA carriers had increased insulin resistance compared to -2518GG carriers (23). Alternatively, in an adult population of western Mexico, it was found that subjects without insulin resistance presented the -2518A allele more frequently than their counterparts with IR (25). In light of these contradictory results, it is important to perform replication studies in different populations to determine the association of this polymorphism with insulin resistance. In the Mexican population, the distributions of genotypic frequencies of this polymorphism in adults and its relations with bladder cancer and tuberculosis have been reported (26,27). Genotypic frequencies and their possible relationship to insulin resistance have not been identified in children. The aim of this study was to investigate whether the -2518 A>G *MCP-1* polymorphism is associated with insulin resistance in Mexican children.

SUBJECTS AND METHODS

Subjects

We analyzed a total of 174 unrelated children (86 girls and 88 boys), with an age range of 6-11 years, who were divided into two groups: 117 children without IR and 57 children with IR. The participants were all born in the State of Guerrero, Mexico, with a family history of ancestors, at least back to the third generation, born in this state. All children with evidence of infectious disease or with any treatment that could influence biochemical or hematological parameters were excluded from the study. Informed written consent was obtained from all parents or guardians before enrollment of children in the study according to the ethical guidelines of the 2008 Declaration of Helsinki. Approval for the study was obtained from the Research Ethics Committee of the University of Guerrero.

Clinical and anthropometric measurements

Body weight was determined in light clothes and without shoes using a body composition monitor (Tanita BC-553, Arlington, USA). Height and body circumferences were measured with a stadiometer and anthropometric tape (Seca, Hamburg, Germany), respectively. The classification of obesity was made using the 2000 Centers for Disease Control and Prevention growth charts, with normal weight defined as the 5th-85th percentiles and obesity as ≥ 95th percentile (28). The four skinfold thicknesses (triceps, biceps, subscapular and suprailiac) were measured with a plicometer

(Dynatronics Co, Salt Lake City, USA) and blood pressure (BP) with an aneroid sphygmomanometer (Riester CE 0124, Jungingen, Germany). Hypertension was defined as systolic or diastolic blood pressure in the 95th percentile or higher for age and sex, using an average of 2 measurements (29).

Laboratory assessment

A fasting blood sample was obtained from each child by antecubital venipuncture. Serum glucose levels were analyzed with semi-automated equipment (COBAS MIRA), and insulin levels were measured using an enzyme-linked immunosorbent assay (GenWay INS-EASIA kit). Intra-assay and inter-assay variation coefficients were 4.8% and 8.1%, respectively, and the detection limit was 0.17 µU/mL. The homeostasis model assessment of insulin resistance was used to determine insulin resistance in children. This score was calculated with the following formula: fasting serum insulin (µU/mL) x fasting plasma glucose (mmol/L)/22.5 (30). Insulin resistance was defined as a HOMA-IR at or above the 75th percentile, which was ≥ 2.4 for all children. Leukocyte and platelet counts were determined using an ADVIA-60 (Bayer Diagnostics). High-sensitivity C-reactive protein (hsCRP) levels were measured by a turbidimetry assay (BioSystems SA) with a sensitivity of 0.06 mg/L and intra-assay and inter-assay variation coefficients of 1.8% and 3.6%, respectively.

Genotyping analysis

Genomic DNA (gDNA) was extracted from peripheral leukocytes obtained from whole blood samples, according to the Miller method. The analysis of the -2518 A>G *MCP-1* (rs1024611) polymorphism was performed by the polymerase chain reaction-restriction fragment length polymorphism (PCR-RFLP) method, using the following primers: 5'CACAGAGAGAGTCTGGCCACGT3' (forward) and 5'CCAACAGAGGACTCTTGGTCT3' (reverse). The reaction was carried out in a final volume of 20 µl, adding buffer 1X to 2.5 mM $MgCl_2$, 0.2 mM dNTPs, 0.2 mM of each primer, 2.0 U/µl Taq polymerase (Invitrogen Life Technologies) and 0.1 µg/mL of gDNA. PCR was performed with an initial denaturation at 94 °C for 5 min, followed by 25 cycles of amplification consisting of 94 °C for 30 s of denaturation, 63 °C for 30 s of annealing and 72 °C for 30 s of extension, and a final extension step at 72 °C for 5 min. The amplified product of 234 bp was digested with PvuII restriction enzyme (New England Biolabs) for 2 hours at 37 °C and analyzed by electrophoresis in 6% polyacrylamide gel (Invitrogen™ life technologies) stained with silver nitrate. The AA genotype lacking the PvII site migrated as a 234 bp fragment, whereas the GG genotype was cleaved and appeared as 159 bp and 75 bp fragments.

Statistical analysis

The analysis was performed with STATA software (V.9.2). Differences in variables between groups were evaluated using a chi-square test for categorical variables, Student's *t* test for continuous variables with symmetrical distributions (data are presented as the mean and standard deviation), and a Mann-Whitney U test for variables without symmetrical distributions (data are presented as median and 5th to 95th percentiles). The genotype and allele frequencies were determined by direct counting, and a chi-square test was used to calculate the Hardy-Weinberg Equilibrium in case and control groups. To evaluate the association between insulin resistance and the polymorphism under investigation, we used a logistic regression model that was adjusted by age, gender, obesity and hypertension. P values < 0.05 were considered significant.

RESULTS

The study was conducted in a total of 174 children, divided into two groups: 117 children without IR were recruited as a control group, and 57 children with IR were the case group. The descriptive characteristics of the participants are summarized in Table 1. The median age of the children was 9 years, without differences between groups in age or gender. The insulin-resistant children had increases in all measures of central and peripheral adiposity and in both systolic and diastolic blood pressure compared to the group with insulin sensitivity. We found a high prevalence of obesity (73.7%) in the insulin-resistant group compared with the insulin-sensitive group (36.8%). The group with IR also showed an increase in serum hsCRP levels but not in leukocyte or platelet counts.

Demographic, clinical and metabolic variables were compared between children grouped according to their genotypes of the -2518 A>G *MCP-1* polymorphism. Although three genetic models were performed,

Table 1. Clinical and laboratory variables of the studied groups

Variables	All children (n = 174)	Group without IR (n = 117)	Group with IR (n = 57)	*P* value
Age (years)‡	9 (6-11)	9 (6-11)	9 (6-11)	0.08
Gender % (n)*				0.36
Male	50.6 (88)	53 (62)	45.6 (26)	
Female	49.4 (86)	47 (55)	54.4 (31)	
Weight (kg)‡	33.2 (20.1-59.1)	30.7 (19.7-48.8)	44.4 (23-68.2)	< 0.001
Height (cm)†	132.6 ± 11.3	131.1 ± 10.6	137.2 ± 12.1	0.001
BMI (kg/m²)‡	18.4 (14.3-27)	17.3 (14.1-24.9)	23.5 (14.9-29.9)	< 0.001
Obesity % (n)*				< 0.001
No	51.1 (89)	63.2 (74)	26.3 (15)	
Yes	48.9 (85)	36.8 (43)	73.7 (42)	
Waist circumference (cm)‡	67 (54-88)	66 (53-84)	80.3 (58-96)	< 0.001
Hip circumference (cm)‡	75 (62-96)	73 (62-89)	85 (66-104)	< 0.001
Waist-to-hip ratio‡	0.9 (0.8-0.97)	0.9 (0.8-0.97)	0.9 (0.8-1.0)	0.001
Arm circumference (cm)‡	21 (16-28)	20 (16-26)	24.5 (17-33)	< 0.001
Biceps skinfold (mm)†	15.5 ± 4.8	14.8 ± 4.8	17.6 ± 4.3	< 0.001
Triceps skinfold (mm)‡	15 (8.5-21.5)	13.5 (8-21.5)	18 (10-22)	< 0.001
Subscapular skinfold (mm)‡	13 (6-22)	12 (5.5-21)	18.5 (8-25)	< 0.001
Suprailiac skinfold (mm)†	17.9 ± 5.5	17.0 ± 5.5	20.7 ± 4.7	< 0.001
SBP (mmHg)‡	98 (81-115)	96 (81-110)	101 (80-124)	< 0.001
DBP (mmHg)‡	58 (48-71)	57 (48-68)	60 (44.5-78)	< 0.001
Glucose (mg/dL)‡	96 (74-112)	95 (72-112)	98 (78-114)	0.06
Insulin (µU/mL)‡	6.9 (0.8-22.4)	4.7 (0.6-9.2)	13.7 (9.9-31.9)	< 0.001
HOMA-IR‡	1.2 (0.-4.9)	0.6 (0-2.1)	3.1 (2.5-7.3)	< 0.001
hsCRP (mg/L)‡	0.8 (0.1-6.5)	0.6 (0.1-6.0)	1.6 (0.1-8.3)	0.004
Leukocytes (10³/mm³)‡	7.7 (5.0-12.3)	7.6 (5.0-12.5)	7.9 (5-11.5)	0.08
Platelets (10³/mm³)‡	308 (219-413)	306 (219-440)	316 (218-410)	0.22

* Values are expressed as percentages and *n*. Chi-square test. † Values are expressed as the means ± SD. Student's *t* test. ‡ Values are expressed as median (p5-p95). Mann-Whitney test.
IR: insulin resistance; BMI: body mass index; SBP: systolic blood pressure; DBP: diastolic blood pressure; HOMA-IR: homeostasis model of assessment-insulin resistance; hsCRP: high sensitivity C-reactive protein.

the table only includes the comparison that shows significant differences. All children were divided into two groups, carriers and non-carriers of the A allele (AA+AG vs. GG). Interestingly, the G allele was the most frequent in children with insulin resistance (69%). However, we found that some A allele carriers also had insulin resistance (31%) (Table 2).

The -2518 A>G *MCP-1* polymorphism was found in Hardy Weinberg Equilibrium in the total population ($X^2 = 0.57$, P = 0.45), in cases ($X^2 = 1.03$, P = 0.31) and in controls ($X^2 = 0.014$, $P = 0.91$). The comparative analysis of genotype and allele frequencies between groups did not show significant differences; however, we found an association of the GG genotype with insulin resistance (OR = 2.2, 95% CI, 1.1-4.5; P = 0.03), determined by an adjusted genetic model (Table 3).

DISCUSSION

In this study, an association between the -2518 A>G *MCP-1* polymorphism and insulin resistance is shown in a sample of Mexican children. Our results indicate that children with the GG genotype have a 2.2-fold higher risk of developing IR in comparison to those with the AA or AG genotype.

In contrast, a study in a German population found a low prevalence of insulin resistance and type 2 diabetes in carriers of the G allele compared with subjects homozygous for the A allele (24). In another study in a Chinese population, the G allele proved to be protective (adjusted OR=0.49, 95% CI, 0.32-0.77; P < 0.0001) against type 2 diabetes compared with subjects homozygous for allele A (31). These results

Table 2. Clinical and laboratory variables according to *MCP-1* genotypes

Variables	All children (n = 174)	AA+AG (n = 104)	GG (n = 70)	*P* value
Age (years)‡	9 (6-11)	9 (6-11)	9 (6-11)	0.39
Gender % (n)*				0.42
Male	50.6 (88)	48.1 (50)	54.3 (38)	
Female	49.4 (86)	51.9 (54)	45.7 (32)	
Weight (kg)‡	34.1 (20.1-59.2)	32.1 (20.3-59.1)	36.2 (20.1-64.9)	0.13
Height (cm)†	133.4 ± 11.5	132.6 ± 11.1	134.6 ± 12.2	0.26
BMI (kg/m^2)‡	18.9 (14.3-28.2)	18.4 (14.3-25.9)	19.7 (14.5-29.1)	0.08
Obesity % (n)*				0.57
No	51.1 (89)	53 (55)	49 (34)	
Yes	48.9 (85)	47 (49)	51 (36)	
Waist circumference (cm)‡	67.5 (54-90)	67 (54-89)	70 (56-94)	0.10
Hip circumference (cm)‡	76 (62-96.5)	74 (62-96)	79 (62-96.5)	0.15
Waist-to-hip ratio‡	0.9 (0.8-0.97)	0.9 (0.8-0.97)	0.9 (0.8-0.97)	0.24
Arm circumference (cm)‡	21 (16-29)	21 (16.5-28)	22 (16-30)	0.20
Biceps skinfold (mm)†	15.6 ± 4.6	15.7 ± 4.9	15.5 ± 4.1	0.76
Triceps skinfold (mm)‡	15 (8.5-21.5)	15 (8.5-21)	15 (7.5-22)	0.97
Subscapular skinfold (mm)‡	13 (6-22.5)	12.8 (5.5-21.5)	13.5 (6-23)	0.65
Suprailiac skinfold (mm)†	18.2 ± 5.6	18.1 ± 5.5	18.2 ± 5.9	0.95
SBP (mmHg)‡	98 (80-115)	98 (80-117)	98 (81-110)	0.82
DBP (mmHg)‡	58 (49-71)	58 (49-72)	58.5 (50-70)	0.83
Hypertension % (n)*				0.47
No	92.5 (161)	91.3 (95)	94.3 (66)	
Yes	7.5 (13)	8.7 (9)	5.7 (4)	
Glucose (mg/dL)‡	96 (73-109)	96.5 (72-109)	95.5 (78-112)	0.71
Insulin (µU/mL)‡	6.9 (0.8-22.4)	6.6 (1.0-21.5)	8.2 (0.8-22.4)	0.17
HOMA-IR‡	1.7 (0.2-5.5)	1.5 (0.2-4.8)	1.9 (0.2-5.8)	0.15
Insulin resistance % (n)*				0.04
No	67.2 (117)	73.1 (76)	58.6 (41)	
Yes	32.8 (57)	26.9 (28)	41.4 (29)	
hsCRP (mg/L)‡	0.8 (0.1-6.5)	0.8 (0.1-8.0)	0.9 (0.1-6.3)	0.99
Leukocytes (10^3/mm^3)‡	7.6 (4.8-11.5)	7.7 (4.8-12.3)	7.6 (5.1-11.2)	0.64
Platelets (10^3/mm^3)‡	308 (219-412)	310.5 (224-413)	306 (205-410)	0.66

* Values are expressed as percentages and *n*. Chi-square test. † Values are expressed as the means ± SD. Student's t test. ‡ Values are expressed as median (p5-p95). Mann-Whitney test.
IR: insulin resistance; BMI: body mass index; SBP: systolic blood pressure; DBP: diastolic blood pressure; HOMA-IR: homeostasis model of assessment-insulin resistance; hsCRP: high sensitivity C-reactive protein.

suggest a protective role of the G allele for the development of insulin resistance and type 2 diabetes in the Chinese population. These differences may be attributed to the ancestry of the population; it is known that the Mexican population originated from mixed racial ancestry consisting of individuals from Europe (mainly Spain) or Africa who migrated to America where Native Americans of this region were living, giving origin to the Mexican mestizo population, who present a greater genetic diversity. This diversity can cause marked differences in allelic frequencies and patterns of linkage disequilibrium across their genome (32).

There are few studies reporting an association of -2518 A>G polymorphism with insulin resistance and type 2 diabetes, but other investigators have found associations of the GG genotype with high serum MCP-1 levels, hypertension, lupus nephritis and tuberculosis (27,33,34).

Table 3. Association of insulin resistance with genotype and allele frequencies of *MCP-1* polymorphism

Genotype/allele	Group without IR (n = 117) % (n)	Group with IR (n = 57) % (n)	*P*†	OR crude (95% CI); *P*	OR adjusted (95% CI); *P*‡
Frequencies			0.13		
AA*	17 (20)	12 (7)		1	
AG	48 (56)	37 (21)		1.1 (0.4-2.9); 0.89	
GG	35 (41)	51 (29)		2.0 (0.8-5.4); 0.16	
Frequencies			0.08		
A*	41 (96)	31 (35)		1	
G	59 (138)	69 (79)		1.6 (1.0-2.6); 0.06	
Dominant model			0.41		
AA*	17 (20)	12 (7)		1	1
AG+GG	83 (97)	88 (50)		1.5 (0.6-3.7); 0.41	1.6 (0.6-4.3); 0.37
Recessive model			0.04		
AA+AG*	65 (76)	49 (28)		1	
GG	35 (41)	51 (29)		1.9 (1.0-3.6); 0.04	2.2 (1.1-4.5); 0.03
Additive model	-	-	-	1.5 (0.96-2.5); 0.07	1.7 (0.98-2.7); 0.05

* Reference category; † Chi square test. ‡ Genetic model adjusted by age, gender, obesity and hypertension.
IR: insulin resistance; OR: odds ratio.

We found that the GG genotype was associated with an increased risk for developing IR when compared with children carrying other genotypes, which suggest that IR may also be related to increased serum *MCP-1* levels. In other studies, it was observed that insulin induces substantial expression and secretion of MCP-1, both *in vitro* in insulin-resistant 3T3-L1 adipocytes and *in vivo* in insulin-resistant obese mice; thus, MCP-1 was identified as an insulin-response gene (6). This result should be considered with caution, as it is necessary to perform a replication study in a larger sample to confirm these results.

Obesity and IR are characterized by chronic systemic low-grade inflammation. Markers of inflammation, such as tumor necrosis factor alpha (TNF-α), interleukin-6 (IL-6), CRP and MCP-1, are increased in peripheral blood levels in obesity and are associated with IR and may predict the development of type 2 diabetes (35). In this study, the children with IR showed increased hsCRP levels but not leukocyte or platelet counts. The GG genotype carriers did not present an increase in these markers, which could be an indicator of systemic inflammation not related to the development of insulin resistance in the studied children.

We observed that children with IR showed increases in all measures of central and peripheral adiposity compared to children without IR. Insulin resistance is a hallmark of obesity, emerging early in the metabolic syndrome, and is highly associated with increased visceral adipose tissue mass (36). Adipose tissue in obese subjects is characterized by macrophage infiltration, which is an early event contributing to the development of systemic insulin resistance. Indeed, transgenic mice that overexpress MCP-1 specifically in adipocytes develop adipose tissue inflammation and insulin resistance without obesity (37). This finding indicates that the subcutaneous adiposity may be an important predictor of IR in children.

Two main limitations should be considered in our investigation. First, the small sample size limited the statistical power. Second, MCP-1 levels were not measured, therefore the association of -2518 A>G polymorphism with MCP-1 levels remains uncertain in our population. Thus, future studies in Mexican children are necessary to determine MCP-1 levels.

In conclusion, the -2518 A>G *MCP-1* gene polymorphism may be related to the development of insulin resistance in Mexican children.

REFERENCES

1. Silink M. Childhood diabetes: a global perspective. Horm Res. 2002;57(Suppl. 1):1-5.

2. Invitti C, Guzzaloni G, Gilardini L, Morabito F, Viberti G. Prevalence and concomitants of glucose intolerance in European obese children and adolescents. Diabetes Care. 2003;26(1):118-24.
3. Caprio S. Insulin resistance in childhood obesity. J Pediatr Endocrinol Metab. 2002;15(Suppl. 1):487-92.
4. Sun SS, Liang R, Huang TT, Daniels SR, Arslanian S, Liu K, et al. Childhood obesity predicts adult metabolic syndrome: the Fels Longitudinal Study. J Pediatr. 2008;152(2):191-200.
5. Samaan MC, Obeid J, Nguyen T, Thabane L, Timmons BW. Chemokine (C-C motif) Ligand 2 is a potential biomarker of inflammation & physical fitness in obese children: a cross-sectional study. BMC Pediatr. 2013;13:47.
6. Sartipy P, Loskutoff DJ. Monocyte chemoattractant protein 1 in obesity and insulin resistance. Proc Natl Acad Sci USA. 2003;100(12):7265-70.
7. Kim CS, Park HS, Kawada T, Kim JH, Lim D, Hubbard NE, et al. Circulating levels of MCP-1 and IL-8 are elevated in human obese subjects and associated with obesity-related parameters. Int J Obes. 2006;30(9):1347-55.
8. Breslin WL, Johnston CA, Strohacker K, Carpenter KC, Davidson TR, Moreno JP, et al. Obese Mexican American children have elevated MCP-1, TNF-α, monocyte concentration, and dyslipidemia. Pediatrics. 2012;129(5):e1180-6.
9. Younce CW, Azfer A, Kolattukudy PE. MCP-1 (monocyte chemotactic protein- 1) induced protein, a recently identified zinc finger protein, induces adipogenesis in 3T3-L1 pre-adipocytes without peroxisome proliferator activated receptor gamma. J Biol Chem. 2009;284(40):27620-8.
10. Weisberg SP, Hunter D, Huber R, Lemieux J, Slaymaker S, Vaddi K, et al. CCR2 modulates inflammatory and metabolic effects of high-fat feeding. J Clin Invest. 2006;116(1):115-24.
11. Salcedo R, Ponce ML, Young HA, Wasserman K, Ward JM, Kleinman HK, et al. Human endothelial cells express CCR2 and respond to MCP-1: direct role of MCP-1 in angiogenesis and tumor progression. Blood. 2000;96(1):34-40.
12. Panee J. Monocyte Chemoattractant Protein 1 (MCP-1) in obesity and diabetes. Cytokine. 2012;60(1):1-12.
13. Dragomir E, Simionescu M. Monocyte chemoattractant protein-1 a major contributor to the inflammatory process associated with diabetes. Arch Physiol Biochem. 2006;112(4-5):239-44.
14. Deshmane SL, Kremlev S, Amini S, Sawaya BE. Monocyte chemoattractant protein-1 (MCP-1): an overview. J Interferon Cytokine Res. 2009;29(6):313-26.
15. Kanda H, Tateya S, Tamori Y, Kotani K, Hiasa K, Kitazawa R, et al. MCP-1 contributes to macrophage infiltration into adipose tissue, insulin resistance, and hepatic steatosis in obesity. J Clin Invest. 2006;116(6):1494-505.
16. Kamei N, Tobe K, Suzuki R, Ohsugi M, Watanabe T, Kubota N, et al. Overexpression of monocyte chemoattractant protein-1 in adipose tissues causes macrophage recruitment and insulin resistance. J Biol Chem. 2006;281(36):26602-14.
17. Zineh I, Beitelshees AL, Silverstein JH, Haller MJ. Serum monocyte chemoattractant protein-1 concentrations associate with diabetes status but not arterial stiffness in children with type 1 diabetes. Diabetes Care. 2009;32(3):465-7.
18. Mine S, Okada Y, Tanikawa T, Kawahara C, Tabata T, Tanaka Y. Increased expression levels of monocyte CCR2 and monocyte chemoattractant protein-1 in patients with diabetes mellitus. Biochem Biophys Res Commun. 2006;344(3):780-5.
19. Zietz B, Büchler C, Herfarth H, Müller-Ladner U, Spiegel D, Schölmerich J, et al. Caucasian patients with type 2 diabetes mellitus have elevated levels of monocyte chemoattractant protein-1 that are not influenced by the -2518 A/G promoter polymorphism. Diabetes Obes Metab. 2005;7(5):570-8.
20. Rovin BH, Lu L, Saxena R. A novel polymorphism in the MCP-1 gene regulatory region that influences MCP-1 expression. Biochem Biophys Res Commun. 1999;259(2):344-8.
21. Yuasa S, Maruyama T, Yamamoto Y, Hirose H, Kawai T, Matsunaga-Irie S, et al. MCP-1 gene A-2518G polymorphism and carotid artery atherosclerosis in patients with type 2 diabetes. Diabetes Res Clin Pract. 2009;86(3):193-8.
22. Gustafson B, Hammarstedt A, Andersson CX, Smith U. Inflamed adipose tissue: a culprit underlying the metabolic syndrome and atherosclerosis. Arterioscler Thromb Vasc Biol. 2007;27(11):2276-83.
23. Kouyama K, Miyake K, Zenibayashi M, Hirota Y, Teranishi T, Tamori Y, et al. Association of serum MCP-1 concentration and MCP-1 polymorphism with insulin resistance in Japanese individuals with obese type 2 diabetes. Kobe J Med Sci. 2008;53(6):345-54.
24. Simeoni E, Hoffmann MM, Winkelmann BR, Ruiz J, Fleury S, Boehm BO, et al. Association between the A-2518G polymorphism in the monocyte chemoattractant protein-1 gene and insulin resistance and type 2 diabetes mellitus. Diabetologia. 2004;47(9):1574-80.
25. Guzmán-Ornelas MO, Petri MH, Vázquez-Del Mercado M, Chavarría-Ávila E, Corona-Meraz FI, Ruíz-Quezada SL, et al. CCL2 Serum Levels and Adiposity Are Associated with the Polymorphic Phenotypes -2518A on CCL2 and 64ILE on CCR2 in a Mexican Population with Insulin Resistance. J Diabetes Res. 2016;2016:5675739.
26. Vázquez-Lavista LG, Lima G, Gabilondo F, Llorente L. Genetic association of monocyte chemoattractant protein 1 (MCP-1) -2518 polymorphism in Mexican patients with transitional cell carcinoma of the bladder. Urology. 2009;74(2):414-8.
27. Flores-Villanueva PO, Ruiz-Morales JA, Song CH, Flores LM, Jo EK, Montaño M, et al. A functional promoter polymorphism in monocyte chemoattractant protein-1 is associated with increased susceptibility to pulmonary tuberculosis. J Exp Med. 2005;202(12):1649-58.
28. Centers for Disease Control and Prevention, National Center for Health Statistics. 2000 CDC growth charts: United States. Available from: www.cdc.gov/growthcharts. Accessed on: March 20, 2008.
29. National High Blood Pressure Education Program Working Group on High Blood Pressure in Children and Adolescents. The fourth report on the diagnosis, evaluation, and treatment of high blood pressure in children and adolescents. Pediatrics. 2004;114(2 Suppl):555-76.
30. Matthews DR, Hosker JP, Rudenski AS, Naylor BA, Treacher DF, Turner RC. Homeostasis model assessment: insulin resistance and beta-cell function from fasting plasma glucose and insulin concentrations in man. Diabetologia. 1985;28(7):412-9.
31. Jing Y, Zhu D, Bi Y, Yang D, Hu Y, Shen S. Monocyte chemoattractant protein 1 -2518 A/G polymorphism and susceptibility to type 2 diabetes in a Chinese population. Clin Chim Acta. 2011;412(5-6):466-9.
32. Price AL, Patterson N, Yu F, Cox DR, Waliszewska A, McDonald GJ, et al. A genomewide admixture map for Latino populations. Am J Hum Genet. 2007;80(6):1024-36.
33. Gonzalez E, Rovin BH, Sen L, Cooke G, Dhanda R, Mummidi S, et al. HIV-1 infection and AIDS dementia are influenced by a mutant MCP-1 allele linked to increased monocyte infiltration of tissues and MCP-1 levels. Proc Natl Acad Sci USA. 2002;99(21):13795-800.
34. Jemaa R, Ben Ali S, Kallel A, Omar S, Feki M, Elasmi M, et al. Association between the -2518G/A polymorphism in the monocyte chemoattractant protein-1 (MCP-1) gene and hypertension in Tunisian patients. Clin Biochem. 2009;42(1-2):34-7.
35. Cai K, Qi D, Hou X, Wang O, Chen J, Deng B, et al. MCP-1 upregulates amylin expression in murine pancreatic β cells through ERK/JNK-AP1 and NF-κB related signaling pathways independent of CCR2. PLoS One. 2011;6(5):e19559.

Outcomes of patients with bone metastases from differentiated thyroid cancer

Inés Califano[1], Susana Deutsch[2], Alicia Löwenstein[3], Carmen Cabezón[4], Fabián Pitoia[5], on behalf of the Thyroid Department, Sociedad Argentina de Endocrinología y Metabolismo

[1] Service of Endocrinology, Instituto de Oncología A. H. Roffo, Universidad de Buenos Aires, Ciudad Autónoma de Buenos Aires, Argentina
[2] Endocrine Unit, Hospital General de Agudos J. A. Fernández, Ciudad Autónoma de Buenos Aires, Argentina
[3] Division of Endocrinology, Hospital General de Agudos J. M. Ramos Mejía, Ciudad Autónoma de Buenos Aires, Argentina
[4] Service of Endocrinology and Nuclear Medicine, Hospital Italiano de Buenos Aires, Ciudad Autónoma de Buenos Aires, Argentina
[5] Division of Endocrinology, Hospital de Clínicas, Universidad de Buenos Aires, Ciudad Autónoma de Buenos Aires, Argentina

Correspondence to:
Inés Califano
Instituto A. H. Roffo,
San Martín 5481, CP 1407,
Ciudad Autónoma de
Buenos Aires, Argentina
ines.m.califano@gmail.com

ABSTRACT

Objective: Bone metastases (BM) from differentiated thyroid cancer (DTC) are associated with poor survival rates. Due to the low frequency of this entity, we performed a multicentric retrospective study that aimed to evaluate the presentation, outcome and causes of death in this population. Subjects and methods: We reviewed file records from 10 databases. BM were diagnosed by: i) biopsy and/or ii) radioiodine (RAI) bone uptake + elevated thyroglobulin (Tg) levels and/or c) bone uptake of 18-FDG in the PET-CT scan + elevatedTg levels. Results: Fifty-two patients with DTC were included (44% male, mean age 54 years); 58% had papillary histology. BM were synchronous with DTC diagnosis in 46% of the participating cases. BM were symptomatic in 65% of the cases. Multiple BM were present in 65% of patients, while simultaneous metastatic disease in additional sites was found in 69%. Ninety-eight percent of patients received treatment for the BM, which included RAI therapy in 42 patients; 30 of them received cumulative RAI doses that were larger than 600 mCi ^{131}I. The mean follow-up after a BM diagnosis was 34 months. The 2- and 5-year survival rates after diagnosis of the first BM were 64% and 38%, respectively. The status on the last evaluation was DTC-related death in 52% of the patients; 26% of them died from direct complications of BM or their treatments. Conclusion: BM are usually radioiodine-refractory and are associated with a short overall survival, although most of the patients died of causes not directly related to the BM. Arch Endocrinol Metab. 2018;62(1):14-20

Keywords
Thyroid cancer; distant metastases; bone metastases

INTRODUCTION

In most published series, patients with differentiated thyroid cancer (DTC) have a 10-year overall survival rate of 85-93% (1). However, when distant metastases occur, the overall survival may decrease to 50% at 5 years of follow-up (1-4).

Among cases, the most frequent localizations of DTC metastases are the lungs in 50%, bones in 25 to 30% and both sites in 20% (5-8).

The treatment of distant metastases usually involves the use of radioactive iodine (RAI), which may be administered several times during follow-up. Nevertheless, once DTC is no longer amenable to RAI therapy or surgery, the expected survival declines rapidly, and death from thyroid carcinoma within 3 years is common (8,9).

Bone metastases (BM) may severely reduce the quality of life (QoL) in patients with disseminated thyroid cancer, causing pain, fractures and spinal cord compression, among other complications (10). BM is a difficult clinical problem that requires a multidisciplinary approach.

Cancer is generally incurable once it has metastasized to the bone. It has been suggested that bone marrow can serve as reservoir for dormant tumor cells, thereby rendering them resistant to RAI and conventional chemotherapeutic agents (11).

However, the causes of death in patients with DTC and BM have not been widely evaluated, probably due to the low frequency of this entity. Therefore, we decided to perform a retrospective review of patients with DTC and BM that were followed up in 10 referral endocrinology units in Argentina in order to evaluate the epidemiology, forms of presentation, treatments modalities and outcome, including overall survival and causes of death.

SUBJECTS AND METHODS

We reviewed the file records of patients with DTC whom were treated at 10 hospitals. Since this was a retrospective study, written consent was deemed unnecessary. Confidentiality of patients' data was maintained in accordance with each institution's standards. We included patients who were treated with total thyroidectomy (either with or without lymph node dissection) and remnant ablation. The patients were classified according to the TNM staging system (AJCC/UICC; 7 ed) (12) and to the risk of recurrence classification from the American Thyroid Association (13). The baseline characteristics of the patients who were included are shown in Table 1.

Table 1. The baseline characteristics of 52 patients with bone metastases and differentiated thyroid cancer who were included in the study

Characteristics	Number of patients (%)
Age at diagnosis of thyroid cancer, median (years)	54.5
Range	15-54
> 45 years	42 (80.7)
Male/female	23/29 (44.3/55.7)
Pathological diagnosis	
Papillary thyroid cancer	30 (57.6)
Classic	17
Follicular variant	9
Tall cell	3
Oncocytic	1
Follicular thyroid cancer	19 (36.5)
Hürthle cell carcinoma	3 (5.7)
Stage (AJCC/UICC7[a]ed)	
I	4 (8)
II	6 (12.5)
III	7 (15)
IVa	7 (15)
IVb	1 (1.5)
Ivc	23 (48)
Risk of recurrence (ATA 2009) (n = 47)	
Intermediate	14 (29.7)
High	33 (70.2)

BM were diagnosed by: i) biopsy and/or ii) after ^{131}I bone uptake associated with elevated thyroglobulin (Tg) levels and/or iii) abnormal bone uptake of ^{18}fluordeoxyglucose in the positron emission tomography (PET/CT) scan associated with elevated Tg levels.

The following clinical-pathological features of the BM were considered for the analysis: methodology for the diagnosis of the BM, the number and localization of the BM foci, the symptoms generated by the BM, the sites of RAI radioiodine uptake after the administration of the ^{131}I dose and the presence of loco-regional disease and/or other non-skeletal metastatic sites.

BM were classified as synchronous if they were detected within the first 6 months after the diagnosis of the DTC and metachronous if they were found later in the follow-up.

Clinical management during follow-up

After the initial approach, the patients were followed by assessing their clinical status in response to initial therapy by using thyroid hormone withdrawal (THW)-stimulated Tg, along with diagnostic or post-treatment whole body scans (WBS) and neck ultrasonography. All patients underwent morphological imaging, including computed tomography (CT) and/or PET/CT. The response to treatment was defined as follows: i) remission: undetectable stimulated Tg levels with negative post-dose WBS associated to the absence of structural images in CT and or PET/CT); ii) biochemical persistence: detectable Tg levels under thyroid hormone suppressive therapy or after THW, or persistent/increasing levels of TgAb with negative post dose WBS associated to the lack of structural images in CT and/or PET/CT); and iii) incomplete structural response.

Patients with BM received RAI treatments (mean cumulative activity: 391 mCi ^{131}I, median 200 mCi, range 100-1500 mCi) until i) adverse events related to RAI appeared or ii) no response to treatment was observed due to progressive disease. Different modalities for the treatment of BM were also evaluated.

We considered the causes of death due to DTC and classified them as secondary to BM when they could be attributed to a direct complication of BM (such as pulmonary thromboembolism caused by immobilization, decubitus ulcer infections in bedridden patients or complications of their treatment, pathological fracture or due to disseminated DTC).

Statistical analyses were performed using SPSS software (version 21: SPSS Inc., Chicago Il). Quantitative variables are expressed as means ± SD; qualitative data are expressed in percentages. Continuous variables were compared using Fisher's exact test and the x^2 test was used to compare categorical variables. Kaplan-Meier curves are used to present survival times. Values were considered statistically significant at $p < 0.05$.

RESULTS

Out of a total of 3810 patients with DTC, 52 (1.3%) were found to have BM and were included in the study (Table 1). BM were diagnosed synchronously (at the moment of the diagnosis of the DTC) in 46.2% of patients (n = 24) and metachronously in 53.8% (n = 28). Metachronous metastases were diagnosed 7-240 months after the initial diagnosis (median: 72 months).

BM were symptomatic in 65.4% of the cases (n = 34). Pain was the most frequent clinical presentation (73.5%, n = 25), while fractures and neurological symptoms were each reported in 8.8% of the cases (n = 3). The characteristics of BM can be observed in Table 2. Either as a presenting symptom or as a later event, spinal cord compression was noted in 6 cases (11,5%).

Simultaneous metastatic disease in sites other than bone was found in 69.2% of the patients (n = 36). The lung was the most frequently affected site in 94.4% of the cases (n = 34), followed by the brain, retroperitoneum, adrenal glands and skin (6.6%).

Table 2. Radioiodine uptake, localization and extent of disease in 52 patients with bone metastases from differentiated thyroid cancer

Characteristics	Number of patients (%)
Radioiodine uptake at metastatic site	
Positive	30 (57.6)
Negative	22 (42.3)
Number of BM	
Solitary	18 (34.6)
Multiple	34 (65.3)
Metastatic site	
Spine	38 (29.2)
Pelvis	25 (19.2)
Ribs	24 (18.4)
Limbs	19 (14.6)
Skull	13 (10)
Clavicle	8 (6.1)
Sternum	3 (2.3)
Extent of disease at the time of BM diagnosis	
Isolated BM	12 (23)
BM+ other metastatic sites	22 (42.3)
BM+ locoregional disease	4 (7.6)
BM+ locoregional + other metastases	14 (26.9)

The blood calcium levels were normal in all cases.

Stimulated Tg levels at the time of diagnosis of BM (excluding two patients with positive TgAb) were available in 43 cases. They were < 100 ng/mL in 16% of patients, between 100-1000 ng/mL in 39.5% and > 1000 ng/mL in the remaining 46.5%.

Only one patient was not treated due to advanced disease and poor performance status. The remaining patients received treatment for their BM.

The treatment modalities included RAI therapy in 80.7% (n = 42; 30 of them received cumulative RAI doses larger than 600 mCi ^{131}I), intravenous monthly bisphosphonates in 57.6 % (n = 30) and 19 of them received pamidronate, while the remaining 11 were treated with zoledronate, surgery in 50% (n = 26), external beam radiotherapy 50% (n = 26), other therapies in 13.4% (sorafenib n = 4, doxorubicin n = 2, thalidomide and radiofrequency ablation, one patient each).

The mean follow-up after diagnosis of first BM was 34.4 ± 33.7 months (median: 24 months, range: 1-67 months). More than 50% of patients died of causes related to the DTC. Hürthle cell carcinoma (30 vs 0%, p 0,005) and fracture as a presenting symptom (20 vs 2.4%, p 0,007) were more frequent in patients who died of DTC-related causes. Radioiodine uptake was found less frequently in patients who died from DTC, although it did not reach statistical significance (40 vs. 61%, p ns). The status on last evaluation can be observed in Figure 1. All of the patients who were alive with persisting disease at the end of the follow-up period had an incomplete structural response.

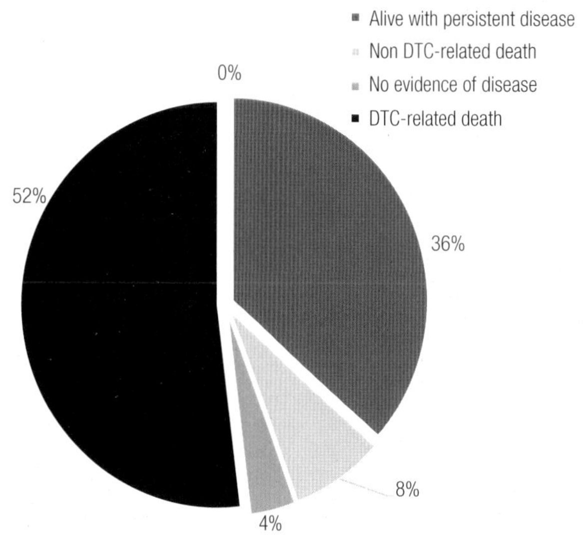

Figure 1. Status of patients with bone metastases from differentiated thyroid cancer at the end of follow-up.

When DTC-related causes of death (n = 27) were analyzed, 25.9% of the patients (n = 7) died of direct complications of BM or their treatment. The remaining 20 died of other complications related to other localizations of DTC (Table 3).

Table 3. Causes of death in 27 patients with bone metastases from differentiated thyroid cancer

Cause of death	Number of patients (%)
Non-BM related	20 (74.1)
Respiratory insufficiency	11
Airway obstruction	2
Central nervous system progression	2
Sepsis	2
Treatment complications	1
Other	4
Secondary to complications of BM	7 (25.9)
Pulmonary thromboembolism	3
Sepsis	1
Treatment complications	1
Other	2

The 2- and 5-year survival rates after the diagnosis of the first BM were 63.5% and 38%, respectively; the overall survival is depicted by the Kaplan-Meier curve in Figure 2.

The median overall survival was 24 months (range 1-120 months).

When we analyzed mortality related to BM (Table 4), the presence of papillary thyroid cancer and painful BM were more frequent in patients who died from causes not related to the BM.

Table 4. Analysis of variables related to mortality in patients who died from bone metastasis compared to those who died from other causes

	Death related to BM (n = 10)	Death related to other causes (n = 19)	P
< 45 years old	2 (20%)	4 (21.1%)	NS
≥ 45 years old	8 (80%)	15 (78.9%)	
Female	4 (40%)	9 (47.4%)	NS
Male	6 (60%)	10 (52.6%)	
Histology			
Papillary	3 (30%)	15 (78.9%)	0.02
Follicular	4 (40%)	4 (21.1%)	NS
Hürthle	3 (30%)	-	0.003
Synchronous	5 (50%)	6 (31.6%)	NS
Metachronous	4 (40%)	13 (68.4%)	
Asymptomatic	4 (40%)	7 (36.8%)	NS
Pain	1 (10%)	10 (52.6%)	0.03
Fracture	2 (20%)	1 (5.3%)	NS
Tumor	2 (20%)	-	
Other	1 (10%)	1 (5.3%)	NS
Positive RAI uptake	4 (40%)	14 (73.7%)	0.08
Solitary	4 (40%)	4 (21.1%)	NS
Multiple	6 (60%)	15 (78.9%)	

RAI: radioiodine; NS: non-significant.

DISCUSSION

Local or distant metastases occur in nearly 10% of patients with DTC (14). In this setting, therapeutic options may include the use of RAI, surgery, and/or the use of external beam radiotherapy (EBRT), among others (15). Nevertheless, between one-third to two-thirds of patients with metastatic DTC will become RAI

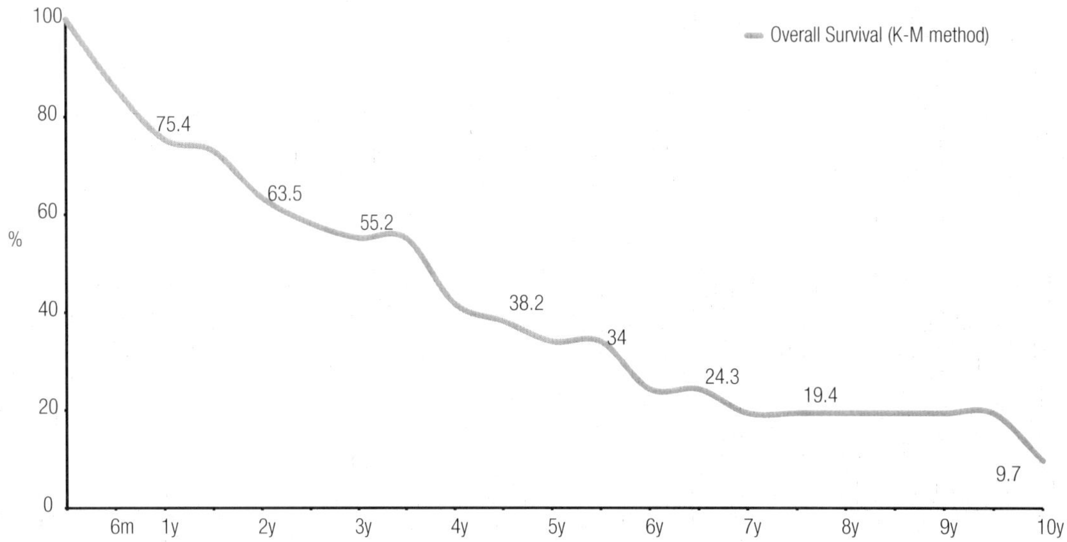

y: year; K-M: Kaplan-Meier.

Figure 2. Overall survival after the development of the first bone metastasis in patients with differentiated thyroid cancer (n = 52).

refractory, and this situation is often seen in patients with BM (8). As we observed in our study, most patients fulfill the current criteria for RAI refractoriness (16).

This subgroup of patients generally has a poor overall prognosis, with 10-year survival rates of only 10% and median survival from the discovery of metastases of only 3 to 5 years (8).

DTC has a high tendency to metastasize to bone compared to other tumors; it was reported to be the third most frequent solid tumor after breast and prostate cancer (17), although the physiopathology of BM from DTC is largely uncharacterized.

Follicular thyroid cancer and papillary thyroid cancer show different patterns of spread. The former has a higher propensity to disseminate to bones (7-28% versus 1.4-7% for with papillary thyroid cancer), probably due to a higher frequency of haematogenous dissemination (10,18). However, in absolute terms, in our study we found a greater number of patients with papillary carcinoma and BM, similar to that reported in other series (19). This finding is probably related to the overall higher incidence of papillary thyroid cancer compared to follicular thyroid cancer that, in most current series, comprises only 4 to 7% of the cases.

Skeletal related events (SRE), such as pathological fractures, spinal cord compression, pain and hypercalcemia, are frequent events that adversely affect the QoL of DTC patients with BM (20). As expected, in the present series, 65% of the patients presented symptoms related to BM.

Most of the BM are located in the spine (21) and, as a consequence, spinal cord compression may occur in 14 to 50% of the cases (22,23). In the present series, it was found in 11% of the cases.

Nearly half of the patients in our study presented with pain as the initial symptom. Osseous pain was more frequent in those patients who died due to causes not related to BM (52.6% vs. 10%). It is possible that pain may have led to an earlier BM diagnosis before severe complications occur.

The incidence of hypercalcemia in BM from DTC is variable and has been reported to be as low as 0-4% (19,20,23) to 25-37% (24). We found no cases of hypercalcemia in the present series. Tumoral hypercalcemia is mainly caused by parathyroid-hormone-related peptide secretion (25). Nevertheless, the physiopathology of hypercalcemia occurring in patients with DTC remains to be elucidated.

Considering the treatment modalities, a combination of multiple strategies is generally recommended for patients with BM from DTC (19). Nearly 90% of our patients received more than one option of treatment. In addition to ^{131}I therapy (81%), surgery (50%), EBRT (50%) and bisphophonates (60%) were frequently used. In selected cases, chemotherapy, sorafenib and radiofrequency ablation were also indicated.

RAI was used in 81% of patients in our series; 60% of them showed uptake of ^{131}I in BM. However, only one patient achieved remission after RAI as the only modality of treatment (cumulative activity of 400 mCi ^{131}I). Sabra and cols. demonstrated the lack of oncological benefit in the majority of patients treated with I-131 for distant metastases (9), highlighting that RAI therapy is rarely curative in these patients when used as a solitary therapy. However, an impact on the survival of patients treated with RAI was shown by some authors (19,22,26). Moreover, the complete surgical resection approach followed by RAI therapy has been related to better overall survival (19,27-29).

The complete resection of BM can rarely be achieved when bone disease comprises multiple sites (as was the case in 63% of our series) and the palliative resection of BM has less of an impact on survival (84.4% vs. 55.3%) (29). It should only be considered to obtain a better QoL (30). The mean 5-year survival in DTC patients with BM ranges from 41% to 87% (20,26,28,31). Accordingly, we found that 38% of patients in our series were alive 5 years after the diagnosis of the first BM.

Prognostic factors for cancer-specific mortality in patients with distant metastases from DTC have been widely studied (8,32-34). Most series consistently report that follicular carcinoma, poorly differentiated histology, a lack of radioiodine uptake, advanced age, widespread disease and BM *per se* are predictors of a worse prognosis and shorter overall survival. Poorly differentiated thyroid cancer patients were excluded from the present study; however, all of the remaining risk factors were found in the majority of our population. In this setting, other metastatic sites (such as the lung) or local recurrences are often the immediate causes of death. In the study by Kitamura and cols. (32), the causes of death were respiratory insufficiency (43%), circulatory failure (15%), hemorrhage (15%) and airway obstruction (13%). Nevertheless, in some cases it was not possible to identify the specific cause, due to the simultaneous compromise of several organs.

In the existing literature, the rates of mortality due exclusively to BM are variable and they are usually low (0 to 24%) (6,35,36). In our study, less than one-third of the deaths were directly related to BM. In the remaining cases, death was caused by other complications of advanced DTC, mainly related to respiratory events.

In conclusion, to our knowledge, this is the first multicentric study performed in Latin America on this topic. BM cause significant morbidity and should be managed with a multidisciplinary approach that aims to improve the QoL. Patient selection is important to tailor therapy to individual needs. Further studies with bone targeted agents are needed to assess the utility of these therapeutic modalities in DTC patients. BM are usually RAI refractory and are associated with a decrease in overall survival, although the causes of death are mainly related to complications of non-BM localizations of DTC.

Acknowledgements: members of Thyroid Department of the Sociedad Argentina de Endocrinología y Metabolismo: Abalovich Marcos, Alcaraz Graciela, Brenta Gabriela, Calabrese María, Castro Jozami Lorena, Cavallo Andrea, Corino Mirta, Fassi Juliana, Faure Eduardo, Frascaroli Genoveva, Gauna Alicia, Gutiérrez Silvia, Ilera Verónica, Iorcansky Sonia, Jaeger Mónica, Kjiezik María, Martínez María, Orlandi Ana, Puscar Ana, Russo Picasso María, Sala Mónica, Sartorio Gerardo, Schnitman Marta, Silva Croome María, Sklate Rosana, Storani María, Vazquez Adriana, Zunino Anabela. The authors would like to thank Marta Alarcón for her collaboration with data analysis.

REFERENCES

1. Hundahl SA, Fleming ID, Fremgen AM, Menck HR. A National Cancer Data Base report on 53,856 cases of thyroid carcinoma treated in the U.S., 1985-1995. Cancer. 1998;83(12):2638-48.
2. Ruegemer JJ, Hay ID, Bergstralh EJ, Ryan JJ, Offord KP, Gorman CA. Distant metastases in differentiated thyroid carcinoma: a multivariate analysis of prognostic variables. J Clin Endocrinol Metab. 1988;67(3):501-8.
3. Hoie J, Stenwig AE, Kullmann G, Lindegaard M. Distant metastases in papillary thyroid cancer. A review of 91 patients. Cancer. 1988;61:1-6.
4. Tickoo SK, Pittas AG, Adler M, Fazzari M, Larson SM, Robbins RJ, et al. Bone metastases from thyroid carcinoma: a histopathologic study with clinical correlates. Arch Pathol Lab Med. 2000;124(10):1440-7.
5. Schlumberger M, Tubiana M, De Vathaire F, Hill C, Gardet P, Travagli JP, et al. Long-term results of treatment of 238 patients with lung and bone metastases from differentiated thyroid carcinoma. J Clin Endocrinol Metab. 1986;63(4):960-67.
6. Samaan NA, Schultz PN, Hickey RC, Goepfert H, Haynie TP, Johnston DA, et al. The results of various modalities of treatment of well differentiated thyroid carcinomas: a retrospective review of 1599 patients. J Clin Endocrinol Metab. 1992;75(3):714-20.
7. Mazzaferri E. Thyroid carcinoma; papillary and follicular. In: Mazzaferri E, Saaman NA. Endocrine Tumors. Cambridge, MA: Blackwell Scientific; 1993. p. 278-333.
8. Durante C, Haddy N, Baudin E, Leboulleux S, Hartl D, Travagli JP, et al. Long term outcome of 444 patients with distant metastases from papillary and follicular thyroid carcinoma: benefits and limits of radioiodine therapy. J Clin Endocrinol Metab. 2006;91(8): 2892-9.
9. Sabra MM, Dominguez JM, Grewal RK, Larson SM, Ghossein RA, Tuttle RM, et al. Clinical outcomes and molecular profile of differentiated thyroid cancers with radioiodine-avid distant metastases. J Clin Endocrinol Metab. 2013;98(5):E829-36.
10. Wexler JA. Approach to the thyroid cancer patient with bone metastases. J Clin Endocrinol Metab. 2011;96(8):2296-307.
11. Weilbaecher KN, Guise TA, McCauley LK. Cancer to bone: a fatal attraction. Nat Reviews Cancer. 2011;11:411-25.
12. Edge S, Byrd D, Compton C, Fritz AG, Greene FL, Trotti A. Thyroid. In: American Joint Committee Cancer Staging Manual TNM Classsification 7Th Ed. New York, NY: Springer; 2010. p. 87-96.
13. Cooper DS, Doherty GM, Haugen BR, Kloss RT, Lee SL, Mandel SJ, et al. Revised American Thyroid Association management guidelines for patients with thyroid nodules and differentiated thyroid cancer. Thyroid. 2009;19:1167-214.
14. Muresan MM, Olivier P, Leclere J, Sirveaux F, Brunaud L, Klein M, et al. Bone metastases from differentiated thyroid carcinoma. Endocr Relat Cancer. 2008;15:37-49.
15. Haugen BR, Alexander EK, Bible KC, Doherty GM, Mandel SJ, Nikiforov YE, et al. 2015 American Thyroid Association management Guidelines for adult patients with thyroid nodules and differentiated thyroid cancer. Thyroid. 2016;26(1):1-133.
16. Schlumberger M, Brose M, Elisei R, Leboulleux S, Luster M, Pitoia F, et al. Definition and management of radioactive iodine-refractory differentiated thyroid cancer. Lancet Diabetes Endocrinol. 2014;2(5):356-8.
17. Coleman R. Clinical features of metastatic bone disease and risk of skeletal morbidity. Clin Cancer Res. 2006;12 (20 suppl):6243-9.
18. Kuschayeva YS, Kuschayev SV, Carroll NM, Felger EA, Links TP, Teytelboym OM, et al. Spinal metastases due to thyroid carcinoma: an analysis of 202 patients. Thyroid. 2014;24(10):1488-500.
19. Orita Y, Sugitani I, Matsuura M, Ushijima M, Tsukahara K, Fujimoto Y, et al. Prognostic factors and the therapeutic strategy for patients with bone metastasis from differentiated thyroid carcinoma. Surgery. 2010;147:424-31.
20. Farooki A, Leung V, Tala H, Tuttle RM. Skeletal-related events due to bone metastases from differentiated thyroid cancer. J Clin Endocrinol Metab. 2012;97(7):2433-9.
21. Zhang W, Liu D, Feng C, Zhou C, Zhan C, Que R, et al. Management of differentiated thyroid carcinoma with bone metastasis: a case report and review of the Chinese literature. J Zhejiang Univ Sci B. 2014;15(12):1081-7.
22. Pittas AG, Adler M, Fazzari M, Tickoo S, Rosai J, Larson SM, et al. Bone metastases from thyroid carcinoma: clinical characteristics and prognostic variables in one hundred forty-six patients. Thyroid. 2000;10(3):261-8.
23. Orita Y, Sugitani I, Takao S, Toda K, Manabe J, Miyata S. Prospective evaluation of zoledronic acid in the treatment of bone metastases from differentiated thyroid carcinoma. Ann Surg Oncol. 2015;22(12):4008-13.
24. Wu K, Hou S, Huang T, Yang R. Thyroid carcinoma with bone metastases: a prognostic factor study. Clin Med Oncol. 2008;2:129-34.

25. Mirrakhimov A. Hypercalcemia of malignancy: an update on pathogenesis and management. N Am J Med Sci. 2015;7:483-93.
26. Bernier MO, Leenhardt L, Hoang K, Aurengo A, Mary JY, Menegaux F, et al. Survival and therapeutic modalities in patients with bone metastases of differentiated thyroid carcinoma. J Clin Endocrinol Metab. 2001;86(4):1568-73.
27. Zettinig G, Fueger BJ, Passler C, Kaserer K, Pirich C, Dudczak R, et al. Long-term follow-up of patients with bone metastases from differentiated thyroid carcinoma – surgery or conventional therapy? Clin Endocrinol (Oxf). 2002;56(3):377-82.
28. Qiu Z-L, Song H-j, Xu Y-Hong, Luo Q-Y. Efficacy and survival analysis of I131 therapy for bone metastases from differentiated thyroid cancer. J Clin Endocrinol Metab. 2011;96(10):3078-86.
29. Nakayama R, Horiuchi K, Susa M, Watanabe I, Watanabe K, Tsuji T, et al. Clinical outcome after bone metastasis surgery in patients with differentiated thyroid carcinoma: a retrospective study of 40 cases. Jpn J Clin Oncol. 2014;44(10):918-25.
30. George R, Jeba J, Ramkumar G, Chacko AG, Tharyan P. Interventions for the treatment of metastatic extradural spinal cord compression in adults. Cochrane Database Syst Rev. 2015;(9):CD006716.
31. Do M, Rhee Y, Kim D, Kim C, Nam K, Ahn C, et al. Clinical features of bone metastasis resulting from thyroid cancer: a review of 28 patients over a 20-year period. Endocr J. 2005;52(6):701-7.
32. Kitamura Y, Shimizu K, Nagahama M, Sugino K, Ozaki O, Mimura T, et al. Immediate causes of death in thyroid carcinoma: clinicopathological analysis of 161 fatal cases. J Clin Endocrinol Metab. 1999;84(11):4043-9.
33. Eustatia-Rutten C, Corssmit E, Biermasz N, Pereira A, Romijn J, Smit J. Survival and death causes in differentiated thyroid carcinoma. J Clin Endocrinol Metab. 2006;91(1):313-9.
34. Lang BH, Wong KP, Cheung CY, Wan KY, Lo C. Evaluating the prognostic factors associated with cancer-specific survival of differentiated thyroid carcinoma presenting with distant metastasis. Ann Surg Oncol. 2013;20:1329-35.
35. Tollefsen HR, Decosse JJ, Hutter RV. Papillary carcinoma of the thyroid. A clinical and pathological study of 70 fatal cases. Cancer. 1964;17:1035-44.
36. Smith SA, Hay ID, Goellner JR, Ryan JJ, McConahey WM. Mortality from papillary thyroid carcinoma. A case-control study of 56 lethal cases. Cancer. 1988;62:1381-8.

Influence of the use of testosterone associated with physical training on some hematologic and physical parameters in older rats with alloxan-induced diabetes

Romeu Paulo Martins Silva[1,2], Rodrigo Otávio dos Santos[2], Nelson Eurípedes Matildes Junior[2], Antônio Vicente Mundim[3], Mario da Silva Garrote-Filho[3], Pâmella Ferreira Rodrigues[2], Nilson Penha-Silva[3]

[1] Centro de Ciências da Saúde e Desporto, Universidade Federal do Acre (UFAC), Rio Branco, AC, Brasil
[2] Centro Universitário do Planalto de Araxá (Uniaraxá), Araxá, MG, Brasil
[3] Instituto de Genética e Bioquímica, Universidade Federal de Uberlândia (UFU), Uberlândia, MG, Brasil

Correspondence to:
Romeu Paulo Martins Silva
Universidade Federal do Acre
Instituto de Genética e Bioquímica
BR 364, km 04
69920-900 – Rio Branco, AC, Brasil
romeupms@gmail.com

ABSTRACT

Objective: This study investigated the possible blood changes in wistar rats elderly with and without treatment with anabolic steroids submitted physical training. **Materials and methods:** Elderly rats (32) were divided into four groups: normal (N), treated normal (NT), diabetic (D) and treated diabetic (DT). They were submitted to 20 sessions of swimming with overload (5% body weight), 40 min/day for four weeks. The NT and DT groups received application of testosterone twice a week. At the end of the sessions, the animals were subjected to swimming until exhaustion and then killed for removal of blood and visceral fat. We evaluated maximum swim time, weight of visceral fat, erythrogram, leukogram, lipidogram and serum levels of glucose, lactate, aspartate aminotransferase and creatine kinase. The results were compared using one-way ANOVA followed by the *post hoc* Tukey test. **Results:** In elderly diabetic rats, the use of anabolic associated with physical training in older rats resulted in improvement in erythrogram, lipidogram and physical performance for high-intensity aerobic exercise. However, it was related to changes in leukocyte count, probably associated with inflammation. **Conclusion:** The combination of the use of testosterone with physical training, followed by maximal effort test caused changes hematological and biochemical can be associated with improvement in physiological characteristics, with increase of the swimming time and decrease of visceral fat levels, improvement in aerobic metabolism of fatty acids and glucose in normal and diabetic animals. Arch Endocrinol Metab. 2017;61(1):62-9

Keywords
Anabolic steroid; aging; diabetes; physical training

INTRODUCTION

Diabetes mellitus is characterized by a deficiency in the production or action of insulin, or both, resulting in increased blood glucose in untreated individuals (1).

Diabetes can be induced in experimental animals by chemical substances such as alloxan or streptozotocin. These substances cause irreversible lesions in the pancreatic cells producing insulin. This causes a large reduction in the production of insulin, which results in diabetes (2).

The deficiency of insulin causes loss of muscle mass due to exacerbation of the decline of proteolysis and protein anabolism.

Besides insulin, protein anabolism is also stimulated by testosterone, androgen steroid hormone produced by the testes and the adrenal (3). Testosterone promotes increased mass (4) and muscle strength (5).

There is evidence that treatment with these compounds can improve the resistance of skeletal muscle against fatigue, which increases the tolerance of experimental animals to physical activity (6).

The intense physical exercise can alter the concentration of blood cells and increase the use of glycogen, resulting in glucose fall (7,8) and increased production of lactic acid.

Testosterone can also assist in modulating the body's immune response (9), by changing the activity of leukocytes and other cells of defense (10).

Physical exercise causes numerous physiological and metabolic adjustments in the immediate or long term so that the body can supply a higher energy demand and to remain in homeostasis (11).

Although it is known that anabolic steroids can increase the tolerance to physical activity (6), the effects of the combination of many synthetic anabolic steroids with the exercise still need to be better known (12).

The purpose of this study was to analyze the effects of anabolic steroids on physical, hematological and biochemical variables in diabetic rats under aerobic physical training.

MATERIALS AND METHODS

The study was conducted in accordance with the recommendations of the Brazilian College of Animal Experimentation (COBEA), with the National Council for Animal Experiments Control (CONCEA) and with the Federal Law guidelines, 11,794, October 8, 2008 – Brazil.

Induction of diabetes by alloxan

Induction of experimental diabetes mellitus followed the protocols described in literature (13). After 24 hours of fasting, animals received intravenous injections (tail vein) of alloxan monohydrate (Sigma, St Louis, MO, USA) in 0.01 M citrate buffer, pH 4.5 (35 mg/kg body weight). The control rats underwent similar handling but only with injection of a citrate buffer solution. Two weeks after that treatment, rats that had levels of fasting glucose greater than or equal to 126 mg/dL were considered diabetic and used in the study (1).

Experimental groups

For this study we used 32 male albino rats (12 months) from Wistar race (*Rattus norvegicus*), distributed randomly into four groups (eight rats in each): normal animals without treatment (N), untreated diabetic animals (D) normal animals with treatment (NT) and diabetic animals with treatment (DT).

Containment and nutrition

The animals were kept in collective cages (100 x 50 x 30 cm) with an average of 3 rats per cage. The temperature inside the chamber of the vivarium was maintained between 22-25 °C in a room with controlled photoperiod set to 12 h of light and 12 h of darkness. All animals were fed with standard balanced diet and water *ad libitum*.

Adaptation and physical training

The animals were subjected to an adjustment period of two weeks. During this period, the animals were subjected to physical exercise with initial duration of 10 min. Every three days the duration of exercise increased by 10 min until reach 40 min at the end of two weeks, with rest on Saturdays and Sundays.

After the adjustment period, the animals maintained the 40 min of physical exercise for six weeks, Monday to Friday, between 2 and 5 PM. This period of training was higher than achieved in other studies. The exercises consisted of sessions of swimming with moderate intensity, with 5% body weight tied to the tail. The animals swam in an adapted tank with depth of 48 cm and water temperature maintained between 30 and 36 °C (14).

Treatment with anabolic

During the six weeks of physical training, the animals of the NT and DT groups received intramuscular injections of the mixture of esters of testosterone (testosterone propionate, 30 mg; testosterone phenyl propionate, 60 mg; testosterone isocaproate, 60 mg; testosterone decanoate, 100 mg; benzyl alcohol, 0.1 mL; and peanut oil, qs 1 mL) (Durateston™, Organon, Brazil), with syringes of 1 mL (15 mg/kg body weight) twice a week (on Tuesdays and Fridays at 4h30min PM).

Animals not treated with the anabolic (groups N and D) received intramuscular injections of peanut oil (15).

Test of maximum effort and sacrifice of animals

At the end of six weeks of training, the animals were subjected to intense physical exercise until exhaustion. It was considered that the exhaustion was achieved when the animal could not keep their noses out of the water for more than 10 s. Once the exhaustion was reached, the animals were removed from the water and placed on a bench. Body and tail were carefully dried with sterile paper towels. After the last session of exercise until exhaustion, the animals were anesthetized with ketamine and xylazine and sacrificed by decapitation in guillotine. Laparotomy was performed to collect the retroperitoneal fat, mesenteric and epididymal in analytical balance.

Collection of blood samples

The blood samples were taken at the end of six weeks of treatment. Before and after the exhaustion test, samples of 25 μl of blood were transferred from the tail of each animal, using heparinized capillary glass, directly into vials containing 50 μl of 1% sodium fluoride for inhibition of glycolytic activity. These samples were used for determination of glucose and lactate. After the exhaustion test, two blood aliquots were collected by cardiac puncture. The first sample (1 mL), collected in tubes containing K_3EDTA as anticoagulant, was used to perform the hematologic analyses. The second sample (3 mL), collected in tubes without anticoagulant, was centrifuged at 720 x *g* and the serum was transferred to sealed vials and stored under refrigeration until the time of biochemical analysis.

Dosage of glucose and lactate

The blood glucose was determined using the Accu-Chek apparatus (Roche, São Paulo, SP, Brazil). The blood lactate was analyzed by electro-enzymatic method in an automatic analyzer (YSI 1500 Sport L-Lactate, USI, Yellow Springs, Ohio, USA).

Erythrogram

The erythrogram, including the determination of the erythrocyte indices [mean corpuscular volume (MCV), mean corpuscular hemoglobin (MCH) and the mean corpuscular hemoglobin concentration (MCHC)], were performed in automated cell counter ABC Vet (ABX Diagnostics, Montpellier, France) using card specific to rats.

Leukogram

The leukometry was also carried out in the automatic cell counter ABC Vet (ABX Diagnostics, Montpellier, France). The identification and differential counting of leukocyte were performed with preparations stained by the method May-Grünwald-Giemsa in optical microscope.

Lipidogram and determination of serum activities of AST and CK

The activities of creatine kinase (CK) and aspartate aminotransferase (AST) and levels of total cholesterol, triacylglycerols (TAG) and cholesterol of high density lipoprotein (HDL-C) were determined by automated methods, using specific commercial kits (Labtest) in automatic multichannel analyzer (ChemWell, USA) previously calibrated and measured with calipers (Calibra 1H) and control serum (Qualitrol 1H). The cholesterol of lipoprotein, low-(LDL-C) was calculated using the equation LDL-C = total cholesterol - (HDL + TAG / 5) (16).

Statistical analysis

The results between the different groups were compared with use of ANOVA, with *post hoc* Tukey test, and were considered significantly different when $p < 0.05$. The tests were conducted using the application GraphPad Prism 5 (GraphPad Software, San Diego, CA, USA).

RESULTS

Table 1 presents the average values obtained in the erythrogram of different groups. The concentration of hemoglobin, the red cell count and hematocrit values were higher in treated groups NT and DT in relation to non-treated groups N and D ($p < 0.05$). But there was no difference in these parameters between diabetic and normal groups in the absence and in presence of treatment with anabolic ($p > 0.05$). The mean corpuscular volume (MCV) was also higher in treated groups (NT and DT) than in groups that were not treated with testosterone (N and D), being higher in DT group than in NT ($p < 0.05$). The mean corpuscular hemoglobin (MCH) was higher in treated groups (NT and DT) than in group N ($p < 0.05$). The mean corpuscular hemoglobin concentration (MCHC) was higher in the group of treated normal rats than in the other groups ($p < 0.05$).

Table 2 presents the results of leukocyte counts in different groups. The treated groups showed higher values of leukocytes in relation to the untreated animals ($p < 0.05$). But no difference was observed between diabetic and normal groups in both the absence and in presence of treatment with anabolic ($p > 0.05$). In relation to total neutrophils, the DT group had the highest count among all groups studied ($p < 0.05$). The situation was reversed in the count of lymphocytes, since it was lower in the DT group compared with group N ($p < 0.05$). The values of band neutrophils were lower in DT than in D ($p < 0.05$). The segmented neutrophils were higher only in the DT when compared with group N ($p < 0.05$). Regarding eosinophils there was no difference between groups ($p > 0.05$). For monocytes, the counts were lower in the DT group in comparison with D ($p < 0.05$).

Figure 1 shows the results obtained in lipidogram of rats of different groups. The concentrations of triacylglycerols (TAG) were significantly higher in group D than in all the other groups (N, NT and DT), for a ($p < 0.05$). The concentration of total cholesterol was higher in group D in relation to groups treated with the anabolic (DT and NT), for a ($p < 0.05$), but not in relation to the healthy rats without treatment (N), for a ($p > 0.05$). The values of HDL-C showed no changes resulting from physical training and treatment with testosterone ($p > 0.05$). The concentration of LDL-C was higher in group D only in relation to group NT ($p < 0.05$).

Table 1. Erythrogram of rats subjected to six weeks of regular exercise followed by maximal effort test

Variables	Without treatment		With treatment	
	Normal	Diabetic	Normal	Diabetic
Hemoglobin (g/dL)	12.67 ± 1.62[a]	12.63 ± 1.15[a]	14.61 ± 0.80[b]	14.61 ± 0.83[b]
Erythrocytes (10^6/µl)	8.09 ± 0.19[a]	7.78 ± 0.45[a]	8.85 ± 0.44[b]	8.69 ± 0.40[b]
Hematocrit (%)	45.50 ± 3.59[a]	44.85 ± 4.40[a]	51.32 ± 3.07[b]	51.77 ± 2.20[b]
MVC (µm^3)	52.57 ± 1.71[a]	55.62 ± 2.38[a]	57.25 ± 2.18[b,c]	59.62 ± 3.50[c]
MCH (pg)	16.50 ± 0.38[a]	17.60 ± 0.55[a,b]	17.86 ± 0.67[b]	17.93 ± 0.44[b]
MCHC (%)	30.21 ± 0.50[a]	31.30 ± 0.91[a]	32.61 ± 0.84	30.70 ± 1.24[a]

Averages followed by same letter are not different (Tukey) at a significance level of 0.05. MCV: mean corpuscular volume; MCH: mean corpuscular hemoglobin; MCHC: mean corpuscular hemoglobin concentration.

Table 2. Leucogram of Wistar rats submitted to six weeks of regular exercise followed by maximal effort test

Variables	Without treatment		With treatment	
	Normal	Diabetic	Normal	Diabetic
Leukocytes (cells/µl)	4100.0 ± 486.5[a]	4612.5 ± 458.0[a]	6025.0 ± 384.5[b]	6000.0 ± 1192.0[b]
Total neutrophils (%)	37.6 ± 7.7[a]	45.8 ± 11.15[a]	41.3 ± 7.0[a]	52.9 ± 5.2
Band neutrophils (%)	2.9 ± 0.9[a,b]	7.0 ± 5.6[a]	2,0 ± 1.4[b]	2.51 ± 0.9[b]
Segmented neutrophils (%)	34.7 ± 7.4[b]	38.8 ± 12.0[a,b]	39.3 ± 7.7[a,b]	50.4 ± 5.5[a]
Lymphocytes (%)	58.6 ± 5.4[b]	46.1 ± 12.1[a]	55.6 ± 5.6[a,b]	47.5 ± 5.1[a]
Eosinophils (%)	1.6 ± 0.5[a]	0.8 ± 0.7[a]	1.4 ± 0.5[a]	1.3 ± 0.7[a]
Basophils	0	0	0	0
Monocytes (%)	5.6 ± 1.5[a,b]	6.9 ± 3.9[a]	5.8 ± 3.5[a,b]	2.2 ± 2.0[b]

Averages followed by same letter are not different (Tukey) at a significance level of 0.05.

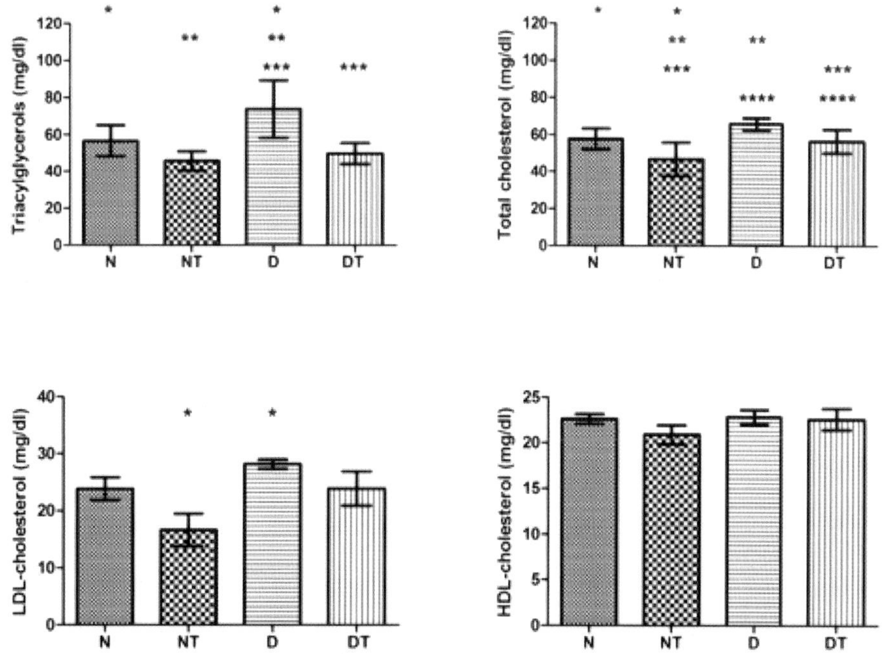

Figure 1. Plasma concentrations of triacylglycerols, total cholesterol, LDL-cholesterol and HDL-cholesterol after the maximal exercise test. The symbols N, NT, D and DT represent normal, treated normal, diabetic and treated diabetic rats, respectively. Values with the same symbol are significantly different (p < 0.05) when compared by Tukey test.

Figure 2 shows the values of glycemia and lactatemia before and after the test of maximal effort for rats of different groups. Before the test, blood glucose was higher in the D group, followed by the DT group ($p < 0.05$). The blood glucose values dropped significantly after the maximal effort test in all experimental groups, but still remained higher in group D ($p < 0.05$).

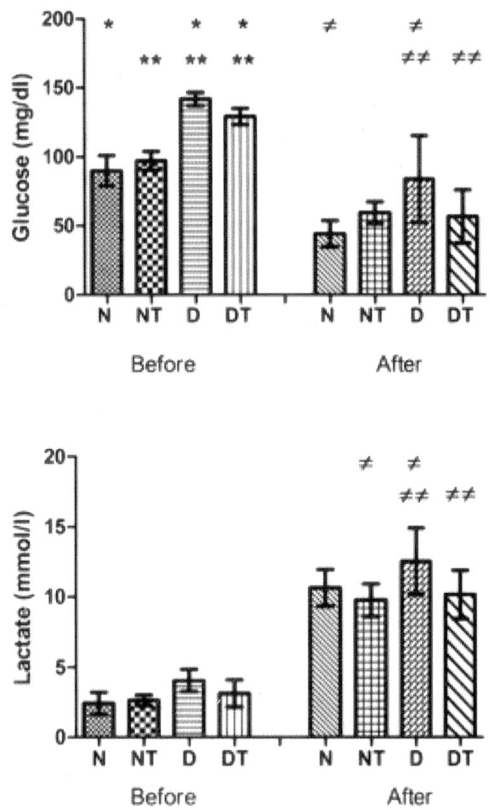

Figure 2. Plasma concentrations of glucose and lactate before and after the maximal exercise test. The symbols N, NT, D and DT represent normal, treated normal, diabetic and treated diabetic rats, respectively. Values with the same symbol are significantly different (p < 0.05) when compared by Tukey test.

Regarding lactatemia, there was no difference between groups before the effort test (Figure 2), for a ($p > 0.05$). After the test of maximum effort, the blood lactate concentration increased in all groups ($p < 0.05$). It increased more in group D compared to groups NT and DT ($p < 0.05$).

Figure 3 shows the activity values of AST and CK after the effort test in all experimental groups. The activity of AST was lower in animals of group NT compared to animals in groups D and DT. The activity of CK was higher in group D when compared to groups NT and DT.

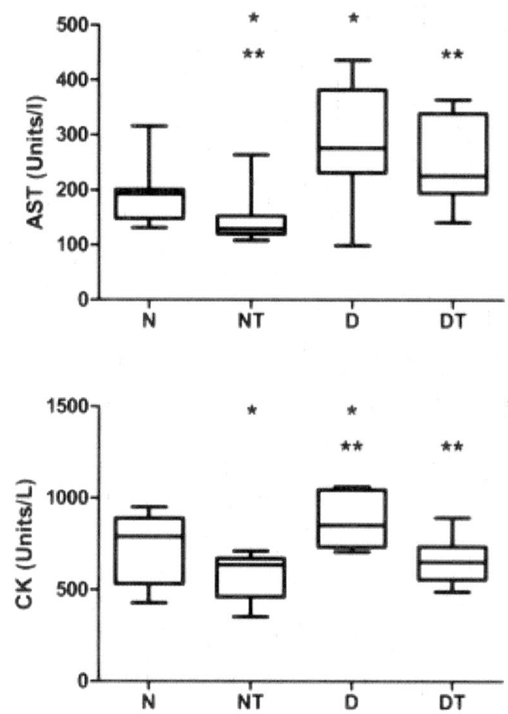

Figure 3. Plasma levels of activities of the enzymes aspartate aminotransferase (AST) and creatine kinase (CK) after the maximal exercise test. The symbols N, NT, D and DT represent normal, treated normal, diabetic and treated diabetic rats, respectively. Values with the same symbol are significantly different (p < 0.05) when compared by Tukey test.

Table 3 shows time of forced swim and weight of the visceral fat in rats of different groups. Animals treated with testosterone (NT and DT) had longer times of forced swimming than their respective non-treated controls (N and D), for a ($p < 0.05$). The amount of visceral fat was lower in groups treated with anabolic (NT and DT) in relation to their respective untreated controls (N and D), for a ($p < 0.05$).

Table 3. Swimming time and mass of visceral fat of rats submitted to six weeks of regular exercise followed by maximal effort test

Parameter	Without treatment		With treatment	
	Normal (n = 8)	Diabetic (n = 8)	Normal (n = 8)	Diabetic (n = 8)
Swimming time (min)	203.75 ± 71.92	119.16 ± 55.34	305.80 ± 34.36	163.80 ± 67.51
Visceral fat (g)	4.22 ± 1.84 (1.34%)	2.27 ± 1.72 (0.69%)	1.68 ± 0.93[a] (0.55%)	1.57 ± 0.65[a] (0.48%)

Averages followed by same letter are not different (Tukey) at a significance level of 0.05. Values between parentheses represent the percentage of visceral fat in relation to the body mass.

DISCUSSION

In the conditions considered in this study, treatment with testosterone produced an increase in the time of forced swimming in normal and diabetic rats in relation to their respective untreated controls. The hematological and biochemical records presented in this work should probably reflect some of the reasons that led to the change in performance of animals and any problems associated with treatment.

The decrease of CK in the diabetic rats treated with testosterone (Figure 3) seems a remarkable fact, since elevations in blood activities of CK and AST from the liver have been reported in athletes using anabolic steroids (17,18) and even in athletes who do not use these substances (19). It seems reasonable to admit, then, that the anabolic might have increased the resistance of skeletal muscle fibers against injury in the diabetic group.

Although elevation in CK had been also attributed to increased permeability of the sarcolemma during exercise (20,21), the activity levels of serum CK are good markers of muscle injury (22). The blood levels of CK are associated to the intensity of exercise when duration is kept constant (20). The metabolic stress and the actions of contraction and relaxation can cause mechanical stress to the point of damaging the muscle tissue (23). In fact, a suitable training program for the physical fitness should not lead to sharp increase in the activities of AST and CK in plasma or serum (24).

The swimming by longer time in the treated group could also be due to increased availability of fatty acids in plasma, due to the mobilization of fat stores, since visceral fat actually fell in the animals treated with the anabolic. Testosterone might be associated with reduction in visceral fat content (25,26), since that aged rats have more visceral fat and produce less testosterone.

The metabolism of fatty acids involves higher consumption of oxygen than metabolism of glycogen associated with anaerobic glycolysis. It is well known that an increased necessity of oxygen stimulates the release of erythropoietin and, consequently, the production of red blood cells. Indeed, the quantity of erythrocytes, the concentration of hemoglobin and hematocrit values were higher in treated animals. In fact, it was reported that testosterone causes increased erythropoiesis in mice (27). This improvement in the erythrogram of the treated group would favor the consumption of oxygen and would increase the energetic efficiency of the aerobic catabolism. Indeed, after the exhaustion test, the amount of lactate in the blood of the diabetic rats was lower in the treated group than in non-treated (Figure 2). This indicates that use of anabolic steroid associated to physical training was effective in aerobic conditioning of the animals.

Furthermore, the use of anabolic was associated with reduction in blood glucose, especially in the diabetic group (Figure 2), as would be desirable. This could be due to the action of testosterone in the increase of Glut4 transcription and enzymatic activities of hexokinase and phosphofructokinase (28).

Further evidence of better utilization of fat induced by treatment with testosterone is a decrease in blood levels of TAG in diabetic rats (Figure 1). The use of steroids combined with the practice of exercise increases the demand for fatty acids in energy metabolism, which certainly must be the factor responsible for decreased levels of TAG in this work.

The concentration of total cholesterol decreased significantly in healthy animals and in diabetic animals treated with testosterone, without association with changes in levels of HDL-cholesterol (Figure 1), what agrees with the results reported by (29,30). Unlike that article, however, there was no decrease in levels of LDL-cholesterol in our work.

Some differences between the responses associated with our experimental design in relation to the literature should be the result of the complexity of the system. Undoubtedly, there must be differences and antagonisms in the results of the combination of time, nature and intensity of exercises with the nature, dose and duration of treatment with anabolic steroids.

Although the acute exercise is associated with elevated levels of cortisol and catecholamines, which would decrease the amount of leukocytes (31,33), and predominantly with elevation in the blood levels of white cells (34), studies in rats with alloxan-induced diabetes have shown that physical exercise causes changes in the immune system and decrease in serum glucose (35,36).

In our study the combination of anabolic with the program of exercise, followed by the exhaustion test, was associated with increased number of leukocytes in healthy and diabetic rats (Table 2). This change should not be a consequence of the exhaustion test, but certainly of the use of anabolic, because the levels of leucocytes were higher in the groups treated with testosterone. These alterations could be due to decrease of oxygen in the blood or increase in mitotic activity of bone marrow cells, which may reflect exacerbation of the inflammatory processes, especially in the diabetic rats (29,37).

In conclusion, the combination of the use of testosterone with physical training during four weeks, followed by maximal effort test, produced elevations of hemoglobin, hematocrit and erythrocytes in healthy elderly rats and in elderly rats with alloxan-induced diabetes. Although these elevations had been greater in normal rats, they were associated with improvement in aerobic metabolism of fatty acids and glucose in diabetic animals. The hematological and biochemical changes were also associated with improvement in physiological characteristics, with increase of the swimming time and decrease of visceral fat levels in normal and diabetic animals. However, treatment with testosterone produced leukogram changes that may indicate exacerbation of inflammatory processes, especially among diabetic rats.

Financial source: this study was supported by grants from the funding agency *Fundação de Amparo à Pesquisa do Estado de Minas Gerais* (Fapemig).

Acknowledgment: this study was supported by federal Univesity of Uberlândia, especially the Institute of Genetics and Biochemistry.

REFERENCES

1. ADA. Diagnosis and classification of diabetes mellitus. Diabetes Care. 2013;36 Suppl 1:S67-74.
2. Elliott JI, Dewchand H, Altmann DM. Streptozotocin-induced diabetes in mice lacking alphabeta T cells. Clin Exp Immunol. 1997;109(1):116-20.
3. Shahidi NT. A review of the chemistry, biological action, and clinical applications of anabolic-androgenic steroids. Clin Ther. 2001;23(9):1355-90.
4. Bardin CW. The anabolic action of testosterone. N Engl J Med. 1996;335(1):52-3.
5. Bhasin S, Woodhouse L, Storer TW. Proof of the effect of testosterone on skeletal muscle. J Endocrinol. 2001;170(1):27-38.
6. Tamaki T, Uchiyama S, Uchiyama Y, Akatsuka A, Roy RR, Edgerton VR. Anabolic steroids increase exercise tolerance. Am J Physiol Endocrinol Metab. 2001;280(6):E973-81.
7. Cumming D. Influence of aerobic versus anaerobic exercise on male reproductive hormones. Clin J Sport Med. 1996;6(2):141.
8. Mackinnon LT. Immunity in athletes. Int J Sports Med. 1997;18 Suppl 1:S62-8.
9. Chao TC, Van Alten PJ, Walter RJ. Steroid sex hormones and macrophage function: modulation of reactive oxygen intermediates and nitrite release. Am J Reprod Immunol. 1994;32(1):43-52.
10. Mooradian AD, Morley JE, Korenman SG. Biological actions of androgens. Endocr Rev. 1987;8(1):1-28.
11. Koivisto V, Soman V, Nadel E, Tamborlane WV, Felig P. Exercise and Insulin – Insulin Binding, Insulin Mobilization, and Counterregulatory Hormone-Secretion. Federation Proceedings. 1980;39(5):1481-6.
12. Kennedy MC, O'Sullivan AJ. Do anabolic-androgenic steroids enhance sporting performance? Med J Aust. 1997;166(2):60-1.
13. Hegde PS, Rajasekaran NS, Chandra TS. Effects of the antioxidant properties of millet species on oxidative stress and glycemic status in alloxan-induced rats. Nutr Res. 2005;25(12):1109-20.
14. Ostman-Smith I. Adaptive changes in the sympathetic nervous system and some effector organs of the rat following long term exercise or cold acclimation and the role of cardiac sympathetic nerves in the genesis of compensatory cardiac hypertrophy. Acta Physiol Scand Suppl. 1979;477:1-118.
15. Trifunovic B, Norton GR, Duffield MJ, Avraam P, Woodiwiss AJ. An androgenic steroid decreases left ventricular compliance in rats. Am J Physiol. 1995;268(3 Pt 2):H1096-105.
16. Friedewald WT, Levy RI, Fredrickson DS. Estimation of the concentration of low-density lipoprotein cholesterol in plasma, without use of the preparative ultracentrifuge. Clin Chem. 1972;18(6):499-502.
17. Maravelias C, Dona A, Stefanidou M, Spiliopoulou C. Adverse effects of anabolic steroids in athletes – A constant threat. Toxicol Lett. 2005;158(3):167-75.
18. Alen M. Androgenic steroid effects on liver and red cells. Br J Sports Med. 1985;19(1):15-20.
19. Hough DO. Anabolic steroids and ergogenic aids. Am Fam Physician. 1990;41(4):1157-64.
20. Harris PA, Marlin DJ, Gray J. Plasma aspartate aminotransferase and creatine kinase activities in thoroughbred racehorses in relation to age, sex, exercise and training. Vet J. 1998;155(3):295-304.
21. Noakes TD. Effect of exercise on serum enzyme activities in humans. Sports Med. 1987;4(4):245-67.
22. Mujika I, Padilla S, Pyne D, Busso T. Physiological changes associated with the pre-event taper in athletes. Sports Med. 2004;34(13):891-927.
23. Lieber RL, Shah S, Friden J. Cytoskeletal disruption after eccentric contraction-induced muscle injury. Clin Orthop Relat Res. 2002(403 Suppl):S90-9.
24. Bogin E, Otto F, Ibañez A. Patologia Clínica Veterinária. Assunción: Maknografic; 1989. 192 p.
25. Tsai EC, Boyko EJ, Leonetti DL, Fujimoto WY. Low serum testosterone level as a predictor of increased visceral fat in Japanese-American men. Int J Obes Relat Metab Disord. 2000;24(4):485-91.
26. Kalinchenko SY, Tishova YA, Mskhalaya GJ, Gooren LJ, Giltay EJ, Saad F. Effects of testosterone supplementation on markers of the metabolic syndrome and inflammation in hypogonadal men with the metabolic syndrome: the double-blinded placebo-controlled Moscow study. Clin Endocrinol (Oxf). 2010;73(5):602-12.
27. Gordon AS, Zanjani ED, Levere RD, Kappas A. Stimulation of mammalian erythropoiesis by 5beta-H steroid metabolites. Proc Natl Acad Sci U S A. 1970;65(4):919-24
28. Sato K, Iemitsu M, Aizawa K, Ajisaka R. Testosterone and DHEA activate the glucose metabolism-related signaling pathway in skeletal muscle. Am J Physiol Endocrinol Metab. 2008;294(5):E961-8.
29. Ebenbichler CF, Sturm W, Ganzer H, Bodner J, Mangweth B, Ritsch A, et al. Flow-mediated, endothelium-dependent vasodilatation

is impaired in male body builders taking anabolic-androgenic steroids. Atherosclerosis. 2001;158(2):483-90.

30. Ginzburg E, Klimas N, Parvus C, Life J, Willix R, Barber MJ, et al. Long-term Safety of Testosterone and Growth Hormone Supplementation: A Retrospective Study of Metabolic, Cardiovascular, and Oncologic Outcomes. J Clin Med Res. 2010;2(4):159-66.
31. Nieman DC. Exercise effects on systemic immunity. Immunol Cell Biol. 2000;78(5):496-501.
32. Pyne DB, Gleeson M. Effects of intensive exercise training on immunity in athletes. Int J Sports Med. 1998;19 Suppl 3:S183-91; discussion S91-4.
33. Rowbottom DG, Green KJ. Acute exercise effects on the immune system. Med Sci Sports Exerc. 2000;32(7):S396-405.
34. Peake J, Nosaka K, Suzuki K. Characterization of inflammatory responses to eccentric exercise in humans. Exerc Immunol Rev. 2005;11:64-85.
35. Crespilho DM, de Almeida Leme JA, de Mello MA, Luciano E. Effects of physical training on the immune system in diabetic rats. Int J Diabetes Dev Ctries. 2010;30(1):33-7.
36. Paula FM, Leite NC, Vanzela EC, Kurauti MA, Freitas-Dias R, Carneiro Em, et al. Exercise Increases pancreatic β-cell viability in a model of type 1 diabetes through IL-6 signaling. FASEB. 2015;29(5):1805-16.
37. Puerta M, Nava MP, Venero C, Veiga JP. Hematology and Plasma Chemistry of House Sparrows (Passer-Domesticus) Along the Summer Months and after Testosterone Treatment. Comp Biochem Physiol A Physiol. 1995;110(4):303-7.

Controversial issues in the management of hyperprolactinemia and prolactinomas - An overview by the Neuroendocrinology Department of the Brazilian Society of Endocrinology and Metabolism

Lucio Vilar[1], Julio Abucham[2], José Luciano Albuquerque[1], Luiz Antônio Araujo[3], Monalisa F. Azevedo[4], Cesar Luiz Boguszewski[5], Luiz Augusto Casulari[4], Malebranche B. C. Cunha Neto[6], Mauro A. Czepielewski[7], Felipe H. G. Duarte[8], Manuel dos S. Faria[9], Monica R. Gadelha[10,11], Heraldo M. Garmes[12], Andrea Glezer[8], Maria Helane Gurgel[13], Raquel S. Jallad[8], Manoel Martins[13], Paulo A. C. Miranda[14], Renan M. Montenegro[13], Nina R. C. Musolino[6], Luciana A. Naves[4], Antônio Ribeiro-Oliveira Júnior[15], Cíntia M. S. Silva[10], Camila Viecceli[7], Marcello D. Bronstein[8]

[1] Serviço de Endocrinologia, Hospital das Clínicas, Universidade Federal de Pernambuco (UFPE), Recife, PE, Brasil
[2] Unidade de Neuroendócrino, Escola Paulista de Medicina, Universidade Federal de São Paulo (Unifesp/EPM), São Paulo, SP, Brasil [3] Centro de Endocrinologia e Diabetes de Joinville (Endoville), Joinville, SC, Brasil
[4] Serviço de Endocrinologia do Hospital Universitário de Brasília, Universidade de Brasília (UnB), Brasília, DF, Brasil
[5] Serviço de Endocrinologia e Metabologia, Hospital de Clínicas, Universidade Federal do Paraná (SEMPR), Curitiba, PR, Brasil
[6] Divisão de Neurocirurgia Funcional, Instituto de Psiquiatria do Hospital das Clínicas, Faculdade de Medicina da Universidade de São Paulo (IPq-HC-FMUSP), São Paulo, SP, Brasil [7] Serviço de Endocrinologia, Hospital de Clínicas de Porto Alegre, PPG Endocrinologia, Faculdade de Medicina, Universidade Federal do Rio Grande do Sul (UFRGS), Porto Alegre, RS, Brasil
[8] Serviço de Endocrinologia, Hospital das Clínicas, Faculdade de Medicina da Universidade de São Paulo (FMUSP), São Paulo, SP, Brasil [9] Serviço de Endocrinologia, Hospital Universitário Presidente Dutra, Universidade Federal do Maranhão (UFMA), São Luís, MA, Brasil
[10] Serviço de Endocrinologia, Hospital Universitário Clementino Fraga Filho, Universidade Federal do Rio de Janeiro (HUCFF-UFRJ), Rio de Janeiro, RJ, Brasil
[11] Unidade de Neuroendocrinologia, Instituto Estadual do Cérebro Paulo Niemeyer, Rio de Janeiro, RJ, Brasil
[12] Departamento de Clínica Médica, Faculdade de Ciências Médicas, Universidade Estadual de Campinas (FCM/Unicamp), Campinas, SP, Brasil
[13] Serviço de Endocrinologia, Hospital Universitário Walter Cantídio, Universidade Federal do Ceará (UFCE), Fortaleza, CE, Brasil
[14] Serviço de Endocrinologia e Metabologia, Santa Casa de Belo Horizonte, Belo Horizonte, MG, Brasil
[15] Serviço de Endocrinologia, Hospital das Clínicas, Universidade Federal de Minas Gerais (UFMG), Belo Horizonte, MG, Brasil

ABSTRACT

Prolactinomas are the most common pituitary adenomas (approximately 40% of cases), and they represent an important cause of hypogonadism and infertility in both sexes. The magnitude of prolactin (PRL) elevation can be useful in determining the etiology of hyperprolactinemia. Indeed, PRL levels > 250 ng/mL are highly suggestive of the presence of a prolactinoma. In contrast, most patients with stalk dysfunction, drug-induced hyperprolactinemia or systemic diseases present with PRL levels < 100 ng/mL. However, exceptions to these rules are not rare. On the other hand, among patients with macroprolactinomas (MACs), artificially low PRL levels may result from the so-called "hook effect". Patients harboring cystic MACs may also present with a mild PRL elevation. The screening for macroprolactin is mostly indicated for asymptomatic patients and those with apparent idiopathic hyperprolactinemia. Dopamine agonists (DAs) are the treatment of choice for prolactinomas, particularly cabergoline, which is more effective and better tolerated than bromocriptine. After 2 years of successful treatment, DA withdrawal should be considered in all cases of microprolactinomas and in selected cases of MACs. In this publication, the goal of the Neuroendocrinology Department of the Brazilian Society of Endocrinology and Metabolism (SBEM) is to provide a review of the diagnosis and treatment of hyperprolactinemia and prolactinomas, emphasizing controversial issues regarding these topics. This review is based on data published in the literature and the authors' experience. Arch Endocrinol Metab. 2018;62(2):236-63

Keywords

Hyperprolactinemia; prolactinomas; pseudoprolactinomas; macroprolactin; hook-effect; dopamine agonists; pituitary surgery; temozolomide

Correspondence to:
Lucio Vilar Hospital das Clínicas, Departamento de Medicina Clínica Av. Prof. Moraes Rego, 1235, Cidade Universitária 50670-901 – Recife, PE, Brasil lvilarf@gmail.com

INTRODUCTION

Hyperprolactinemia has multiple etiologies (Table 1) and is the most common endocrine disorder of the hypothalamic-pituitary axis (1-3). A prolactinoma is the most common cause of chronic hyperprolactinemia once pregnancy, primary hypothyroidism, and drugs that raise serum prolactin (PRL) levels have been ruled out (4-6).

Prolactinomas are the most common hormone-secreting pituitary tumors,accounting for approximately 40% of all pituitary tumors (2,6) In adults, prolactinomas have an estimated prevalence of 60-100 per million population (7,8), and in a population from three different districts of Belgium, prolactinomas have been reported to represent 73.3% of all pituitary adenomas, with a higher prevalence in women (78.2%) (9). Between the age of 20 and 50 years, the ratio between women and men is estimated to be 10:1, whereas after the fifth decade of life, both genders are equally affected (10,11). Although prolactinomas are rare at the pediatric and adolescent ages, they account for approximately half of all pituitary adenomas in that population (12). PRL-secreting carcinomas are extremely rare (13).

Table 1. Causes of hyperprolactinemia

Physiologic

- Pregnancy; lactation; stress; sleep; coitus; exercise

Pathologic

- Systemic diseases – Primary hypothyroidism; adrenal insufficiency; renal insufficiency; cirrhosis; pseudocyesis; epileptic seizures
- Hypothalamic diseases – tumors (craniopharyngiomas, dysgerminomas, meningiomas, etc.); infiltrative disorders (histiocytosis, sarcoidosis, etc.), metastasis; cranial radiation; Rathke's cleft cysts, etc.
- Pituitary diseases – Prolactinomas; acromegaly; thyrotropinomas; Cushing's disease; infiltrative disorders; metastasis; lymphocytic hypophysitis; empty sella syndrome, etc.
- Stalk disorders – Hastitis; seccion; traumatic brain injury
- Neurogenic – Chest wall lesions (burns; breast surgery; thoracotomy; nipple rings; herpes zoster, etc.); spinal cord injury (cervical ependymoma; tabes dorsalis; extrinsic tumors, etc.), breast stimulation, etc.
- Idiopathic
- Ectopic prolactin production – Renal cell carcinoma; ovarian teratomas; gonadoblastoma; non-Hodgkin lymphoma, uterine cervical carcinoma; colorectal adenocarcinoma, etc.)

Macroprolactinemia

Drug-induced (Table 3)

Adapted from Ref. 1.

The most characteristic signs and symptoms found in patients with hyperprolactinemia are those related to hypogonadotropic hypogonadism and galactorrhea (1,3,7). Increased PRL levels decrease gonadotropin pulsatile secretion through inhibition of hypothalamic GnRH release (14). In addition, there may be direct effects of hyperprolactinemia on testes and ovaries. Hypogonadism can cause menstrual irregularity and amenorrhea in women, sexual dysfunction, infertility, and loss of bone mineral mass in both genders (15,16). Hyperprolactinemia can also reduce the libido independently of testosterone levels (17). In patients harboring macroprolactinomas, tumor mass effect symptoms, such as headache, visual changes, and, more rarely, cerebrospinal fluid (CSF) rhinorrhea, hydrocephalus and seizures, can also occur (1-3). Hypopituitarism beyond hypogonadism can occur if there is compression of the pituitary stalk or destruction of normal pituitary tissue (3,6,7). It is worth commenting that some women present with non-puerperal galactorrhea in the presence of regular menstrual cycles and normal PRL levels (18,19). This so-called "idiopathic galactorrhea" is estimated to be present in up to 40-50% of all women with non-puerperal galactorrhea (19,20). In contrast, the finding of galactorrhea in men is highly suggestive of a prolactinoma (2,18).

In this publication, the goal of the Neuroendocrinology Department of the Brazilian Society of Endocrinology and Metabolism (SBEM) is to provide a review on the diagnosis and treatment of hyperprolactinemia and prolactinomas, emphasizing controversial issues regarding these topics.

PROLACTIN SERUM ISOFORMS

The PRL size is heterogeneous in terms of circulating molecular forms. The predominant form in healthy subjects and in patients with prolactinomas is monomeric PRL (molecular weight of 23 kDa), while dimeric or big PRL (45-60 kDa) and big-big PRL or macroprolactin (150-170 kDa) correspond to less than 20% of the total PRL (20,21). When the serum of a patient with hyperprolactinemia contains mostly macroprolactin, the condition is termed macroprolactinemia (22,23). In up to 90% of cases, macroprolactin is composed of a complex formed by an IgG and monomeric PRL (2,24-29).

DIAGNOSTIC EVALUATION

For the correct identification of the etiology of hyperprolactinemia, some parameters must be taken into account: medical history, physical examination, clinical features, laboratory findings (especially PRL serum levels), and imaging studies of the pituitary and sella turcica (1,3,5). Furthermore, the screening for macroprolactinemia should often be considered, particularly in cases of asymptomatic hyperprolactinemia (3-5).

In addition to PRL determination, TSH, free T_4, and creatinine levels should be obtained to rule out secondary causes of hyperprolactinemia (1,3,6). Moreover, acromegaly must be investigated by measuring IGF-1 in all patients with a macroadenoma, even when there are no manifestations of this disease (30). Finally, β-hCG measurement is mandatory in any woman of childbearing age with amenorrhea (1,3).

1. CONTROVERSIAL ISSUES REGARDING DIAGNOSIS

1.1. Environmental influences on PRL secretion

Prolactin is secreted in a pulsatile manner, and serum levels can vary greatly throughout the day, with higher levels during sleep, a morning peak and a gradual decline after awakening, but without a typical circadian rhythm. Under normal conditions, ~50% of the total daily production of PRL occurs during the sleep period. Thus, samples should be collected up to 3 hours after awakening, preferably while the patient is fasted (1,4).

Stress from any source, whether psychological, induced by exercise or due to other acute illness, leads to the physiological elevation of PRL levels (2,3,5). However, supine rest is not necessary prior to sampling, contrary to what was believed in the past (31). Venipuncture stress may cause an elevation in the PRL level, but it is usually mild (< 40-60 ng/mL) (32). The same is true for breast stimulation (1,2,33). Moreover, as PRL is secreted episodically, its levels measured during the day may possibly be beyond the upper limit of normality for a particular laboratory in healthy individuals (1,3). Therefore, an elevated PRL level should be confirmed at least once (33) unless the PRL levels are clearly elevated (> 80-100 ng/mL) (1). Nevertheless, according to the guidelines of the Endocrine Society, a single PRL level above the upper limit of normal confirms the diagnosis of hyperprolactinemia, as long as the serum sample was obtained without excessive venipuncture stress (4).

COMMENT 1: As PRL is secreted in a pulsatile manner and as venipuncture stress can increase PRL levels, we suggest that an elevated PRL level should be confirmed at least once, unless the PRL levels are clearly elevated (> 80-100 ng/mL).

COMMENT 2: Vigorous exercise and nipple stimulation should be avoided for at least 30 minutes before checking PRL levels as they may result in PRL elevation.

1.2 Accuracy of prolactin levels

The magnitude of PRL elevation can be useful in determining the etiology of hyperprolactinemia because the highest values are observed in patients with prolactinomas (1-5,33,34). For example, levels > 250 ng/mL are highly suggestive of the presence of a prolactinoma (3-5), although they may occasionally be found in other conditions (1,34), as commented on below. In contrast, most patients with stalk dysfunction (pseudoprolactinomas), drug-induced hyperprolactinemia or systemic diseases present with PRL levels < 100 ng/mL (1,4,34). However, exceptions to these rules are not rare (1,34).

In patients with prolactinomas, circulating PRL levels usually parallel the tumor size (1,4,7). Indeed, microprolactinomas (MIC) (diameter < 10 mm) usually result in PRL levels of 100-200 ng/mL, but not infrequently, they may be < 100 ng/mL, and occasionally reach 500 ng/mL or more (1,33,34). Macroprolactinomas (MACs) (diameter ≥ 10 mm) are typically associated with PRL values > 250 ng/mL (4-7). In the vast majority of patients with giant prolactinomas (maximum diameter ≥ 4 cm), PRL levels will be > 1000 ng/mL (35,36). On the other hand, artificially low PRL levels may result from the so-called "hook effect", which should be considered in all cases of large (≥ 3 cm) pituitary macroadenomas associated with normal or mildly elevated PRL levels (< 200 ng/mL) (1,37-39), as commented on below. Patients harboring cystic MACs may also present with mild PRL elevation (1-3).

The Brazilian Multicenter Study on Hyperprolactinemia (BMSH) analyzed 1234 patients whose results are presented in Figure 1 and Table 2 (34). In this study, only patients harboring prolactinomas presented with PRL values ≥ 500 ng/nL (34).

1.2.1 How do PRL levels behave in cases of pseudoprolactinomas?

In patients with "pseudoprolactinomas", whose main etiology isa nonfunctioning pituitary adenoma (NFPA), hyperprolactinemia results from compression of the pituitary stalk (2,40). In that situation, this so-

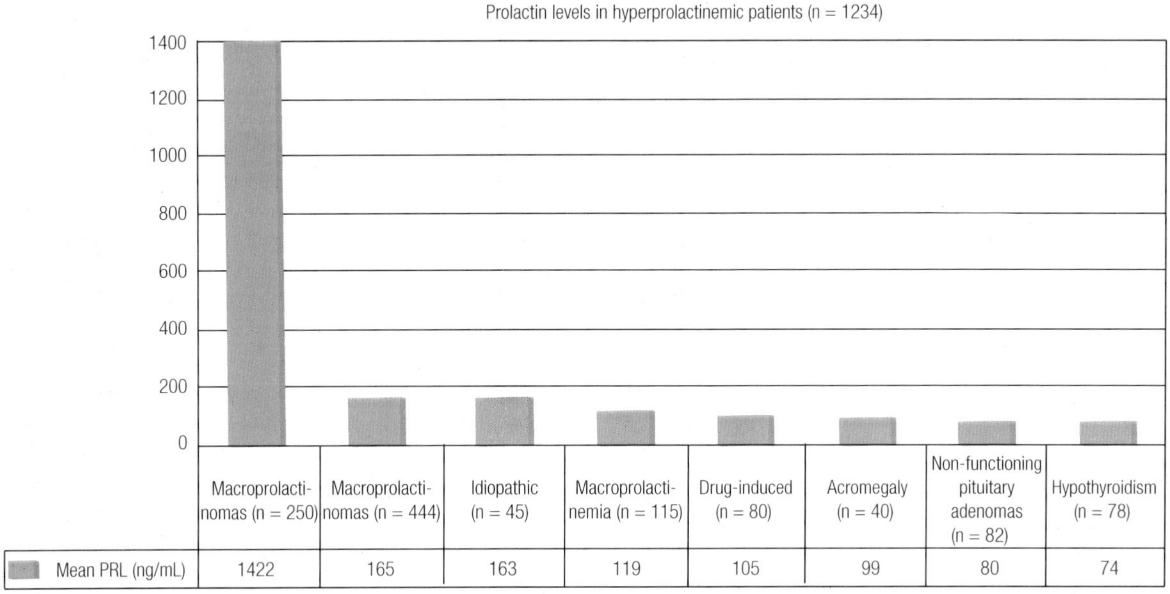

Figure 1. PRL levels according to the etiology of the hyperprolactinemia in the Brazilian multicenter study on hyperprolactinemia (Adapted from Ref. 34).

Table 2. Prolactin levels (ng/mL) according to the etiology of the hyperprolactinemia in the Brazilian Multicenter Study on Hyperprolactinemia

Etiology	N (%)	Mean PRL (range) (ng/mL)
Macroprolactinomas	250 (20.2)	1422.9 ± 3134.7 (108-21,200)
Microprolactinomas	444 (36)	165.6 ± 255.1 (32-525)
Idiopathic	45 (3.6)	163.9 ± 81.8 (46-328)
Macroprolactinemia	115 (9.3)	119.5 ± 112.9 (32.5-404)
Drug-induced	180 (14.6)	105.1 ± 73.2 (28-380)
Acromegaly	40 (3.2)	99.3 ± 57.4 (28-275)
NFPA	82 (6.6)	80.9 ± 54.5 (28-490)
Primary hypothyroidism	78 (6.3)	74.6 ± 42.4 (30-253)

NFPA: Non-functioning pituitary adenomas. Adapted from Ref. 34.

called disconnection hyperprolactinemia is thought to result from loss of the inhibitory effect of dopamine on PRL secretion (19). NFPAs represent the principal differential diagnosis of macroprolactinomas, as they require distinct treatments and have a distinct natural history and prognosis (1,40). The term pseudoprolactinomas also includes other conditions such as craniopharyngiomas, Rathke´s cleft cysts, sarcoidosis, Langerhans-cell histiocytosis and metastasis (19,40).

Based on a large series of histologically confirmed cases (n = 226) with NFPA, serum PRL > 2000 mIU/L (> 95 ng/mL) is almost never (< 2%) encountered in these patients (41). Accordingly, in a recent study, among 64 patients with immunohistochemically confirmed NFPAs, PRL levels ranged from 33 to 250 ng/mL (~80% < 100 ng/mL) (42) By contrast, in BMSH, among 82 patients with NFPA, PRL levels ranged from 28 to 490 ng/mL (< 100 ng/mL in 82%); however, not all patients had been submitted to immunohistochemical evaluation (Table 3) (34).

COMMENT 3: In cases of non-functioning pituitary adenomas, hyperprolactinemia results from stalk compression, and thus, prolactin (PRL) levels are modestly elevated (< 100 ng/mL) in the great majority of cases. Values > 250 ng/mL are exceedingly rare. By contrast, in patients with macroprolactinomas, PRL levels are usually > 250 ng/mL, and not infrequently, they exceed 1000 ng/mL. However, PRL levels may be misleadingly low due to the hook effect or in patients with cystic macroprolactinomas.

1.2.2 How do PRL levels behave in cases of drug-induced hyperprolactinemia?

The most common cause of non-physiological hyperprolactinemia is the use of drugs, which act through different mechanisms: increased transcription of the PRL gene (*estrogens*), antagonism of the dopamine receptor (*risperidone, haloperidol, metoclopramide, domperidone, sulpiride, etc.*), dopamine depletion (*reserpine, methyldopa*), inhibition of hypothalamic dopamine production (*verapamil, heroin, morphine, enkephalin analogs, etc.*), inhibition of dopamine reuptake (*tricyclic antidepressants, cocaine, amphetamine, monoamine oxidase inhibitors*), inhibition of serotonin reuptake (opiates, fenfluramine, fluoxetine, sibutramine), etc. (1,2,42-47) (Table 3).

Table 3. Drug-induced hyperprolactinemia

Antipsychotics
- Typical – Phenothiazines; butirophenones; thyoxanthenes
- Atypical – Risperidone; molindone; amisulpride; quetiapine; olanzapine

Antidepressants
- Tricyclics – Amitriptyline; desipramine; clomipramine
- MAO inhibitors – Pargyline; clorgyline
- SSRIs – Fluoxetine; citalopram; paroxetine

Antihypertensive drugs
- Verapamil; α-methyldopa; reserpine; labetolol

Anticonvulsivants
- Phenytoin

Prokinetic agents
- Metoclopramide; domperidone; bromopride

Others
- Estrogens; anesthetics; cimetidine; ranitidine; opiates; methadone; morphine; apomorphine; heroin; cocaine; marijuana; alcohol; sibutramine, etc.

MAO: monoamine oxidase; SSRIs: selective serotonin re-uptake inhibitors. Adapted from Refs. 1, 2, and 3.

In the Brazilian Multicenter Study on Hyperprolactinemia (BMSH), antidepressants and neuroleptics (in monotherapy or in combination) were the culprits in a large majority of the cases (82.2%) (34). Among antipsychotics, the most frequently involved drugs were haloperidol, phenothiazines, and risperidone, while tricyclic drugs were the main representants among the antidepressants (34). Other studies found the following rates of hyperprolactinemia associated with each therapeutic drug class: 31% for neuroleptics, 28% for neuroleptic-like drugs, 26% for antidepressants, 5% for H2-receptor antagonists, and 10% for other drugs (45). In one group of 106 patients receiving antipsychotics, hyperprolactinemia was present in 81%, 35%, 29%, and 38% of patients taking risperidone, olanzapine, ziprasidone, and typical antipsychotics, respectively (46).

The newer atypical antipsychotics (AAPs) are characterized by increased antipsychotic efficacy and fewer neurological and endocrine related side-effects compared to classical antipsychotic drugs (45,46). With the exception of risperidone, amisulpride and molindone, which are often associated with high PRL levels (45), most of the AAPs elicit a poor hyperprolactinemic response or no hyperprolactinemia at all (43,45,46). Furthermore, the use of drugs such as quetiapine and aripiprazole (a dopamine partial agonist) was shown to be associated with resolution of the hyperprolactinemia induced by other AAPs (48). Moreover, decreased PRL levels were also reported when aripiprazole was used as adjunct therapy to risperidone (49).

Antidepressants induce hyperprolactinemia in a small proportion of patients, but they rarely elevate PRL to a significant degree (46). Among 80 patients treated with fluoxetine, only 10 (12.5% developed hyperprolactinemia, with 38 ng/mL being the highest PRL level (50). Atypical antidepressants, including bupropion and mirtazapine, appear to have no effect on PRL levels (44,47).

Although PRL elevation is usually mild (25-100 ng/mL) in cases of drug-induced hyperprolactinemia, it is also highly variable. Indeed, metoclopramide, risperidone, and phenothiazines can lead to prolactin levels > 200 ng/mL (1,43-46). Among 180 cases enrolled in the BMSH, most (64%) presented with PRL levels < 100 ng/mL, but in 5%, they exceeded 250 ng/mL (range, 28-380; mean, 105.1 ± 73.2) (Table 3) (34). Interestingly, PRL levels of 720 ng/mL were recently reported in a young lady who had been treated with domperidone for 3 months. Following domperidone discontinuation, PRL fell to the normal range (51).

COMMENT 4: Although drug-induced hyperprolactinemia is usually associated with PRL levels < 100 ng/mL, they are largely variable and may overlap those found in patients with prolactinomas.

1.2.3 How do the hook effect and linearity issues in PRL assays impact our practice?

Immunometric assays have greatly improved the sensitivity of PRL and other hormone measurements. They are usually performed through capture antibodies that are immobilized in a solid phase, and a second antibodyis labeled a signal generator. These antibodies bind to different epitopes of the PRL to be quantified, thus forming a "sandwich" test using either a fluorescent or chemiluminescent marker. The relative antigen-to-antibody proportion influences its interaction and may compromise the appropriate formation of the immunocomplexes. Thus, extremely high concentrations of PRL can simultaneously saturate both the capture and the labeled antibody when only a few PRL molecules are actually bound in a sandwich complex to be quantified by the test. In that situation, most of the PRL molecules are bound to just one antibody instead and are subsequently washed away (Figure 2). Therefore, falsely low results are reported, and the correct result for the PRL concentration is much higher than reported. This artifact is called a high-dose hook effect, also known as the prozone phenomenon, and the reported results are usually within or, more often, slightly above the manufacturer´s reference range (52,53).

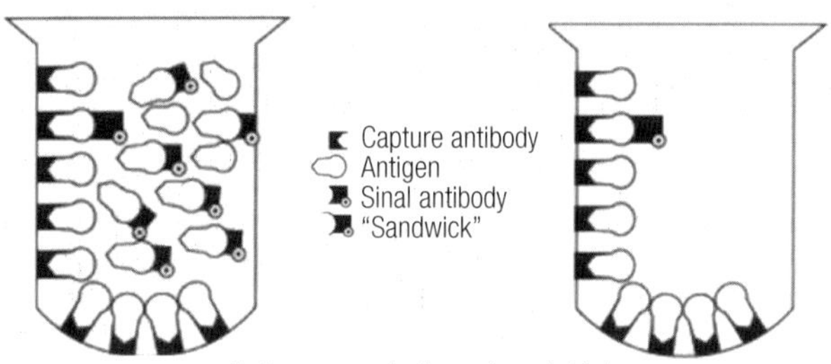

Figure 2. Schematic depiction of "hook effect." *Left*, Extremely high antigen concentrations saturate both capture and signal antibodies and prevent "sandwich" formation. *Right*, When liquid phase is discarded, most of the antigen is lost with the signal antibody; thus, antigen concentration is measured as low (Adapted from Ref. 39).

The hook effect differs between the different assay systems used in clinical practice. Dilution of the sample at 1:100 is the test of choice to unmask this hook effect (1,4). Indeed, this step will result in a dramatic rise in PRL levels if the patient has a macroprolactinoma, remaining low in cases of non-functioning pituitary adenomas (1,4,37,38).

Physicians should keep in mind that laboratories cannot dilute all samples on a routine basis to rule out the hook effect. Thus, it is extremely important that they are aware of the phenomenon so they do not forget to order dilution for all PRL samples suspected to be overconcentrated. In clinical practice, this means that dilutions must be ordered for PRL measurements in all patients with macroadenomas ³ 3 cm and initial PRL levels < 200 ng/mL, even if the PRL levels are normal (1,2,38). However, it is relevant to mention that dilutions ordered by physicians are performed at the discretion of laboratory workers. This means that, according to the reportable reference range of an assay and its reported levels of hook effect by the respective manufacturer, dilutions may occasionally start at 1:10. For instance, considering an assay in which, according to its manufacturer, the hook effect is not supposed to be induced up to a PRL value of 20,680 ng/mL, this theoretically means that a starting dilution of 1:10 should be sufficient enough to detect the phenomenon, as it is very improbable to have a PRL value higher than 200,680 ng/mL (53). In this regard, it is noteworthy that unnecessary dilutions usually cause a loss of accuracy in measurements. Fortunately, with the newer assays, extremely high levels of PRL are usually necessary to hook the assay, and this fact has dramatically decreased the incidence of this phenomenon (53,54).

Interestingly, the hook effect has often been confused with assay linearity problems by clinicians (54). In a given assay with a reportable PRL ranging from 0.25-200 ng/mL according to the manufacturer, PRL samples coming from patients with untreated macroprolactinomas may often fall out of this reportable range, even when an automatic dilution of 1:10 is superimposed. In this case, it is common that the laboratory releases a result of "> 2000 ng/mL", and it seems that they are not aware of the importance of exact quantification of the result. Therefore, clinicians must refrain from starting treatment until the laboratory re-assays the sample at further dilutions, even if it has to be performed manually, and up to the point that the linear range of the assay is reached. Otherwise, the observed effect of a treatment may be misled due to an inexact reported measurement (53,54).

COMMENT 5: The hook effect should be considered in every patient presenting with a large (≥ 3 cm) pituitary macroadenoma and prolactin levels within the normal range or only modestly elevated.

1.3 Macroprolactinemia screening: routinely or just in asymptomatic individuals?

Macroprolactinemia is a condition where more than 60% of circulating PRL is made up of macroprolactin (1,29). In most of the *in vitro* studies, macroprolactin was shown to display low biological activity (28,29,55). This is corroborated by the finding that in most series with macroprolactinemia, individuals are pauci- or asymptomatic (56,57), with no need to perform sellar imaging (58) or specific treatments (58,59). Others argued that the binding of PRL to their receptor could be blocked by modification of the tertiary structure of the original molecule (60).

However, there are individuals who, despite increased macroprolactin, also present with high levels of monomeric PRL, leading to "true" hyperprolactinemia with clinical symptoms and the need foran etiologic diagnosis for the proper management of hyperprolactinemia (59). Moreover, the presence of symptoms could result from the concomitance of macroprolactinemia with other conditions, such as polycystic ovary syndrome (61), idiopathic galactorrhea (1,2), or psychogenic erectile dysfunction (62).

Assaying serum PRL before and after precipitation with polyethylene glycol (PEG) is the most used method for screening macroprolactinemias due to its low cost and easy workability (63). Theoretically, macroprolactin is precipitated with PEG, and only monomeric PRL will be recovered in the supernatant. However, some monomeric PRL also suffers precipitation, hence the need for the standardization of normal monomeric PRL values after PEG precipitation (58,60). Recoveries < 40% are indicative of the predominance of macroprolactin, whereas recoveries > 60% point to the diagnosis of monomeric hyperprolactinemia (56,58). Overall, PEG precipitation enables the correct diagnosis of macroprolactinemia in at least 80% of cases (56,63). The gold standard diagnostic test is the separation of isoforms by gel filtration, which correlates well with the PEG precipitation and is the only way of assessment when screening with PEG is inconclusive (58,63). However, it is an expensive and time-consuming method that cannot be used routinely.

It is noteworthy that different assays recognize macroprolactin differently (64). It has been demonstrated that some of the new assays show lower cross-reactivity with macroprolactin; however, the number of samples defined as macroprolactin is still significant (65).

Hyperprolactinemia related to macroprolactin may be due to its lower renal clearance, longer half-life and lower capability to activate hypothalamic dopaminergic tone, which negatively regulates the secretion of pituitary prolactin (5). The frequency of macroprolactinemia in the general population was shown to be 0.2% in women from Scandinavia (66) and 3.7% in a total of 1330 Japanese hospital workers of both genders (67), whereas among hyperprolactinemic individuals, it ranged from 8 to 42%, with a mean of 19.6%, in 8 European series (56,68-75). The study population may explain the variation in the frequency of macroprolactinemia in hyperprolactinemic individuals. As an example, two Brazilian studies have shown frequencies of 16.5% in 115 consecutive patients with hyperprolactinemia (76) and 46% in 113 cases from a reference laboratory (58). This high frequency of macroprolactinemia becomes an important issue in clinical practice: what is the probability with an additional assessment and treatment in an individual presenting with macroprolactinemia? Should all individuals with hyperprolactinemia be actively investigated for the presence of macroprolactinemia?

The request for serum PRL assessment occurs in two scenarios. At first, there are complaints related to hyperprolactinemia, such as galactorrhea, hypogonadism and infertility, leading to serum PRL measurement. If laboratory tests confirm the clinical suspicion of monomeric hyperprolactinemia, macroprolactinemia screening is not indicated, and it is recommended to proceed to the usual investigation of physiological, pharmacological and pathological causes of hyperprolactinemia for proper handling of the case. In the second scenario, serum PRL evaluation is requested in the absence of complaints related to hyperprolactinemia. In this situation, facing hyperprolactinemia in an asymptomatic individual, macroprolactinemia screening is always indicated. If positive and monomeric PRL levels are normal, it should guide the patient that there is no need for further investigation, follow-up or treatment, due to the benign nature of the condition. If the screening with PEG is inconclusive, one may proceed to gel-filtration chromatography, or if the latter is unavailable, be guided by the clinical picture. If the macroprolactin result is negative, investigate hyperprolactinemia as usual. A flowchart for the management of macroprolactinemic individuals is proposed in Figure 3.

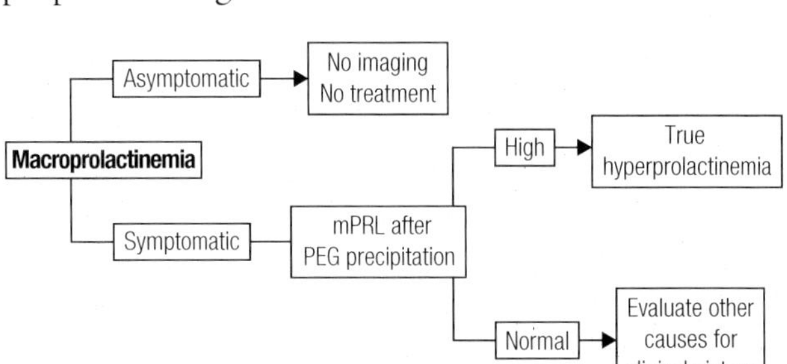

Figure 3. Flowchart to the management of patients with macroprolactinemia (mPRL: monomeric prolactin) (Adapted from Ref. 6).

Some authors advocate routine macroprolactin screening as a cost-effective procedure (56,76-78), and others allow screening to rule out macroprolactinemia and investigate other conditions that justify symptoms (79). In a study conducted in a Brazilian reference laboratory, there was more cost in searching for individuals with true hyperprolactinemia, but screening macroprolactinemia did not prevent investigation and inappropriate treatment, pointing to the need for the dissemination of medical knowledge about macroprolactinemia (80). By contrast, according to some studies, the detection of macroprolactin may change the initial diagnosis in a significant proportion of patients. Indeed, in three series (73,74,81), macroprolactinemia was encountered in 25 to 68.3% (mean, 42.3%) of patients with apparent idiopathic hyperprolactinemia (IH). Moreover, the diagnosis of PRL-secreting pituitary microadenoma shifted to non-secreting pituitary microadenoma in 10 of 49 patients (20%) reported by Donadio and cols. (73). Thus, macroprolactinemia may occasionally represent a relevant cause of misdiagnosis, unnecessary investigation and inappropriate treatment (73,74,81). Conversely, PRL should never be measured in asymptomatic patients, in order to avoid the unnecessary detection of macroprolactinemia cases (1,5).

Concerning the natural history of macroprolactinemia, macroprolactinemic subjects usually display persistent macroprolactinemia without the development of raised free PRL (82). However, during follow-up, hyperprolactinemia may develop in macroprolactinemic subjects who were initially normoprolactinemic along with an increase in anti-PRL autoantibody titers (82).

Overall, symptoms related to hyperprolactinemia (galactorrhea, menstrual disorders and sexual dysfunction) have been reported in up to 45% of patients with macroprolactinemia (56,58,69,70,73,74,76,83,84). As mentioned, this would mostly result from the concomitance with monomeric hyperprolactinemia (74,75,85) or other disorders, such as polycystic ovary syndrome (1,61,62). Of note, the finding of both galactorrhea and menstrual disorders is rare in macroprolactinemia (83,84).

In most patients with macroprolactinemia, PRL levels are < 100 ng/mL, but they are highly variable: from 20-663 ng/mL (mean, 61 ± 66; < 100 ng/mL in approximately 91% of cases) (83), to 119.5 ± 112.9 (range, 32.5-404; < 100 mg/L in 74%) among 115 patients in the BMSH (33). In most studies, PRL levels were lower in macroprolactinemic patients than in those with monomeric hyperprolactinemia, but there was a great overlap between groups (34,56,63,69,83). Moreover, MRI abnormalities (e.g., macroadenomas and, mostly, microadenomas or an empty sella) may be found in approximately 20-25% of macroprolactinemic patients (69,70,73,74,84).

COMMENT 6: Macroprolactinemia is, in most cases, a laboratory diagnostic pitfall, with a mean frequency of ~20% among hyperprolactinemic subjects. Clinical, radiological and laboratory features cannot be used reliably to differentiatemonomeric hyperprolactinemia from macroprolactinemia. The screening for macroprolactin is mostly indicated for asymptomatic hyperprolactinemic patients, subjects with apparent idiopathic hyperprolactinemia, and any patient without an obvious cause for the hyperprolactinemia.

TREATMENT OF HYPERPROLACTINEMIA AND PROLACTINOMAS

The ideal treatment of hyperprolactinemia depends on its etiology and may include, for instance, L-thyroxine replacement in patients with primary hypothyroidism, dopamine agonists (DAs) for prolactinomas, and drug withdrawal in cases of drug-induced hyperprolactinemia (2-7). By contrast, macroprolactinemia does not need to be treated (5,24,25).

Current available therapeutic options for prolactinomas include surgery, pituitary radiation therapy and pharmacotherapy with dopamine agonists (DAs) (19). DAs are the gold standard treatment for prolactinomas, as their use controls hormonal secretion and tumor growth in approximately 80% of cases (8). Among DAs, bromocriptine (BRC) and cabergoline (CAB), both of which are ergot derivatives, are the most commonly used worldwide. Quinagolide is available in some European countries. Cabergoline (CAB), a specific agonist of the dopamine receptor type 2 (D_2R), is the first choice because of its better tolerability and greater efficacy in inducing PRL normalization and tumor shrinkage (Figures 4 and 5) (Table 4) (19,86-89). Bromocriptine use leads to normal serum PRL levels in 80% of microprolactinomas and 70% of macroprolactinomas, whereas with CAB, this goal is achieved in 85% of patients (3,86-88). CAB effectiveness is higher in naïve patients, but the drug is also very effective in patients with intolerance or resistance to BCR (Figures 6 and 7) (34,88). The better performance of CAB probably results from its better tolerance and higher affinity for D_2R (10,19,88).

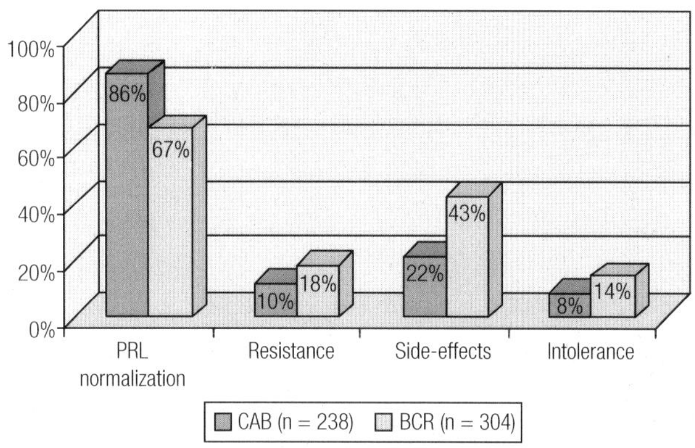

Figure 4. Comparison of cabergoline (CAB) and bromocriptine (BCR), concerning efficacy and tolerability (Adapted from Ref. 34).

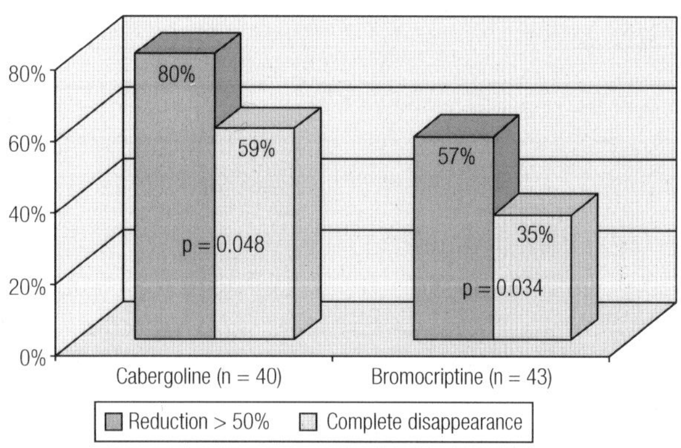

Figure 5. Comparative efficacy of CAB and BCR in inducing tumor shrinkage in naïve patients with macroprolactinomas (Adapted from Ref. 34).

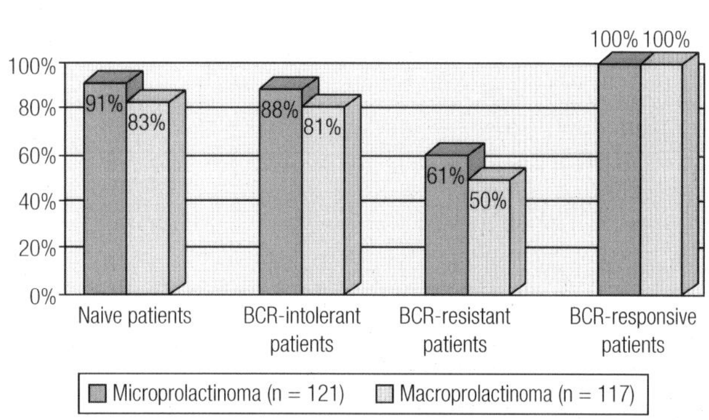

Figure 6. Efficacy of cabergoline on the normalization of PRL levels in 238 patients with prolactinomas. BCR: bromocriptine (Adapted from Ref. 34).

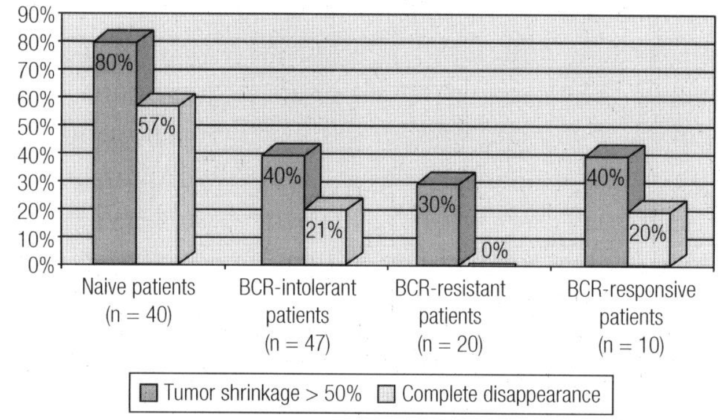

Figure 7. Concerning macroprolactinoma shrinkage, cabergoline is effective not only in naive patients but also in those previoiusly treated with bromocriptine (BCR) (Adapted from Ref. 34).

Table 4. Comparative efficacy of cabergoline (CAB) and bromocriptine (BCR) among patients with macroprolactinomas from the Brazilian Multicenter Study on Hyperprolactinemia

Outcome	CAB (n = 117)	BCR (n = 133)	p-value
PRL normalization	77.8%	59.4%	0.042
Tumor reduction > 50%	80%	58.7%	0.048
Complete tumor disappearance	57.5%	34.7%	0.034

Adapted from Ref. 34.

2. CONTROVERSIAL ISSUES REGARDING TREATMENT

In this topic, we will cover challenging or controversial aspects related to the treatment of prolactinomas and the management of psychotropic-induced hyperprolactinemia.

2.1 How to manage the resistance to dopamine agonists?

Different arbitrary concepts have been proposed for the definition of resistance to dopamine agonist (DA) therapy (2,4,88-91). Currently many experts have adopted the definition suggested by Molitch, which includes failure to normalize PRL levels and to decrease macroprolactinoma size by ≥ 50% with maximal conventional doses of medication (7.5 mg/day of bromocriptine or 2.0 mg/week of cabergoline) (89,90). Bromocriptine (BCR) fails to normalize prolactin levels in approximately one-quarter of patients; cabergoline (CAB), in 10-15%. BCR fails to decrease prolactinoma size by at least 50% in approximately one-third of the patients; CAB, in 10-15% (34,88-91).

Pathogenetic mechanisms

There are a number of potential mechanisms to explainresistance to DAs. Drug absorption or drug affinity to D_2R are not involved (90). DA resistance is rather associated with a decrease in D_2R gene transcription, resulting in a 4-fold decrease in the number of D_2Rs on the cell membrane (92,93). Moreover, there is a decrease in the G protein that couples the D_2R to adenylyl cyclase, further decreasing the ability of dopamine to inhibit PRL secretion (90).

Patients who initially respond to a DA may rarely become resistant to these drugs at a later point in time (90). Most commonly, this is due to noncompliance. Rarely, there may be malignant transformation of a prolactinoma (94). In some cases, the development of DA resistance is due to the concomitant use of hormone replacement therapy with estrogen or testosterone (95).

Treatment

The approaches for patients with resistance to DA therapy include (1) switching to another DA; (2) raising the dose of the DA beyond conventional doses if the patient continues to respond and tolerate; (3) surgical tumor resection; (4) radiotherapy; and (5) experimental treatments with other drugs (34,88,90,96,97).

Switching to another DA

Most of the data regarding switching dopamine agonists in resistant patients address switching from BCR to CAB. CAB is effective in normalizing PRL levels in approximately 50-80% of patients resistant to BCR, and up to 70% respond with some tumor size change (30,90,96,97). It is not clear why CAB should be so effective in patients resistant to BCR, but this may be due to cabergoline's possessing a higher affinity for dopamine binding sites, a longer time occupying the receptor, and a slower elimination from the pituitary (90,97). By contrast, the response to BCR in a patient resistant to CAB is much more rare and has only been reported twice (90,98).

Raising the dose of the DA beyond conventional doses

As long as there is a continued response and no adverse effects from higher doses, there is no reason not to continue to increase the CAB dose (90). There is, however, a concern regarding the risk of cardiac valvulopathy induced by high doses of CAB (see below) (88,90).

Using an individualized, stepwise approach of dose titration of CAB, Ono and cols. (99) documented that 25 of 26 patients (96.1%) considered to have DA resistance, achieved normalization of the PRL levels within 12 months, with a mean dose of CAB of 5.2 ± 0.6 mg per week (range 3-12 mg/week). The rate of PRL normalization gradually increased to 35, 73, and 89% at 3, 6, and 9 mg/week, respectively, finally reaching 96% at the highest dose of 12 mg/week (99). DiSarno and cols. (100) found that doses > 2.0 mg/week (up to 7 mg/week) of CAB werestill unable to normalize PRL levels in 18% of patients with macroadenomas and 10% of those with microadenomas. More recently, Vilar and cols. (101) prospectively evaluated the management of 25 prolactinomas refractory to CAB 3 mg/week by progressively increasing the CAB dose as needed and tolerated, every 3 months, up to 9 mg/week. Overall, normalization of PRL levels was achieved in 18 patients (72%), as follows: in 3 (12%) patients, with up to 4 mg/week; in 9 (36%) patients, with 5 mg/week; and in 6 (24%) patients, with 6-7 mg/week. No patients benefitted from doses > 7 mg/week. CAB was well tolerated, and no significant echocardiographic valve abnormalities were detected (101).

Debulking surgery

Patients can always undergo transsphenoidal surgery if their tumor is potentially resectable and an experienced neurosurgeon is available (4,90). There is also some evidence that debulking surgery may improve the response to DA (6,102-104). Of 61 patients resistant to either BCR or CAB, Hamilton and cols. (102) reported that surgery resulted in a normalization of PRL in 36% without dopamine agonist medication and in 15% with medication. Similarly, Primeau and cols. (102) found in 26 patients resistant to BCR, quinagolide or CAB that surgery resulted in a normalization of PRL in 42% without medication and in 27% with medication. In the European Multicenter Study, the rate of postoperative normalization of PRL was only 7.8% without medication and 5.3% with medication (104).

Radiotherapy

Among the functioning pituitary tumors, prolactinomas seem to be the less responsive to radiotherapy (see below). Indeed, although it can also be effective in controlling tumor growth, its efficacy in restoring PRL levels to normal is limited (4,89,90).

Other drugs

Of note, if one is dealing with microprolactinomas resistant to DAs, hormonal replacement therapy is often all that is necessary for men and premenopausal women not willing to conceive (4,19,90).

Estrogens may cause a decrease in the effectiveness of dopamine agonists through multiple mechanisms, including direct effects on PRL gene transcription (105), stimulation of mitotic activity (106), and a decrease in the number of D_2 receptors on the lactotroph cell membrane (107). Moreover, estrogen may block apoptosis (108). Thus, reducing endogenous estrogens in resistant prolactinomas through the use of SERMs in women or aromatase inhibitors in men might be an interesting experimental approach. Accordingly, a few patients with "bromocriptine resistant" invasive macroprolactinomas have been shown to respond with a decrease in tumor size and a lowering of PRL levels when tamoxifen was added (90,109). The use of the SERM clomiphene was also shown to be effective in the recovery of hypogonadism in prolactinoma patients who persisted with low testosterone levels despite maximal doses of DA (110,111). In addition, the successful use of anastrozole, an aromatase inhibitor, was recently reported in two males with DA-resistant prolactinomas (90,112).

Somatostatin analogs generally are not useful for PRL-secreting tumors (90), and there have been few reports on the successful combination therapy of octreotide (113) or lanreotide (114) and cabergoline in cases of DA-resistant tumors. The somatostatin receptor subtype 5 (SSTR5) is the most important with respect to the regulation of PRL secretion (115). Therefore, as pasireotide only has substantial activity at SSTR5 (116), it would be potentially more useful than the SSTR2-agonists octreotide and lanreotide in patients with aggressive DA-resistant prolactinomas (90).

Temozolomide, an oral alkylating agent, has been successfully used in the treatment of aggressive or malignant pituitary tumors since 2006 (117,118). It has also been found to be moderately successful in some very aggressive, large DA-resistant prolactinomas. Reviewing such cases, Whitelaw and cols. (119) found that 12 of 20 (75%) resistant PRL-secreting macroadenomas responded to temozolomide. Given the toxicity of the drug, its use is generally regarded as the therapy of last resort and should only be performed after the failure of DAs, surgery and radiotherapy for tumor control (90,119). Unfortunately, many of these very aggressive tumors escape from the suppressive effects of temozolomide after 0.5-2.5 years (90,119).

Other treatment strategies undergoing clinical trials are the use of chimeric molecules (somatostatin analogues and dopamine D_2 receptors) (2,3), PRL receptor antagonists (3), and antiblastic drugs, such as mTOR and tyrosine kinase inhibitors (3,120).

COMMENT 7: Patients with resistance to bromocriptine should be switched to treatment with cabergoline (CAB), which leads to prolactin normalization in at least 50% of cases. Facedwith resistance to CAB, a stepwise increase in the dose should be performed first, as long as there is a continued response and no adverse effects. This approach is successful in at least 70% of patients. In our experience, doses > 7 mg/week do not provide additional benefits. Debulking surgery may improve a response to the dopamine agonist (DA) when the medical treatment has failed.Radiation and temozolomide can be indicated to control aggressive tumor growth even under DA therapy.

2.2 Are there differences in the safety profile of DAs?

DA therapy often precipitates a broad spectrum of side effects, more frequently gastrointestinal symptoms (e.g., constipation, nausea, vomiting, etc.) but also postural hypotension, dizziness and headaches, which may range from mild to severe (34,88,121). The most common adverse events include nausea or vomiting (~35%), headache (~30%), and dizziness or vertigo (~25%) (121). The safety profile of CAB is similar to that reported for BRC, but CAB adverse effects are generally less frequent, less severe, and of shorter duration (34,88), and they resolve with dose reduction or continued use in many patients (34,88,121). The rate of treatment discontinuation due to complete intolerance is also significantly higher with BCR, compared to CAB (~12% vs ~4%) (87).

Whether CAB is associated with an increased risk of clinically relevant cardiac valvulopathy in patients with prolactinomas as in those with Parkinson's disease is still debated (see below) (10,121).

2.3 Do dopamine agonists cause psychiatric disorders?

Dopamine antagonists (e.g., haloperidol, olanzapine, quetiapine, sulpiride) are classically used for the treatment of psychiatric disorders such as psychosis and schizophrenia due to the supposed dopaminergic hyperactivity that occurs in these cases (43,46,47). DA treatment exerts the opposite effect to that of the dopamine antagonists (7). These agents can rarely cause psychiatric adverse side effects, including depression, somnolence, anorexia, anxiety, insomnia, impaired concentration, nervousness, hallucinations, nightmares, psychosis, impulsive control disorders (ICDs), and mania (3,5,122-125). The exact incidence of these side effects in DA-treated patients is not known but is thought to range from less than 1% to 3% (122,123).

ICDs are characterized by difficulties in resisting urges to engage in behaviors that are excessive and/ or ultimately harmful to oneself or others and can include gambling, kleptomania, intermittent explosive disorder, compulsive sexual behavior and compulsive buying (126).

Few reports have been published focusing on ICDs and other psychiatric disorders in prolactinoma patients treated with CAB (123-133). These reports have described disorders such as a first episode of mania (123,129); mania with psychotic features in a subject with bipolar disorder after starting CAB (125); psychosis in a patient with undiagnosed depression (126); compulsive gambling one year after starting CAB (130); gambling and compulsive sexual behavior just after starting CAB (131); psychosis in a patient without a previous history of psychiatric disorder three months after starting CAB (132); and depression and compulsive buying (133).

In 2011, Martinkova and cols. (128) published a review reporting a 10% prevalence of ICD in patients on CAB for prolactinoma treatment. In another study, males with prolactinomas treated with DAs have been reported to be 9.9 times more likely to develop an impulse control disorder compared to their counterparts with nonfunctioning pituitary adenomas (134). More recently, Barake and cols. (135) conducted the only randomized study aiming to assess the impact of CAB on the appearance of ICDs and concluded that patients on CAB (particularly with higher dosages) were more susceptible to impulsivity disorders than those not taking the drug.

Psychiatric effects of CAB can be modulated by P-glycoprotein (P-gp). This protein, encoded by the *ABCB1* gene (136), is a membrane transporter expressed in tumor cells and in normal tissues that acts as an efflux transporter in order to transport certain substances out of the brain and protect it against harmful substances. A recent study showed that CAB is a P-gp substrate (137). This study demonstrated that *ABCB1* gene polymorphisms (with loss of function) could explain individual differences in the occurrence of central nervous system side-effects, demonstrating a future perspective to select patients for CAB treatment based on this gene study (137).

COMMENT 8: In susceptible subjects, psychotic symptoms and impulsive control disorders may be triggered or aggravated by dopamine agonist (DA) therapy. It seems therefore important to exclude psychiatric disorders before prescribing DAs and to carefully follow up patients prone to or with a history of psychiatric disorders.

2.4 Risk of heart valvular disease associated with dopamine agonists – what is its relevance?

The main warning signs that cause concerns among endocrinologists about a possible association between the therapeutic use of dopamine agonists (DAs) with heart valvular disease (HVD) emerged from two articles published in 2007 involving patients with Parkinson's disease (138,139). In this group of patients, there is now strong evidence that treatment with high doses of CAB and pergolide (PGL) is associated with a higher risk of cardiac valvular regurgitation and moderate evidence that treatment with CAB, and the non-ergot-derived DAs pramipexole is associated with a higher risk of heart failure (140). The underlying mechanism involves the activation of the 5-hydroxytryptamine 2B (5-HT2B) receptors, abundantly expressed on heart valves, which induces a cascade of events involving mitogenesis, fibroblast proliferation, valve thickening and, finally, valvular dysfunction (141,142). DAs bind to 5-HT2B receptors with different affinities; for instance, CAG and PGL show high affinity and act as a potent agonist, whereas bromocriptine (BRC) has a lower affinity compared to other DAs (141,142). However, there have been case reports and clinical studies in Parkinson's disease reporting on an increased risk of abnormal valvular regurgitation and cardiac and non-cardiac fibrotic reactions in patients treated with BRC (143,144).

As expected, the findings in patients with Parkinson's disease brought an immediate concern about the risk of HVD in endocrine patients treated with DAs, especially CAB, despite the striking differences between these groups that must be highlighted. First, the daily and cumulative doses of DAs used in neurology (at least 3 mg of CAB per day) are approximately 10-fold higher than those used in endocrinology (rarely more than 3 mg of CAB per week) (145). Moreover, most studies in Parkinson's disease predominantly include men older than 60 years of agewho are usually on therapy with multiple drugs, while patients with endocrine abnormalities treated with DAs are predominantly young or middle-age women (146). This is important because the prevalence of valvular regurgitation increases with age and is influenced by gender, body mass index and hypertension (146,147). Another factor to be considered is the impact of examiner bias in the results, as shown in the study by Gu and cols. (148).

In patients with hyperprolactinemia, most cross-sectional studies were dedicated to investigating the role of CAB in HVD. A meta-analysis of seven observational studies with 1,398 individuals found an increased risk of mild-to-moderate tricuspid valve regurgitation in hyperprolactinemic patients taking CAB. No significant differences were observed in mitral or aortic valve regurgitation (149). Another recent systematic review analyzed data from 21 studies and from 40 patients followed by the authors (150). Utilizing the precise definition of CAB-associated valvulopathy as the triad of moderate or severe regurgitation associated with a restricted and thickened valve, clinically relevant disease was identified in only two out of 1,811 patients, resulting in a prevalence of 0.11% (150). The authors of this study also prospectively assessed 40 patients with prolactinoma taking cabergoline. Cardiovascular examination before echocardiography detected an audible systolic murmur in 10% of cases (all were functional murmurs), and no clinically significant valvular lesion was shown on echocardiogram in the 90% of patients without a murmur (150).

A Brazilian study by Boguszewski and cols. (151) was the first to include a group of prolactinoma patients treated with BRC for comparison. Notably, a higher prevalence of trace tricuspid regurgitation was observed in patients taking BRC, while more prevalent trace-to-mild tricuspid and trace mitral regurgitation and a higher mitral tent area were observed in CAB users; nevertheless, all these echocardiographic findings were not clinically significant (151). This observation was confirmed in a subsequent study in which an increased prevalence of subclinical HVD in patients with prolactinomas on long-term treatment with either BRC or CAB was reported (152).

Beyond the cross-sectional investigations, longitudinal studies have shed light on the potential damage caused by DAs to cardiac valves. Delgado and cols. (153) followed patients with prolactinomas treated (n = 45) or not treated (n = 29) with CAB for 2 years and found an increased prevalence of valvular calcification in CAB users that was not accompanied by a higher prevalence of valvular dysfunction. Auriemma and cols. (154) concluded that 5 years of CAB therapy in prolactinomas does not increase the risk of significant cardiac valve regurgitation. Similarly, 19 patients with prolactinomas were followed in Curitiba, Brazil, during 5 years of continuous treatment with DAs. Neither a significant change in valvular regurgitation grades nor symptomatic disease was observed in the follow-up (155). Population-based studies have also confirmed the safety of CAB in endocrine patients. A nationwide cohort study carried out in Denmark did not support that hyperprolactinemia or its treatment is associated with an increased risk of clinically significant HVD (156). In a multi-country, nested case-control study involving data from the United Kingdom, Italy, and the Netherlands, CAB was associated with an increased risk of HVD in Parkinson's disease but not in hyperprolactinemia (157), confirming the role of high cumulative doses in the development of valvular dysfunction and the safety of long-term use of low cumulative doses.

In two studies involving 51 prolactinoma patients considered to be resistant to standard doses of CAB, no significant echocardiographic valve abnormalities were detected despite the use of doses ranging from 3 to 12 mg/week (99,110).

The absence of a detrimental effect of CAB therapy on cardiac valves has also been noticed in a longitudinal study in patients with acromegaly (158).

The findings of the abovementioned studies challenge the US Food and Drug Administration (FDA) advice that patients with prolactinoma treated with CAB should have an annual echocardiogram to screen for valvular heart disease. Of note, with conventional doses of cabergoline, i.e., up to 2 mg/week, usually used in patients with prolactinomas, there does not appear to be any increased risk of cardiac valve abnormalities (90,145,156). However, as it is uncertain at what dose level these valve effects become significant, some experts recommend assessing all patients receiving > 2 mg/week with an echocardiogram on a yearly basis (90). More recently, based on the findings of their systematic review, Caputo and cols. (150) proposed that such patients should be screened by a clinical cardiovascular examination and that echocardiograms should be reserved for patients with an audible murmur, those treated for more than 5 years at a dose of more than 3 mg per week, or those who maintain cabergoline treatment after the age of 50 years. Nevertheless, special attention should be given in interpreting echocardiographic findings in older individuals, as highlighted by some authors (146,147).

Subclinical valvular abnormalities detected by echocardiography are not an indication for cessation of the therapy (121,154). Importantly, if valve lesions are detected or progress during follow-up, further evaluation is indicated to distinguish CAB-induced etiologies from other causes of valvulopathies. In such cases, therapy may be interrupted, reduced or maintained based on clinical judgment and discussion with the patient (121,150,154).

COMMENT 9: Current available data do not support major concerns about the risk of valvulopathy in patients with hyperprolactinemia or other endocrine diseases who are chronically treated with DAs in standard doses. Thus, an echocardiogram evaluation would not be recommended for patients receiving cabergoline at doses up to 2 mg/week.

2.5 Withdrawal of the dopamine agonist – Why, when, how and how often?

Why, when and how?

Although it is well known that prolactinomas respond very well to DAs, the optimal duration of treatment is still not clear (4,6,10). Despite the need for long-term therapy, withdrawal of treatment should be considered because of the adverse effects of medical treatment, potential long-term consequences in cardiac valves, and treatment costs (4,6,88).

Studies on persistent normoprolactinemia after DA withdrawal have been published since 1979 (159). In 2002, a Brazilian study by Passos and cols. (160) showed a remission rate of 20.6% after BCR discontinuation. In 2003, a landmark prospective study by Colao and cols. (161) demonstrated that CAB could be successfully withdrawn in 70% of patients with a MIC and 64% of those harboring a MAC (161). An extension of this study to 8 years documented remission rates of 66 and 47%, respectively (162). The higher success rates of this study were attributed to stricter selection criteria for CAB withdrawal, including a prolonged period of normoprolactinemia during treatment and a significant tumor size reduction (161,162). Since 2003, several studies have evaluated the recurrence rates of hyperprolactinemia after DA withdrawal with variable results (162-170).

In a meta-analysis of 19 studies with a total of 743 patients, the overall remission rate after the withdrawal of DA therapy was only 21%, 32% for idiopathic hyperprolactinemia, 21% for microadenoma and 16% for macroprolactinomas (171). Furthermore, a higher rate of remission was found in studies in which CAB was used (35% in 4 studies) versus BRC (20% in 12 studies) ($p = 0.07$) (171). In studies lasting over 24 months of treatment, the remission was higher (34%) in comparison to studies with a shorter treatment duration (16%) ($p = 0.01$) (153). The remission rate was also higher in studies in which agreater than 50% reduction of the tumor was achieved in all patients prior to discontinuation of therapy (171).

The guidelines provided by the Endocrine Society in 2011 recommended that patients who have attained normoprolactinemia for at least 2 years and who have no visible tumor remnant on MRI may be candidates for a gradual DA withdrawal (4).

A meta-analysis from 2015 that only evaluated patients submitted to CAB withdrawal found that the hyperprolactinemia recurrence rate was 65% by a random effects meta-analysis (172). In a random effects meta-regression adjusting for optimal withdrawal strategies, a CAB dose reduced to the lowest level before withdrawal was associated with treatment success ($p = 0.006$), whereas CAB treatment longer than 2 years showed no trend of effect ($p = 0.587$). Patients who received the lowest CAB dose and presented a significant reduction in tumor size before withdrawal were more likely to benefit from CAB withdrawal ($p < 0.001$) (172).

In three recent studies, the recurrence rates after CAB withdrawal ranged from 27% to 54% (168-170). Among 74 patients (19 MACs and 55 MICs) treated with CAB for ≥ 3 years, recurrences occurred within 12 months in 34 (45.9%), regardless of the previous duration of CAB therapy (up to 3 yrs, 3 to 5 yrs or > 5 yrs) or initial adenoma size (168). Among 67 patients (23 MACs and 44 MICs), the overall recurrence rate was 54% (35% in cases of MIC and 64% in subjects with MAC) (169). A higher remission rate was found with CAB, compared to BCR (55% vs. 36%) (169). More recently, treatment discontinuation was evaluated in 11 patients with macroprolactinomas treated with CAB for at least 5 years (170). Recurrences of hyperprolactinemia were observed in 3 (27%) post-withdrawal patients at a median time of 3.0 (range; 2.9-11.2) months, indicating that a high percentage (73%) maintained remission for at least 12 months after CAB cessation (170).

How often?

Two independent studies (173,174) have investigated the outcome of a second attempt at CAB withdrawal in patients with recurrence of hyperprolactinemia after the first withdrawal, receiving additional CAB therapy for at least 2 years. The results of these studies have demonstrated that a second attempt at CAB withdrawal after 2 additional years of therapy may be successful in approximately 30% of patients (173,174).

What are the predictors of remission?

Several studies in the literature sought the predictors of remission after stopping DAs, but the results of these studies have been contradictory (4,6,10,19). Overall, parameters more often associated with a successful DA withdrawal include suppressed PRL levels, the use of low doses of CAB, and lack of a visible tumor on MRI before withdrawal. However, hyperprolactinemia recurrence was observed even in patients who presented with these parameters (168-172).

In the great majority of studies, patients harboring MACs presented a lower risk of hyperprolactinemia remission than those with MICs when treatment is discontinued (161-169). The same was true when CAB and BCR were compared (167-169). In the series by Dogansen and cols. (169), the overall remission rate was 46% (65% in cases of MIC and 36% in subjects with MAC). A higher remission rate was experienced by patients treated with CAB vs. BCR, for both MIC (86% vs. 56%) and MAC (45% vs. 27%), respectively (169).

Menopause might be considered a factor that influences the reduction of PRL levels (175). Nevertheless, Colao and cols. (163) showed that the rate of recurrence of hyperprolactinemia was similar among premenopausal and postmenopausal patients.

There are few studies showing that some patients may spontaneously normalize serum PRL concentrations after pregnancy. Auriemma and cols. (176) reported that pregnancy was associated with normalization of PRL levels in 68% of patients. Moreover, breastfeeding did not increase the recurrence rate of hyperprolactinemia (177). Thus, DA withdrawal has been suggested after pregnancy to assess the possibility of hyperprolactinemia remission (176,177). Previous pituitary surgery and radiotherapy also favor persistent normal PRL levels after DA withdrawal (4,6,88).

How long should patients be followedup after withdrawal?

The follow-up after DA withdrawal has varied in different studies. Generally, the patients have been observed for 1 to 5 years after cessation of treatment (171,172). Most patients relapse within the first year, during which the patient should be subjected to a stricter monitoring of PRL levels (e.g., every 3 months) (164-169). In virtually all studies, all recurrences were observed within 24 months of DA discontinuation (162-173). In cases of hyperprolactinemia recurrence, the risk of tumor growth is very low (< 10%) (88,160,162,169).

COMMENT 10: Following two years of treatment, cabergoline (CAB) withdrawal should be strongly considered in all patients with microprolactinomas and those with macroprolactinomas without visible tumor or harboring small tumor remnants, in the presence of PRL levels < 10 ng/mL and the use of the lowest dose of CAB. Before drug withdrawal, it is recommended to gradually taper the CAB dose.

2.6 What is the role of surgery for prolactinomas?

Transsphenoidal surgery (TSS) represents the golden standard of surgical approach for both microprolactinomas and most macroprolactinomas (88), whereas craniotomy must be reserved for tumors inaccessible via the transsphenoidal approach and currently is indicated in extremely rare cases (6,88,178).

Additional indications for TSS surgery are complications of the prolactinomas, particularly the management of symptomatic apoplexy (178) and the surgical repair of CSF leaks (179). The latter can occur spontaneously due to tumor invasion of the sphenoid sinus or result from a rapid tumor shrinkage induced by DA therapy (180-182). In a recent review, more than 90% of cases of cerebrospinal fluid leakage were related to the use of DA, with a mean time of 3.3 months between the start of drug administration and the diagnosis of rhinorrhea (182). However, this complication can also occur during long-term treatment (183). An additional strategy to CSF leakage would be the withdrawal of DA to allow tumor re-growth to stop the leak (181). As β2-transferrin is only found in CSF, its detection in nasal secretions is a very accurate tool for confirming the diagnosis of CSF rhinorrhea (179,184).

Table 5. Indications for surgery in prolactinomas

Increasing tumor size despite optimal medical therapy
Pituitary apoplexy
Intolerance to dopamine agonists
Resistance to dopamine-agonists
Persistent optic chiasm compression
Cerebrospinal fluid leak during administration of dopamine agonists

Adapted from Refs. 6, 10, and 19.

Efficacy

The most important determinants of successful surgery for prolactinoma treatment are the experience of the neurosurgeon, moderately increased serum PRL levels (< 200 ng/mL), and tumor size and invasiveness (6,121). In a literature review involving more than 50 series, initial surgical remission, defined as the normalization of PRL levels, occurred on average in 74.7% and 34% of patients with microprolactinomas (MICs) and macroprolactinomas (MACs), with a recurrence rate of 18% and 23%, respectively (88). More recently, the analysis of surgical results from 13 published series, including at least 100 patients, has shown the control of PRL levels to be achieved in approximately 73% of 1211 microprolactinomas and 38% of 1480 macroprolactinomas (185).

Notably, as shown in two recent studies (102,104), many patients with partial resistance to CAB achieve PRL normalization after surgical debulking, using a lower dose of CAB than the presurgical one.

Safety

Complications from TSS for MIC are infrequent, the mortality rate being at most 0.6% and the major morbidity rate being approximately 3.4% (88,121). In patients with large tumors, particularly those with giant prolactinomas, the mortality rate ranges from 3.3% to 31.2% (88,121). Visual loss, stroke/vascular injury, meningitis/abscess, oculomotor palsy and cerebrospinal fluid rhinorrhea have been reported to occur in 0.1%, 0.2%, 0.1%, 0.1% and 1.9% of cases, respectively (121,186-188). Transient diabetes insipidus (DI) is quite common with TSS for both micro- and macroadenomas (121). In contrast, permanent DI is rare and has been reported to occur in approximately 1% of surgeries on MACs (121,187,188). Hypopituitarism, commonly found in patients with macroadenomas before surgery as a consequence of mass effects, has been reported either to further worsen or to improve after surgery (102-104).

COMMENT 11: Surgery, usually by the transsphenoidal approach, is indicated for patients with resistance or intolerance to dopamine agonists; macroprolactinomas with chiasmal compression and visual impairment without fast improvement by medical treatment; and acute tumor complications, such as symptomatic apoplexy or cerebrospinal fluid leakage.

2.7 What is the role of radiotherapy for prolactinomas?

As prolactinomas are among the most radioresistant pituitary tumors, PRL normalization occurs in only approximately one-third of patients submitted to radiotherapy (RT) (88,189,190). Moreover, it is associated with a high risk of radiation-induced hypopituitarism at 10-20 years (121,191). Therefore, RT is only indicated to control tumor growth in DA-resistant cases not controlled by surgery, as well as in the very rare cases of malignant prolactinomas (4,6,88).

Historically, patients have been treated with both external beam radiotherapy and stereotactic techniques (189). External beam radiotherapy, also referred to as "conventional radiotherapy" (CRT), involves the use of multiple non-overlapping beams of X-rays that intersect over the target area (191). Stereotactic RT is a form of RT that uses stereotactic guidance to deliver high doses of radiation in a single fraction (radiosurgery) or in multiple fractions (191).

Efficacy

A comprehensive review of the literature regarding hormonal normalization in patients with prolactinomas treated with CRT or radiosurgery concluded that the overall normalization rate of both approaches seems to be similar (34.1% for CRT vs. 31.4% for radiosurgery) (88). In the series by Wan and cols. (190), of the 176 patients with prolactinomas submitted to gamma-knife radiosurgery, 23.3% achieved PRL normalization, whereas in 90.3%, the tumor volume decreased or remained unchanged.

Stereotactic techniques deliver less radiation to normal brain and nerve tissue in the tumor vicinity. Thus, radiation-induced complications are thought to be less frequent with radiosurgery than with CRT (88,189,190). Moreover, a shorter time to hormonal normalization with radiosurgery has been reported in some series (189,191), but not in all (192).

Currently, radiosurgery has been the recommended treatment option unless the tumor is larger than 3-4 cm, or within 3 mm of the optic nerves, chiasm or tracts (192). In this situation, patients should be offered CRT or, whenever possible, stereotactic RT in multiple fractions (88,189-191).

Safety

The use of convention radiotherapy (CRT) is associated with the development of several severe complications (121). More than 50% of patients receiving pituitary radiotherapy will develop at least one anterior pituitary hormone deficiency within the following decade (193,194). Although hypopituitarism tends to arise in the first 5 years after radiation treatment, new deficiencies can appear even 20 years later (103,176,177). Additional complications of CRT include cerebrovascular accidents (CVAs), a second brain tumor and optic nerve injury. The incidence of CVA has been found to increase from the time of radiation, from 4% at 5 years to 11% at 10 years and 21% at 20 years (121,195). The cumulative risk of second brain tumors has been demonstrated to range from 2.0% at 10 yr, to 2.4% at 20 yr, and 8.5% at 30 yr (196). The rate of presumed radiation-induced optic neuropathy has been estimated to be 0.8% at 10 years (197). Another rare complication is radiation-induced necrosis of the surrounding brain tissue, with a prevalence of approximately 0.2-0.8% (88,121).

In patients receiving radiosurgery, hypopituitarism has been found to be the most common complication, occurring in approximately one-third of patients (121,198). Clinical deterioration due to visual field loss and worsened facial sensory loss, as well as a handful of cases of second brain malignancies have also been reported (88,191,199).

These data suggest the greater safety of radiosurgery compared to CRT. However, further studies of large series and with long follow-ups are required to draw definitive conclusions (121).

COMMENT 12: Due to its low efficacy and potentially severe side-effects, radiation therapy is only indicated to control tumor growth in DA-resistant cases not controlled by surgery. Whenever possible, preference should be given to stereotactic techniques.

2.8 How giant prolactinomas should be managed?

Although there is no consensus on the definition of giant prolactinomas (GPs), they are usually defined as tumors with a maximum diameter greater than or equal to 4 cm (200-202).

GPs represent only 2-3% of all prolactinomas, and they are more commonly found in middle-aged men (200,201). These tumors are usually more aggressive in men than in women (203). GPs often cause visual field defects and/or ophthalmoplegia due to compression of the optic chiasm and/or cranial nerves, respectively, and headaches, as well as other neurological alterations and other atypical manifestations for a pituitary adenoma, such as orbital invasion, epistaxis or obstructive hydrocephalus (204-207). Panhypopituitarism may also be present. Therefore, formal visual testing is usually necessary, and pituitary function evaluation is mandatory (200,203).

Different therapeutic approaches, such as dopamine agonists (DAs) alone or in combination with surgery and radiotherapy, may be necessary to reach the therapeutic goals in patients with GPs, which include tumor volume control, normalization of the PRL level and restoration of eugonadism (200). Temozolomide (TMZ) has been used in aggressive prolactinomas that are unresponsive to the abovementioned therapies

(117-119). Due to the large tumor volume and commonly invasive behavior, control of mass effects should be a priority in the management of patients with giant prolactinomas (88).

Dopamine agonists

As medical therapy in most cases causes a marked and rapid reduction of the tumor size, it is considered the first-line treatment option in patients with GPs, even in the presence of visual abnormalities. However, close monitoring of the visual field is mandatory (200-202). In this setting, early surgery (e.g., within 15 to 30 days) may occasionally be necessary if the tumors do not shrink and if severe visual field defects do not improve or even get worse (200-202).

The use of DA for GPs seems to reduce significantly the tumor mass (> 30% decrease in tumor diameter or > 65% reduction in tumor volume) in 74% of the cases and to normalize the PRL level in 60% of the cases (200). Cabergoline (CAB) is the preferred DA for the medical management of GPs due to its greater efficacy and better tolerability compared to BCR (34,88). In the series by Espinosa and cols. (208), CAB treatment resulted in the normalization of PRL levels in 68% and in the reduction of > 50% in tumor volume in 87% of the GP patients. The composite goal of PRL normalization and > 50% tumor reduction was achieved by 55% of patients with GPs (n = 26) and by 66% of patients with no giant macroprolactinomas (n = 100) (p = 0.19) (208). Among GPs ≥ 6 cm, DA treatment achieved PRL normalization in 11/18 (61%) patients within a median interval of 20 months (209). In the series by Vilar and cols. (210), 10 of 16 patients (62.5%) reached PRL normalization at weekly doses ranging from 2.5 to 7 mg. Regarding DA withdrawal, there are no data in the literature about CAB withdrawal in patients with GPs. Concerning BRC withdrawn in these patients, some authors described the persistence of normoprolactinemia and tumor volume shrinkage in only a minority of patients (211-213).

Surgery

Neurosurgery should be considered as part of the multidisciplinary approach to patients with DA-resistant prolactinoma (debulking surgery) or should be restricted to some acute complications such as apoplexy or leakage of cerebrospinal fluid during DA therapy (4,206,214). Neurosurgery could also be considered for patients with severe visual field defects that do not show any improvement or even worsen during DA treatment. The transsphenoidal approach is usually the first choice, even for GPs (200). In patients with giant and invasive prolactinomas, surgery is hardly curative, regardless of the surgical technique employed or the neurosurgeon's experience. Therefore, in these cases, the goal of surgery is to debulk the tumor in order to improve the symptoms related to mass effects (88,121). Debulking surgery may also improve the tumor response to DA therapy (102,104).

Radiotherapy

Radiotherapy should be used in patients with GPs who do not achieve disease control with DA therapy and surgery, particularly regarding mass effects (200-202).

Temozolomide

Temozolomide is an oral alkylating chemotherapeutic agent that exerts cytotoxic effects through methylation of DNA and can be used in aggressive giant prolactinomas that remain uncontrolled in terms of mass effects despite the multiple treatment modalities previously mentioned. The standard dose is 150–200 mg/m^2 for 5 days, repeated every 28-days in a cycle (117,119).

COMMENT 13: Cabergoline is the therapy of choice for patients with giant prolactinomas (GPs), as this drug enables normalization of prolactin levels and significant tumor reduction in the majority of cases, but higher doses are often required, compared to those for smaller macroprolactinomas. Surgery should be considered as part of the management of these patients, especially in patients who still have a large tumor load despite dopamine agonist therapy. Radiotherapy and/or temozolomide should be reserved for the subgroup of GPs that are not controlled in terms of mass effects regardless of the multiple conventional treatment modalities.

2.9 How to manage the challenges involving prolactinomas and pregnancy?

Chronic anovulation and infertility are very frequent among women with prolactinomas, mostly due to the hypogonadotropic hypogonadism related to hyperprolactinemia (6,10,88). Hyperprolactinemia decreases the luteinizing hormone (LH) pulse amplitude and frequency through the suppression of GnRH (14). This effect appears to be mediated by an earlier step of suppressing the generation of kisspeptin, a protein made by neurons in the arcuate and periventricular nuclei of the hypothalamus, which stimulates GnRH release (215). PRL can also decrease estrogen and progesterone production through direct effects on the ovaries (216). Fertility is, however, restored in most women with the use of DA. In the absence of hormonal control in cases with microprolactinomas, clomiphene citrate or recombinant gonadotropins may be used for ovulation induction (216,217).

During pregnancy, the primary concern is growth of the tumor because of high levels of estrogens, leading to visual disturbances and headache. The second point of concern is the fetal exposure to DA in early embryogenesis and the potential risk of malformations (216,217).

Tumor growth

Prolactinomas can enlarge during pregnancy as a result of both the stimulatory effect of these high estrogen levels and the discontinuation of the dopamine agonist that might have caused tumor shrinkage (216). In microprolactinomas, the chance of clinically significant tumor growth is less than 5%; therefore, after pregnancy confirmation, DA can be withdrawn, and the patient should be monitored clinically every trimester. In contrast, in patients with macroadenomas, the risk of tumor growth with clinical repercussion is up to 35% (217). However, Holmgren and cols. (218) noted a reduced risk of tumor growth during pregnancy in patients treated with BRC for at least 12 months. Thus, in patients with expansive macroprolactinomas, it is mandatory to observe a tumor within the sellar boundaries and usually to wait at least 1 year under treatment with a DA (217,219).

DAs safety in the fetus

BRC has been shown to cross the placenta in human studies (103); CAB has been shown to do so in animal models, but such data are lacking in humans (121,216). As a general approach in pregnancy, DAsare discontinued as soon as pregnancy is confirmed (216). Nevertheless, taking into account that CAB has a long half-life and can be detected in the circulation within 30 days after drug withdrawal, early fetal exposure is unavoidable (217). Moreover, the experience with this drug is still limited compared to BRC: ~950 vs. ~6200 pregnancies induced by CAB and BRC, respectively (216). These facts are the rational for BRC preference in hyperprolactinemic women willing to become pregnant (217), as recommended by the Guidelines of the Endocrine Society, with BRC being the only authorized DA for pregnancy induction (4). However, in clinical practice, CAB has often been used for this purpose with no apparent damage to the fetus (216).

The potential fetal malformation and impairment of the dopaminergic brain circuitry under DA use are a concern (216,217,219). Addressing this issue, Molitch (216) has compared outcomes data from 6239 pregnancies induced by BCR with 968 pregnancies induced by CAB and pregnancies in the US general population, regarding miscarriages, births at term, premature births, multiple pregnancies, and malformed newborns. Overall, no difference was found among the three groups (216).

In the vast majority of cases, the DA was withdrawn at up to 6 weeks of pregnancy. In the literature, there are only data on approximately 100 cases of BRC use throughout pregnancy, which have disclosed one case of undescended testis and one case of talipes deformity (217,220,221). Recently, a compilation of 15 pregnancies with the use of CAB during the entire pregnancy has shown 12 healthy babies and one fetal death by severe pre-eclampsia (222).

Concerning the long follow-up of children conceived during BRC treatment, Bronstein followed up 70 children, during 12 to 240 months, and there was one case of idiopathic hydrocephalus, one child with tuberous sclerosis and another one with precocious puberty (223). In two other studies (217,224), no impairment of physical development was observed.

In four studies, the follow-ups of children conceived on CAB were described. Bronstein (223) and Ono and cols. (225) did not find any abnormalities in five and 83 children followed for 41 months and 12 years, respectively. Lebbe and cols. (226) following 88 children described two cases of slight delay in verbal fluency and one case of difficulty in achieving complete continence. Moreover, Stalldecker and cols. (227) followed 61 children and found two cases of seizures and two cases of pervasive developmental disorder.

In summary, BCR and CAB seem to be equally safe for the fetus; none of these drugs are apparently associated with increased risk for abortions or malformations, when used for pregnancy induction in infertile hyperprolactinemic women. Ideally, CAB should be discontinued 30 days before the conception (216,218,223).

The best approach

An algorithm proposed by Glezer and cols. (217) for the management of prolactinoma during pregnancy is shown is Figure 8. The DA should be withdrawn as soon as pregnancy is confirmed in patients with microadenomas or enclosed macroadenomas. Assessment of tumor shrinkage in macroadenomas is mandatory before pregnancy allowance. In previously expanded or invasive tumors, the choice of BRC maintenance throughout pregnancy or its reintroduction if needed, or else the indication of previous surgical debulking, depends on the physician's and patient's decision (217).

Patients with microprolactinomas (MICs) or enclosed macroprolactinomas (MACs) should be followed each trimester, with attention to headache and visual impairment (217). In the presence of those complaints, sellar MRI without contrast, preferably after the first trimester, should be performed, and BRC reintroduction is indicated if tumor growth is related to the clinical findings (217). In cases of BCR intolerance, CAB, although off-label, could be used instead (217,219,222). On the other hand, in patients with expanding MACs, DA maintenance throughout pregnancy should be evaluated by an expert (217,219). Clinical evaluation monthly and neuroophthalmological evaluation each trimester are indicated. In patients with MICs or MACs experiencing symptoms related to mass effects and without improvement with clinical treatment, neurosurgery should be performed, preferably during the second trimester (216,217). An alternative approach might be delivery of the baby, if the pregnancy is sufficiently advanced (e.g., > 37 weeks) (216,217,219).

Notably, during pregnancy, periodic checking of PRL levels is of no diagnostic benefit and can be misleading (216,217). Indeed, in normal women, PRL levels rise with gestation, but PRL levels do not always rise with tumor enlargement, and tumor enlargement can occur without a change in the PRL concentration (216). A rise in PRL may well not indicate tumor enlargement and therefore may cause unnecessary worry. By contrast, the lack of a rise in PRL may be falsely reassuring in a patient with headaches or other evidence of tumor enlargement (216).

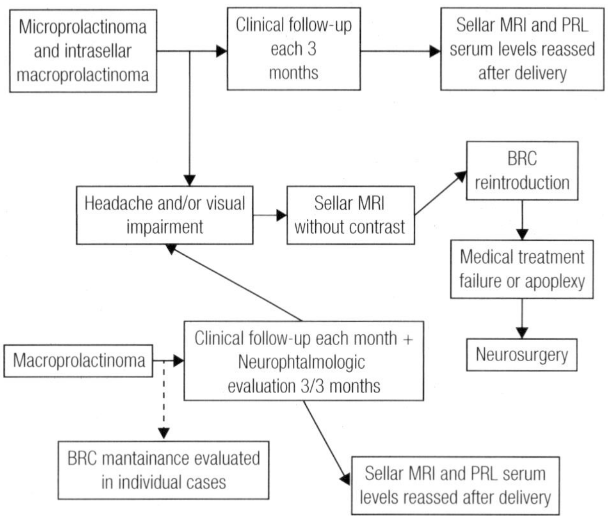

Figure 8. Algorithm suggested for the prolactinoma management during pregnancy (PRL: prolactin; BCR: bromocriptine; MRI: magnetic resonance imaging) (Adapted from Ref. 217).

Follow-up

After pregnancy, PRL levels and tumor size should be reassessed because reduction, or even complete tumor disappearance, after pregnancy may occur. Moreover, asymptomatic tumor enlargement may occur during pregnancy (216,217). It has been suggested that high levels of estrogen during pregnancy can induce areas of tumor necrosis and apoptosis. The median rate of hyperprolactinemia remission after pregnancy in eight studies was 27%, ranging from 10 to 68% (217).

Breastfeeding does not seem to be associated with tumor growth risk, and it is allowed in patients who did not require DA during pregnancy (216-219).

COMMENT 14: In the large majority of cases, a dopamine agonist is only necessary to induce pregnancy and should be discontinued as soon as pregnancy is confirmed. Nevertheless, in selected cases harboring invasive macroprolactinomas or in patients with marked growth and visual and/or headache complaints, the drug may be used throughout pregnancy.

COMMENT 15: Bromocriptine and cabergoline seem to be equally safe for the fetus, when used for pregnancy induction. Indeed, short-term exposure to these drugs for less than 6 weeks of gestation has not been found to cause any increase in spontaneous abortions, ectopic pregnancies, trophoblastic disease, multiple pregnancies, or congenital malformations.

2.10 How to manage the psychotropic-induced hyperprolactinemia?

It should always be kept in mind that patients with apparent psychotropic-induced hyperprolactinemia may have an alternative etiology for the PRL elevation, such prolactinomas, primary hypothyroidism, macroprolactinemia, or pseudo-prolactinoma (1). Ideally, a baseline PRL level should be obtained before starting psychotropic medications known to increase PRL, but in the majority of cases, this is not practically possible, particularly when these medications are started urgently (4,44). Endocrine Society Guidelines suggest discontinuing the drug for 3 days or substituting with an alternative drug if psychotropic-induced hyperprolactinemia is suspected and then remeasuring PRL (4). Nevertheless, the decision to withdraw or substitute the medication should always be made in consultation with the patient's psychiatrist (4,46). If the drug cannot be safely withdrawn due to the risk of a relapse of psychiatric symptoms and if the onset of hyperprolactinemia does not coincide with the initiation of therapy, then pituitary MRI should be performed to exclude or diagnose a sellar region lesion (4,46).

The different approaches proposed for symptomatic patients with confirmed psychotropic-induced hyperprolactinemia include (i) switching the offending drug to aripiprazole or other atypical antipsychotics (AAPs) with a low effect on PRL levels (41,209-211) and (ii) adding DA therapy (41).

Switching to aripiprazole or other AAPs

Because the atypical antipsychotic aripiprazole is a partial D2 receptor agonist, it has a neutral effect on PRL levels and may often decrease them (46, 228). Thus, it may be used as alternative therapy for patients with antipsychotic-induced hyperprolactinemia (46,228). Other atypical antipsychotics, such as quetiapine, olanzapine, lurasidone, asenapine, or clozapine, cause only a mild elevation in PRL levels, and only in a subgroup of those treated (43,46). Therefore, these drugs may also serve as alternatives to antipsychotics with robust effects on PRL (e.g., risperidone) (43,46).

However, in patients who are clinically very stable on antipsychotic treatment, switching to a different antipsychotic such as aripiprazole or other atypical antipsychotics may be inappropriate (46-48). In these cases, using aripiprazole as adjunctive therapy may be useful. Indeed, in a placebo-controlled trial, adjunctive aripiprazole normalized drug-induced hyperprolactinemia in more than 80% of patients with schizophrenia (229). More recently, in a double-blind, randomized, placebo-controlled trial involving patients with risperidone-induced hyperprolactinemia, normalization of PRL levels was encountered in 46% of patients who received adjunctive aripiprazole therapy (49).

Very interestingly, aripiprazole therapy was recently shown to be effective in normalizing PRL levels and in reducing tumor size in two patients with microprolactinomas and psychotic symptoms (230,231).

Adding DA therapy

The use of DA in the treatment of antipsychotic-induced hyperprolactinemia is not well studied (46,47). DA and antipsychotic medications may have opposing mechanisms of action. Indeed, the therapeutic effects of most antipsychotics come from D_2 receptor antagonism (232,233). Thus, there is a concern that DA therapy may reduce the effectiveness of antipsychotic drugs and trigger relapse or exacerbation of psychosis (46). There is, however, little evidence to support this concern. For instance, Chang and cols. (234) reported a cabergoline-induced psychotic exacerbation in three schizophrenic patients when CAB was introduced for the treatment of the hyperprolactinemic symptoms. Likewise, Santos Andrade and cols. (235) described a similar situation when BCR was added for macroprolactinoma treatment in a patient with schizophrenia on haloperidol. By contrast, in 5 studies that involved 174 schizophrenic and bipolar patients and had a duration ranging from 8 weeks to 6 months, the association of dopamine antagonists with low doses of CAB or BCR for the treatment of hyperprolactinemic symptoms apparently did not impair the underlying psychiatric disorder (236-240).

DA therapy should therefore be reserved for patients with severe hyperprolactinemia who fail to respond to aripiprazole as an alternative or adjunctive treatment. Due to its higher specificity for the D_2 receptor, CAB would be preferable to BCR in the management of antipsychotic-induced hyperprolactinemia. Nevertheless, it should be used cautiously, in doses as low as possible (46).

COMMENT 16: The best approach for symptomatic antipsychotic-induced hyperprolactinemia would be the use of aripiprazole as an alternative or adjunctive therapy. DA therapy at low doses can be used cautiously in patients who do not respond to the first approach.

REFERENCES

1. Vilar L, Fleseriu M, Bronstein MD. Pitfalls in the diagnosis of hyperprolactinemia. Arq Bras Endocrinol Metab. 2014;58(1):9-22.
2. Vilar L, Naves LA, Fleseriu M. Avaliação diagnóstica da hiperprolactinemia (Diagnostic evaluation of hyperprolactinemia). In: Vilar L, editor. Endocrinologia Clínica, 6a ed. (Clinical Endocrinology, 6th ed.). Rio de Janeiro: Guanabara Koogan; 2016. p. 3-14.
3. Bronstein MD. Disorders of prolactin secretion and prolactinomas. In: DeGroot LJ, Jameson JL, editors. Endocrinology. 6th ed. Philadelphia: Saunders/Elsevier; 2010. p. 333-57.
4. Melmed S, Casanueva FF, Hoffman AR, Kleinberg DL, Montori VM, Schlechte JA, et al. Diagnosis and treatment of hyperprolactinemia: An Endocrine Society clinical practice guideline. J Clin Endocrinol Metab. 2011;96(2):273-88.
5. Glezer A, Bronstein MD. Approach to the patient with persistent hyperprolactinemia and negative sellar imaging. J Clin Endocrinol Metab. 2012;97(7):2211-6.
6. Glezer A, Bronstein MD. Prolactinomas. Endocrinol Metab Clin N Am. 2015;44(1):71-8.
7. Colao A, Lombardi G. Growth hormone and prolactin excess. Lancet. 1998;352:1455-61.
8. Ciccarelli A, Daly AF, Beckers A. The epidemiology of prolactinomas. Pituitary 2005;8(1):3-6.
9. Daly AF, Rixhon M, Adam C, Dempegioti A, Tichomirowa MA, Beckers A. High prevalence of pituitary adenomas: a cross-sectional study in the province of Liege, Belgium. J Clin Endocrinol Metab. 2006;91(12):4769-75.
10. Auriema R, Pivonello R, Colao A. Prolactinomas. In: Vilar L (editor). In: Vilar L, editor. Endocrinologia Clínica, 6a ed. (Clinical Endocrinology, 6th ed.). Rio de Janeiro: Guanabara Koogan; 2016. p. 15-29.
11. Colao A, Sarno AD, Cappabianca P, Briganti F, Pivonello R, Di Somma C, et al. Gender differences in the prevalence, clinical features and response to cabergoline in hyperprolactinemia. Eur J Endocrinol. 2003;148(3):325-31.
12. Fideleff HL, Boquete HR, Suárez MG, Azaretzky M. Prolactinoma in children and adolescents. Horm Res. 2009;72(4):197-205.
13. Heaney AP. Pituitary carcinoma: difficult diagnosis and treatment. J Clin Endocrinol Metab. 2011;96(12):3649-60.
14. Milenković L, D'Angelo G, Kelly PA, Weiner RI. Inhibition of gonadotropin hormone-releasing hormone release by prolactin from GT1 neuronal cell lines through prolactin receptors. Proc Natl Acad Sci USA. 1994;91(4):1244-7.
15. Buvat J, Lemaire A, Buvat-Herbaut M, Fourlinnie JC, Racadot A, Fossati P. Hyperprolactinemia and sexual function in men. Horm Res. 1985;22(3):196-203.
16. Corona G, Mannucci E, Fisher AD, Lotti F, Ricca V, Balercia G, et al. Effect of hyperprolactinemia in male patients consulting for sexual dysfunction. J Sex Med. 2007;4(5):1485-93.
17. Huang W, Molitch M. Evaluation and management of galactorrhea. Am Fam Physician. 2012;85(11):1073-80.
18. Sakiyama R, Quan M. Galactorrhea and hyperprolactinemia. Obstet Gynecol Surv. 1983;38(12):689-700.
19. Romijn JA. Hyperprolactinemia and prolactinoma.Handb Clin Neurol. 2014;124:185-95.
20. Suh HK, Frantz AG. Size heterogeneity of human prolactin in plasma and pituitary extracts. J Clin Endocrinol Metab. 1974;39(5):928-35.
21. Sinha YN. Structural variants of prolactin: occurrence and physiological significance. Endocr Rev. 1995;16(3):354-69.
22. Jackson RD, Wortsman J, Malarkey WB. Characterization of a large molecular weight prolactin in women with idiopathic hyperprolactinemia and normal menses. J Clin Endocrinol Metab. 1985;61(2):258-64.
23. Jackson RD, Wortsman J, Malarkey WB. Macroprolactinemia presenting like a pituitary tumor. Am J Med. 1985;78(2):346-50.
24. Hattori N. The frequency of macroprolactinemia in pregnant women and the heterogeneity of its etiologies. J Clin Endocrinol Metab. 1996;81(2):586-90.
25. Cavaco B, Leite V, Santos MA, Arranhado E, Sobrinho LG. Some forms of big big prolactin behave as a complex of monomeric prolactin with an immunoglobulin G in patients with macroprolactinemia or prolactinoma. J Clin Endocrinol Metab. 1995;80(8):2342-6.
26. Hattori N, Ikekubo K, Nakaya Y, Kitagawa K, Inagaki C. Immunoglobulin G subclasses and prolactin (PRL) isoforms in macroprolactinemia due to anti-PRL autoantibodies. J Clin Endocrinol Metab. 2005;90(5):3036-44.
27. Heffner LJ, Gramates LS, Yuan RW. A glycosylated prolactin species is covalently bound to immunoglobulin in human amniotic fluid. Biochem Biophys Res Commun. 1989;165(1):299-305.
28. Thirunavakkarasu K, Dutta P, Sridhar S, Dhaliwal L, Prashad GR, Gainder S, et al. Macroprolactinemia in hyperprolactinemic infertile women. Endocrine. 2013;44(3):750-5.
29. Kasum M, Oreskovic S, Zec I, Jezek D, Tomic V, Gall V, et al. Macroprolactinemia: new insights in hyperprolactinemia. Biochem Med (Zagreb). 2012;22(2):171-9.
30. Vilar L, Czepielewski MA, Naves LA, Rollin GA, Casulari LA, Coelho CE. Substantial shrinkage of adenomas cosecreting growth hormone and prolactin with use of cabergoline therapy. Endocr Pract. 2007;13(4):396-402.
31. Vieira JGH, Oliveira JH, Tachihana T, Maciel RMB, Hauache OM. Evaluation of plasma prolactin levels: is it necessary to rest before the collection? Arq Bras Endocrinol Metab. 2006;50(3):569-70.
32. Ferriani RA, Sá MFS. Effect of venipuncture stress on plasma prolactin levels. Int J Gynaecol Obstet. 1985;23(6):459-62.
33. Molitch ME. Disorders of prolactin secretion. Endocrinol Metab Clin North Am. 2001;30(3):585-610.
34. Vilar L, Freitas MC, Naves LA, Casulari LA, Azevedo M, Montenegro R Jr, et al. Diagnosis and management of hyperprolactinemia: results of a Brazilian multicenter study with 1234 patients. J Endocrinol Invest. 2008;31(5):436-44.
35. Rahmanian M, Meybodi HA, Larijani B, Mohajeri-Tehrani MR. Giantprolactinoma: case report and review of literature.J Diabetes Metab Disord. 2013;12(1):3.
36. Acharya SV, Gopal RA, Menon PS, Bandgar TR, Shah NS. Giantprolactinoma and effectiveness of medical management. Endocr Pract. 2010;16(1):42-6.
37. Fleseriu M, Lee M, Pineyro MM, Skugor M, Reddy SK, Siraj ES, et al. Giant invasive pituitary prolactinoma with falsely low serum prolactin: the significance of 'hook effect'. J Neurooncol. 2006;79(1):41-3.
38. Barkan AL, Chandler WF. Giant pituitary prolactinoma with falsely low serum prolactin: the pitfall of the "high-dose hook effect": case report. Neurosurgery. 1998;42(4):913-5.
39. Frieze TW, Mong DP, Koops MK. "Hook effect" in prolactinomas: case report and review of literature. Endocr Pract. 2002;8(4):296-303.
40. Randall RV, Scheithauer BW, Laws, ER Jr, Abboud CF. Pseudoprolactinomas. Trans Am Clin Climatol Assoc. 1983; 94:114-21.

41. Karavitaki N, Thanabalasingham G, Shore HC, Trifanescu R, Ansorge O, Meston N, et al. Do the limits of serum prolactin in disconnection hyperprolactinaemia need re-definition? A study of 226 patients with histologically verified non-functioning pituitary macroadenoma. Clin Endocrinol (Oxf). 2006;65(4):524-9.
42. Vilar L, Albuquerque JL, Vilar CF, Ferreira LA, Cardoso IRA, Inacio IS, et al. Demographic, clinical, and laboratorial features of 770 patients with hyperprolactinemia. Arch Endocrinol Metab. 2017; 61 (Suppl. 3):S11.
43. Voicu V, Medvedovici A, Ranetti AE, Rădulescu FŞ. Drug-induced hypo- and hyperprolactinemia: mechanisms, clinical and therapeutic consequences. Expert Opin Drug Metab Toxicol. 2013;9(8):955-68.
44. La Torre D, Falorni A. Pharmacological causes of hyperprolactinemia. Ther Clin Risk Manag. 2007;3(5):929-51.
45. Petit A, Piednoir D, Germain ML, Trenque T. Drug-induced hyperprolactinemia: a case-non-case study from the national pharmacovigilance database. Therapie. 2003;58(2):159-63.
46. Johnsen E, Kroken RA, Abaza M, Olberg H, Jørgensen HA. Antipsychotic- induced hyperprolactinemia: a cross-sectional survey. J Clin Psychopharmacol. 2008;28(6):686-90.
47. Ajmal A, Joffe H, Nachtigall LB. Psychotropic-induced hyperprolactinemia: a clinical review. Psychosomatics. 2014;55(1):29-36
48. Kunwar AR, Megna JL. Resolution of risperidone-induced hyperprolactinemia with substitution of quetiapine. Ann Pharmacother. 2003;37(2):206-8.
49. Shim JC, Shin JG, Kelly DL, Jung DU, Seo YS, Liu KH, et al. Adjunctive treatment with a dopamine partial agonist, aripiprazole, for antipsychotic-induced hyperprolactinemia:a placebo-controlled trial. Am J Psychiatry. 2007;164(9):1404-10.
50. Papakostas GI, Miller KK, Petersen T, Sklarsky KG, Hilliker SE, Klibanski A, et al. Serum prolactin levels among outpatients with major depressive disorders during the acute phase of treatment with fluoxetine. J Clin Psychiatry. 2006;67(6):952-7.
51. Vilar L, Lyra R, Albuquerque JL, Lyra R, Vilar CF, Diniz ET, et al. Very high prolactin levels associated to chronic therapy with domperidone. Arch Endocrinol Metab. 2016;60 (Suppl. 3):S22.
52. St-Jean E, Blain F, Comtois R. High prolactin levels may be missed by immunoradiometric assay in patients with macroprolactinomas. Clin Endocrinol (Oxf). 1996;44(3):305-9.
53. Stenman UH. Pitfalls in hormone determinations. Best Pract Res Clin Endocrinol Metab. 2013;27(6):743-4.
54. do Carmo Dias Gontijo M, de Souza Vasconcellos L, Ribeiro-Oliveira A Jr. Hook effect and linear range in prolactin assays: distinct confounding entities. Pituitary. 2016;19(4):458-9.
55. Glezer A, Soares CR, Vieira JG, Giannella-Neto D, Ribela MT, Goffin V, et al. Human macroprolactin displays low biological activity via its homologous receptor in a new sensitive bioassay. J Clin Endocrinol Metab. 2006;91(3):1048-55.
56. Gibney J, Smith TP, McKenna TJ. The impact on clinical practice of routine screening for macroprolactin.J Clin Endocrinol Metab. 2005;90(7):3927-32.
57. Leite V, Cosby H, Sobrinho LG, Fresnoza MA, Santos MA, Friesen HG. Characterization of big, big prolactin in patients with hyperprolactinaemia. Clin Endocrinol (Oxf). 1992;37(4):365-72.
58. Hauache OM, Rocha AJ, Maia AC Jr, Maciel RM, Vieira JG. Screening for macroprolactinaemia and pituitary imaging studies. Clin Endocrinol (Oxf). 2002;57(3):327-31.
59. Bronstein MD. Editorial: is macroprolactinemia just a diagnostic pitfall? Endocrine. 2012;41(2):169-70.
60. Hattori N, Nakayama Y, Kitagawa K, Ishihara T, Saiki Y, Inagaki C. Anti-prolactin (PRL) autoantibody-binding sites (epitopes) on PRL molecule in macroprolactinemia. J Endocrinol. 2006;190(2):287-93.
61. Hayashida SA, Marcondes JA, Soares JM Jr, Rocha MP, Barcellos CR, Kobayashi NK, et al. Evaluation of macroprolactinemia in 259 women under investigation for polycystic ovary syndrome. Clin Endocrinol (Oxf). 2014;80(4):616-8.
62. Guay AT, Sabharwal P, Varma S, Malarkey WB. Delayed diagnosis of psychological erectile dysfunction because of the presence of macroprolactinemia. J Clin Endocrinol Metab. 1996;81(7):2512-4.
63. Vieira JGH, Tachibana TT, Obara LH, Maciel RMB. Extensive experience and validation of polyethylene glycol precipitation as a screening method for macroprolactinemia. Clin Chem. 1998;44(8):1758-9.
64. Smith TP, Suliman AM, Fahie-Wilson MN, McKenna TJ. Gross variability in the detection of prolactin in sera containing big big prolactin (macroprolactin) by commercial immunoassays. J Clin Endocrinol Metab. 2002;87(12):5410-5.
65. Vieira JGH, Tachibana TT, Ferrer CM, de Sá J, Biscolla RP, Ana Hoff AO, et al. Hyperprolactinemia: new assay more specific for the monomeric form does not eliminate screening for macroprolactin with polyethylene glycol precipitation. Arq Bras Endocrinol Metab. 2010;54(9):856-62.
66. Bjøro T, Mørkrid L, Wergeland R, Turter A, Kvistborg A, Sand T, Torjesen P. Frequency of hyperprolactinaemia due to large molecular weight prolactin (150-170 kD PRL).Scand J Clin Lab Invest. 1995;55(2):139-47.
67. Hattori N, Ishihara T, Saiki Y. Macroprolactinaemia: prevalence and aetiologies in a large group of hospital workers. Clin Endocrinol (Oxf). 2009;71(5):702-8.
68. Fahie-Wilson MN, Soule SG. Macroprolactinemia contribution to hyperprolactinemia in a district general hospital and evaluation of a screening test based on precipitation with polyethylene glycol. Ann Clin Biochem. 1997;34:252-8.
69. Vallette-Kasic S, Morange-Ramos I, Selim A, Gunz G, Morange S, Enjalbert A, et al. Macroprolactinemia revisited: a study on 106 patients. J Clin Endocrinol Metab. 2002;87(2):581-8.
70. Strachan MW, Teoh WL, Don-Wauchope AC, Seth J, Stoddart M, Beckett GJ. Clinical and radiological features of patients with macroprolactinaemia. Clin Endocrinol (Oxf). 2003;59(3):339-46.
71. Theunissen C, De Schepper J, Schiettecatte J, Verdood P, Hooghe-Peeters EL, Velkeniers B. Macroprolactinemia: clinical significance and characterization of the condition. Acta Clin Belg. 2005;60(4):190-7.
72. Bağdatoğlu C, Bağdatoğlu OT, Muslu N, Köseoğlu A, Dağtekin A, Polat G, et al. The importance of macroprolactinemia in the differential diagnosis of hyperprolactinemic patients. Turk Neurosurg. 2008;18(3):223-7.
73. Donadio F, Barbieri A, Angioni R, Mantovani G, Beck-Peccoz P, Spada A, et al. Patients with macroprolactinaemia: clinical and radiological features. Eur J Clin Invest. 2007;37(7):552-7.
74. Isik S, Berker D, Tutuncu YA, Ozuguz U, Gokay F, Erden G, et al. Clinical and radiological findings in macroprolactinemia. Endocrine. 2012;41(2):327-33.
75. Parlant-Pinet L, Harthé C, Roucher F, Morel Y, Borson-Chazot F, Raverot G, et al. Macroprolactinaemia: a biological diagnostic strategy from the study of 222 patients. Eur J Endocrinol. 2015;172(6):687-95.
76. Vilar L, Moura E, Canadas V, Gusmão A, Campos R, Leal E, et al. Prevalence of macroprolactinemia among 115 patients with hyperprolactinemia. Arq Bras Endocrinol Metab. 2007;51(1):86-91.
77. Fahie-Wilson M. The macroprolactinemiaproblem and its solution. South Med J. 2006;99(11):1206.
78. Shimatsu A, Hattori A. Macroprolactinemia: diagnostic, clinical, and pathogenic significance. Clin Dev Immunol. 2012;2012:167132.
79. Leaños-Miranda A, Ramírez-Valenzuela KL, Campos-Galicia I, Chang-Verdugo R, Chinolla-Arellano LZ. Frequency of

macroprolactinemia in hyperprolactinemic women presenting with menstrual irregularities, galactorrhea, and/or infertility: etiology and clinical manifestations. Int J Endocrinol. 2013;2013:478282.

80. de Soárez PC, Souza SC, Vieira JG, Ferraz MB. The effect of identifying macroprolactinemia on health-care utilization and costs in patients with elevated serum prolactin levels. Value Health. 2009;12(6):930-4.

81. Vilar L, Gadelha PS, Rangel Filho F, Siqueira A, Viana KF, Fonseca MM, et al. Prevalence of macroprolactinemia among patients with idiopathic hyperprolactinemia. Arq Bras Endocrinol Metab. 2014;58 (Suppl 1):S17-18.

82. Hattori N, Adachi T, Ishihara T, Shimatsu A. The natural history of macroprolactinaemia. Eur J Endocrinol. 2012;166(4):625-9.

83. Vilar L, Naves LA, Freitas MC, Lima M, Canadas V, Albuquerque JL, et al. Clinical and laboratory features greatly overlap in patients with macroprolactinemia or monomeric hyperprolactinemia. Minerva Endocrinol. 2007;2(2):79-86.

84. Vilar L, Vilar CF, Albuquerque JL, Gadelha PS, Thé AC, Trovão E, et al. Clinical and MRI findings among 120 patients with macroprolactinemia: results from a prospective study. Arch Endocrinol Metab. 2017;61 (Suppl. 3):S8.

85. Elenkova A, Genov N, Abadzhieva Z, Kirilov G, Vasilev V, Kalinov K, et al. Macroprolactinemia in patients with prolactinomas: prevalence and clinical significance. Exp Clin Endocrinol Diabetes. 2013;121(4):201-5.

86. dos Santos Nunes V, El Dib R, Boguszewski CL, Nogueira CR. Cabergoline versus bromocriptine in the treatment of hyperprolactinemia: a systematic review of randomized controlled trials and meta-analysis. Pituitary. 2011;14(3):259-65.

87. Webster J, Piscitelli G, Polli A, Ferrari CI, Ismail I, Scanlon MF. A comparison of cabergoline and bromocriptine in the treatment of hyperprolactinemic amenorrhea. Cabergoline Comparative Study Group. N Engl J Med. 1994;331(14):904-9.

88. Gillam MP, Molitch MP, Lombardi G, Colao A. Advances in the treatment of prolactinomas. Endocr Rev. 2006;27(5):485-534.

89. Molitch ME. Pharmacologic resistance in prolactinoma patients. Pituitary. 2005;8(1):43-52.

90. Molitch ME. Management of medically refractory prolactinoma.J Neurooncol. 2014;117(3):421-8.

91. Vilar L, Burke CW. Quinagolide efficacy and tolerability in hyperprolactinaemic patients who are resistant to or intolerant of bromocriptine. Clin Endocrinol (Oxf). 1994;41(6):821-6.

92. Passos VQ, Fortes MAHZ, Giannella-Neto D, Bronstein MD. Genes differentially expressed in prolactinomas responsive and resistant to dopamine agonists. Neuroendocrinology. 2009;89(2):163-70.

93. Shimazu S, Shimatsu A, Yamada S, Inoshita N, Nagamura Y, Usui T, et al. Resistance to dopamine agonists in prolactinoma is correlated with reduction of dopamine D2 receptor long isoform mRNA levels. Eur J Endocrinol. 2012;166(3):383-90.

94. Hurel SJ, Harris PE, McNicol AM, Foster S, Kelly WF, Baylis PH. Metastatic prolactinoma: effect of octreotide, cabergoline, carboplatin and etoposide; immunocytochemical analysis of proto-oncogene expression. J Clin Endocrinol Metab. 1997;82(9):2962-5.

95. Prior JC, Cox TA, Fairholm D, Kostashuk E, Nugent R. Testosterone-related exacerbation of a prolactin-producing macroadenoma: possible role for estrogen. J Clin Endocrinol Metab. 1987;64(2):391-4.

96. Olafsdottir A, Schlechte J. Management of resistant prolactinomas. Nat Clin Pract Endocrinol Metab. 2006;2(10):552-61.

97. Colao A, DiSarno A, Sarnacchiaro F, Ferone D, DiRenzo G, Merola B, et al. Prolactinomas resistant to standard dopamine agonists respond to chronic cabergoline treatment. J Clin Endocrinol Metab. 1997;82(3):876-83.

98. Iyer P, Molitch ME. Positive prolactin response to bromocriptine in two patients with cabergoline resistant prolactinomas. Endocr Pract. 2011;17(3):e55-8.

99. Ono M, Miki N, Kawamata T, Makino R, Amano K, Seki T, et al. Prospective study of high-dose cabergoline treatment of prolactinomas in 150 patients. J Clin Endocrinol Metab. 2008; 93(12):4721-7.

100. Di Sarno A, Landi ML, Marzullo P, Di Somma C, Pivonello R, Cerbone G, et al. The effect of quinagolide and cabergoline, two selective dopamine receptor type 2 agonists, in the treatment of prolactinomas. Clin Endocrinol (Oxf). 2000; 53(1):53-60.

101. Vilar L, Vilar C, Albuquerque JL, Gadelha P, Thé AC, Trovão E, et al. The use of increasing doses of cabergoline in the management of cabergoline-resistant prolactinomas. Endocrine Abstracts. 2017;49:EP975.

102. Primeau V, Raftopoulos C, Maiter D.Outcomes of transsphenoidal surgery in prolactinomas: improvement of hormonal control in dopamine agonist-resistant patients. Eur J Endocrinol. 2012;166(5):779-86.

103. Hamilton DK, Vance ML, Roulos PT, Laws ER. Surgical outcomes in hyporesponsive prolactinomas: analysis of patients with resistance or intolerance to dopamine agonists. Pituitary. 2005;8(1):53-60.

104. Vrooner L, Jaffrain-Rea M-L, Petrossians P, Tamagno G, Chanson P, Vilar L, et al. Prolactinomas resistant to standard doses of cabergoline: a multicenter study of 92 patients. Eur J Endocrinol. 2012;167(5):651-62.

105. Maurer RA. Estradiol regulates the transcription of the prolactin gene. J Biol Chem. 1982;257(5):2133-6.

106. Lloyd GM, Meares JD, Jacobi J. Effects of oestrogen and bromocriptine on in vivo secretion and mitosis in prolactin cells. Nature. 1975;255(5508):497-8.

107. Pasqualini C, Bojda F, Kerdelhue B. Direct effect of estradiol on the number of dopamine receptors in the anterior pituitary of ovariectomized rats. Endocrinology. 1986;119(6):2484-9.

108. Aoki MDP, Aoki A, Maldonado CA. Sexual dimorphism of apoptosis in lactotrophs induced by bromocryptine. Histochem Cell Biol. 2001;116(3):215-22.

109. Lamberts SWJ, Verleun T, Oosterom R. Effect of tamoxifen administration on prolactin release by invasive prolactin-secreting pituitary adenomas. Neuroendocrinology. 1982;34(5):339-42.

110. Vilar L, Vilar CF, Aroucha PT, Albuquerque JL, Gadelha PS, Thé AC, et al. The role ofclomiphene citrate in the resolution of hypogonadism in male patients with prolactinomas under cabergoline therapy. Arch Endocrinol Metab. 2017;61 (Suppl. 3):S28.

111. Ribeiro RS, Abucham J. Recovery of persistent hypogonadism by clomiphene in males with prolactinomas under dopamine agonist treatment. Eur J Endocrinol. 2009;161(1):163-9.

112. Gillam MP, Middler S, Freed DJ, Molitch ME.The novel use of very high doses of cabergoline and a combination of testosterone and an aromatase inhibitor in the treatment of a giant prolactinoma. J Clin Endocrinol Metab. 2002;87(10):4447-51.

113. Fusco A, Lugli F, Sacco E, Tilaro L, Bianchi A, Angelini F, et al. Efficacy of the combined cabergoline and octreotide treatment in a case of a dopamine-agonist resistant macroprolactinoma. Pituitary. 2011;14(4):351-7.

114. Vilar L, Vilar C, Albuquerque JL, Gadelha P, Thé AC, Trovão E, et al. Effect of the addition of lanreotide autogel to the treatment of an aggressive prolactinoma – a case report. Endocrine Abstracts. 2017;49:EP841.

115. Jaquet P, Qouafik L, Saveanu A, Gunz G, Fina F, Dufour H, et al. Quantitative and functional expression of somatostatin receptor subtypes in human prolactinomas. J Clin Endocrinol Metab. 1999;84(9):3268-76.
116. Bruns C, Lewis I, Briner U, Meno-Tetang G, Weckbecker G. SOM230: a novel somatostatin peptidomimetic with broad somatotropin release inhibiting factor (SRIF) receptor binding and a unique antisecretory profile. Eur J Endocrinol. 2002;146(5):707-16.
117. Halevy C, Whitelaw BC. How effective is temozolomide for treating pituitary tumours and when should it be used? Pituitary.2017;20(2):261-6.
118. Ji Y, Vogel RI, Lou E. Temozolomide treatment of pituitary carcinomas and atypical adenomas: systematic review of case reports. Neurooncol Pract. 2016;3(3):188-95.
119. Whitelaw BC, Dworakowska D, Thomas NQ, Barazi S, Riordan-Eva P, King AP, et al. Temozolomide in the management of dopamine agonist-resistant prolactinomas. Clin Endocrinol (Oxf). 2012;76(6):877-86.
120. Jouanneau E, Wierinckx A, Ducray F, Favrel V, Borson-Chazot F, Honnorat J, et al. New targeted therapies in pituitary carcinoma resistant to temozolomide. Pituitary. 2012;15(1):37-43.
121. Auriemma RS, Grasso LF, Pivonello R, Colao A. The safety of treatments for prolactinomas. Expert Opin Drug Saf. 2016;15(4):503-12.
122. National Library of Medicine. Daily Med Current Medication Information. 2010 Available from: http://dailymed.nlm.nih.gov/dailymed/drugInfo.cfm?id=31309. Accessed on: April 7, 2017.
123. Yüksel RN, Elyas Kaya Z, Dilbaz N, Cingi Yirün M. Cabergoline-induced manic episode: case report. Ther Adv Psychopharmacol. 2016;6(3):229-23.
124. Voon V, Reynolds B, Brezing C, Gallea C, Skaljic M, Ekanayake V, et al. Impulsive choice and response in dopamine agonist-related impulse control behaviors. Psychopharmacology (Berl). 2010;207(4):645-59.
125. Rovera C, Cremaschi L, Thanju A, Fiorentini A, Mauri MC, Serati M. Cabergoline can induce mania with psychotic features in bipolar I disorder: a case report. Asian J Psychiatr. 2016;22:94-5.
126. Bilal L, Ching C. Cabergoline-induced psychosis in a patient with undiagnosed depression.J Neuropsychiatry Clin Neurosci. 2012;24(4):E54.
127. Samuel M, Rodriguez-Oroz M, Antonini A, Brotchie JM, Ray Chaudhuri K, Brown RG, et al. Management of impulse control disorders in Parkinson's disease: Controversies and future approaches. Mov Disord. 2015;30(2):150-9.
128. Martinkova J, Trejbalova L, Sasikova M, Benetin J, Valkovic P. Impulse control disorders associated with dopaminergic medication in patients with pituitary adenomas. Clin Neuropharmacol. 2011;34(5):179-81.
129. Harris YT, Harris AZ, Deasis JM, Ferrando SJ, Reddy N, Young RC. Cabergoline associated with first episode mania. Psychosomatics. 2012;53(6):595-600.
130. Davie M. Pathological gambling associated with cabergoline therapy in a patient with a pituitary prolactinoma. J Neuropsychiatry Clin Neurosci. 2007;19(4):473-4.
131. Falhammar H, Yarker JY. Pathological gambling and hypersexuality in cabergoline-treated prolactinoma. Med J Aust. 2009;190(2):97.
132. Bilal L, Ching C. Cabergoline-induced psychosis in a patient with undiagnosed depression. J Neuropsychiatry Clin Neurosci. 2012;24(4):E54.
133. Almanzar S, Zapata-Vega MI, Raya JA. Dopamine agonist-induced impulse control disorders in a patient with prolactinoma. Psychosomatics. 2013;54(4):387-91.
134. Bancos I, Nannenga MR, Bostwick JM, Silber MH, Erickson D, Nippoldt TB. Impulse control disorders in patients with dopamine agonist-treated prolactinomas and nonfunctioning pituitary adenomas: a case-control study. Clin Endocrinol (Oxf). 2014;80(6):863-8.
135. Barake M, Evins AE, Stoeckel L, Pachas GN, Nachtigall LB, Miller KK, et al. Investigation of impulsivity in patients on dopamine agonist therapy for hyperprolactinemia: a pilot study. Pituitary. 2014;17(2):150-6.
136. 136.Hoffmeyer S, Burk O, von Richter O, Arnold HP, Brockmoller J, Johne A, et al. Functional polymorphisms of the human multidrug-resistance gene: multiple sequence variations and correlation of one allele with P-glycoprotein expression and activity in vivo. Proc Natl Acad Sci U S A. 2000;97(7):3473-8.
137. Athanasoulia AP, Sievers C, Ising M, Brockhaus AC, Yassouridis A, Stalla GK, et al. Polymorphisms of the drug transporter gene ABCB1 predict side effects of treatment with cabergoline in patients with PRL adenomas. Eur J Endocrinol. 2012;167(3):327-35.
138. Zanettini R, Antonini A, Gatto G, Gentile R, Tesei S, Pezzoli G. Valvular heart disease and the use of dopamine agonists for Parkinson's disease. N Engl J Med. 2007;356(1):39-46.
139. Schade R, Andersohn F, Suissa S, Haverkamp W, Garbe E. Dopamine agonists and the risk of cardiac-valve regurgitation. N Engl J Med. 2007;356(1):29-38.
140. Tran T, Brophy JM, Suissa S, Renoux C. Risks of cardiac valve regurgitation and heart failure associated with ergot- and non-ergot-derived dopamine agonist use in patients with Parkinson's disease: asystematic review of observational studies. CNS Drugs. 2015;29(12):985-98.
141. Roth BL. Drugs and valvular heart disease. N Engl J Med. 2007;356(1):6-9.
142. Elangbam, C.S. Drug-induced valvulopathy: an update. Toxicol Pathol. 2010;38(6):837-48.
143. Serratrice J, Disdier P, Habib G, Viallet F, Weiller PJ. Fibrotic valvular heart disease subsequent to bromocriptine treatment. Cardiol Rev. 2002;10(6):334-6.
144. Tan LC, Ng KK, Au WL, Lee RK, Chan YH, Tan NC. Bromocriptine use and the risk of valvular heart disease. Mov Disord. 2009;24(3):344-9.
145. Valassi E, Klibanski A, Biller BM. Potential cardiac valve effects of dopamine agonists in hyperprolactinemia. J Clin Endocrinol Metab. 2010;95(3):1025-33.
146. Choong CY, Abascal VM, Weyman J, Levine RA, Gentile F, Thomas JD, et al. Prevalence of valvular regurgitation by Doppler echocardiography in patients with structurally normal hearts by two-dimensional echocardiography. Am Heart J. 1989;117(3):636-42.
147. Okura H, Takada Y, Yamabe A, Ozaki T, Yamagishi H, Toda I, et al. Prevalence and correlates of physiological valvular regurgitation in healthy subjects. Circ J. 2011;75(11):2699-704.
148. Gu H, Luck S, Carroll PV, Powrie J, Chambers J. Cardiac valve disease and low-dose dopamine agonist therapy: an artefact of reporting bias? Clin Endocrinol (Oxf). 2011;74(5):608-10.
149. De Vecchis R, Esposito C, Ariano C. Cabergoline use and risk of fibrosis and insufficiency of cardiac valves. Meta-analysis of observational studies. Herz. 2013;38(8):868-80.
150. Caputo C, Prior D, Inder WJ. The need for annual echocardiography to detect cabergoline-associated valvulopathy in patients with prolactinoma: a systematic review and additional clinical data. Lancet Diabetes Endocrinol. 2015;3(11):906-13.
151. Boguszewski CL, dos Santos CM, Sakamoto KS, Marini LC, de Souza AM, Azevedo M. A comparison of cabergoline and bromocriptine on the risk of valvular heart disease in patients with prolactinomas. Pituitary. 2012;15(1):44-9.

152. Elenkova A, Shabani R, Kalinov K, Zacharieva S. Increased prevalence of subclinical cardiac valve fibrosis in patients with prolactinomas on long-term bromocriptine and cabergoline treatment. Eur J Endocrinol. 2012;167(1):17-25.

153. Delgado V, Biermasz NR, van Thiel SW, Ewe SH, Marsan NA, Holman ER, et al. Changes in heart valve structure and function in patients treated with dopamine agonists for prolactinomas, a 2-year follow-up study. Clin Endocrinol (Oxf). 2012;77(1):99-105.

154. Auriemma RS, Pivonello R, Perone Y, Grasso LF, Ferreri L, Simeoli C, et al. Safety of long-term treatment with cabergoline on cardiac valve disease in patients with prolactinomas. Eur J Endocrinol. 2013;169(3):359-66.

155. Zaccaron BA, Sena RH, Souza AM, Boguszewski CL. Safety of long-term treatment with dopamine agonists on valvular heart disease in patients with prolactinomas. Arq Bras Endocrinol Metab. 2014;58(Suppl 5):S172.

156. Steffensen C, Maegbaek ML, Laurberg P, Andersen M, Kistorp CM, Norrelund H, et al. Heart valve disease among patients with hyperprolactinemia: a nationwide population-based cohort study. J Clin Endocrinol Metab. 2012;97(5):1629-34.

157. Trifirò G, Mokhles MM, Dieleman JP, van Soest EM, Verhamme K, Mazzaglia G, et al. Risk of cardiac valve regurgitation with dopamine agonist use in Parkinson's disease and hyperprolactinaemia: a multi-country, nested case-control study. Drug Saf. 2012;35(2):159-71.

158. Maione L, Garcia C, Bouchachi A, Kallel N, Maison P, Salenave S, et al. No evidence of a detrimental effect of cabergoline therapy on cardiac valves in patients with acromegaly. J Clin Endocrinol Metab. 2012;97(9):E1714-E19.

159. Eversmann T, Fahlbusch R, Rjosk HK, von Werder K. Persisting suppression of prolactin secretion after long-term treatment with bromocriptine in patients with prolactinomas. Acta Endocrinol (Copenh). 1979;92(3):413-27.

160. Passos VQ, Souza JJ, Musolino NR, Bronstein MD. Long-term follow-up of prolactinomas: normoprolactinemia after bromocriptine withdrawal. J Clin Endocrinol Metab. 2002; 87(8):3578-82.

161. Colao A, Di Sarno A, Cappabianca P, Di Somma C, Pivonello R, Lombardi G. Withdrawal of long-term cabergoline therapy for tumoral and nontumoral hyperprolactinemia. N Engl J Med. 2003;349(21):2023-33.

162. Colao A, Di Sarno A, Guerra E, Pivonello R, Cappabianca P, Caranci F, et al. Predictors of remission of hyperprolactinaemia after long-term withdrawal of cabergoline therapy. Clin Endocrinol (Oxf). 2007;67(3):426-33.

163. Biswas M, Smith J, Jadon D, McEwan P, Rees DA, Evans LM, et al. Long-term remission following withdrawal of dopamine agonist therapy in subjects with microprolactinomas. Clin Endocrinol (Oxf). 2005;63(1):26-31.

164. Kharlip J, Salvatori R, Yenokyan G, Wand GS. Recurrence of hyperprolactinemia after withdrawal of long-term cabergoline therapy. J Clin Endocrinol Metab. 2009;94(7):2428-36.

165. Huda MS, Athauda NB, Teh MM, Carroll PV, Powrie J. Factors determining the remission of microprolactinomas after dopamine agonist withdrawal. Clin Endocrinol (Oxf). 2010;72(4):507-11.

166. Barber TM, Kenkre J, Garnett C, Scott RV, Byrne JV, Wass JA. Recurrence of hyperprolactinaemia following discontinuation of dopamine agonist therapy in patients with prolactinoma occurs commonly especially in macroprolactinoma. Clin Endocrinol (Oxf). 2011;75(6):819-24.

167. Anagnostis P, Adamidou F, Polyzos SA, Efstathiadou Z, Karathanassi E, Kita M. Long term follow-up of patients with prolactinomas and outcome of dopamine agonist withdrawal: a single center experience. Pituitary. 2012;15(1):25-9.

168. Sala E, Bellaviti Buttoni P, Malchiodi E, Verrua E, Carosi G, et al. Recurrence of hyperprolactinemia following dopamine agonist withdrawal and possible predictive factors of recurrence in prolactinomas. J Endocrinol Invest. 2016;39(12):1377-82.

169. Dogansen SC, Selcukbiricik OS, Tanrikulu S, Yarman S. Withdrawal of dopamine agonist therapy in prolactinomas: In which patients and when? Pituitary. 2016;19(3):303-10.

170. Watanabe S, Akutsu H, Takano S, Yamamoto T, Ishikawa E, Suzuki H, et al. Long-term results of cabergoline therapy for macroprolactinomas and analysis of factors associated with remission after withdrawal. Clin Endocrinol (Oxf). 2017;86(2):207-13.

171. Dekkers OM, Lagro J, Burman P, Jørgensen JO, Romijn JA, Pereira AM. Recurrence of hyperprolactinemia after withdrawal of dopamine agonists: systematic review and meta-analysis. J Clin Endocrinol Metab. 2010; 95(1):43-51.

172. Hu J, Zheng X, Zhang W, Yang H. Current drug withdrawal strategy in prolactinoma patients treated with cabergoline: a systematic review and meta-analysis. Pituitary. 2015;18(5):745-51.

173. Vilar L, Albuquerque JL, Gadelha PS, Rangel Filho F, Siqueira AM, da Fonseca MM, et al. Second attempt of cabergoline withdrawal in patients with prolactinomas after a failed first attempt: is it worthwhile? Front Endocrinol (Lausanne). 2015;6:11.

174. Kwancharoen R, Auriemma RS, Yenokyan G, Wand GS, Colao A, Salvatori R. Second attempt to withdraw cabergoline in prolactinomas: a pilot study. Pituitary. 2014;17(5):451-6.

175. Karunakaran S, Page RC, Wass JA. The effect of the menopause on prolactin levels in patients with hyperprolactinaemia. Clin Endocrinol (Oxf). 2001;54(3):295-300.

176. Auriemma RS, Perone Y, Di Sarno A, Grasso LF, Guerra E, Gasperi M, et al. Results of a single-center observational 10-year survey study on recurrence of hyperprolactinemia after pregnancy and lactation. J Clin Endocrinol Metab. 2013;98(1):372-9.

177. Domingue ME, Devuyst F, Alexopoulou O, Corvilain B, Maiter D. Outcome of prolactinoma after pregnancy and lactation: a study on 73 patients. Clin Endocrinol (Oxf). 2014;80(5):642-8.

178. Smith TR, Hulou MM, Huang KT, Gokoglu A, Cote DJ, Woodmansee WW, Laws ER Jr. Current indications for the surgical treatment of prolactinomas. J Clin Neurosci. 2015;22(11):1785-91

179. Lund VJ. Endoscopic management of cerebrospinalfluid leaks. Am J Rhinol. 2002;16(1):17-23.

180. Mankia SK, Weerakkody RA, Wijesuriya S, Kandasamy N, Finucane F, Guilfoyle M, et al. Spontaneous cerebrospinalfluid rhinorrhoea as the presenting feature of an invasive macroprolactinoma. BMJ Case Rep. 2009;2009. pii: bcr12.2008.1383

181. Leong KS, Foy PM, Swift AC, Atkin SL, Hadden DR, MacFarlane IA. CSF rhinorrhoea following treatment with dopamine agonists for massive invasive prolactinomas. Clin Endocrinol (Oxf). 2000;52(1):43-9.

182. Lam G, Mehta V, Zada G. Spontaneous and medically induced cerebrospinal fluid leakage in the setting of pituitary adenomas: review of the literature. Neurosurg Focus. 2012;32(6):E2.

183. Bronstein MD, Musolino NR, Benabou S, Marino R Jr. Cerebrospinal fluid rhinorrhea occurring in long-term bromocriptine treatment for macroprolactinomas. Surg Neurol. 1989;32(5):346-9.

184. Anani WQ, Ojerholm E, Shurin MR. Resolving transferrin isoforms via agarose gel electrophoresis. Lab Med. 2015;46(1):26-33.

185. Colao A. The prolactinoma. Best Pract Res Clin Endocrinol Metab. 2009;23(5):575-96.

186. Barker 2nd FG, Klibanski A, Swearingen B. Transsphenoidal surgery for pituitary tumors in the United States, 1996–2000: mortality, morbidity, and the effects of hospital and surgeon volume. J Clin Endocrinol Metab. 2003;88(10):4709-19.

187. Sudhakar N, Ray A, Vafidis JA. Complications after trans-sphenoidal surgery: our experience and a review of the literature. Br J Neurosurg. 2004;18(5):507-12.

188. Nelson Jr AT, Tucker Jr HS, Becker DP. Residual anterior pituitary function following transsphenoidal resection of pituitary macroadenomas. J Neurosurg 1984;61(3):577-80.

189. 189.Sheplan Olsen LJ, Robles Irizarry L, Chao ST, Weil RJ, Hamrahian AH, Hatipoglu B, Suh JH. Radiotherapy for prolactin-secreting pituitary tumors.Pituitary. 2012;15(2):135-45.

190. Wan H, Chihiro O, Yuan S. MASEP gamma knife radiosurgery for secretory pituitary adenomas: experience in 347 consecutive cases. J Exp Clin Cancer Res. 2009;28:36.

191. Kong DS, Lee JI, Lim do H, Kim KW, Shin HJ, Nam DH, et al. The efficacy of fractionated radiotherapy and stereotactic radiosurgery for pituitary adenomas: long-term results of 125 consecutive patients treated in a single institution. Cancer. 2017;110(4):854-60.

192. Castinetti F, Nagai M, Morange I, Dufour H, Caron P, Chanson P, et al. Long-term results of stereotactic radiosurgery in secretory pituitary adenomas. J Clin Endocrinol Metab. 2009;94(9):3400-7.

193. Tsang RW, Brierley JD, Panzarella T, Gospodarowicz MK, Sutcliffe SB, Simpson WJ. Radiation therapy for pituitary adenoma: treatment outcome and prognostic factors. Int J Radiat Oncol Biol Phys. 1994;30(3):557-65.

194. Littley MD, Shalet SM, Beardwell CG, Robinson EL, Sutton ML Radiation-induced hypopituitarism is dose-dependent. Clin Endocrinol (Oxf). 1989;31(3):363-73.

195. Brada M, Burchell L, Ashley S, Traish D. The incidence of cerebrovascular accidents in patients with pituitary adenoma. Neurooncol Pract. 2014;1(1):22-8.

196. Minniti G, Traish D, Ashley S, Gonsalves A, Brada M. Risk of second brain tumor after conservative surgery and radiotherapy for pituitary adenoma: update after an additional 10 years. J Clin Endocrinol Metab. 2005;90(2):800-4.

197. Erridge SC, Conkey DS, Stockton D, Strachan MW, Statham PF, Whittle IR, et al. Radiotherapy for pituitary adenomas: long-term efficacy and toxicity. Radiother Oncol. 2009;93(3):597-601.

198. Cohen-Inbar O, Xu Z, Schlesinger D, Vance ML, Sheehan JP. Gamma Knife radiosurgery for medically and surgically refractory prolactinomas: long-term results. Pituitary. 2015;18(6):820-30.

199. Liu X, Kano H, Kondziolka D, Park KJ, Iyer A, Shin S, et al. Gamma knife stereotactic radiosurgery for drug resistant or intolerant invasive prolactinomas. Pituitary. 2013;16(1):68-75.

200. Moraes AB, Silva CM, Vieira Neto L, Gadelha MR. Giant prolactinomas: the therapeutic approach. Clin Endocrinol (Oxf). 2013;79(4):447-56.

201. Delgrange E, Raverot G, Bex M, Burman P, Decoudier B, Devuyst F, et al. Giant prolactinomas in women. Eur J Endocrinol. 2013;170(1):31-8.

202. Maiter D, Delgrange E. Therapy of endocrine disease: the challenges in managing giant prolactinomas. Eur J Endocrinol. 2014;170(6):R213-27.

203. Delgrange E, Trouillas J, Maiter D, Donckier J, Tourniaire J. Sex-related difference in the growth of prolactinomas: a clinical and proliferation marker study.J Clin Endocrinol Metab. 1997;82(7):2102-7.

204. Shrivastava RK, Arginteanu MS, King WA, Post KD. Giant prolactinomas: clinical management and long-term follow up. J Neurosurg. 2002;97(2):299-306.

205. Levy RA, Quint DJ. Giant pituitary adenoma with unusual orbital and skull base extension. AJR Am J Roentgenol. 1998;170(1):194-6.

206. Chaurasia PK, Singh D, Meher S, Saran RK, Singh H. Epistaxis as first clinical presentation in a child with giant prolactinoma: Case report and review of literature. J Pediatr Neurosci. 2011;6(2):134-7.

207. Alkatari S, Aljohani N. Obstructive hydrocephalus, fifth nerve and hypothalamus involvement: acute presentation of a giant prolactinoma. Clin Med Insights Case Rep. 2012;5:115-8.

208. Espinosa E, Sosa E, Mendoza V, Ramírez C, Melgar V, Mercado M. Giant prolactinomas: are they really different from ordinary macroprolactinomas? Endocrine. 2015;52(3):652-9.

209. Shimon I, Sosa E, Mendoza V, Greenman Y, Tirosh A, Espinosa E et al. Giant prolactinomas larger than 60 mm in size: a cohort of massive and aggressive prolactin-secreting pituitary adenomas. Pituitary. 2016;19(4):429-36.

210. Vilar L, Albuquerque JL, Gomes B, Gadelha PS, Lopes IGA, Thé AC , et al. Giant prolactinomas: clinical manifestations and response to treatment in 16 cases. Arch Endocrinol Metab. 2015; 59 (Suppl. 1):S21.

211. Saeki N, NakamuraM, Sunami K, Yamaura A. Surgical indication after bromocriptine therapy on giant prolactinomas: effects and limitations of the medical treatment. Endocr J. 1998;45(4):529-37.

212. Sieck JO, Niles NL, Jinkins JR, Al-Mefty O, el-Akkad S, Woodhouse N. Extrasellar prolactinomas: successful management of 24 patients using bromocriptine. Horm Res.1986;23(3):167-76.

213. Kyung Rae C, Kyung-Il J, Hyung Jin S. Bromocriptine therapy for the treatment of invasive prolactinoma: the single institute experience. Brain Tumor Res Treat. 2013 ; 1(2):71–7

214. Komotar RJ, Starke RM, Raper DM, Anand VK, Schwartz TH. Endoscopic endonasal compared with microscopic transsphenoidal and open transcranial resection of giant pituitary adenomas. Pituitary. 2012;15(2):150-9.

215. Brown RS, Herbison AE, Grattan DR. Prolactin regulation of kisspeptin neurons in the mouse brain and its role in the lactation-induced suppression of kisspeptin expression. J Neuroendocrinol. 2014:26(12):898-908.

216. Molitch ME. Endocrinology in pregnancy: management of the pregnant patient with a prolactinoma. Eur J Endocrinol. 2015;172(5):R205-13.

217. Glezer A, Jallad RS, Machado MC, Fragoso MC, Bronstein MD. Pregnancy and pituitary adenomas. Minerva Endocrinol. 2016;41(3):341-50.

218. Holmgren U, Bergstrand G, Hagenfeldt K, Werner S. Women with prolactinoma--effect of pregnancy and lactation on serum prolactin and on tumour growth. Acta Endocrinol (Copenh). 1986;111(4):452-9.

219. Bronstein MD, Paraiba DB, Jallad RS. Management of pituitary tumors in pregnancy.Nat Rev Endocrinol. 2011;7(5):301-10.

220. Raymond JP, Goldstein E, Konopka P, Leleu MR, Merceron LE, Loria Y..Follow-up of children born of bromocriptine-treated mothers. Horm Res. 1985;22(3):239-46.

221. Canales ES, Garcia IC, Ruiz JE, Zárate A. Bromocriptine as prophylactic therapy in prolactinoma during pregnancy. Fertil Steril. 1981;36(4):524-6.

222. Glezer A, Bronstein MD. Prolactinomas, cabergoline, and pregnancy. Endocrine. 2014;47(1):64-9.

223. Bronstein MD. Prolactinomas and pregnancy. Pituitary. 2005;8(1):31-8.

224. Krupp P, Monka C, Richter K. The safety aspects of infertility treatments. Program of the Second World Congress of Gynecology and Obstetrics 1988. Rio de Janeiro, Brazil. p. 9.

225. Ono M, Miki N, Amano K, Kawamata T, Seki T, Makino R, et al. High-dose cabergoline therapy for hyperprolactinemic infertility in women with micro- and macroprolactinomas. J Clin Endocrinol Metab. 2010;95(6):2672-9.

226. Lebbe M, Hubinont C, Bernard P, Maiter D. Outcome of 100 pregnancies initiated under treatment with cabergoline in hyperprolactinaemic women. Clin Endocrinol (Oxf). 2010;73(2):236-42.

227. Stalldecker G, Gil MSM, Guitelman MA, Alfieri A, Ballarino MC, Boero L, et al. Effects of cabergoline on pregnancy and embryo-fetal development: retrospective study on 103 pregnancies and a review of the literature. Pituitary. 2010;13(4):345-50.

228. Yoon HW, Lee JS, Park SJ, Lee SK, Choi WJ, Kim TY, et al. Comparing the effectiveness and safety of the addition of and switching to aripiprazole for resolving antipsychotic-induced hyperprolactinemia: a multicenter, open-label, prospective study. Clin Neuropharmacol. 2016;39(6):288-94.

229. Raghuthaman G, Venkateswaran R, Krishnadas R. Adjunctive aripiprazole in risperidone-induced hyperprolactinaemia: double-blind, randomised, placebo-controlled trial. B J Psych Open. 2015;1(2):172-7.

230. Burback L. Management of a microprolactinoma with aripiprazole in a woman with cabergoline-induced mania. Endocrinol Diabetes Metab Case Rep. 2015;2015:150100.

231. Bakker IC, Schubart CD, Zelissen PM. Successful treatment of a prolactinoma with the antipsychotic drug aripiprazole. Endocrinol Diabetes Metab Case Rep. 2016;2016:160028.

232. Yanofski J. The dopamine dilemma. Psychiatry (Edgmont). 2010;7(6):18-23.

233. Owen R, Owen F, Poulter M, Crow TJ. Dopamine D2 receptors in substantia nigra in schizophrenia. Brain Res. 1994;299(1):152-4.

234. Chang SC, Chen CH, Lu ML. Cabergoline-induced psychotic exacerbation in schizophrenic patients. Gen Hosp Psychiatry. 2008;30(4):378-80.

235. Santos Andrade EH, Pan PM, da Silva PF, Gadelha A. New insights in the management of antipsychotics in the treatment of schizophrenia in a patient with prolactinoma: a case report and review of the literature. Case Rep Med. 2010;2010:573252.

236. Pollice R, Di Giovambattista E, Tomassini A, Di Pucchio A, Mazza M, Di Michele V, et al. Risperidone-induced symptomatic hyperprolactinemia in youth with schizophrenia: efficacy and tolerability of cabergoline treatment. Clin Ter. 2007;158(2):121-6.

237. Tollin SR. Use of the dopamine agonists bromocriptine and cabergoline in the management of risperidone-induced hyperprolactinemia in patients with psychotic disorders. J Endocrinol Invest. 2000;23(11):765-70.

238. Cavallaro R, Cocchi F, Angelone SM, Lattuada E, Smeraldi E. Cabergoline treatment of risperidone-induced hyperprolactinemia: a pilot study. J Clin Psychiatry. 2004;65(2):187-90.

239. Kalkavoura CS, Michopoulos I, Arvanitakis P, Theodoropoulou P, Dimopoulou K, Tzebelikos E, Lykouras L. Effects of cabergoline on hyperprolactinemia, psychopathology, and sexual functioning in schizophrenic patients. Exp Clin Psychopharmacol. 2013;21(4):332-41.

240. Lee MS, Song HC, Na H, Yang J, Ko YH, Jung IK, Joe SH. Effect of bromocriptine on antipsychotic drug-induced hyperprolactinemia: eight-week randomized, single-blind, placebo-controlled, multicenter study. Psychiatry Clin Neurosci. 2010;64 (1):19-27.

Increased insulin sensitivity in individuals with neurofbromatosis type 1

Aline Stangherlin Martins[1], Ann Kristine Jansen[2], Luiz Oswaldo Carneiro Rodrigues[1], Camila Maria Matos[1], Marcio Leandro Ribeiro Souza[1], Débora Marques Miranda[3], Nilton Alves de Rezende[1]

[1] Centro de Referência de Neurofibromatose, Universidade Federal de Minas Gerais (UFMG), Belo Horizonte, MG, Brasil
[2] Departamento de Nutrição, Universidade Federal de Minas Gerais (UFMG), Belo Horizonte, MG, Brasil
[3] Departamento de Clínica Médica, Universidade Federal de Minas Gerais (UFMG), Belo Horizonte, MG, Brasil

Correspondence to:
Nilton Alves de Rezende
Centro de Referência de Neurofibromatose,
Departamento de Medicina Interna,
Universidade Federal de Minas Gerais
Alameda Álvaro Celso, 55
30150-260 – Belo Horizonte,
MG, Brasil
narezende@terra.com

ABSTRACT

Objects: To compare insulin resistance (IR) and metabolic aspects of patients with neurofibromatosis type 1 (NF1) and individuals without the disease. Subjects and methods: Forty patients with NF1 were matched by sex, age, and body mass index (BMI) to 40 controls from the community. Blood samples were collected for biochemical assessment. Homeostasis model assessment adiponectin (HOMA-AD), Homeostasis model assessment insulin resistance (HOMA-IR), and adiponectin/leptin ratio (ALR) were used to identify IR. Results: The median HOMA-IR values were similar between the groups. However, the HOMA-AD value was significantly lower and the ALR significantly higher in the NF1 group. Fasting blood glucose (FBG), leptin, and visfatin levels of patients with NF1 were significantly lower, although adiponectin levels were significantly higher than those in the controls. Fasting insulin and blood glucose levels 2 hours after administration of 75 g of dextrose, glycated hemoglobin, and resistin showed no significant differences between groups.The HOMA-AD correlated with BMI, FBG, blood glucose levels 2 hours after administration of 75 g of dextrose, fasting insulin, glycated hemoglobin, adiponectin, leptin, visfatin, ALR, and HOMA-IR. The ALR correlated with BMI leptin, visfatin, and adiponectin. Conclusions: Lower levels of FBG, leptin, visfatin, and HOMA-AD, and higher adiponectin levels and ALR may be related to increased insulin sensitivity and lower occurrence of type 2 diabetes mellitus in patients with NF1. Arch Endocrinol Metab. 2018;62(1):34-9

Keywords
Blood glucose; neurofibromatosis 1; diabetes mellitus; type 2; insulin resistance

INTRODUCTION

A rare disease is generally defined as a disease with a very low prevalence (1). Although considered individually rare, as a group, these diseases affect a significant percentage of the population and present a relevant health problem (2). Therefore, research is needed to better understand these diseases.

Neurofibromatosis type 1 (NF1) is a rare, autosomal-dominant disorder caused by inherited or new mutations on chromosome 17. These mutations result in dysfunction of the neurofibromin protein, which is involved in growth control and behavior of various tissues (3). It is one the most common human monogenic diseases, with an estimated prevalence of approximately 1: 3,500 births (4).

The clinical NF1 criteria include *café-au-lait* spots, neurofibromas, axillary and/or inguinal freckling, Lisch nodules in the iris, optical gliomas, specific bone dysplasia, and familial history (5). NF1 is a multisystem disease, affecting the musculoskeletal, cardiovascular, endocrine, and central and peripheral nervous systems as well as learning skills (6).

Data suggest a lower prevalence of type 2 diabetes mellitus (T2DM) in patients with NF1 (7,8). Madubata and cols. (9) showed that patients with NF1 had a lower chance of having DM compared to healthy individuals. Moreover, Martins and cols. (10) reported that patients with NF1 showed significantly lower fasting blood glucose (FBG) levels compared to controls without the disease.

T2DM (90% to 95% of all cases of diabetes) is associated with insulin resistance (IR) (11). The hyperinsulinemic euglycemic clamp technique is considered the gold standard to assess IR; however, it is a complex and expensive method that is often not available for studies and clinical practice (12). Another

IR validated index is the homeostasis model assessment for insulin resistance (HOMA-IR) (13). This index shows a strong correlation with hyperinsulinemic euglycemic clamp findings (14). However, there is some debate regarding its ability to detect IR in individuals with normal glucose or impaired glucose tolerance (15).

Matsuhisa and cols. (16) developed a modified HOMA index, the HOMA-adiponectin (HOMA-AD), by including adiponectin levels in the denominator. This modification makes the HOMA index a more sensitive marker of IR (16,17).

Mediators produced by adipose tissue, called adipocytokines (leptin, visfatin, resistin, and adiponectin) affect glucose homeostasis, appetite regulation, inflammation, and atherosclerosis and are associated with IR (18). Studies have shown increased levels of leptin, visfatin, and resistin in individuals with T2DM (18). In contrast, adiponectin levels are reportedly lower in patients with DM and metabolic syndrome (19) and studies have shown that their levels may be markers of the risk of prediabetes (20).

In addition, some studies have suggested that the adiponectin-leptin ratio (ALR) may be an effective parameter for the assessment of IR in individuals with or without diabetes (21).

The results of previous studies lead us to hypothesize that patients with NF1 may have (1) genetic differences that modify glucose utilization and cellular control and/or (2) phenotypic characteristics that result in increased insulin sensitivity, favoring the maintenance of lower levels of FBG and reducing the risk of developing T2DM. Thus, this study aimed to evaluate IR and metabolic aspects of patients with NF1 compared with control individuals without the disease.

MATERIALS AND METHODS

Population

The study included patients over 20 years of age with NF1 followed at the Reference Center on Neurofibromatoses at the Federal University of Minas Gerais (CRNF-UFMG) who met at least three criteria for the diagnosis of disease according to the National Institute of Health (22).

The control group consisted of volunteers from the community (e.g., university students, CRNF-UFMG officials, and companions of patients seen at the clinic) who were similar in terms of sex, age, and BMI to the included patients with NF1.

Individuals diagnosed with diabetes, liver disease or malignancy, and infection as well as those using steroids, antibiotics, statins, insulin, and oral hypoglycemic agents were excluded from both groups.

Sample

The sample size was calculated based on the results of the study by Martins and cols. (10), and we used a standard deviation of 13 units, a least significant difference of 10 units, and power of 90%, resulting in the requirement for a minimum of 37 participants in each group.

Ethical aspects

The study was approved by the Ethics and Human Research of the UFMG (number 258.325, year 2013) and all participants signed an informed consent form.

Procedures

Weight and height of the participants were measured, and BMI calculated based on protocols established by the World Health Organization (23).

We assessed the physical activity level by the International Physical Activity Questionnaire (24) and the diet by means of a 3-day non-consecutive dietary record. For each record, the total amounts of the following components were calculated using the food composition tables: calories, carbohydrates, lipids, proteins, fiber, cholesterol, saturated fatty acids, monounsaturated and polyunsaturated fatty acids, zinc, magnesium, selenium, and vitamin D.

Blood samples were collected from the participants for analysis of FBG, blood glucose 2 hours after administration of 75 g of dextrose, glycated hemoglobin (HbA1c), and fasting insulin, adiponectin, leptin, visfatin, and resistin according to the protocol used at the CRNF-UFMG.

Blood glucose and glycosylated hemoglobin (HbA1c) levels were measured using the Vitros equipment and reagents from Ortho-Clinical Diagnostics® (blood glucose coefficient of variation [CV] inter-assay, level 1: 2.24% and level 2: 2.23%; HbA1c CV, level 1: 5.11% and level 2: 6.04%). Insulin levels were measured using the Architect-Abbott® equipment, with Abbott® reagents (CV inter-assay, level 1: 4.4, level 2: 2.9, and level 3: 3.2).

The leptin assay was performed using the human leptin enzyme-linked immunoassay (ELISA) kit from Millipore (CV inter-assay: 3.7%; CV intra-assay: 4.4%, respectively). Resistin levels were measured using the human resistin ELISA from eBioscience® (CV inter-assay: 8.1%; CV intra-assay: 5.1%). Adiponectin levels were measured using the human adiponectin ELISA kit from eBioscience® (CV inter-assay: 3.1%; CV intra-assay: 4.2%, respectively). Visfatin was assayed using the human visfatin ELISA kit from MyBioSource® (CV < 10%). The assays were performed according to the kit protocols.

FBG, HbA1c, and glucose levels 2 hours after administration of 75 g of dextrose were categorized according to the cutoff values established by the American Diabetes Association (11).

The markers of IR included the HOMA-IR (HOMA-IR = fasting insulin (U/mL) × FBG (mmol/L)/22.5), HOMA-AD (HOMA-AD = fasting insulin (U/mL) × FBG (mmol/L)/Adiponectin (μ/mL) and ALR.

Statistical analysis

Continuous variables were described as means and standard deviations or as medians and 25th and 75th percentiles as appropriate. Categorical variables were described as absolute and relative frequencies.

The Kolmogorov-Smirnov test was used to test the normality of the variables. Paired t-tests were used to compare groups with normally distributed variables. The Wilcoxon test was used to compare groups with non-normal variables distribution. McNemar's test was used to compare proportions between two groups. When McNemar's test could not be used, we used chi-square or Fisher's exact tests.

The Spearman correlation test was used to verify the correlations between HOMA-AD and ALR and other variables.

To determine whether the differences and associations were statistically significant, we used a 5% level of significance. Thus, P-values ≤ 0.05 were considered to represent statistically significant differences.

Data were analyzed using the Statistical Package for Social Science (SPSS) version 13.0.

RESULTS

We evaluated 47 patients with NF1 and 47 controls. Seven individuals were excluded from the NF1 group (one because of the use of corticosteroids, one because of suspicion of malignancy, and five owing to unavailability of blood test results). The respective controls were also excluded, finally amounting to 40 participants in each group.

The general characteristics of patients with NF1 and controls are described in Table 1. The average weight and the median height were significantly lower in the NF1 group.

Table 1. General characteristics of patients with NF1 and controls

Variables	NF1 (n = 40)	Controls (n = 40)	P-value
Sex[a]			
Female	28 (70.0)	28 (70.0)	1.000[d]
Male	12 (30.0)	12 (30.0)	
Age[b]	40.7 (11.8)	40.4 (12.1)	0.390[e]
Weight (kg)[b]	60.6 (13.1)	68.5 (14.5)	< 0.001[e]
Height (m)[c]	1.57 (1.51–1.63)	1.62 (1.57–1.74)	< 0.001[f]
BMI (kg/m^2)[c]	24.2 (21.6–26.2)	24.6 (22.3–26.5)	0.096[f]
Physical activity level*			
Not active	9 (22.5)	14 (35)	
Not very active	3 (7.5)	5 (12.5)	0.343[d]
Moderately active	28 (70)	21 (52.5)	

[a] n (%); [b] Mean (standard deviation); [c] Median (percentiles 25-75); [d] McNemar's test; [e] Paired t-test; [f] Wilcoxon Test; BMI: body mass index. *According to the International Physical Activity Questionnaire (25).

There were no statistically significant differences between the NF1 and control groups regarding the intake of any of the evaluated nutrients.

Table 2 shows the IR markers and metabolic characteristics of patients with NF1 and controls. The HOMA-IR values were similar between groups. However, the HOMA-AD value was significantly lower and ALR was significantly higher in the NF1 group. The FBG, leptin, and visfatin levels in patients with NF1 were significantly lower than those in controls. The adiponectin levels was significantly higher in the NF1 group. No significant differences were observed between groups in the levels of resistin, post dextrose glucose, HbA1c, and fasting insulin.

The HOMA-AD values were correlated with BMI, FBG, post dextrose glucose, fasting insulin HbA1c, adiponectin, leptin, and visfatin levels, as well as ALR and HOMA-IR values (Table 3).

The ALR correlated with BMI ($r = -0.239$, $p = 0.033$), adiponectin ($r = 0.652$, $p < 0.001$), leptin ($r = -0.869$, $p < 0.001$) and visfatin levels ($r = -0,329$, $p = 0,003$).

Table 2. Insulin resistance markers and metabolic characteristics of patients with NF1 and controls

Variables	NF1 (n = 40)	Controls (n = 40)	P-value
HOMA-IR[a]	1.1 (0.7-1.6)	1.3 (0.9–2.3)	0.147[c]
HOMA-AD[a]	1.0 (0.5–1.7)	1.9 (1.0–4.1)	0.001[c]
ALR[a]	3.8 (2.1–12.6)	1.2 (0.7–2.1)	< 0.001[c]
FBG (mg/dL)[a]	83.5 (78.0–90.0)	86.0 (83.0–94.0)	0.008[c]
FBG classification[b]			
Normal (< 100 mg/dL)	40 (100.0)	35 (87.5)	0.027[d]
Impaired (≥ 100 mg/dL)	0	5 (12.5)	
Glucose level postdextrose administration (mg/dL)[a]	96.5 (85.3–112.5)	99.5 (88.0–118.3)	0.255[c]
Glucose level postdextrose administration classification[b]			
Normal (< 140 mg/dL)	38 (95.0)	34 (85.0)	0.219[e]
Impaired (≥ 140 mg/dL)	2 (5.0)	6 (15.0)	
HbA1c (%)[a]	5.2 (5.0–5.5)	5.4 (5.0–5.7)	0.100[c]
HbA1c classification[b]			
< 5.7%	30 (75.0)	26 (65.0)	
5.7–6,4%	10 (25.0)	14 (35.0)	0.503[e]
≥ 6.5%	0	0	
Fasting insulin (µU/mL)[a]	4.9 (3.6–11.6)	6.0 (4.4–15.7)	0.357[c]
Adiponectin (µg/mL)[a]	23.7 (17.0–39.4)	15.3 (11.3–20.9)	0.001[c]
Leptin (ng/mL)[a]	5.7 (3.1–11.7)	11,9 (6.8–20.7)	0.042[c]
Resistin (ng/mL)[a]	6.8 (3.4–9.0)	5,8 (2.4–9.8)	0.490[c]
Visfatin (ng/mL)[a]	118.2 (105.8–124.8)	138.2 (125.5–147.7)	< 0.001[c]

[a] Median (percentiles 25 and 75); [b] n (%); [c] Wilcoxon test; [d] Fisher's exact test; [e] McNemar's test. HOMA-IR: Homeostasis Model Assessment Insulin Resistance; HOMA-AD: Homeostasis Model Assessment Adiponectin; FBG: fasting blood glucose; HbA1c: glycated hemoglobin; ALR: adiponectin-leptin ratio.

Table 3. Variables significantly correlated with HOMA-AD values in all study participants (n = 80)

Variable	Correlation coefficient[a]	P-value
BMI	0.349	0.002
FBG	0.448	< 0.001
Fasting insulin	0.667	< 0.001
Post dextrose glucose	0.388	< 0.001
HbA1c	0.315	0.004
Adiponectin	-0.662	< 0.001
Leptin	0.300	0.007
Visfatin	0.269	0.016
ALR	-0.547	< 0.001
HOMA-IR	0.700	< 0.001

[a] Spearman correlation coefficient; FBG: fasting blood glucose; HbA1c: glycated hemoglobin; HOMA-IR: Homeostasis Model Assessment-Insulin Resistance; ALR: adiponectin-leptin ratio; HOMA-AD: Homeostasis Model Assessment-Adiponectin.

DISCUSSION

The results of the present study revealed that HOMA-IR was similar between the NF1 and control groups. However, the HOMA-AD values were significantly lower in patients with NF1 than those in the control group. FBG, leptin, and visfatin levels were significantly lower and adiponectin levels and ALR were significantly higher in patients with NF1 than those in the control group.

While the HOMA-IR is the most widely used index for the determination of IR, some authors have reported that this index fails to identify IR in individuals with normal glucose levels and impaired glucose tolerance (15). In this study, 100% of patients with NF1 showed FBG within normal levels and only 12.5% of controls had impaired FBG levels. Thus, the HOMA-IR may not be the most appropriate method for identifying IR in patients with NF1, in this sample.

HOMA-AD has been reported to be a suitable method for identifying IR in specific populations, and some authors consider it a more sensitive marker of IR (16,17). The results of this study revealed a significantly lower median HOMA-AD level in the NF1 group, suggesting that these patients may have greater insulin sensitivity than controls.

The ALR has also been reported to be a more efficient marker of IR than HOMA-IR, showing an inverse correlation with IR markers (21). In the present study, ALR was significantly higher in patients with NF1, also suggesting a greater sensitivity to insulin in this group of patients.

The mechanisms to explain increased insulin sensitivity in individuals with NF1 are unknown. It is known that excess adipose tissue plays an essential role in the development of IR. However, Pal and cols. (25) demonstrated that patients with mutations in the tumor suppressor phosphatase and tensin homologue, which causes a syndrome of predisposition to cancer, have increased insulin sensitivity and excess weight compared to controls. The authors have also shown that the excess weight found in the patients was not due to increased lean or bone mass, but rather to increased adiposity, and suggest that the excess weight may be due to the improved action of insulin in the adipose tissue.

Studies have shown that suppression of lipolysis is highly sensitive to insulin (26). This way, considering the conclusions of these studies, patients with NF1 who exhibit insulin sensitivity could be obese. However, our patients had BMI within the normal range, and other studies have already demonstrated a lower BMI in NF1 patients, contradicting the findings of Pal and cols. Two hypotheses could explain these findings, insulin sensitivity in individuals with NF1 may be mild, and it may not be sufficient to induce obesity or insulin sensitivity that is specific to non-fat tissues.

We believe that the characteristics of body composition in NFI patients, demonstrated in other studies (27) and associated with increased adiponectin and lower visfatin and leptin levels, may be related to higher insulin sensitivity found in this group of individuals.

Regarding metabolic characteristics, the median values of FBG in patients with NF1 were significantly lower than those in control individuals; the number of individuals with impaired FBG was also significantly lower in the NF1 group than in the control group. These data agree with a previous study by our group (10), which evaluated 57 patients with NF1 and 171 controls and found significantly lower levels of FBG in patients with NF1.

HbA1c, blood glucose 2 hours after administration of dextrosol, and fasting insulin levels were also similar between the groups, suggesting that some mechanism involved in the control of fasting glucose may be responsible for the lower levels of FBG in the NF1 group. After a prolonged period of fasting, glucose levels in the blood decline, stimulating the pancreatic alpha cells to release glucagon. The result is hepatic glycogenolysis and gluconeogenesis to increase blood glucose levels (28). Thus, we hypothesize that the lower levels of FBG in NF1 could be a result of a change in the glycogenolysis or gluconeogenesis process.

Neurofibromin plays a role in the regulation of the hypothalamus and pituitary gland (29), which are involved in the regulation of energy balance (30). Neurofibromin could play a role in glucose metabolism, and its deficiency may cause reduced gluconeogenesis in patients with NF1. Moreover, the modified pathways resulting in insulin changes related to neurofibromin are not clear.

A second hypothesis to explain the lower levels of FBG in patients with NF1 is derivate of the production of insulin-like growth factor 2 (IGF2) by neurofibromas. Studies have shown that tumors produce IGF2, which increases the consumption of peripheral glucose and decreases the glucose production in the liver, resulting in hypoglycemia (31). However, further studies are needed to verify if the FBG levels in patients with NF1 can be accounted for by IGF2 produced by neurofibromas.

A third hypothesis that could explain the lower fasting glucose levels in patients with NF1 is related to adipocytokine levels. The results of this study showed that adiponectin levels in patients with NF1 were significantly higher and levels of visfatin and leptin were significantly lower than in controls. According to Yamauchi and cols. (32) one of the mechanisms through which adiponectin may decrease the risk of T2DM is the suppression of hepatic gluconeogenesis. Leptin can reduce hepatic glucose production by decreasing the synthesis of phosphoenolpyruvate carboxylase, which is the key enzyme in gluconeogenesis (33). However, Gutiérrez-Juárez and cols. (34) showed that administration of leptin in rats stimulated gluconeogenesis. Visfatin, in turn, appears to stimulate gluconeogenesis (35).

Thus, differences in the levels of these adipocytokines may contribute to lower hepatic gluconeogenesis and lower levels of FBG in patients with NF1. However, further studies are needed to validate this hypothesis. The reason for the changes in the levels of these adipocytokines in patients with NF1 remains unknown. No other studies have evaluated adipocytokine levels in NF1.

The correlation of HOMA-AD values with diabetes mellitus markers, FBG, post dextrose glucose, and HbA1c in addition to HOMA-IR values, levels of adiponectin, leptin, and visfatin, and ALR reinforce the hypothesis that the characteristics observed in patients with NF1 (lower levels of FBG, visfatin, and leptin and higher adiponectin and adiponectin/leptin levels) may explain the lower incidence of T2DM in these patients.

This study has several limitations, including the small number of patients involved, although NF1 is a rare disease for which surveys are usually performed with even fewer participants. In addition, IR was not evaluated using the gold-standard techniques.

In conclusion, the results of this matched case-control study suggested for the first time that NF1 individuals have increased insulin sensitivity, as well as lower levels of FBG, visfatin, and leptin and higher adiponectin levels, than those without the disease. These characteristics may be associated with the lower occurrence of T2DM in this group of patients.

Acknowledgments: we thank the patients of CRNF-UFMG, the volunteers who participated in the study, the researchers, and students of the Molecular Medicine Laboratory of University Federal of Minas Gerais, and the employees of CRNF-MG for their collaboration.

Funding: this work was funded by National Council of Technological and Scientific Development, CNPq (No. 471725/2013-7), and Fapemig (No. APQ-00928-11 and No. PPM-00120-14). ASM received a grant from Coordination for Improvement of Personnel with Higher Education.

REFERENCES

1. Denis A, Simoens S, Fostier C, Mergaert L, Cleemput I. Policies for rare diseases and orphan drugs. Health Technology Assessment (HTA). Brussels: Belgian Health Care Knowledge Centre (KCE) 2009. KCE reports 112C (D/2009/10.273/32).
2. Brasil. Ministério da Saúde. Diretrizes para Atenção Integral às Pessoas com Doenças Raras no Sistema Único de Saúde. Ministério da Saúde; 2014.
3. Riccardi VM. Neurofibromatosis type 1 is a disorder of dysplasia: the importance of distinguishing features, consequences, and complications. Birth Defects Res A Clin MolTeratol. 2010;88(1):9-14.
4. Radtke HB, Sebold CD, Allison C, Haidle JL, Schneider G. Neurofibromatosis type 1 in genetic counseling practice: recommendations of the National Society of Genetic Counselors. J Genet Couns. 2007;16(4):387-407.
5. Rodrigues LO, Batista PB, Goloni-Bertollo EM, de Souza-Costa D, Eliam L, Eliam M, et al. Neurofibromatoses: part 1 - diagnosis and differential diagnosis. Arq Neuropsiquiatr. 2014;72(3):241-50.
6. Souza JF, Toledo LL, Ferreira MC, Rodrigues LO, Rezende NA. Neurofibromatosis type 1: more frequent and severe then usually thought. Rev Assoc Med Bras (1992). 2009;55(4):394-9.
7. Rasmussen SA, Yang Q, Friedman JA. Mortality in neurofibromatosis 1: an analysis using U.S. death certificates. Am J Hum Genet. 2001;68(5):1110-8.
8. Masocco M, Kodra Y, Vichi M, Conti S, Kanieff M, Pace M, et al. Mortality associated with neurofibromatosis type 1: a study based on Italian death certificates (1995-2006). Orphanet J Rare Dis. 2011 Mar 25;6:11.
9. Madubata CC, Olsen MA, Stwalley DL, Gutmann DH, Johnson KJ. Neurofibromatosis type 1 and chronic neurological conditions in the United States: an administrative claims analysis. Genet Med. 2015;17(1):36-42.
10. Martins AS, Jansen AK, Rodrigues LO, Matos CM, Souza ML, de Souza JF, et al. Lower fasting blood glucose in neurofibromatosis type 1. Endocr Connect. 2016;5(1):28-33.
11. American Diabetes Association. Standards of medical care in diabetes. Diabetes Care. 2016;39:S1-S112.
12. Ausk KJ, Boyko EJ, Ioannou GN. Insulin resistance predicts mortality in nondiabetic individuals in the U.S.A. Diabetes Care. 2010;33(6):1179-85.
13. Matthews DR, Hosker JP, Rudenski AS, Naylor BA, Treacher DF, Turner RC. Homeostasis model assessment: insulin resistance and beta-cell function from fasting plasma glucose and insulin concentrations in man. Diabetologia. 1985;28(7):412-9.
14. Vasques AC, Rosado L, Rosado G, Ribeiro RC, Franceschini S, Geloneze B. Anthropometric Indicators of Insulin Resistance. Arq Bras Cardiol. 2010;95:e14-e23.
15. Kang ES, Yun YS, Park SW, Kim HJ, Ahn CW, Song YD, et al. Limitation of the validity of the homeostasis model assessment as an index of insulin resistance in Korea. Metabolism. 2005;54(2):206-11.
16. Matsuhisa M, Yamasaki Y, Emoto M, Shimabukuro M, Ueda S, Funahashi T, et al. A novel index of insulin resistance determined from the homeostasis model assessment index and adiponectin levels in Japanese subjects. Diabetes Res Clin Pract. 2007;77(1):151-4.
17. Vilela BS, Vasques AC, Cassani RS, Forti AC, Pareja JC, Tambascia MA, et al. The HOMA-Adiponectin (HOMA-AD) Closely Mirrors the HOMA-IR Index in the Screening of Insulin Resistance in the Brazilian Metabolic Syndrome Study (BRAMS). PLoS One. 2016;11(8):e0158751.
18. Guzik TJ, Mangalat D, Korbut RJ. Adipocytokines - novel link between inflammation and vascular function? J Physiol Pharmacol. 2006;57(4):505-28.
19. Whitehead JP, Richards AA, Hickman IJ, Macdonald GA, Prins JB. Adiponectin--a key adipokine in the metabolic syndrome. Diabetes Obes Metab. 2006;8(3):264-80.
20. Jiang Y, Owei I, Wan J, Ebenibo S, Dagogo-Jack S. Adiponectin levels predict prediabetes risk: the Pathobiology of Prediabetes in A Biracial Cohort (POP-ABC) study. BMJ Open Diabetes Res Care. 2016;4(1):e000194.
21. Jung CH, Rhee EJ, Choi JH, Bae JC, Yoo SH, Kim WJ, et al. The relationship of adiponectin/leptin ratio with homeostasis model assessment insulin resistance index and metabolic syndrome in apparently healthy korean male adults. Korean Diabetes J. 2010;34(4):237-43.
22. National Institutes of Health Neurofibromatosis. NIH Consensus Statement Online. Available from: https://consensus.nih.gov/1987/1987neurofibromatosis064html.htm; 1987. Accessed on 10 May, 2015.
23. World Health Organization. Physical status: the use and interpretation of anthropometry. Geneva: World Health Organization; 1995.
24. Matsudo S, Araujo T, Matsudo V, Andrade D, Andrade E, Oliveira LC, et al. Questionário Internacional de Atividade Física: Estudo de Validade e Reprodutibilidade no Brasil. Rev Bras Ativ Fis Saude. 2001;6:5-18.
25. Pal A, BarberTM, Van de Bunt M, Rudge SA, Zhang Q, Lachlan KL, et al. PTEN mutations as a cause of constitutive insulin sensitivity and obesity. N Engl J Med. 2012;367(11):1002-11.
26. Karpe F, Tan GD. Adipose tissue function in the insulin-resistance syndrome. Biochem SocTrans. 2005;33(Pt 5):1045-8.
27. Souza M, Jansen A, Martins A, Rodrigues L, Rezende N. Body composition in adults with neurofibromatosis type 1. Rev Assoc Med Bras (1992). 2016;62(9):831-6.
28. Röder PV, Wu B, Liu Y, Han W. Pancreatic regulation of glucose homeostasis. Exp Mol Med. 2016;48:e219.
29. Hegedus B, Yeh TH, Lee DY, Emnett RJ, Li J, Gutmann DH. Neurofibromin regulates somatic growth through the hypothalamic-pituitary axis. Hum Mol Genet. 2008;17(19):2956-66.
30. Van de Sande-Lee SV, Velloso LA. Hypothalmic dysfunction in obesity. Arq Bras Endocrinol Metabol. 2012;56(6):341-50.
31. Iglesias P, Diez JJ. Management of endocrine disease: a clinical update on tumor-induced hypoglycemia. Eur J Endocrinol. 2014;170(4):R147-57.
32. Yamauchi T, Kamon J, Minokoshi Y, Ito Y, Waki H, Uchida S, et al. Adiponectin stimulates glucose utilization and fatty-acid oxidation by activating AMP-activated protein kinase. Nat Med. 2002;8(11):1288-95.
33. Anderwald C, Müller G, Koca G, Fürnsinn C, Waldhäusl W, Roden M. Short-term leptin-dependent inhibition of hepatic gluconeogenesis is mediated by insulin receptor substrate-2. Mol Endocrinol. 2002;16(7):1612-28.
34. Gutiérrez-Juárez R, Obici S, Rossetti L. Melanocortin-independent effects of leptin on hepatic glucose fluxes. J Biol Chem. 2004;279(48):49704-15.
35. ChoiYJ, Choi SE, Ha ES, KangY, Han SJ, Kim DJ, et al. Extracellular visfatin activates gluconeogenesis in HepG2 cells through the classical PKA/CREB-dependent pathway. Horm Metab Res. 2014;46(4):233-9.

15

Maternal hypothyroxinemia in the first trimester of gestation and association with obstetric and neonatal outcomes and iron deficiency: a prospective Brazilian study

Pedro Weslley Rosario[1], Luis Fernando Faria Oliveira[2], Maria Regina Calsolari[1]

[1] Programa de Pós-Graduação e Serviço de Endocrinologia, Santa Casa de Belo Horizonte, Belo Horizonte, MG, Brasil
[2] Fundação Universidade de Itaúna, Itaúna, MG, Brasil

Correspondence to:
Pedro Weslley Rosario
Instituto de Ensino e Pesquisa, Santa Casa de Belo Horizonte
Rua Domingos Vieira, 590
30150-240 – Belo Horizonte, MG, Brasil
pedrowsrosario@gmail.com

ABSTRACT

Objective: To evaluate the association of isolated hypothyroxinemia in the first trimester with obstetric and neonatal outcomes and iron deficiency. Subjects and methods: The study was prospective. Women who had become pregnant spontaneously were initially selected. Next, anti-thyroid peroxidase antibodies (TPOAb), free T4 (FT4), total T4 (TT4), TSH, and ferritin were measured. TPOAb-positive women were excluded. The final sample consisted of 596 women with serum TSH between 0.1 and 2.5 mIU/l. Hypothyroxinemia was defined as FT4 < 0.86 ng/dL and < 0.92 ng/dL, corresponding to the 5th and 10th percentiles, respectively, and TT4 < 7.8 ng/dL. None of the pregnant women was treated with levothyroxine until the end of pregnancy. Results: The women ranged in age from 18 to 36 years, with a median gestation of 9 weeks. T4 levels were not correlated with BMI or maternal TSH. Isolated hypothyroxinemia was observed in 4.3% (FT4 < 0.86 ng/dL), 9% (FT4 < 0.92 ng/dL), and 7% (TT4 < 7.8 ng/dL) of the pregnant women. The frequencies of obstetric and neonatal outcomes were similar in women with versus without hypothyroxinemia. In women without iron deficiency, 8.4%, 3.9%, and 6.5% had FT4 < 0.92 ng/dl, FT4 < 0.86 ng/dL and TT4 < 7.8 μg/dL, respectively. These frequencies of hypothyroxinemia were significantly higher among women with iron deficiency (20.7%, 14.8% and 17.2%, respectively). Conclusions: This prospective Brazilian study found no association between isolated hypothyroxinemia in the first trimester of gestation and obstetric or neonatal outcomes, but an association was demonstrated with iron deficiency. Arch Endocrinol Metab. 2018;62(3):332-6

Keywords
Pregnancy; first trimester; hypothyroxinemia; iron deficiency; obstetric and neonatal outcomes

INTRODUCTION

When screening for thyroid dysfunction in pregnancy is indicated, it should be performed in the first prenatal visit, which usually occurs in the first trimester. Possible consequences of subclinical hypothyroidism and isolated maternal hypothyroxinemia also appear to be more worrisome when they occur in the first trimester of gestation, a period when the fetus still does not produce thyroid hormone and depends on maternal thyroxine (T4) (1). It is therefore more important to know the impact of these conditions when diagnosed in the early stages of pregnancy (1,2).

Isolated hypothyroxinemia is diagnosed in the presence of serum TSH within the normal range associated with T4 concentrations below the 2.5th, 5th or 10th percentile (2-4). Regarding TSH, except when the assay- and population-specific references values are available, the range of 0.1 to 2.5 mIU/l has been accepted for the definition of maternal euthyroidism in the first trimester (2,3,5-7). It is worth noting that this range does also seem to be adequate for our population (8). Iodine deficiency appears to the most important factor in the etiology of isolated hypothyroxinemia, but other factors have also been implicated, such as environmental disruptors, obesity, and iron deficiency (4). No consensus exists regarding the consequences and need for levothyroxine (L-T4) replacement therapy in isolated hypothyroxinemia (4). The American College of Obstetricians and Gynecologists (ACOG) does not consider this condition in its guidelines (9). The American Thyroid Association (ATA) does not recommend its treatment (3), while the Endocrine

Society proposes partial replacement therapy (5). According to the European Thyroid Association (ETA), treatment can be considered when hypothyroxinemia is detected in the first trimester, but not when it is detected in the second or third trimester (2). A large recent study found no benefit of L-T4 replacement therapy in isolated hypothyroxinemia, but one limitation of that study is that this therapy was generally initiated only in the 18th week of gestation (10,11).

In view of the lack of consensus regarding the management of isolated hypothyroxinemia, notably when detected in the first trimester, the objective of this study was to evaluate the association of this condition with obstetric and neonatal outcomes. The association with iron deficiency was also explored. To our knowledge, no Brazilian study has so far evaluated these associations.

SUBJECTS AND METHODS

The study was prospective and was approved by the local Research Ethics Committee (8).

Selection

The population studied was from the metropolitan region of Belo Horizonte (Minas Gerais, Brazil). One thousand and eighty two pregnant women who underwent prenatal exams at a clinical analysis laboratory and who had become pregnant spontaneously were initially interviewed and examined (8). Women who met the clinical criteria shown in Table 1 (n = 748) were first selected. Next, anti-thyroid peroxidase antibodies (TPOAb), free T4 (FT4), total T4 (TT4), TSH, and ferritin were measured. TPOAb-positive pregnant women (n = 38) were excluded. Women with hyperemesis gravidarum, twin pregnancy or trophoblastic disease (n = 50) were also excluded. The sample consisted of 660 women and 596 with serum TSH between 0.1 and 2.5 mIU/l (2,3,5-7,8) were selected.

Protocol

At the time of the study, and still today, T4 measurement is not necessary in women with TSH ≤ 2.5 mIU/L without TPOAb. There was also, and continues to be, no consensus recommendation regarding the treatment of hypothyroxinemia. Hence, in order to avoid interference with the results, the protocol was approved foreseeing the non-repetition of thyroid function tests during pregnancy and was thus executed. None of the pregnant women was treated with L-T4 until the end of pregnancy. Regarding iron supplementation, the women only received the recommended daily doses in all pregnant women without additional supplementation in those with iron deficiency.

Outcomes

Obstetric and neonatal outcomes were compared between women with FT4 < 0.86 ng/dL and < 0.92 ng/dL and those with FT4 ≥ 0.92 ng/dL. These values correspond, respectively, to the 5th and 10th percentiles of FT4 concentrations obtained for the initially selected 660 TPOAb-negative women (8). We also compared women with TT4 < 7.8 ng/dL and ≥ 7.8 ng/dL. This value is provided by the assay as the lower limit of normal for the first trimester of gestation and corresponds exactly to 1.5 times the lower limit of the reference range for non-pregnant healthy adults (12). The outcomes (reported in Table 2) were predefined before the start of the study based on those used in the largest series that evaluated the association between hypothyroxinemia and pregnancy outcomes (13). The definitions of hypothyroxinemia were also pre-established.

Laboratory

Iron deficiency was defined as a ferritin concentration < 15 ng/mL (14). TSH, FT4, TT4 and TPOAb were measured with a chemiluminescent assay (Diagnostic Products Corporation, Los Angeles, CA). Serum samples were obtained from the women in the morning (at about 8 a.m.) after an 8- to 10-h fast (8).

Table 1. Inclusion criteria

Clinical criteria
Absence of thyroid disease, no current or previous treatment with antithyroid drugs or L-T4, no history of ^{131}I therapy or thyroidectomy
No use of potentially interfering medications such as dopaminergic agonists or antagonists, neuroleptics, corticosteroids, estrogen, amiodarone, interferon, lithium, anticonvulsants, metformin, octreotide; or recent (in the past 8 weeks) exposure to iodinated contrast agents
No history of head and neck external radiotherapy
Absence of type 1 diabetes or other autoimmune diseases
No family history of thyroid disease
Absence of goiter or any palpable thyroid anomaly
Absence of ophthalmopathy
Complementary criteria: ≤ 12 weeks gestation

Table 2. Obstetric outcomes

Obstetric outcomes	FT4 (ng/dL)			TT4 (μg/dL)	
	< 0.86* (n = 26)*	< 0.92** (n = 54)**	≥ 0.92* ** (n = 542)* **	< 7.8*** (n = 42)***	≥ 7.8*** (n = 554)***
Hypertensive disease of pregnancy	2 (7.7%)*	5 (9.2%)**	47 (8.6%)* **	4 (9.5%)***	50 (9%)***
Gestational mellitus diabetes	3 (11.5%)*	6 (11.1%)**	56 (10.3%)* **	5 (12%)***	60 (10.8%)***
Placental abruption	0*	0**	2 (0.3%)* **	0***	2 (0.3%)***
Delivery before 34 weeks of gestation	0*	1 (1.8%)**	5 (0.9%)* **	1 (2.4%)***	5 (0.9%)***
Delivery before 37 weeks of gestation	1 (3.8%)*	2 (3.7%)**	15 (2.7%)* **	2 (4.7%)***	16 (2.8%)***
Fetal loss (after initial evaluation)	0*	2 (3.7%)**	16 (2.9%)* **	2 (4.7%)***	16 (2.8%)***

FT4: free T4; TT4: total T4.

* FT4 < 0.86 ng/dL versus ≥ 0.92 ng/dL: p ≥ 0.5 in all comparisons.

** FT4 < 0.92 ng/dL versus ≥ 0.92 ng/dL: p ≥ 0.65 in all comparisons.

*** TT4 < 7.8 mg/dL versus TT4 ≥ 7.8 μg/dL: p ≥ 0.35 in all comparisons.

Statistical

The Spearman or Pearson correlation test was used to analyze the correlation between T4 and body mass index (BMI) and TSH. The t-test or Mann-Whitney test and Fisher's exact test or the χ^2 test were used for comparison between groups. A P value < 0.05 was considered statistically significant.

RESULTS

The characteristics of the 596 patients are shown in Table 3.

FT4 levels were not correlated with BMI (p = 0.6) or maternal TSH (p = 0.1). TT4 levels were also not correlated with BMI (p = 0.7) or maternal TSH (p = 0.15).

Tables 2 and 4 show the obstetric and neonatal outcomes, respectively, according to maternal T4 concentrations in the first trimester of gestation. The groups were similar in terms of age, BMI and maternal TSH levels. No difference in the frequencies of obstetric or neonatal outcomes was observed, regardless of the definition of isolated hypothyroxinemia.

Table 3. Characteristics of the 596 patients

Age [range, median (years)]	18-36 (27)
Body mass index [range, median (kg/m²)]	18-30 (22.6)
Gestational age [range, median (weeks)]	7-12 (9)
Primigravidae	312 (52.3%)
TSH [range, median (mIU/L)]	0.1-2.5 (0.98)
Hypothyroxinemia	Free T4 < 0.86 ng/dL: 26 (4.3%) Free T4 < 0.92 ng/dL: 54 (9%) Total T4 < 7.8 μg/dL: 42 (7%)
Iron deficiency	29 (4.8%)

Iron deficiency was diagnosed in 29 (4.8%) pregnant women. This frequency was 4.2% in women with FT4 ≥ 0.92 ng/dL. The frequencies of iron deficiency were significantly higher in women with FT4 < 0.86 ng/dL and < 0.92 ng/dL (hypothyroxinemia), 15.4% (p = 0.03) and 11.1% (p = 0.04), respectively. Women with TT4 < 7.8 μg/dL (hypothyroxinemia) also exhibited a higher frequency of iron deficiency than women with TT4 ≥ 7.8 μg/dL (12% versus 4.3%, p = 0.045). In women without iron deficiency, 8.4%, 3.9% and 6.5% had FT4 < 0.92 ng/dL, FT4 < 0.86 ng/dL and TT4 < 7.8 μg/dL respectively. These frequencies of hypothyroxinemia were significantly higher among women with iron deficiency, 20.7% (p = 0.038), 14.8% (p = 0.032) and 17.2% (p = 0.045), respectively.

DISCUSSION

Some characteristics of the present study should be highlighted. This was a prospective study. Hypothyroxinemia was defined using three different criteria of T4 concentration. Regarding TSH, a cutoff of 2.5 mIU/l was used since it is still the most accepted value for the first trimester of gestation (2,3,5-7) and is compatible with the normal range for our population (8). In addition, an overestimated TSH cutoff may compromise the conclusions because of the inclusion of women with subclinical hypothyroidism. Women with TPOAb were excluded to rule out the possible interference of thyroid autoimmunity with the outcomes. The women were evaluated in the first trimester since eventual repercussions of isolated hypothyroxinemia would be greater during this period (1,2,11) and treatment is particularly considered in this stage of pregnancy (2). None of

Table 4. Neonatal outcomes

Neonatal outcomes	FT4 (ng/dL)			TT4 (μg/dL)	
	< 0.86* (n = 26)*	< 0.92** (n = 54)**	≥ 0.92* ** (n = 542)* **	< 7.8*** (n = 42)***	≥ 7.8*** (n = 554)***
Birth weight < 2,500 g	1 (3.8%)*	2 (3.7%)**	32 (5.9%)* **	2 (4.7%)***	33 (5.9%)***
Birth weight < 1,500 g	0*	1 (1.8%)**	8 (1.4%)* **	1 (2.3%)***	8 (1.6%)***
Need for intensive therapy	0*	1 (1.8%)**	11 (2%)* **	1 (2.3%)***	11 (2%)***
Need for mechanical ventilation > 24 h	0*	1 (1.8%)**	11 (2%)* **	1 (2.3%)***	11 (2%)***
Necrotizing enterocolitis[a]	0*	0**	1 (0.2%)* **	0***	1 (0.2%)***
Intraventricular hemorrhage grade 3 or 4	0*	0**	0* **	0***	0
Major congenital malformations	0*	1 (1.8%)**	5 (0.9%)* **	0***	6 (1%)***
Neonatal death (< 28 days)	0*	0**	3 (0.5%)* **	0***	3 (0.5%)***

FT4: free T4; TT4: total T4. [a] With need for surgery.
* FT4 < 0.86 ng/dL versus ≥ 0.92 ng/dL: p ≥ 0.8 in all comparisons.
** FT4 < 0.92 ng/dL versus ≥ 0.92 ng/dL: p ≥ 0.45 in all comparisons.
*** TT4 < 7.8 μg/dL versus TT4 ≥ 7.8 μg/dL: p ≥ 0.5 in all comparisons.

the women was treated with L-T4 during pregnancy. Finally, few studies have investigated the relationship between hypothyroxinemia and iron deficiency. To our knowledge, this is the first Brazilian study analyzing the association of hypothyroxinemia with obstetric and neonatal outcomes and iron deficiency.

Regarding the association of hypothyroxinemia with iron deficiency, our results confirm the data of a Chinese observational study, which also evaluated women in the first trimester of gestation from an iodine-sufficient area (15). Since it would be more than a coincidence that iron and iodine deficiencies are the consequence of broad nutritional deficiency or that isolated hypothyroxinemia (in the absence of hypothyroidism) causes iron deficiency, iron deficiency is more likely to contribute to hypothyroxinemia (15). It is possible that iodine sufficiency influences the consequence of iron deficiency in terms of thyroid dysfunction, whether it is predominantly hypothyroxinemia (without TSH elevation) in an iodine-sufficient population (15) like ours, or subclinical hypothyroidism in an iodine-deficient population (16). However, further clinical studies involving pregnant women are necessary to consistently confirm this association.

We found no association between isolated hypothyroxinemia in the first trimester of gestation and obstetric or neonatal outcomes. Casey and cols., comparing 16,011 women with normal TSH and T4 and 233 with hypothyroxinemia before 20 weeks of gestation, also observed no association between this alteration and any of the obstetric or neonatal outcomes analyzed (13). Cleary-Goldman and cols. evaluated 10,021 pregnant women with normal TSH and T4 and 232 with hypothyroxinemia (17). In the first trimester, hypothyroxinemia was associated with preterm labor (adjusted odds ratio [aOR] 1.62; 95% confidence interval [CI] 1.00-2.62) and macrosomia (aOR 1.97; 95% CI 1.37-2.83) (17). In the second trimester, it was associated with gestational diabetes (aOR 1.7; 95% CI 1.02-2.84) (17). Finally, a third study involving more than 5,000 women revealed an association of hypothyroxinemia with preterm labor (18), but not with hypertensive disease in pregnancy (19). A meta-analysis that included these and other smaller studies found only a statistically significant increased risk of placental abruption (OR 2.3; 95% CI: 1.1–4.8) compared to euthyroid controls (20). Taken together, these findings show that the association of hypothyroxinemia with obstetric and neonatal outcomes is still inconsistent (4). In fact, there is no reproducibility of the results in the different studies and no cause-effect relationship could be established.

We recognize some limitations of the study. First, the number of women with hypothyroxinemia may have been insufficient to obtain statistical significance of small differences compared to euthyroid women. Second, since this was not an intervention study, the objective was limited to demonstrating the association between iron deficiency and hypothyroxinemia, but we did not evaluate the effect of iron supplementation on T4 concentrations. Finally, we analyzed obstetric and neonatal outcomes but not parameters of fetal brain development, which could also be compromised by isolated hypothyroxinemia (3). Although an association between hypothyroxinemia at the beginning of pregnancy and some impairment of fetal brain development has been reported in some series (3,20), two randomized studies found no beneficial effect of L-T4 therapy on this aspect (10,21).

In conclusion, this prospective Brazilian study found no association of isolated hypothyroxinemia in the first trimester of gestation with obstetric or neonatal outcomes. Despite the need for confirmation in larger series, this result weakens the concern regarding serum T4 in pregnant women with normal TSH, i.e., with isolated hypothyroxinemia. In contrast, an association was demonstrated between hypothyroxinemia and iron deficiency. This finding suggests the importance of iron and possible repercussions of its deficiency on thyroid function and the need for intervention studies evaluating the effects of iron supplementation on thyroid status in pregnant women.

Funding: this work was supported by "National Council for Scientific and Technological Development – CNPq".

REFERENCES

1. Haddow JE, Palomaki GE, Allan WC, Williams JR, Knight GJ, Gagnon J, et al. Maternal thyroid deficiency during pregnancy and subsequent neuropsychological development of the child. N Engl J Med. 1999;341(8):549-55.
2. Lazarus J, Brown RS, Daumerie C3 Hubalewska-Dydejczyk A, Negro R, Vaidya B. 2014 European thyroid association guidelines for the management of subclinical hypothyroidism in pregnancy and in children. Eur Thyroid J. 2014;3(2):76-94.
3. Alexander EK, Pearce EN, Brent GA, Brown RS, Chen H, Dosiou C, et al. 2017 Guidelines of the American Thyroid Association for the Diagnosis and Management of Thyroid Disease During Pregnancy and the Postpartum. Thyroid. 2017;27(3):315-89.
4. Dosiou C, Medici M. Management of Endocrine Disease: Isolated maternal hypothyroxinemia during pregnancy: knowns and unknowns. Eur J Endocrinol. 2017;176(1):R21-R38.
5. De Groot L, Abalovich M, Alexander EK, Amino N, Barbour L, Cobin RH, et al. Management of Thyroid Dysfunction during Pregnancy and Postpartum: An Endocrine Society Clinical Practice Guideline. J Clin Endocrinol Metab. 2012;97(8):2543-65.
6. Brenta G, Vaisman M, Sgarbi JA, Bergoglio LM, Andrada NC, Bravo PP, et al.; Task Force on Hypothyroidism of the Latin American Thyroid Society (LATS). Clinical practice guidelines for the management of hypothyroidism. Arq Bras Endocrinol Metabol. 2013;57(4):265-91.
7. Sgarbi JA, Teixeira PF, Maciel LM, Mazeto GM, Vaisman M, Montenegro Junior RM, et al.; Brazilian Society of Endocrinology and Metabolism. The Brazilian consensus for the clinical approach and treatment of subclinical hypothyroidism in adults: recommendations of the thyroid Department of the Brazilian Society of Endocrinology and Metabolism. Arq Bras Endocrinol Metabol. 2013;57(3):166-83.
8. Rosario PW, Carvalho M, Calsolari MR. TSH reference values in the first trimester of gestation and correlation between maternal TSH and obstetric and neonatal outcomes: a prospective Brazilian study. Arch Endocrinol Metab. 2016;60(4):314-8.
9. American College of Obstetricians and Gynecologists. Practice Bulletin No. 148: Thyroid disease in pregnancy. Obstet Gynecol. 2015;125(4):996-1005.
10. Casey BM, Thom EA, Peaceman AM, Varner MW, Sorokin Y, Hirtz DG, et al.; Eunice Kennedy Shriver National Institute of Child Health and Human Development Maternal–Fetal Medicine Units Network. Treatment of Subclinical Hypothyroidism or Hypothyroxinemia in Pregnancy. N Engl J Med. 2017;376(9):815-25.
11. Cooper DS, Pearce EM. Subclinical Hypothyroidism and Hypothyroxinemia in Pregnancy – Still No Answers. N Engl J Med. 2017;376(9):876-7.
12. IMULITE® and IMMULITE® 2000 Reference Range Compendium.
13. Casey BM, Dashe JS, Spong CY, McIntire DD, Leveno KJ, Cunningham GF. Perinatal significance of isolated maternal hypothyroxinemia identified in the first half of pregnancy. Obstet Gynecol. 2007;109(5):1129-35.
14. Daru J, Allotey J, Peña-Rosas JP, Khan KS. Serum ferritin thresholds for the diagnosis of iron deficiency in pregnancy: a systematic review. Transfus Med. 2017;27(3):167-74.
15. Yu X, Shan Z, Li C, Mao J, Wang W, Xie X, et al. Iron deficiency, an independent risk factor for isolated hypothyroxinemia in pregnant and nonpregnant women of childbearing age in China. J Clin Endocrinol Metab. 2015;100(4):1594-601.
16. Zimmermann MB, Burgi H, Hurrell RF. Iron deficiency predicts poor maternal thyroid status during pregnancy. J Clin Endocrinol Metab. 2007;92(9):3436-40.
17. Cleary-Goldman J, Malone FD, Lambert-Messerlian G, Sullivan L, Canick J, Porter TF, et al. Maternal thyroid hypofunction and pregnancy outcome. Obstet Gynecol. 2008;112(1):85-92.
18. Korevaar TI, Schalekamp-Timmermans S, de Rijke YB, Visser WE, Visser W, de Muinck Keizer-Schrama SM, et al. Hypothyroxinemia and TPO-antibody positivity are risk factors for premature delivery: the generation R study. J Clin Endocrinol Metab. 2013;98(11):4382-90.
19. Medici M, Korevaar TI, Schalekamp-Timmermans S, Gaillard R, de Rijke YB, Visser WE, et al. Maternal early-pregnancy thyroid function is associated with subsequent hypertensive disorders of pregnancy: the generation R study. J Clin Endocrinol Metab. 2014;99(12):E2591-8.
20. Chan S, Boelaert K. Optimal management of hypothyroidism, hypothyroxinaemia and euthyroid TPO antibody positivity preconception and in pregnancy. Clin Endocrinol (Oxf). 2015;82(3):313-26.
21. Lazarus JH, Bestwick JP, Channon S, Paradice R, Maina A, Rees R, et al. Antenatal thyroid screening and childhood cognitive function. N Engl J Med. 2012;366:493-501.

Higher fber intake is associated with lower blood pressure levels in patients with type 1 diabetes

Mileni Vanti Beretta[1,2], Fernanda R. Bernaud[1], Ciglea Nascimento[1], Thais Steemburgo[2], Ticiana C. Rodrigues[1,3]

[1] Divisão de Endocrinologia, Hospital de Clínicas de Porto Alegre (HCPA), Porto Alegre, RS, Brasil
[2] Programa de Pós-graduação em Alimentação, Nutrição e Saúde, Departamento de Nutrição, Universidade Federal do Rio Grande do Sul (UFRGS), Porto Alegre, RS, Brasil
[3] Departamento de Medicina Interna, Faculdade de Medicina, Universidade Federal do Rio Grande do Sul (UFRGS), Porto Alegre, RS, Brasil

Correspondence to:
Ticiana C. Rodrigues
Divisão de Endocrinologia, Hospital de Clínicas de Porto Alegre
Rua Ramiro Barcelos, 2350, Prédio 12, 4° andar
90035-003 – Porto Alegre, RS, Brasil
ticianacr@yahoo.com.br

ABSTRACT

Objective: The present investigation sought to evaluate the potential association between dietary fiber intake and blood pressure (BP) in adult patients with type 1 diabetes (T1D). Subjects and methods: A cross-sectional study was carried out in 111 outpatients with T1D from Porto Alegre, Brazil. Patients were predominantly male (56%) and white (88%), with a mean age of 40 ± 10 years, diabetes duration of 18 ± 9 years, BMI 24.8 ± 3.85 kg/m², and HbA1c 9.0 ± 2.0%. After clinical and laboratory evaluation, dietary intake was evaluated by 3-day weighed-diet records, whose reliability was confirmed by 24-h urinary nitrogen output. Patients were stratified into two groups according to adequacy of fiber intake in relation to American Diabetes Association (ADA) recommendations: below recommended daily intake (< 14g fiber/1000 kcal) or at/above recommended intake (≥ 14g/1000 kcal). Results: Patients in the higher fiber intake group exhibited significantly lower systolic (SBP) (115.9 ± 12.2 vs 125.1 ± 25.0 mmHg, p = 0.016) and diastolic blood pressure (DBP) (72.9 ± 9.2 vs 78.5 ± 9.3 mmHg, p = 0.009), higher energy intake (2164.0 ± 626.0 vs 1632.8 ± 502.0 kcal, p < 0.001), and lower BMI (24.4 ± 3.5 vs 26.2 ± 4.8, p = 0.044). Linear regression modelling, adjusted for age, energy intake, sodium intake, and BMI, indicated that higher fiber intake was associated with lower SBP and DBP levels. No significant between-group differences were observed with regard to duration of diabetes, glycemic control, insulin dosage, or presence of hypertension, nephropathy, or retinopathy. Conclusion: We conclude that fiber consumption meeting or exceeding current ADA recommendations is associated with lower SBP and DBP in patients with T1D. Arch Endocrinol Metab. 2018;62(1):40-7

Keywords
Fiber; type 1 diabetes; blood pressure; hypertension

The American Diabetes Association has specific dietary recommendations for individuals with type 1 diabetes (T1D) (1), which include: preferring whole grains and fiber; preferring fructose naturally current in fruits; restricted intake of saturated fats, trans fats, and cholesterol; and keeping daily sodium intake under 2,300 mg. In addition, regarding fiber in particular, the recommended intake is 14 g total fiber per 1000 kcal of energy intake, or approximately 25 g/day for adult women and 38 g/day for adult men. However, most studies evaluating fiber intake in persons with diabetes have been limited by short observation periods and small sample sizes, and by assessing combinations of fiber-rich diets and foods with low glycaemic index, which may have hindered analysis of the isolated effect of fiber as a determinant of improved glycaemic control in patients with diabetes (2,3).

Some observational studies have demonstrated an inverse relationship between total fiber intake and blood pressure (BP) levels (4,5). Intake of fiber from natural dietary sources, such as whole grains, fruits, and pulses, appears to have a beneficial effect on BP and on serum cholesterol levels in individuals with type 2 diabetes (T2D) (6,7). Furthermore, in patients with T1D and T2D, a high-fiber diet (40 g/day) was associated with significant reductions in fasting and post-prandial blood sugar levels (8). In T1D, dietary fiber plays important roles in lipid profile, glyceamic control, several parameters related to obesity, risk of cardiovascular disease (CVD), endothelial dysfunction, and markers of inflammation (9-12).

Current recommendations for the dietary treatment of hypertension in patients with diabetes, although evidence-based, are largely drawn from studies not conducted in diabetic populations. In fact, the effects of dietary fiber on BP in patients with T1D has been the subject of little research. One recent study of patients with T1D demonstrated a protective effect of fiber, especially soluble fiber, against CVD and all-cause mortality (9).

The role of fiber in the presence of hypertension in patients with T1D has yet to be established definitively. Within this context, the aim of the present study was to evaluate a potential association between dietary fiber intake (in accordance with American Diabetes Association recommendations) and BP levels in adults with T1D.

SUBJECTS AND METHODS

Participants

This cross-sectional study was carried out on a cohort of patients with T1D recruited consecutively from the outpatient endocrinology clinic of Hospital de Clínicas de Porto Alegre, a large teaching hospital in Porto Alegre, Brazil. T1D was defined as diabetes with onset before 40 years of age, ketonuria or ketonaemia at the time of diagnosis, and dependence on insulin therapy to sustain life. Patients were selected on the basis of the following criteria: dietary counselling by a dietitian during the 6 months preceding study enrolment; age > 18 years; and duration of diabetes > 5 years. Patients with renal failure, symptomatic heart failure (NYHA class III or IV), acute cardiovascular events in the 6 months preceding study enrolment (stroke, myocardial infarction, or acute pulmonary oedema), or inability to complete weighed dietary records were excluded from the cohort. All ongoing medications were maintained, except for statins.

The recruitment process took place from January 2011 to December 2012, and all participants provided written informed consent for inclusion in the study. The study protocol was approved by the Hospital de Clínicas de Porto Alegre Research Ethics Committee (number 08-470).

Clinical evaluation

All patients were evaluated by an endocrinologist and interviewed on past medical history, demographic data, medication use, and current lifestyle. Patients were classified by ethnicity as white or non-white. Smoking status was classified dichotomously (as smoker or non-smoker), as was current alcohol intake (present or absent). The frequency of physical exercise was graded into four levels using a standardised questionnaire, based on activities carried out during a typical day (13); level 1 corresponded to a sedentary lifestyle.

Sitting BP was measured in triplicate, in the left arm, after a 10-minute rest, using a digital sphygmomanometer (Omron® HEM-705 CP). Hypertension was defined as BP readings ≥ 140/90 mmHg on two separate occasions, or current antihypertensive therapy (14). All patients underwent a full physical examination.

The presence of diabetic nephropathy (DN) was classified according to the results of a random spot urine sample or 24-hour timed urinary collection (at least two samples obtained 6 months apart). Patients were considered normoalbuminuric when the urinary albumin excretion (UAE) rate was < 17 mg/L or < 20 µg/min; microalbuminuric when the UAE was 17-174 mg/L or 20-199 mg/min; and macroalbuminuric when the UAE was > 176 mg/L or > 199 mg/min on at least two occasions during a 2-month period (15).

Diabetic retinopathy (DR) was assessed by an ophthalmologist. DR was detected by dilated-pupil direct and indirect ophthalmoscopy, and graded by severity using the Global Diabetic Retinopathy Project Group scale (16) as 'absence of DR', 'mild non-proliferative DR' (NPDR), 'moderate NPDR', 'severe DR', or 'proliferative DR' (PDR). For purposes of analysis, patients were divided into two groups (absence or presence of DR, regardless of severity).

Nutritional evaluation

Nutritional evaluation was carried out as described previously (11). Briefly, dietary habits were assessed by means of 3-day weighed food records (two non-consecutive weekdays and one weekend day), as previously standardised (17,18).

The adequacy of dietary records was evaluated by comparing reported protein intake to protein intake estimated from 24-hour urinary urea nitrogen, collected on the third day of dietary records (17). The ratio of reported protein intake to estimated protein intake was considered acceptable when in the range of 0.79 to 1.26 (18).

The nutrient contents of dietary records were analised in NutriBase 2007 Clinical Nutrition Manager (Cybersoft, Phoenix, AZ, USA), version 7.14 (19). Nutrient intake was expressed as the percentage of total daily energy intake (%) and in grams amounts (g/day or mg/day). Nutrition facts for frequently consumed foods were updated and/or supplemented as necessary with data obtained from local manufacturers of specific industrialized foods.

The total, soluble, and insoluble fiber content was estimated according to data provided in the CRC Handbook of Dietary Fiber in Human Nutrition (20). Dietary sources of fiber were based on the foods described by patients in their 3-day weighed food records. The main sources of dietary fiber consumed by the cohort were pulses (beans, lentils, peas), wholegrain foods (granola, wholemeal bread, wholegrain biscuits/crackers, flaxseed, sesame seeds, sunflower seeds, quinoa, amaranth), rice, barley, potatoes, sweet potatoes, cassava (manioc), eddoes, taro, wheat, and fruits such as apple, banana, clementine, grape, mango, orange, papaya, peach, and pineapple. Vegetables were grouped in two categories on the basis of carbohydrate content (% of grams weight), with group A vegetables containing up to 5% and group B vegetables containing up to 10% carbohydrate (21).

Laboratory evaluation

HbA1c was measured by high-performance liquid chromatography (Merck-Hitachi 9100; Merck®, Darmstadt, Germany) (reference range 4.7-6.0%). Fasting plasma glucose was measured by the glucose-peroxidase enzymatic colorimetric method (Biodiagnostica®). Total serum cholesterol and triglycerides were measured by enzymatic colorimetric methods (ADVIA 1800® Autoanalyzer, Germany), and HDL cholesterol by the homogeneous direct method (ADVIA 1800® Autoanalyzer, Germany). High-sensitivity C-reactive protein (hs-CRP) was quantitated by the turbidimetric method (ADVIA 1800® Autoanalyzer, Germany), and fibrinogen was determined by the Clauss clotting method, which measures the rate of fibrinogen conversion to fibrin in a diluted sample under the influence of excess thrombin. Urinary urea was measured by an enzymatic ultraviolet assay (ADVIA 1800® Autoanalyzer, Germany).

Statistical analyses

Data are presented as mean ± standard deviation (SD), n (%), or median (interquartile range). Baseline characteristics were compared by fiber intake status by means of Student's *t*-test and Mann–Whitney *U* test. Patients were stratified into two groups on the basis of fiber intake in relation to American Diabetes Association recommendations: intake below recommendations (< 14 g/1000 kcal/day) or intake meeting/exceeding recommendations (≥ 14 g/1000 kcal/day). To determine the association between blood pressure and higher fiber intake (≥ 14 g/1000 kcal/day), a linear regression model was constructed with systolic (SBP) and diastolic (DBP) blood pressure values as the dependent variables. The multivariate model was adjusted for age, total calorie intake, BMI and sodium intake. All analyses were carried out in SPSS 18.0 (Chicago, IL, USA).

RESULTS

Of the 111 patients evaluated, 56% were male and 88% were white. The mean age was 40.0 ± 10.0 years, and mean duration of diabetes was 18.0 ± 9.0 years. Mean BMI was 24.8 ± 3.85 kg/m^2 and mean HbA1c was 9.0 ± 2.0%. Table 1 describes the clinical and laboratory characteristics of the sample stratified by fiber intake. There were no significant differences between the lower and higher fiber intake groups in terms of age, gender, ethnicity, duration of diabetes, physical activity level, or alcohol consumption. Patients in the high fiber intake group had a lower mean BMI than did those in the low fiber intake group (24.4 ± 3.5 vs 26.2 ± 4.8 kg/m^2, p = 0.044). There were no between-group differences in waist circumference or presence of hypertension. Regarding BP, patients in the higher fiber intake group (≥ 14 g/1000 kcal/day) had lower SBP (115.9 ± 12.2 vs 125.1 ± 25.0 mmHg, p = 0.016) and DBP (73.0 ± 9.2 vs 78.5 ± 9.3 mmHg, p = 0.009) than patients who consumed less fiber per day than recommended (< 14 g/1000 kcal/day). In addition, patients in the higher fiber intake group used lower doses of insulin. A similar, significant difference was found regarding antihypertensive therapy: fewer patients were on angiotensin-converting enzyme (ACE) inhibitors in the higher fiber intake group than in the lower fiber intake group (11.5% vs 20.8%, p < 0.001). There were no between-group differences in glycaemic control (HbA1c or serum glucose levels), presence of DN or DR, or lipid profile (total cholesterol, HDL cholesterol, LDL cholesterol, and triglycerides).

Daily macronutrient intake values, according to adequacy of fiber intake, are described in Table 2. Patients in the adequate fiber intake group had higher intakes of total energy, carbohydrates, protein, and fat than did patients who consumed less than the recommended adequate intake of fiber. Significant between-group differences were also found in terms of fat fractions (saturated, monounsaturated, and polyunsaturated). Furthermore, patients in the higher fiber intake group had a significantly higher daily intake of sodium (2360.64 ± 919,81 vs 1676.59 ± 688.01 mg/day; p = 0.004). There were no between-group differences in intake of trans fats or cholesterol.

Table 3 describes the daily fiber intake, stratified by type and source, in our sample. As expected, patients in the high fiber intake group (≥ 14g/1000 kcal) consumed more total, soluble, and insoluble fiber than did their counterparts in the below-adequate fiber intake group. Analysis of the main sources of dietary

Table 1. Clinical and laboratory profile of patients with type 1 DM, stratified by adequacy of fiber intake (American Diabetes Association) (1)

	Below recommended fiber intake (< 14 g/1000 kcal/day)	At or above recommended fiber intake (≥ 14 g/1000 kcal/day)	P
N	24	87	-
Age (years)	37 ± 13	40 ± 11	0.161†
Sex (male)	29.2%	56.3%	0.180‡
Ethnicity (white)	91.7%	83.9%	0.451‡
Duration of diabetes (years)	19.4 ± 11.0	17.6 ± 8.6	0.394†
Physical activity: level 1* (%)	54.2	46.0	0.811‡
Alcohol intake (%)	54.5	56.2	0.893‡
BMI (kg/m²)	26.2 ± 4.8	24.4 ± 3.5	0.044†
Weight (kg)	70.40 ± 12.92	69.02 ± 10.73	0.632†
Height (cm)	162.95 ± 9.15	169.21 ± 9.21	0.004†
Waist circumference (cm)	83.0 ± 8.5	83.3 ± 9.8	0.856†
Males	78.40 ± 6.22	86.51 ± 9.14	0.059†
Females	83.30 ± 8.08	79.54 ± 9.44	0.210†
Hypertension (%)	40.9	38.2	0.815‡
SBP (mmHg)	125.1 ± 25.0	115.9 ± 12.2	0.016†
DBP (mmHg)	78.5 ± 9.3	72.9 ± 9.2	0.009†
Under treatment for hypertension	58.3%	32.2%	0.161
ACE inhibitor	20.8%	11.5%	< 0.001
ACE inhibitor + diuretic	12.5%	12.6%	0.813
Diuretic	4.2%	1.1%	0.250
Calcium channel blocker	4.2%	0.0%	< 0.001
ACE inhibitor + beta blocker + diuretic	8.3%	2.3%	0.043
Insulin dosage			
IU/kg body weight	53.88 ± 21.91	47.80 ± 19.34	0.240†
Diabetic nephropathy (%)	0.80 ± 0.26	0.67 ± 0.25	0.061†
Diabetic retinopathy (%)	20.8	12.6	0.312‡
HbA1c (%)	10.7	9.7	0.472‡
Plasma glucose (mg/dL)	90.7 ± 2.5	90.0 ± 1.8	0.079†
Cholesterol, total (mg/dL)	241.33 ± 160.0	193.0 ± 107.0	0.084†
Cholesterol, HDL (mg/dL)	194.2 ± 30	187.3 ± 37	0.408†
Cholesterol, LDL (mg/dL)	60.0 ± 17.0	59.5 ± 16.3	0.884†
Triglycerides (mg/dL)	116.6 ± 31.0	111.5 ± 35.0	0.511†
hs-CRP (mg/L)	98.5 (49-207)	88.1 (34.0-223.0)	0.315†
Fibrinogen (mg/dL)	2.5 (0.1-7.3)	2.1 (0.1-8.4)	0.566†
Urinary sodium excretion (mg/24h)	408.1 (225-672)	364.3 (208-667.0)	0.088†

Data expressed as mean ± SD, median (IQR), or n (%). † Student's *t* test. ‡ chi-square test. * Level 1: sedentary.

ACE: angiotensin-converting enzyme; BMI: body mass index; DBP: diastolic blood pressure; HbA1c: glycated haemoglobin; HDL: high-density lipoprotein; hs-CRP: high-sensitivity C-reactive protein; LDL: low-density lipoprotein; SBP: systolic blood pressure.

fiber revealed a significant between-group difference in the intake of fiber from pulses. Patients in the high fiber intake group consumed a greater amount of total fiber from pulses than did patients in the below-adequate fiber intake group (7.8 vs 1.6 g/day; $p < 0.001$). There were no significant between-group differences in terms of total fiber intake from vegetables (groups A+B), tubers, and whole grains.

Furthermore, we observed inverse correlations between total fiber, soluble fiber, and insoluble fiber intake with BP levels ($r = -0.219$, $p = 0.021$; $r = -0.221$, $p = 0.02$; and $r = -0.215$, $p = 0.02$ respectively).

Linear regression models (Table 4 and Table 5) were constructed to evaluate potential associations between BP levels and higher fiber intake (≥ 14g/1000 kcal). The models were adjusted for age, total energy intake, BMI and sodium intake. Analysis revealed that lower SBP and DBP levels were associated with higher fiber intake (beta -11.11, $p = 0.01$ and -6.21, $p = 0.005$ respectively), independent of the adjustments.

DISCUSSION

The present study demonstrated an association between increased dietary fiber intake and lower BP levels in patients with T1D. Patients whose daily fiber intake met or exceeded American Diabetes Association recommendations (≥ 14g/1000 kcal) exhibited lower SBP and DBP levels. These associations remained significant after adjustment for potential confounding factors (age, total energy intake, sodium intake, and BMI). Furthermore, we observed an association between fiber type and BP. Increased intake of soluble and insoluble fiber was negatively associated with BP levels. In this patient group, the mean total fiber intake was 19.8 ± 7.2 g/day (5.8 ± 2.4 g from soluble and

Table 2. Daily nutrient intake of patients with type 1 DM, stratified by adequacy of fiber intake (American Diabetes Association) (1)

	Below recommended fiber intake (< 14 g/1000 kcal/day)	At or above recommended fiber intake (≥ 14 g/1000 kcal/day)	P
n	24	87	-
Total energy intake (kcal/day)	1632.8 ± 502.0	2164.0 ± 626	0.001†
Total energy intake (KJ)	6821.76	9045.52	0.001†
Total energy intake (kcal/body weight/day)	24.09 ± 7.3	31.24 ± 8.0	0.001†
Carbohydrate			
g/day	201.7 ± 71.0	269.6 ± 86.5	0.001†
% of total energy intake	49.5 ± 7.6	50.2 ± 8.6	0.899†
Protein			
g/day	74.9 ± 27.1	98.1 ± 33.0	0.002†
% of total energy intake	18.4 ± 3.5	18.3 ± 3.6	0.742†
Fat, total			
g/day	57.6 ± 22.8	77.5 ± 34.5	0.009†
% of total energy intake	31.6 ± 8.3	31.7 ± 9.4	0.952†
Fat, saturated			
g/day	17.8 ± 9.0	24.2 ± 10.5	0.007†
% of total energy intake	9.5 ± 2.3	10.0 ± 3.1	0.648†
Fat, monounsaturated	21.0 ± 8.6	27.0 ± 12.6	0.031†
g/day	21.0 ± 9.8	27.6 ± 12.2	0.021†
% of total energy intake	9.5 ± 3.1	11.1 ± 3.5	0.627†
Fat, polyunsaturated			
g/day	12.0 (1.98-23.65)	19.0 (2.7-66.1)	0.026§
% of total energy intake	7.0 (1.73-12.78)	7.7 (1.8-27.3)	0.519§
Fat, trans (g/day)	0.2 (0.0-2.58)	0.3 (0.0-4.0)	0.770§
Cholesterol, dietary (mg/day)	224.7 ± 171.9	231.3 ± 109.0	0.818†
Sodium (mg/day)	1676.59 ± 688.01	2360.64 ± 919.81	0.004†

Data expressed as mean ± SD or median (IQR).† *t* test. § Mann-Whitney U.

14.0 ± 5.3 g from insoluble fiber). The main sources of dietary fiber associated with significant differences were pulses (beans, lentils, peas) and fruit (banana, apple, papaya, pineapple, clementine, orange, grape, mango, and peach).

The type of dietary fiber appears to play an important role in the risk of cardiovascular disease (CVD) in patients with T1D. Schoenaker and cols. (9) evaluated 2,108 patients with T1D aged 15 to 60 years and found that those who consumed at least 5 g of soluble fiber per day experienced a 16% reduction in CVD risk. In the present study, we evaluated parameters associated with CVD, such as lipid profile, and found no significant association between increased fiber intake (≥ 14g/1000 kcal/day) and serum levels of total cholesterol, HDL cholesterol, or LDL cholesterol.

Table 3. Daily fiber intake, types of fiber and their main dietary sources in patients with type 1 DM, stratified by adequacy of fiber intake (American Diabetes Association) (1)

	Below recommended fiber intake (< 14 g/1000 kcal/day)	At or above recommended fiber intake (≥ 14 g/1000 kcal/day)	P
n	24	87	-
Fiber (g/day)			
Total	10.4 ± 2.0	22.9 ± 7.4	< 0.001†
Soluble	3.2 ± 1.6	6.5 ± 2.2	< 0.001†
Insoluble	7.6 ± 2.0	15.8 ± 4.5	< 0.001†
Dietary sources (g/day)			
Fiber from fruit[a]	1.2 (0.0 – 3.5)	2.7 (0.0-10.2)	0.010§
Fiber from vegetables (A+B)[b]	1.2 (0.0 – 3.5)	2.8 (0.0-47.2)	0.208§
Fiber from tubers[c]	0.5 (0.0 – 2.2)	0.5 (0.0-3.5)	0.791§
Fiber from whole grains[d]	1.5 (0.0 – 6.5)	2.3 (0.0-12.4)	0.292§
Fiber from pulses[e]	1.6 (0.0 – 5.8)	7.8 (0.0-26.0)	< 0.001§

Data expressed as mean ± SD or median (IQR).† t test. § Mann–Whitney U.
[a] Fruit: apple, banana, clementine, grape, mango, orange, papaya, peach, pineapple.
[b] A vegetables: cabbage, chard, cress, cucumber, kale, lettuce, mustard greens, radish, rocket, spinach, turnip.
[b] B vegetables: aubergine (cooked), beets (cooked), broccoli, carrot (cooked), cauliflower (cooked), chayote (cooked), courgette (cooked), hearts of palm, onion, peppers, runner beans, squash/marrow (cooked).
[c] Tubers: potatoes, sweet potatoes, cassava (manioc), eddoes, taro.
[d] Whole grains: granola, wholemeal bread, wholegrain biscuits/crackers, wholemeal flour, oats, flaxseed, quinoa, amaranth, sunflower seeds.
[e] Pulses: beans, lentils, peas.

Table 4. Linear regression analysis: systolic blood pressure and adequate fiber intake (≥ 14g fiber/1000 kcal). Model adjusted for age, total energy intake, BMI, and sodium intake

Variables	β	P
≥ 14g fiber/1000 kcal	-11.11	0.010
Age (years)	0.03	0.810
Total energy intake (kcal/day)	- 0.004	0.200
BMI (kg/m²)	0.032	0.930
Sodium intake (mg/day)	0.03	0.031

BMI: body mass index.

Table 5. Linear regression analysis: diastolic blood pressure and adequate fiber intake (≥ 14g fiber/1000 kcal). Model adjusted for age, total energy intake, BMI, and sodium intake

Variables	β	P
	-6.21	0.005
≥ 14g fiber/1000 kcal	-0.18	0.040
Age (years)	0.005	0.009
Total energy intake (kcal/day)	0.14	0.550
BMI (kg/m²)	-0.001	0.310
Sodium intake (mg/day)	-6.21	0.005

BMI: body mass index.

In this sample of patients with T1D, the higher fiber intake group (≥ 14 g/1000 kcal/day) was also found to have higher energy and macronutrient (carbohydrate, protein, and fat) intake than patients in the lower fiber consumption group (< 14 g/1000 kcal/day). Interestingly, despite this increased energy and macronutrient intake, patients in the higher fiber intake group also had lower BMI, superior metabolic control of diabetes, and inferior use of medications to treat diabetes (insulin) and hypertension (ACE inhibitors). Patients in the higher fiber intake group also consumed more sodium than their counterparts in the lower fiber intake group, although without exceeding the recommended daily intake of sodium for diabetics (22).

Sacks and cols. (23) evaluated the effect of the Dietary Approaches to Stop Hypertension (DASH) diet in hypertensive and normotensive (but non-diabetic) individuals. Those who followed the DASH diet showed significant reductions in BP as compared with those who did not follow the diet. De Paula and cols. (24) analyzed the impact of fiber intake on the BP of 225 patients with T2D. Patients were stratified by BP tertiles, and patients in the subgroup with the highest BP levels (i.e., the top tertile) were found to consume less fruits and vegetables and fewer portions of dairy than recommended in the DASH diet.

A prospective study evaluated the association between quantity and variety of fruits and vegetables in the diet and incidence of diabetes (25), and found that increased intake of these foods was associated with a lower risk of developing any diabetes (21%). Furthermore, increased consumption of fruits alone, vegetables alone, and both fruits and vegetables was associated with significant reductions in the risk of T2D (30%, 22%, and 39%, respectively). In the present study, we observed that fiber from beans/pulses and from fruit was a particularly important dietary component that may be associated with BP levels in patients with T1D.

The mechanisms by which dietary fibers lead to lower BP levels have not yet been elucidated (26). However, is well established in the literature that both soluble and insoluble fibers exert a protective and preventive effect in some pathologies such as metabolic syndrome, CVD and hyperlipidemia (27), in addition, it has an important role as evidenced in satiety and weight loss (28). Dietary fiber intake appears to improve serum lipids levels (29) and this reduction can be associated with improved endothelial vasodilation and consequently with reduced BP levels (27,29). Based on these findings and our observation that the group of patients with higher fiber intake also consumed more energy, including all macronutrients as well as sodium, we suggest that fiber intake may have a favorable effect on vasodilatation and on oxidative stress. Additional studies are needed to elucidate the mechanisms involved in the proposed beneficial effects of fiber intake on BP levels.

A potential limitation of the present study is that BP was only measured during the first study visit and when patients returned to submit their food records. In an ideal setting, 24-hour ambulatory BP monitoring would have been performed. Nevertheless, given the lack of studies demonstrating specific effects of fiber intake on BP level in patients with T1D, our study is highly relevant to clinical practice.

In conclusion, increased total fiber intake is associated with lower SBP and DBP in patients with T1D. Future studies, including randomized clinical trials should confirm the beneficial effects of dietary fiber (of different types and sources) on BP levels in patients with T1D.

Individual contributions: the authors' contributions were as follows: M. V. B. contributed to data collection and wrote the manuscript; F. R. B. and C. N. contributed to data collection and reviewed the manuscript; T. S. helped draft and review the manuscript; T. C. R. designed the study, contributed to data collection, and reviewed the manuscript.

Fundings and acknowledgements: this study was funded by Fipe (*Fundo de Incentivo à Pesquisa do Hospital de Clínicas de Porto Alegre*) and Fapergs (*Fundação de Amparo à Pesquisa do Estado do Rio Grande do Sul*). M. V. B. was the recipient of a Pibic-Fapergs grant and F. R. B. was the recipient of a Capes (*Coordenação de Aperfeiçoamento de Pessoal de Nível Superior*) scholarship.

REFERENCES

1. American Diabetes Association. Nutrition Therapy Recommendations for the Management of Adults with Diabetes. Diabetes Care. 2014;37(Suppl. 1):120-43.
2. Miller CK, Edwards L, Kissling G, Sanville L. Nutrition education improves metabolic outcomes among older adults with diabetes mellitus: results from a randomized controlled trial. Prev Med. 2002;34:252-9.
3. Norris SL, Zhang X, Avenell A, Gregg E, Bowman B, Schmid CH, et al. Long-term effectiveness of weight-loss interventions in adults with prediabetes: a review. Am J Prev Med. 2005;28:126-39.
4. Ascherio A, Hennekens C, Willett WC, Sacks F, Rosner B, Manson J. Prospective study of nutritional factors, blood pressure, and hypertension among US women. Hypertension. 1996;27(5):1065-72.
5. Sacks FM, Kass EH. Low blood pressure in vegetarians: effects of specific foods and nutrients. Am J Clin Nutr. 1988;48 (Suppl 3):795-800.
6. Franz MJ, Powers MA, Leontos C, Holzmeister LA, Kulkarni K, Monk A, et al.The evidence for medical nutrition therapy for type 1 and type 2 diabetes in adults. J Am Diet Assoc. 2010;110:1852-89.
7. Slavin JL. Position of the American Dietetic Association: health implications of dietary fiber. J Am Diet Assoc. 2008;108(10):1716-31.
8. Rodrigues Silva C, Dutra de Oliveira JE, de Souza RA, Silva HC. Effect of a rice bran fiber diet on serum glucose levels of diabetic patients in Brazil. Arch Latinoam Nutr. 2005;55(1):23-7.
9. Schoenaker DA, Toeller M, Chaturvedi N, Fuller JH, Soedamah-Muthu SS; EURODIAB Prospective Complications Study Group. Prospective Complications Study Group. Dietary saturated fat and fiber and risk of cardiovascular disease and all-cause mortality among type 1 diabetic patients: the EURODIAB Prospective Complications Study. Diabetologia. 2012;55(8):2132-41.
10. Volp ACP, Alfenas RCG, Costa NMB, Minim VPR, Stringuera PC, Bressan J. Capacidade dos biomarcadores inflamatórios em predizer a síndrome metabólica. Arq Bras Endocrinol Metab. 2008;52(3):537-49.
11. Bernaud FS, Beretta MV, do Nascimento C, Escobar F, Gross JL, Azevedo MJ. Fiber intake and inflammation in type 1 diabetes. Diabetol Metab Syndr. 2014;6:66.
12. Li J, Wang J, Kaneko T, Qin LQ, Sato A. Effects of fiber intake on the blood pressure, lipids, and heart rate in Goto Kakizaki rats. Nutrition. 2004;20(11-12):1003-7.
13. Tuomilehto J, Lindström J, Eriksson JG, Valle TT, Hämäläinen H, Ilanne-Parikka P, et al. Prevention of type 2 diabetes mellitus by changes in lifestyle among subjects with impaired glucose tolerance. N Engl J Med. 2001;344(18):1343-50.
14. Chobanian AV, Bakris GL, Black HR, Cushman WC, Green LA, Izzo JL Jr, et al. The Seventh Report of the Joint National committee on Prevention, Detection, Evaluation, and Treatment of high Blood Pressure: the JNC 7 report. JAMA, 2003;289:2560-72.
15. Gross JL, Azevedo MJ, Silveiro SP, Canani LH, Caramori ML, Zelmanovitz T. Diabetic nephropathy: diagnosis, prevention and treatment. Diabetes Care. 2005;28:164-76.

16. Wilkinson CP, Ferris FL 3rd, Klein RE, Lee PP, Agardh CD, Davis M, et al. Proposed international clinical diabetic retinopathy and diabetic macular edema disease severity scales. Ophthalmology. 2003;110:1677-82.
17. Moulin CC, Tiskievicz F, Zelmanovitz T, de Oliveira J, Azevedo MJ, Gross JL. Use of weighed diet records in the evaluation of diets with different protein contents in patients with type 2 diabetes. Am J Clin Nutr. 1998;67:853-7.
18. Vaz JS, Bittencourt M, Almeida JC, Gross JL, De Azevedo MJ, Zelmanovitz T. Protein intake estimated by weighed diet records in patients with type 2 diabetes: Misreporting and intra-individual variability using 24-hour nitrogen output as criterion standard. J Am Diet Assoc. 2008;108(5):867-72.
19. Department of Agriculture USDA SR 17. Research Quality Nutrient Data: The Agricultural Research Service: Composition of Foods. Agricultural Handbook No. 8. Washington, DC: U.S., 2007.
20. Schakel S, Sievert YA, Buzzard IM. Dietary fiber values for common foods. In: Spiller GA (ed): CRC Handbook of Dietary Fiber in Human Nutrition. Boca Raton, FL: CRC Press, 2001. P. 615-648.
21. Ornellas LH. Técnica dietética: seleção e preparo de alimentos. 8.ed. São Paulo: Atheneu; 2006. p. p. 276.
22. American Diabetes Association. Nutrition recommendations and interventions for diabetes: a position statement of the American Diabetes Association. Diabetes Care. 2013;36(Suppl 1):11-66.
23. Sacks FM, Svetkey LP, Vollmer WM, Appel LJ, Bray GA, Harsha D, et al. Effects on blood pressure of reduced dietary sodium and the Dietary Approaches to Stop Hypertension (DASH) diet. DASH-Sodium Collaborative Research Group. N Engl J Med. 2001;344(1):3-10.
24. de Paula TP, Steemburgo T, de Almeida JC, Dall'Alba V, Gross JL, de Azevedo MJ. The role of Dietary Approaches to Stop Hypertension (DASH) diet food groups in blood pressure in type 2 diabetes. Br J Nutr. 2012;108(1):155-62.
25. Cooper AJ, Sharp SJ, Lentjes MA, Luben RN, Khaw KT, Wareham NJ, et al. A Prospective study of the association between quantity and variety of fruit and vegetable intake and incident type 2 diabetes. Diabetes Care. 35(6):1293-300.
26. Aleixandre A, Miguel M. Dietary fiber and blood pressure control. Food Funct. 2016;7(4):1864-71.
27. Anderson JW, Baird P, Davis RH Jr, Ferreri S, Knudtson M, Koraym A, et al. Health benefits of dietary fiber. Nutr Rev. 2009;67(4): 188-205.
28. Babio N, Balanza R, Basulto J, Bulló M, Salas-Salvadó J. Dietary fibre: influence on body weight, glycemic control and plasma cholesterol profile. Nutr Hosp. 2010;25(3):327-40.
29. Brown L, Rosner B, Willett WW, Sacks FM. Cholesterol-lowering effects of dietary fiber: a meta-analysis. Am J Clin Nutr. 1999;69(1):30-42.

Correlation between adipokines and carotid intima media thickness in a group of obese Romanian children: is small for gestational age status an independent factor for cardiovascular risk?

Ramona Stroescu[1,2], Teofana Bizerea[1,2], Gabriela Doroş[1,2], Monica Marazan[1], Maria Lesovici[1], Otilia Mărginean[1,2]

[1] "Louis Turcanu" Emergency Hospital for Children, Timişoara, România
[2] "Victor Babes" University of Medicine and Pharmacy, Timişoara, România

Correspondence to:
Ramona Stroescu
"Louis Turcanu" Emergency Hospital for Children Timişoara
300011 – Iosif Nemoianu 2 Timişoara
ramona.giurescu@gmail.com

ABSTRACT

Objective: To investigate the relationship between markers of adiposity and common carotid artery (CIMT) in obese children born small for gestational age (SGA) *versus* appropriate for gestational age (AGA), to establish cut-off values for CIMT in obese pediatric populations. **Subjects and methods:** A cross-sectional study was carried out over a 1-year period (Jul 2013 – June 2014). We analyzed 122 obese patients aged 4-20 (mean age 14.9 ± 2.28). Twenty-six patients were born SGA. CIMT was measured in all the patients. Using ROC curve, cut-off values were obtained for both groups. **Results:** We demonstrated a correlation between CIMT and adiponectin, leptin and high sensitivity C-reactive protein (hsCRP) ($r = -0.25$, $r = 0.279$, $r = 0.498$) in obese children. CIMT in obese children born SGA were significantly increased as compared with obese children born AGA of similar age, sex and body mass index (BMI) ($p = 0.0035$). A CIMT cut off value of 0.049 cm has been obtained with a high sensitivity and specificity. **Conclusion:** CIMT is a well-known marker of subclinical atherosclerosis and its measurement is a noninvasive and inexpensive method of detecting subclinical atherosclerosis. Being born SGA increases the atherogenic risk. Obese children with CIMT above 0.049 cm should be screened for metabolic syndrome (MetS). Arch Endocrinol Metab. 2017;61(1):14-20

INTRODUCTION

CIMT provides an index of atherosclerosis in other vascular regions (1-5) and has been shown to be associated with most risk factors for atherosclerosis (6-8). Increased values of CIMT determined by B-mode ultrasound have been shown to be directly associated with an elevated risk of myocardial infarction and stroke in older adults without a previous history of cardiovascular disease (9). Thus, CIMT has been proposed as a risk factor that may be included in the algorithms for cardiovascular risk assessment (9).

The pathogenesis of atherosclerosis as identified by the Pathobiological Determinants of Atherosclerosis in Youth trial has endothelial dysfunction as its first step; an accumulation of modified lipoproteins cause a thickening of the intima; macrophages attach to the lipoproteins, resulting in the formation of foam cells, which accumulate in the intima forming a fatty streak; this step is followed by proliferation of smooth muscle cells, developing a fibrous area (10). Atherosclerotic modifications of blood vessels start in childhood, although clinical manifestations of atherosclerosis mainly occur in adults. In children and adolescents, atherosclerosis can present itself as a diffuse thickening of the intima-media space rather than the common structure of fatty streaks and fibrous capsules (11).

CIMT is commonly used as a marker of atherosclerosis; a predictive association with cardiovascular disease has been established. In adults, CIMT > 0.9 mm has been shown as a marker of cardiovascular risk caused by atherosclerosis (12). In children, there are few data regarding reference values for CIMT.

Adipose tissue is an important endocrine organ that produces interleukin-6 (IL–6), tumor necrosis factor alpha (TNF-α), plasminogen activator inhibitor-1 and adipokines (leptin and adiponectin). Adipokines control energy homeostasis and are involved in metabolic, endocrine and immunological processes.

Leptin is a hormone closely linked to adipose tissue and its levels are directly influenced by the amount of body fat mass and size of individual adipocytes; through its actions on the medial and lateral hypothalamus, it controls food intake and energy expenditure. In obesity, however, it was observed that high levels of leptin do not reduce appetite; a possible explanation may be a state of leptin resistance. It also has a pro-inflammatory action, stimulating the secretion of IL-6 and TNF-α (13,14).

Adiponectin, as opposed to leptin, is a hormone inversely correlated with body fat mass. Adiponectin is the most abundant of the adipokines and is an insulin-sensitizing hormone with anti-inflammatory, anti-atherogenic and anti-diabetic properties (15,16).

High sensitivity C-reactive protein (hsCRP) is a biomarker of the low grade chronic inflammation associated with atherosclerosis. Likewise, CRP is one of the most important inflammatory markers in obesity. Several studies showed that hsCRP is a strong independent predictor of cardiovascular risk. It has a role at different phases of atherosclerosis (17). Adults with hsCRP above 0.3 mg/dL have twice the risk of atherosclerosis compared to those with low levels (< 0.1 mg/dL) (18,19). There are also studies indicating the utility of hsCRP in assessing cardiovascular risk in obese children (20).

Chronic inflammation in obesity leads to endothelial dysfunction, followed by further atherosclerotic modifications of blood vessels.

Children and adolescents with risk factors such as obesity, dyslipidemia, high blood pressure and impaired glucose metabolism are at risk for atherosclerosis in adulthood (21-23). Childhood obesity correlates with early onset of cardiovascular disease in adults. Children born small for gestational age (SGA) have a high risk of developing MetS with all its components.

This study aimed to investigate the relationship between markers of adiposity, like leptin, adiponectin, hsCRP and CIMT in obese children, to compare values of CIMT and markers of adiposity between children born SGA and AGA, and to establish cut off values for CIMT in obese pediatric populations.

SUBJECTS AND METHODS

A cross-sectional study was conducted over a period of 1 year, between July 2013 and June 2014, on cases of obesity in children diagnosed at the Emergency Hospital for Children "Louis Ţurcanu" Timişoara, in the departments of Diabetes and Nutritional Diseases, Endocrinology and Cardiology.

Subjects were considered obese on the basis of age-specific BMI reference guidelines from Centers for Disease Control and Prevention Child Growth Standards 2000 (above 95th percentile) (24). When defining SGA, growth nomograms and charts proposed by Niklasson and cols. (25) were used; subjects whose birth weight was more than 2 standard deviations (SD) below the average for gestational age were considered SGA; subjects with birth weight within normal range for gestational age were defined as AGA.

CIMT was measured by B-mode ultrasound using a 10-MHz linear transducer (General Electric). The subjects were examined in the supine position with the neck extended and the probe in the antero-lateral position. All measurements of CIMT were made in the longitudinal plane at the point of maximum thickness on the far wall of the right common carotid artery along a 1 cm section of the artery proximal to the carotid bulb. CIMT was defined as the distance between the intima-blood interface and the adventitia-media junction. After freezing the image, measurements were made using electronic calipers. The maximal thicknesses of the intima-media width were measured to give three readings and the mean value was used for statistical purposes.

hsCRP was determined by immunonephelometry from serum samples and processed in a BN ProSpec® system (Siemens Healthcare Diagnostics Inc.) (undetected if < 0.02 mg/dL).

Quantitative measurements of serum leptin and adiponectin levels were performed using commercially available enzyme-linked immunosorbent assay kits (Antisel and Diamedix).

Exclusion criteria were evidenced for endocrine or syndromal disorders of obesity, systemic disease or acute illness.

We analyzed 122 patients diagnosed with obesity: 96 patients born AGA and 26 patients born SGA. Both groups were matched for age, sex and BMI. CIMT was also measured in members of a control group of 42 nonobese patients matched for age, sex and birth weight with the obese group (SGA+AGA).

The data are expressed as means ± standard deviation or as frequencies. Statistical analysis was performed with MedCalc. Pearson's correlation was used to establish correlations between the parameters in the study group. A $p < 0.05$ was considered statistically significant. ROC curve was used for determining the optimal cut-off value for CIMT in obese children.

Consent was obtained from the parents and the Ethical Committee of the hospital.

RESULTS

CIMT values measured in the nonobese group were significantly lower than those in the obese group (0.035 cm vs 0.046 cm, $p < 0.01$) as shown in Table 1.

The anthropometric and metabolic characteristics and CIMT values of the obese group are shown in Table 2.

The SGA group had significantly higher levels of leptin and hsCRP ($p = 0.036$, $p = 0.017$, respectively) and lower levels of adiponectin ($p = 0.04$). CIMT was significantly increased in the SGA group (mean 0.057 cm vs 0.043 cm) (Figure 1); there were significant differences between the two groups ($p = 0.0035$).

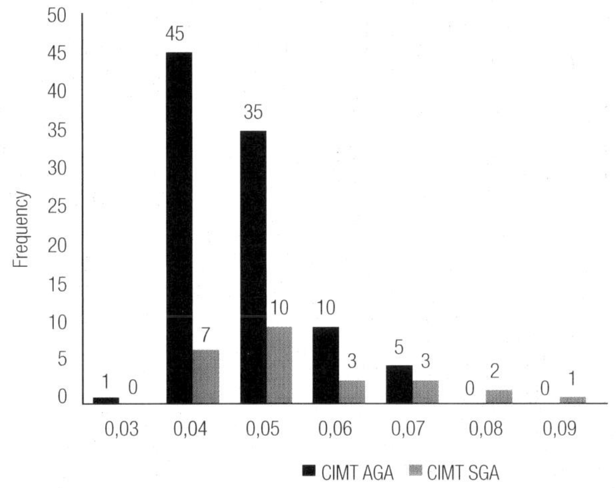

Figure 1. CIMT histogram in SGA and AGA group.

Table 1. The anthropometric characteristics and CIMT values of the nonobese group and of the obese group

Total number	Obese group (SGA+AGA) 122			Non obese group 42			P value
	Mean	SD	Range	Mean	SD	Range	
Age (years)	14.9	2.3	4-20	14.5	2.48	4-18	0.68
Birth weight (grams)	3231.72	610	970-4300	3032.87	388.31	2350-3800	0.57
Sex (%)							0.68
Male		40.3%			36.5%		
Female		59.7%			63.5%		
Antropometric data BMI (kg/m^2)	32.8	7.27	19-54.5	16.09	3.31	7.43-21.85	< 0.01
CIMT (cm)	0.046	0.01	0.03-0.09	0.035	0.005	0.025-0.05	< 0.01

BMI: body mass index; CIMT: carotid intima media thickness.

Table 2. Anthropometric and metabolic characteristics and CIMT values of AGA versus SGA group

Total number	Obese SGA-group I 26			Obese AGA-group II 96			P value
	Mean	SD	Range	Mean	SD	Range	
Age (years)	14.41	3.3	5-17	15.05	2.28	4-20	0.22
Birth weight (grams)	2550	403.5	970-2860	3446.25	461.4	2400-4300	< 0.01
Gestational age (weeks)	38	2.9	30-41	39.368	1.14902	34-41	0.025
Sex (%)							
Male		42.3%			36.5%		
Female		57.7%			63.5%		0.78
Residence urban/rural		57%/43%			60%/40%		0.79
Antropometric data BMI (kg/m^2)	29.6	8.13	19-54.5	30.6	6.3	17-47	0.5
CIMT (cm)	0.057	0.008	0.04-0.09	0.043	0.008	0.03-0.07	< 0.01
Biological data Leptin (ng/mL)	29.5	14.23	15.2-43.7	26	13.08	12.9-39.1	0.036
Adiponectin (ug/mL)	16.4	2.27	1-48	19.9	2.34	2.4-64	0.04
hsCRP (mg/dL)	0.9	0.24	0.6-1.1	0.7	0.32	0.39-1	0.017

BMI: body mass index; CIMT: carotid intima media thickness; hsCRP: high sensitive C reactive protein.

The relationship between CIMT and adypokines

We further aimed to determine correlations between CIMT and the other variables.

CIMT was directly weakly correlated with leptin ($r = 0.279$; $p < 0.05$) and strongly with hsCRP ($r = 0.498$; $p = 0.01$), and inversely and weakly correlated with adiponectin ($r = -0.25$; $p = 0.04$) (Table 3).

Table 3. Correlation between CIMT and other variables

	Leptin	Adiponectin	hsCRP
CIMT Pearson's correlation	0.279	-0.25	0.498
p	0.01	0.04	0.031

hs-CRP: high-sensitivity C-reactive protein.

Establishing cut-off values using ROC curve in obese children

We have determined cut-off values for the SGA group using ROC curve (Figure 2). The limited size of the SGA sample (26 patients) compelled us to establish a cut-off value using CIMT measurements from both groups (Figure 3). This cut-off value of CIMT acts as a designated limit; higher values indicate an increased risk of developing MetS.

Using ROC curve, we obtained for the obese group a cut-off CIMT value of 0.049 cm with a sensitivity of 100% and a specificity of 84%.

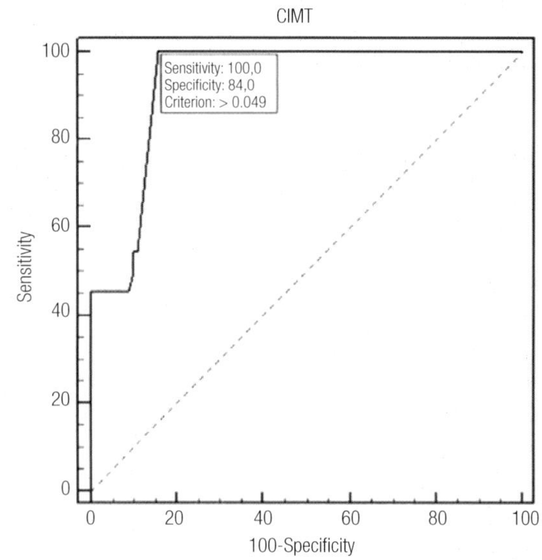

Figure 2. ROC curve SGA group.

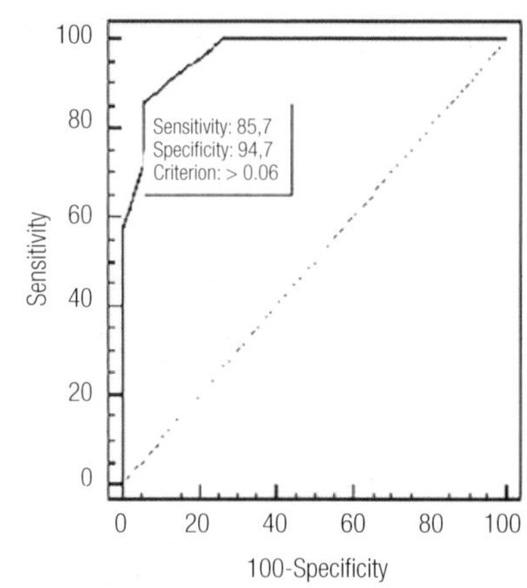

Figure 3. ROC curve SGA+AGA groups.

DISCUSSION

Previous reports indicate that the presence of obesity in childhood is associated with increased adult CIMT (22,23). CIMT is a well-known marker of subclinical atherosclerosis and it can also indicate future cardio-cerebrovascular disease (26-28).

In a recent study, we demonstrated a relationship between CIMT, MetS and its components in obese children (29).

Obesity is a chronic inflammatory disorder in which leptin, adiponectin and CRP play an important role (30). In this study, a correlation between CIMT adiponectin, leptin and hsCRP was observed. In healthy individuals, adiponectin has anti-atherogenic properties and studies have shown that, in adults, a low level of adiponectin correlates with coronary lesions and is an independent risk factor for the progression of type 2 diabetes (31,32). Previous research suggests that elevated leptin levels are involved in cardio-cerebrovascular disorders such as myocardial infarction and stroke (33).

Leptin induces smooth muscle cell hypertrophy and proliferation through endothelin-1 and angiotensin II dependent mechanisms (34). Angiotensin II increases the production of reactive oxygen species and induces the release of the vasoconstrictor endothelin-1 (35,36). Leptin also stimulates the secretion of inflammatory markers such as CRP, TNF-α and IL-6, which are directly involved in the development of endothelial dysfunction and atherosclerosis (37,38).

Winer and cols. established that low levels of adiponectin are associated with higher CRP levels (39). Also, a direct correlation between CIMT and leptin was demonstrated in obese individuals (40). The weak correlation between CIMT, adiponectin and leptin detected in our study was an indicator of further cumulative risk factors leading to changes in CIMT values. A stronger correlation has been observed between CIMT and hsCRP, suggesting an inflammatory process in obesity. Endothelial dysfunction is considered the earliest step in the atherosclerotic process and precedes any morphological changes in the walls of blood vessels.

The catch-up growth in children born SGA has been associated with a high risk of developing MetS with all its components: obesity, impaired glucose tolerance, insulin resistance with subsequent development of diabetes, arterial hypertension and dyslipidemia. There is also a risk of developing adrenal and reproductive disorders (41). These changes have been related to intrauterine life environments and linked to epigenetic fetal programming.

Visentin and cols., in a study examining relationships between levels of adipokines (adiponectin and leptin), inflammatory markers (CRP, TNF-α and IL-6) and vascular remodeling in pregnancies with intrauterine growth restriction, found higher CIMT values, high serum concentrations of proinflamatory cytokines (leptin, hsCRP, TNF-α and IL-6) and low levels of adiponectin in fetuses (42).

In our study, there was a significant statistical difference between AGA and SGA groups regarding CIMT, adiponectin, leptin and hsCRP as shown in Table 1.

Reference values for CIMT in adults are 0.04-0.07 cm (43). An increase in CIMT with each decade of age (0.066 cm/decade) was observed, with CIMT values as high as 0.0733 cm in the 70-79 years group (44). An increase of 0.1 mm in CIMT is known to raise the risk of myocardial infarction by 11% (45).

In children, there are very few studies on CIMT; normal CIMT is considered to be 0.04 cm (46). A study assessing CIMT in children aged 6-14 found a median CIMT of 0.048 cm in nonobese children and 0.055 cm in obese children (47). Another study, which enrolled 128 patients aged 6-18 years, showed a CIMT of 0.043 cm in nonobese children versus 0.051 cm in obese children (48). In our control group – the nonobese group – we obtained a median CIMT value as low as 0.035 cm. A significant difference from previous results can be clearly observed. An explanation might be the number of adolescents enrolled in the study group; as we know, CIMT value increases with age.

We found little literature data regarding reference values for CIMT in obese children; with this study we achieved threshold values of CIMT maintaining high sensitivity and specificity. For both groups we obtained a cut-off value of 0.049 cm, with a sensitivity of 100% and a specificity of 84%.

It is our belief that these cut-off CIMT values for assessing metabolic risk are "pilot" results. In order to refine these values and offer a reliable tool for determining cardiovascular risk in obese children, further extensive population studies are recommended.

Limitation

Data from our small clinical samples and the limited number may not be representative for general populations. CIMT may also be influenced by other risk factors that have not been tested in our study.

CONCLUSION

CIMT is a well-known marker of subclinical atherosclerosis and its measurement is a noninvasive and inexpensive method of detecting subclinical atherosclerosis; it is in relationship to adiponectin, leptin and hsCRP. Being born SGA increases the atherogenic risk. Obese children having CIMT > 0.049 cm should be tested for MetS. Further population studies that look into CIMT values in obese and nonobese children are necessary.

Acknowledgments: this research was supported by a grant at University of Medicine and Pharmacy "Victor Babes" Timisoara PII-C2-TC-2014 ChildObesity-2014 obtained by Ramona Stroescu.

REFERENCES

1. Craven TE, Ryu JE, Espeland MA, Kahl FR, McKinney WM, Toole JF, et al. Evaluation of the association between carotid artery atherosclerosis and coronary artery stenosis: a case-control study. Circulation. 1990;82:1230-42.
2. Wendelhag I, Wiklund O, Wilkstrand J. Atherosclerotic changes in the femoral and carotid arteries in familial hypercholesterolemia. Arterioscler Thromb. 1993;13:1404-11.
3. Burke GL, Evans GW, Riley WA, Sharrett AR, Howard G, Barnes RW, et al. Arterial wall thickness is associated with prevalent cardiovascular disease in middle aged adults: the Atherosclerosis Risk in Communities (ARIC) Study. Stroke. 1995;26:386-91.
4. Allan PI, Mowbray PI, Lee AJ, Fowkes FGR. Relationship between carotid intima-media thickness and symptomatic and

asymptomatic peripheral arterial disease: the Edinburgh Artery Study. Stroke. 1997;28:348-53.

5. Bots ML, Hoes AW, Koudstaal PJ, Hofman A, Grobbee DE. Common carotid intima-media thickness and risk of stroke and myocardial infarction: the Rotterdam Study. Circulation. 1997;96:1432-7.
6. Ebrahim S, Papacosta O, Whincup P, Wannamethee G, Walker M, Nicolaides AN, et al. Carotid plaque, intima media thickness, cardiovascular risk factors, and prevalent cardiovascular disease in men and women: the British Regional Heart Study. Stroke. 1999;30:841-50.
7. Howard G, Manolio TA, Burke GL, Wolfson SK, O'Leary DH. Does the association of risk factors and atherosclerosis change with age? An analysis of the combined ARIC and CHS cohorts. Stroke. 1997;28:1693-701.
8. Mannami T, Konishi M, Baba S, Nishi N, Terao A. Prevalence of asymptomatic carotid atherosclerotic lesions detected by high resolution ultrasonography and its relation to cardiovascular risk factors in the general population of a Japanese city: the Suita Study. Stroke. 1997;28:518-25.
9. O'Leary DH, Polak JF, Kronmal RA, Manolio TA, Burke GL, Wolfson SK Jr. Carotid-artery intima media thickness as a risk factor for myocardial infarction and stroke in older adults. N Engl J Med. 1999;340:14-22.
10. McGill HC Jr, McMahan CA, Zieske AW, Malcom GT, Tracy RE, Strong JP. Effects of nonlipid risk factors on atherosclerosis in youth with a favorable lipoprotein profile. Pathobiological Determinants of Atherosclerosis in Youth (PDAY) Research Group. Circulation. 2001;103(11):1546-50.
11. Groner JA, Joshi M, Bauer JA. Pediatric precursors of adult cardiovascular disease: noninvasive assessment of early vascular changes in children and adolescents. Pediatrics. 2006;118(4):1683-91.
12. Amato M, Montorsi P, Ravani A. Carotid intima-media thickness by B-mode ultrasound as surrogate of coronary atherosclerosis: correlation with quantitative coronary angiography and coronary intravascular ultrasound findings. Eur Heart J. 2007;28:2094-101.
13. Anubhuti, Arora S. Leptin and its metabolic complications-an update. Infam. 2008;10:973-93.
14. Meyers MG, Cowley MA, Munzberg H. Mechanisms of leptin action and leptin resistance. Annu Rev Physiol. 2008;70:537-56.
15. Shehzad A, Iqbal W, Shehzad O, Lee YS. Adiponectin: regulation of its production and its role in human diseases. Hormones. 2012;11:8-20.
16. Aprahamian TR, Sam F. Adiponectin in cardiovascular inflammation and obesity. Int J Infam. 2011;2011:376909.
17. Montero D, Walther G, Perez-Martin A. Endothelial dysfunction, inflammation, and oxidative stress in obese children and adolescents: markers and effect of lifestyle intervention. Obesity Rev. 2012;13:441-55.
18. Ridker PM. High-sensitivity C-reactive protein: potential adjunct for global risk assessment in the primary prevention of cardiovascular disease. Circulation. 2001;103:1813-8.
19. Pearson TA, Mensah GA, Alexander RW, Anderson JL, Cannon RO 3rd, Criqui M, et al. Markers of inflammation and cardiovascular disease: application to clinical and public health practice. A statement for healthcare professionals from the Centers for Disease Control and Prevention and the American Heart Association. Circulation. 2003;107:499-511.
20. Soriano-Guilén L, Hernández-Garcia B, Pita J, Domínguez-Garrido N, Del Río-Camacho G, Rovira A. High-sensitivity C-reactive protein is a good marker of cardiovascular risk in obese children and adolescents. Eur J Endocr. 2008;159:R1-4.
21. Roede MJ, Van Wieringen JC. Growth diagrams 1980. Netherlands third nation-wide survey, Tijdschrift voor Sociale Gezondheidszorg. 1985;63(suppl):1-34.
22. Davis PH, Dawson JD, Riley WA, Lauer RM. Carotid intimal-medial thickness is related to cardiovascular risk factors measured from childhood through middle age: The Muscatine Study. Circulation. 2001;104:2815-9.
23. Raitakari OT, Juonala M, Kähönen M, Taittonen L, Laitinen T, Mäki-Torkko N, et al. Cardiovascular risk factors in childhood and carotid artery intima-media thickness in adulthood: the Cardiovascular Risk in Young Finns Study. JAMA. 2003;290:2277-83.
24. National Center for Health Statistics, Centers for Disease Control and Prevention growth charts: United States National Center for Health Statistics, Hyattsville, MD, United States, 2000. Avaliable from www.cdc.gov/growthcharts.
25. Niklasson A, Ericson A, Fryer JG, Karlberg J, Lawrence C, Karlberg P. An update of the Swedish reference standards for weight, length and head circumference at birth for given gestational age (1977-1981). Acta Paediatr Scand. 1991;80(8-9):756-62.
26. Li S, Chen W, Srinivasan SR, Bond MG, Tang R, Urbina EM, et al. Childhood cardiovascular risk factors and carotid vascular changes in adulthood the Bogalusa Heart Study. JAMA. 2003;290:2271-6.
27. Csiba L. Carotid intima-media thickness measured by ultrasonography: effect of different pharmacotherapies on atherosclerosis progression. Orv Hetil. 2005;146:1239-44.
28. Reinehr T, Kiess W, de Sousa G, Stoffel-Wagner B, Wunsch R. Intima media thickness in children obesity relations to inflammatory marker, glucose metabolism, and blood pressure. Metabolism. 2006;55:113-8.
29. Stroescu R, Micle I, Marginean O, Bizerea T, Marazan M, Puiu M, et al. Is small for gestational age status associated with an increased risk of atherogenesis? Maedica. 2013;8:315-20.
30. Li J, Li F, Zhao A. Inflammation and leptin. Met Dis. 2006;3:387-93.
31. Kumada M, Kihara S, Sumitsuji S, Kawamoto T, Matsumoto S, Ouchi N, et al. Association of hypoadiponectinemia with coronary artery disease in men. Arterioscler Thromb Vasc Biol. 2003;23:85-9.
32. Winer JC, Zern TL, Taksali SE, Dziura J, Cali AM, Wollschlager M, et al. Adiponectin in childhood and adolescent obesity and its association with inflammatory markers and components of the metabolic syndrome. J Clin Endocrinol Metab. 2006;91:4415-23.
33. Beltowski J. Leptin and atherosclerosis. Atherosclerosis. 2006;189:47-60.
34. Zeidan A, Purdham DM, Rajapurohitam V, Javadov S, Chakrabarti S, Karmazyn M. Leptin induces vascular smooth muscle cell hypertrophy through angiotensin II-and endothelin-1-dependent mechanisms and mediates stretch-induced hypertrophy. J Pharmacol Exp Ther. 2005;315:1075-84.
35. Yanagitani Y, Rakugi H, Okamura A, Moriguchi K, Takiuchi S, Ohishi M, et al. Angiotensin II type 1 receptor-mediated peroxide production in human macrophages. Hypertension. 1999;33:335-39.
36. Imai T, Hirata Y, Emori T, Yanagisawa M, Masaki T, Marumo F. Induction of endothelin-1gene by angiotensin and vasopressin in endothelial cells. Hypertension. 1992;19:753-7.
37. Koh KK, Quon MJ, Lee SJ, Han SH, Ahn JY, Kim JA, et al. Efonidipine simultaneously improves blood pressure, endothelial dysfunction, and metabolic parameters in non-diabetic patients with hypertension. Diabetes Care. 2007;30:1605-7.
38. Loffreda S, Yang SQ, Lin HZ, Karp CL, Brengman ML, Wang DJ, et al. Leptin regulates proinflammatory immune responses. FASEB J. 1998;12:57-65.

39. Winer JC, Zern TL, Taksali SE, Dziura J, Cali AMG, Wollschlager M, et al. Adiponectin in childhood and adolescent obesity and its association with inflammatory markers and components of the metabolic syndrome. J Clin Endocrinol Metab. 2006;91:4415-23.

40. Ciccone M, Vettor R, Pannacciulli N, Minenna A, Bellacicco M, Rizzon P, et al. Plasma leptin is independently associated with the intima-media thickness of the common carotid artery. Int J Obes Relat Metab Disord. 2001;25:805-10.

41. Reinehr T, Kleber M, Toschke A. Small for gestational age (SGA) status is associated with metabolic syndrome in over-weight children. Eur J Endocrinol. 2009;20:1-19.

42. Visentin S, Lapolla A, Londero AP, Cosma C, Dalfrà M, Camerin M, et al. Adiponectin levels are reduced while markers of systemic inflammation and aortic remodelling are increased in intrauterine growth restricted mother-child couple. Biomed Res Int. 2014;401595.

43. Mahmoud MZ. Sonography of common carotid arteries' intima: media thickness in the normal adult population in Sudan. N Am J Med Sci 2013;5(2):88-94.

44. Beşir FH, Yazgan S, Celbek G, Aydın M, Yazgan O, Erkan ME, et al. Normal values correlates' of carotid intima-media thickness and affecting parameters in healthy adults. Anadolu Kardiyol Derg. 2012;12(5):427-33.

45. Bots ML, Hoes AW, Koudstaal PJ, Hofman A, Grobbee DE. Common carotid intima-media thickness and risk of stroke and myocardial infarction: the Rotterdam Study. Circulation. 1997;96: 1432-7.

46. Reinehr T, Wunsch R, Pütter C, Scherag A. Relationship between Carotid Intima-Media Thickness and Metabolic Syndrome in Adolescents. J Pediatr. 2013;163(2):327-32.

47. Iannuzzi A, Licenziati MR, Acampora C, Salvatore V. Increased carotid intima-media thickness and stiffness in obese children. Diabetes Care. 2004;27(10):2506-8.

48. Stabouli S, Kotsis V, Karagianni C, Zakopoulos N, Konstantopoulos A. Blood pressure and carotid artery intima-media thickness in children and adolescents: the role of obesity. Hellenic J Cardiol. 2012;53(1):41-7.

Is FGF-23 an early indicator of atherosclerosis and cardiac dysfunction in patients with gestational diabetes?

Dilek Tuzun[1], Ayten Oguz[1], Muhammet Naci Aydin[2], Ergul Belge Kurutas[3], Onder Ercan[4], Murat Sahin[1], Velid Ünsal[3], Imran Ceren[2], Ahmet Akçay[2], Kamile Gul[1]

[1] Kahramanmaras Sutcu Imam University, Faculty of Medicine, Department of Endocrinology and Metabolism, Kahramanmaras, Turkey
[2] Kahramanmaras Sutcu Imam University, Faculty of Medicine, Department of Cardiology, Kahramanmaras, Turkey
[3] Kahramanmaras Sutcu Imam University, Faculty of Medicine, Department of Biochemistry, Kahramanmaras, Turkey
[4] Kahramanmaras Sutcu Imam University, Faculty of Medicine, Department of Obstetric and Gynecology, Kahramanmaras, Turkey

Correspondence to:
Dilek Tuzun
Kayseri Yolu 10 km
Avşar Kampüsü Kahramanmaraş
Sütçü Imam Üniversitesi, 46100,
Kahramanmaras, Turkıye
tuzund@gmail.com

ABSTRACT

Objective: Fibroblast growth factor 23 (FGF-23) is a phosphorus-regulating hormone and plays a role in the pathogenesis of myocardial hypertrophy. The aim of this study was to evaluate the association of FGF-23 levels with echocardiographic parameters and insulin resistance (IR) in patients with gestational diabetes. Subjects and methods: Fifty-four pregnant patients with gestational diabetes mellitus (GDM) (age, 31.12 ± 5.72 years) and 33 healthy pregnant women (age, 29.51 ± 4.92 years) were involved in the study. Fasting insulin, fasting plasma glucose (FPG), lipid profile, oral glucose tolerance test (OGTT), FGF23, echocardiographic parameters, and carotid artery intima-media thickness (CIMT) were evaluated in the two groups. Results: The two groups were not significantly different in age, sex, body mass index, lipid profile, or blood pressure. Insulin, homeostatic model assessment-insulin resistance (HOMA-IR), FGF-23 levels, CIMT, left ventricular (LV) mass, LV mass index and myocardial performance index (MPI) were significantly higher in the GDM group. HOMA-IR was positively correlated with FGF-23, and insulin was positively correlated with FGF-23. Additionally, FGF-23 was positively correlated with CIMT, LV mass index, and MPI. Conclusion: Our findings suggest that monitoring serum FGF-23 may be useful as a non-invasive indicator of subclinical atherosclerosis in patients with GDM. Arch Endocrinol Metab. 2018;62(5):506-13

Keywords
FGF-23; myocardial performance index; gestational diabetes mellitus

INTRODUCTION

Gestational diabetes mellitus (GDM) is defined as a glucose intolerance with onset or first recognition occurring during pregnancy (1). It leads to maternal hyperglycemia, endothelial dysfunction, and abnormal regulation of vascular tone (2). GDM has serious adverse perinatal outcomes and increases long-term risk for the development of type 2 diabetes, obesity, and cardiovascular disease in mother and fetus (3).

Tissue Doppler imaging (TDI) was reported as appropriate for evaluating early changes in systolic and diastolic left ventricle (LV) function (4). The myocardial performance index (MPI) is a sensitive parameter widely used to quantitatively assess global ventricular function in a noninvasive way and combines systolic and diastolic intervals. It is related to morbidity and mortality in many cardiovascular diseases (5). MPI has been studied in several cardiac disorders including heart failure, hypertension, and diabetes, and it has been found to predict worsened morbidity and mortality (6-8). Left ventricular hypertrophy (LVH) is a marker of subclinical cardiovascular disease (CVD) and is associated with cardiovascular morbidity and mortality independent of established risk factors such as age, sex, and diabetes (9). The association between the left ventricular mass index (LVMI) and coronary flow reserve in patients with DM has been investigated in previous studies (10).

Fibroblast growth factor-23 (FGF-23) is a hormone involved in calcium–phosphate homoeostasis, primarily produced and secreted by osteocytes (11). In the renal tubules, FGF-23 binds to the FGF receptor 1c and the klotho coreceptor to promote phosphaturia and lower circulating levels of 1,25-dihydroxyvitamin D (9). FGF-23 may also play a role in some metabolic processes, such as insulin resistance (IR), and may also be a marker of diabetes progression or may increase with diabetes-related complications (12). Moreover, serum FGF-23 was shown to be independently associated with LVH in chronic kidney disease (CKD) (13). It has been investigated in several diseases; however, to the best of our knowledge, the relationship between FGF-23 and myocardial function has not been studied yet in patients with GDM.

Carotid artery intima-media thickness (CIMT) assessment and carotid artery plaque identification using ultrasound are well-recognized tools for identification and monitoring of atherosclerosis. Elevated serum FGF-23 levels have been found to be associated with vascular diseases such as CIMT, arterial stiffness, and coronary atherosclerosis in patients with advanced CKD (14,15).

Therefore, we conducted a cross-sectional study to test the hypothesis that elevated FGF-23 concentrations are independently associated with LVMI, MPI, and CIMT in patients with gestational diabetes and to investigate the correlation between FGF-23 levels and IR in gestational diabetic patients compared to pregnant women with normal glucose tolerance.

SUBJECTS AND METHODS

This prospective study was conducted between 2014 May and 2015 May in the Department of Endocrinology and Metabolism of Kahramanmaras Sutcu Imam University, Kahramanmaras, Turkey. It was approved by the local ethical committee (Date: 01.08.2013, Decision Number: 2013712-10), and written informed consent was obtained from all subjects.

Sixty-four pregnant patients seen and diagnosed with GDM (the patient group) in endocrinology and metabolism outpatient clinics were included in the study. From the patient group, 10 patients were ruled out due to follow-up failure, and the study continued with 54 patients. Thirty-three consecutive healthy pregnant patients seen in an antenatal obstetrics and gynecology outpatient clinic were chosen as the control group.

Exclusion criteria

Patients were excluded if they had moderate to severe valvular heart disease, any rhythm other than the normal sinus rhythm, more than a mild degree of pericardial effusion, abnormal left ventricular systolic function (ejection fraction ≤ 50%), known coronary artery disease, clinical suspicion of coronary artery disease, uncontrolled hypertension, or acute illnesses. The patients who had previous impaired fasting glucose, impaired glucose tolerance or diabetes mellitus, family history of diabetes mellitus, chronic and acute renal failure, or a smoking habit and those who used calcium supplements or a vitamin D treatment were also ruled out from the study.

Study protocol

Fasting plasma glucose (FPG), LDL-cholesterol, HDL-cholesterol, triglycerides (TG), alanine aminotransferase (ALT), calcium, phosphate, insulin, 25 hydroxy vitamin D, parathyroid hormone (PTH), and fibroblast growth factor 23 (FGF-23) were measured at the 24th-28th gestational weeks in all subjects. Blood pressure and anthropometric measurements were performed, and body mass index was calculated. Additionally, an oral glucose tolerance test (OGTT) with 75 g glucose was performed at the 24th–28th gestational weeks in all subjects. Serum glucose levels were evaluated according to American Diabetes Association 2013 criteria (16).

Laboratory parameters

Blood samples for hormones and biochemical parameters were taken after an overnight fast from an antecubital vein between 08:00 a.m. and 09:00 a.m. Glucose was analyzed by the glucose hexokinase method. LDL, HDL, and TG were analyzed by the turbidymetric method (Siemens Dimension, Clinical Chemistry System, Newark, DE, USA), using appropriate commercial kits. Insulin was determined by a two-site chemiluminescent immunometric assay with solid-phase mouse monoclonal anti-insulin antibodies conjugated with calf intestine alkaline phosphatase in buffer solution (Immulite Insulin, Diagnostic Products Corporations, Los Angeles, CA) with 2 IU/mL sensitivity. The estimate of insulin resistance by the homeostasis model assessment (HOMA) score was calculated with the formula fasting serum insulin (lU/mL) x fasting plasma glucose (mmol/L)/ 22.5, as described by Matthews and coworkers (17). A HOMA index ≥ 2.5 indicated IR.

FGF-23 level measurement

Serum FGF-23 levels were determined, and venous blood samples were collected in tubes from the antecubital vein, followed by an overnight fast. The tubes were centrifuged at 2000g (10min) to remove the serum. Aliquots of serum samples were stored at −80°C until FGF-23 assaying. Serum FGF-23 levels were determined using Human FGF-23 ELISA Kit (cat. number EZHFGF-23-32K) purchased from Millipore (USA) according to the manufacturer's instructions. The Millipore Human FGF-23 ELISA Kit employs the quantitative sandwich enzyme immunoassay technique.

Echocardiographic assessment

The echocardiographic examinations, including M-Mode, two-dimensional, SDE, and tissue Doppler echocardiography (TDI) recordings, were performed with Vivid 7 Pro (GE, Horten, Norway, 2–4 MHz phased array transducer). Measurements were made according to the American Society of Echocardiography guidelines by a single cardiologist unaware of the clinical data and averaged from five cardiac cycles.

For all participants, two-dimensional, M-Mode, and TDI echocardiography examinations were performed by the same physician. LV mass was calculated with the Devereux Formula (18) and indexed to body surface area.

In all TDI images, the systolic velocity duration was measured as ejection time (ET, ms), the time between the end of the systolic velocity and the beginning of early diastolic velocity was measured as isovolumetric relaxation time (IRT, ms), and the time between the end of the late diastolic velocity and the beginning of systolic velocity as isovolumetric contraction time (ICT, ms) MPI, which is calculated from systolic and diastolic time intervals, reflects the global left ventricular function with good reproducibility, and is independent from the left ventricle's geometry and heart rate.

The myocardial performance index was calculated using the formula (ICT + IRT)/ET.

Measurement of carotid intima-media thickness

Measurements of all participants' CIMT were performed by the same endocrinologist with the same ultrasound device (Logic P5 System, General Electric Medical Systems, Milwaukee, WI, USA) using a linear transducer of 12 MHz width. The carotid arteries were scanned in longitudinal projection. Intima media is defined as the distance between the beginning of the tunica intima and the beginning of the tunica adventitia. Intima media thickness measurements on the common carotid artery's far wall were bilaterally performed. For reproducible measurements, a high-quality image acquisition was used along a minimum length of 10 mm of an arterial segment. The mean CIMT was calculated from three consecutive examinations.

Statistical analysis

Statistical analysis was conducted with Statistical Package for Social Sciences 15.0 packet program (SPSS Inc., Chicago, IL). Descriptive statistics were shown as mean±standard deviation. The student t test was used to compare continuous variables between two groups. The difference between the groups regarding the qualitative variables was investigated with a Chi-square test. A p value less than 0.05 was considered statistically significant. Similarly, for bivariate correlation coefficients, parametric data was analyzed using Pearson's rho.

RESULTS

Fifty-four pregnant women (age, 31.12 ± 5.72 years) who had GDM and 33 healthy pregnant women (age, 29.51 ± 4.92 years) were involved in the study. The GDM patients' and controls' demographic and biochemical characteristics are presented in Table 1. There was no significant difference in age, sex, lipid parameters, body mass index (BMI), or systolic and diastolic blood pressure. FPG, oral glucose tolerance test first hour glucose ($OGTTglucose_{1}$), oral glucose tolerance test second hour glucose ($OGTTglucose_{2}$), insulin, HOMA-IR, FGF-23 levels, and mean CIMT were significantly higher in the GDM group.

Changes in the patient group's and control group's conventional and Doppler echocardiographic measurements are presented in Table 2. LV mass and LV mass index were significantly higher in the patient group. No significant difference existed between the groups' left ventricular end-diastolic dimensions (LV EDDs), left ventricular end-systolic dimensions (LV ESDs), interventricular septum thickness (IVS), posterior wall thickness (PW), left atrial dimension, left ventricular ejection fraction (LV EF), mitral E and A velocity, E/A, DT, or LA volume index.

Tissue Doppler echocardiographic parameters of the gestational diabetes and control groups are presented in Table 3. MPI was significantly higher in the patient group. HOMA-IR did not show a positive correlation with FGF-23, PW, or IVS (r = 0.309, p = 0.008; r = 0.336, p = 0.004; and r = 0.356, p = 0.002, respectively), but it showed a negative correlation with HOMA-IR and LV EDD (r = -0.242, p = 0.039).

Table 1. Characteristics of patient and control groups

Parameters	Patient group n = 54	Control group n = 33	p
Age (years)	31.12 ± 5.72	29.51 ± 4.92	0.105
BMI (kg/m^2)	32.05 ± 5.84	30.12 ± 4.42	0.183
BSA (m^2)	1.81 ± 0.17	1.78 ± 0.15	0.437
Systolic BP (mmHg)	110.48 ± 10.63	106.36 ± 13.09	0.113
Diastolic BP (mmHg)	69.57 ± 9.06	66.45 ± 8.76	0.055
FPG (mg/dL)	89.70 ± 12.28	75.27 ± 6.25	< 0.001
OGTTglucose$_1$ (mg/dL)	189.53 ± 30.97	126.48 ± 26.22	< 0.001
OGTTglucose$_2$ (mg/dL)	151.68 ± 25.78	103.33 ± 22.36	< 0.001
LDL (mg/dL)	108.98 ± 33.99	117.05 ± 33.11	0.281
HDL (mg/dL)	65.86 ± 21.60	66.21 ± 10.46	0.930
TG (mg/dL)	200.73 ± 61.05	183.21 ± 50.27	0.169
ALT (U/L)	18.64 ± 7.27	18.15 ± 6.13	0.744
Insulin (uIU/L)	12.84 ± 9.10	9.07 ± 4.99	0.032
HOMA-IR	2.71 ± 1.98	1.75 ± 1.04	0.021
Calcium (mg/dL)	8.82 ± 0.30	8.75 ± 0.27	0.284
Phosphate (mg/dL)	3.58 ± 0.41	3.75 ± 0.36	0.069
25 OH D (ng/mL)	34.31 ± 4.25	33.93 ± 3.42	0.669
PTH (pg/mL)	39.06 ± 3.38	38.67 ± 3.39	0.600
CRP	3.13 ± 0.25	3.17 ± 0.23	0.446
FGF 23 (pg/mL)	162.24 ± 22.41	68.36 ± 10.96	< 0.001
CIMT (cm)	0.064 ± 0.009	0.057 ± 0.007	< 0.001

BMI: body mass index; BSA: body surface area; BP: blood pressure; FPG: fasting plasma glucose; OGTTglucose$_1$: oral glucose tolerance test first hour glucose; OGTTglucose$_2$: oral glucose tolerance test second hour glucose; LDL: low density lipoprotein; HDL: high density lipoprotein; TG: triglycerides; ALT: alanine aminotransferase; HOMA-IR: homeostatic model assessment index-insulin resistance; 25 OH D: 25 hydroxy vitamin D; PTH: parathyroid hormone; FGF-23: fibroblast growth factor; CIMT: carotid intima-media thickness.

Table 2. Conventional and Doppler echocardigraphic measurements of the gestational diabetes and control groups

Parameters	Patient group n = 54	Control group n = 33	p
LV EDD (mm)	46.00 ± 3.12	44.88 ± 5.25	0.274
LV ESD (mm)	28.12 ± 6.51	28.21 ± 3.01	0.946
IVS (mm)	9.92 ± 3.83	8.60 ± 1.63	0.063
PW (mm)	13.16 ± 3.60	8.17 ± 1.47	0.384
LV mass (g)	164.75 ± 42.04	139.30 ± 29.37	0.003
LV mass index (g/m^2)	90.47 ± 20.16	77.85 ± 15.87	0.003
Left atrial dimension (mm)	50.16 ± 11.79	48.81 ± 11.02	0.597
LV EF (%)	68.72 ± 4.74	68.63 ± 4.16	0.932
Mitral E velocity (cm/s)	83.11 ± 13.26	87.93 ± 14.59	0.117
Mitral A velocity (cm/s)	68.38 ± 11.13	71.36 ± 13.76	0.273
E/A	1.23 ± 0.24	1.25 ± 0.23	0.704
DT (ms)	170.48 ± 34.59	167.90 ± 35.23	0.739
LA volume index (mL/m^2)	27.81 ± 6.29	27.37 ± 5.67	0.741

LV: left ventricular; LV EDD: LV end-diastolic dimension; LV ESD: LV end-systolic dimension; IVS: interventricular septum thickness; PW: posterior wall thickness; EF: ejection fraction; E: early diastolic velocity; A: late diastolic velocity; DT: mitral E-wave deceleration time; LA: left atrium.

Insulin had a positive correlation with FGF-23, PW, and IVS (r = 0.271, p = 0.011; r = 0.264, p = 0.014; r = 0.282, and p = 0.008, respectively). Additionally, FPG had a positive correlation with BMI, CIMT, FGF-23, LV mass index, PW, IVS, RVL-MPI, IVS-MPI, and LVL-MPI (r = 0.274, p = 0.010; r = 0.209, p = 0.052; r = 0.519, p < 0.001; r = 0.291, p = 0.006; r = 0.312, p = 0.003; r = 0.406, p < 0.001; r = 0.240, p = 0.025; and r = 0.285, p = 0.007, respectively). FGF-23 had a positive correlation with CIMT, LV mass index, RVL-MPI, IVS-MPI, and LVL-MPI (r = 0.400, p < 0.001; r = 0.282, p = 0.008; r = 0.544, p < 0.001; r = 0.310, p = 0.004; and r = 0.268, p = 0.012, respectively) (Table 4).

DISCUSSION

Several previous studies demonstrated that FGF-23 is independently associated with several cardiovascular risk factors, such as endothelial dysfunction, increased arterial stiffness, LVH, left ventricular dilatation impaired vasoreactivity, cardiovascular mortality, and atherosclerosis in hemodialysis patients and healthy subjects (14,15). CIMT assessment and common carotid artery plaque identification by ultrasound are well-recognized tools for identification and monitoring of atherosclerosis. Elevated serum FGF-23 levels have been found to be associated with vascular diseases such as CIMT, arterial stiffness, and coronary atherosclerosis in patients with advanced CKD (16,17). Although Balci and cols. (19) reported a positive correlation between CIMT and FGF-23 in hemodialysis patients, Gungor and cols. (20) did not find any correlation. Several studies have indicated that a pregnancy complicated by GDM has a significant impact on endothelial function during pregnancy (21,22). However, the impact of FGF-23 on the early stages of atherosclerosis in patients with gestational diabetes is not defined. In this study, mean CIMT was significantly higher in patients with GDM, and a positive correlation between FGF-23 and CIMT was found. Association of FGF-23 with CIMT may be another possible mechanism underlying the development and progression of atherosclerosis in patients with GDM.

The myocardial performance index reflects LV systolic and diastolic function. MPI is also abnormal in individuals without overt cardiac disease who have risk factors such as diabetes mellitus and treated and untreated hypertension (17,23,24). In a recent study, MPI was measured by the conventional method and with tissue Doppler echocardiography. It was significantly higher in the diabetic group than in the control group (25). In patients with CKD, FGF-23 supraphysiologic levels were strongly associated with LVMI, left ventricular hypertrophy (LVH), cardiovascular events, and mortality (14,26). High prevalence of preclinical diastolic dysfunction is a well-established fact among diabetic patients. The evidence indicates that myocardial damage in diabetic subjects affects diastolic function before the systolic function (27). Using tissue Doppler and strain/strain rate echocardiography, a recent study showed that LV longitudinal systolic and diastolic functions were impaired in diabetic patients (28). However, limited studies have been conducted on GDM's effect on diastolic functions (29). Caliskan and

Table 3. Tissue Doppler echocardiographic parameters of the gestational diabetes and control groups

Parameters	Patient group n = 54	Control group n = 33	p
Left ventricular lateral wall			
Sm (cm/s)	10.75 ± 2.61	10.42 ±1.71	0.514
Em/Am	1.49 ± 0.42	1.34 ± 0.68	0.211
MPI	0.50 ± 0.94	0.44 ± 0.08	0.004
Interventricular septum			
Sm (cm/s)	8.22 ± 1.65	9.15 ± 2.07	0.024
Em/Am	1.28 ± 0.41	1.13 ± 0.55	0.154
MPI	0.52 ± 0.07	0.42 ± 0.09	0.002
Right ventricular lateral wall			
Sm (cm/s)	16.48 ± 3.73	18.87 ± 5.12	0.014
Em/Am	0.97 ± 0.35	0.84 ± 0.43	0.128
MPI	0.55 ± 0.09	0.41 ± 0.07	< 0.001

Sm: systolic myocardial velocity; Em: myocardial early diastolic velocity; Am: myocardial late diastolic velocity; MPI: myocardial performance index.

cols. (29) found that although LV systolic function and LVMI were similar between the two groups (GDM and control groups), the diastolic function parameters were impaired in the GDM group. In our study, although LVMI was significantly higher in the GDM group than in the control group, no significant difference existed in diastolic function parameters (mitral E/A ratio) between groups. Sm determined by TDI is another measure of LV systolic functions independent from the LV's shape (31). In our study, Sm had fewer patients with GDM, indicating the presence of possible subclinical systolic dysfunction. MPI was significantly higher in patients with GDM than in the control group. Additionally, FGF-23 showed a significant positive correlation with MPI. Therefore, we think MPI, which reflects diastolic and systolic functions, is a more important marker than mitral inflow velocity (E/A) in the evaluation of cardiac functions.

The data concerning the relationship between FGF-23 levels and IR are contradictory. Wahl and cols. (13) have observed that FGF-23 levels are greater in coronary artery disease patients who have diabetes. Garland and cols. (30) reported that increasing HOMA-IR was positively associated with FGF-23 in stage 3-5 chronic kidney disease patients. Holecki and cols. (31) showed increased levels of both circulating FGF-23 forms in elderly subjects are not associated with obesity or IR. Hanks and cols. (32) found that the surrogate marker of IR, HOMA-IR were positively associated with FGF-23. The relationship between

Table 4. Correlation between metabolic parameters, FGF-23, convensional and tissue doppler echocardiographic parameters of the all participants

Parameters		HOMA-IR	Insulin	FPG	OGTTglucose$_1$	OGTTglucose$_2$	FGF-23
BMI (kg/m^2)							
	r	0.048	0.025	0.274	0.075	0.234	0.181
	p	0.686	0.817	0.010	0.489	0.029	0.094
CIMT (cm)							
	r	0.136	0.126	0.209	0.339	0.156	0.400
	p	0.251	0.244	0.052	0.001	0.150	< 0.001
FGF-23							
	r	0.309	0.271	0.519	0.631	0.679	-
	p	0.008	0.011	< 0.001	< 0.001	< 0.001	-
LVMI (g/m^2)							
	r	0.097	0.076	0.291	0.180	0.262	0.282
	p	0.414	0.482	0.006	0.095	0.014	0.008
E/A							
	r	0.045	0.052	-0.086	-0.090	-0.070	-0.030
	p	0.707	0.632	0.430	0.407	0.517	0.783
LV mass (g)							
	r	0.159	0.109	0.312	0.178	0.259	0.298
	p	0.178	0.316	0.003	0.099	0.016	0.005
RVL-MPI							
	r	0.196	0.143	0.406	0.455	0.464	0.544
	p	0.096	0.187	< 0.001	< 0.001	< 0.001	< 0.001
IVS-MPI							
	r	0.087	0.153	0.240	0.230	0.172	0.310
	p	0.462	0.158	0.025	0.032	0.110	0.004
LVL-MPI							
	r	0.032	0.031	0.285	0.244	0.248	0.268
	p	0.788	0.774	0.007	0.023	0.021	0.012

BMI: body mass index; CIMT: carotid intima-media thickness; FGF-23: fibroblast growth factor 23; LVMI: left ventricular mass index; E: mitral early diastolic velocity; A: mitral late diastolic velocity; RVL: right ventricular lateral wall; LVL: left ventricular lateral wall; MPI: myocardial performance index; HOMA-IR: homeostatic model assessment index-insulin resistance; FPG: fasting plasma glucose; OGTTglucose$_1$: oral glucose tolerance test first hour glucose; OGTT glucose$_2$: oral glucose tolerance test second hour glucose

IR and FGF-23 has not been investigated in patients with GDM. This study showed a positive correlation between HOMA-IR and FGF-23. Association of FGF-23 with IR may be another possible mechanism underlying the development and progression of atherosclerosis in DM patients.

In conclusion, the present prospective study is the first in the literature that evaluated the relationship between FGF-23 and MPI in patients with gestational diabetes in the absence of CVD. Plasma FGF-23 levels were shown to be associated with increased LVMI, MPI, and CIMT in patients with GDM. The significant and positive association of FGF-23 plasma level with LVMI and MPI raises the possibility of a specific pathophysiologic effect of FGF-23 on left ventricular mass and function distinct from its effects on serum calcium, phosphorus, and intact parathormone. Additionally, this study showed that FGF-23 may play a role in the development of GDM with IR. Therefore, we believe that FGF-23 plays a role in the pathogenesis and development of preclinical atherosclerosis and cardiac dysfunction in patients with GDM.

Acknowledgments: none.

Disclosure of grants or other funding: we have no direct or indirect commercial, financial incentive associated with publishing this article.

REFERENCES

1. Baz B, Riveline JP, Gautier JF. Endocrinology of Pregnancy: Gestational Diabetes Mellitus: Definition, aetiological and clinical aspects. Eur J Endocrinol. 2016;174(2):R43-51.
2. Muñoz-Hoyos A, Rodriguez-Cabezas T, Molina-Carballo A, Martinez-Sempere JJ, Ruiz-Cosano C, Acuña-Castroviejo D. Melatonin concentration in the umbilical artery and vein in human preterm and term neonates and neonates with acute fetal distress. J Pineal Res. 1992;13(4):184-91.
3. Catalano PM, Kirwan JP, Haugel-de Mouzon S, King J. Gestational diabetes and insulin resistance: role in short- and long-term implications for mother and fetus. J Nutr. 2003;133:1674S-83S.
4. Kibar AE, Pac FA, Ballı S, Oflaz MB, Ece I, Bas VN, et al. Early subclinical left-ventricular dysfunction in obese nonhypertensive children: a tissue Doppler imaging study. Pediatr Cardiol. 2013;34(6):1482-90.
5. Tei C, Ling LH, Hodge DO, Bailey KR, Oh JK, Rodeheffer RJ, et al. New index of combined systolic and diastolic myocardial performance: a simple and reproducible measure of cardiac function--a study in normals and dilated cardiomyopathy. J Cardiol. 1995;26(6):357-66.
6. Karatzis EN, Giannakopoulou AT, Papadakis JE, Karazachos AV, Nearchou NS. Myocardial performance index (Tei index): evaluating its application to myocardial infarction. Hellenic J Cardiol. 2009;50(1):60-5.
7. Orem C, Küçükosmanoğlu M, Hacihasanoğlu A, Yilmaz R, Kasap H, Erdoğan T, et al. Association of Doppler-derived myocardial performance index with albuminuria in patients with diabetes. J Am Soc Echocardiogr. 2004;17(11):1185-90.
8. Mishra RK, Kizer JR, Palmieri V, Roman MJ, Galloway JM, Fabsitz RR, et al. Utility of the myocardial performance index in a population with high prevalences of obesity, diabetes, and hypertension: the strong heart study. Echocardiography. 2007;24(4):340-7.
9. Gosse P. Left ventricular hypertrophy as a predictor of cardiovascular risk. J Hypertens Suppl. 2005;23(1):S27-33.
10. Galderisi M, Capaldo B, Sidiropulos M, D'Errico A, Ferrara L, Turco A, et al. Determinants of reduction of coronary flow reserve in patients with type 2 diabetes mellitus or arterial hypertension without angiographically determined epicardial coronary stenosis. Am J Hypertens. 2007;20(12):1283-90.
11. Hanks LJ, Casazza K, Judd SE, Jenny NS, Gutiérrez OM. Associations of fibroblast growth factor-23 with markers of inflammation, insulin resistance and obesity in adults. PLoS One. 2015;10(3):e0122885.
12. Shimada T, Hasegawa H, Yamazaki Y, Muto T, Hino R, Takeuchi Y, et al. FGF-23 is a potent regulator of vitamin D metabolism and phosphate homeostasis. J Bone Miner Res. 2004;19(3):429-35.
13. Wahl P, Xie H, Scialla J, Anderson CA, Bellovich K, Brecklin C, et al. Earlier onset and greater severity of disordered mineral metabolism in diabetic patients with chronic kidney disease. Diabetes Care. 2012;35(5):994-1001.
14. Gutierrez OM, Januzzi JL, Isakova T, Laliberte K, Smith K, Collerone G, et al. Fibroblast growth factor 23 and left ventricular hypertrophy in chronic kidney disease. Circulation. 2009;119(19):2545-52.
15. Mirza MA, Larsson A, Lind L, Larsson TE. Circulating fibroblast growth factor-23 is associated with vascular dysfunction in the community. Atherosclerosis. 2009;205(2):385-90.
16. American Diabetes Association. Standards of medical care in diabetes-2013. Diabetes Care. 2013;36(1):11-66.
17. Matthews DR, Hosker JP, Rudenski AS, Naylor BA, Treacher DF, Turner RC. Homeostasis model assessment: insulin resistance and beta-cell function from fasting plasma glucose and insulin concentrations in man. Diabetologia. 1985;28(7):412-9.
18. Devereux RB, Alonso DR, Lutas EM, Gottlieb GJ, Campo E, Sachs I, et al. Echocardiographic assessment of left ventricular hypertrophy: comparison to necropsy findings. Am J Cardiol. 1986;57(6):450-8.
19. Balci M, Kirkpantur A, Gulbay M, Gurbuz OA. Plasma fibroblast growth factor-23 levels are independently associated with carotid artery atherosclerosis in maintenance hemodialysis patients. Hemodial Int. 2010;14(4):425-32.
20. Gungor O, Kismali E, Sisman AR, Kircelli F, Carrero JJ, Tatar E, et al. The relationships between serum sTWEAK, FGF-23 levels, and carotid atherosclerosis in renal transplant patients. Ren Fail. 2013;35(1):77-81.
21. Knock GA, McCarthy AL, Lowy C, Poston L. Association of gestational diabetes with abnormal maternal vascular endothelial function. Br J Obstet Gynaecol. 1997;104:229-34.
22. Chirayath HH, Wareing M, Taggart MJ, Baker PN. Endothelial dysfunction in myometrial arteries of women with gestational diabetes. Diabetes Res Clin Pract. 2010;89:134-40.
23. Evrengul H, Dursunoglu D, Kaftan A, et al. Relation of insulin resistance and left ventricular function and structure in non-diabetic patients with essential hypertension. Acta Cardiol 2005;60:191-8.
24. Keser N, Yildiz S, Kurtoğ N, Dindar I. Modified TEI index: a promising parameter in essential hypertension? Echocardiography. 2005;22(4):296-304.

25. Turfan M, Akyel A, Bolayir HA, Vatankulu MA, Aktürk M, Yetkin I, et al. Correlation of the myocardial performance index with plasma B-type natriureticpeptide levels in type 2 diabetes mellitus and impaired glucose tolerance. Kardiol Pol. 2012;70(6):556-62.
26. Isakova T, Xie H, Yang W, Xie D, Anderson AH, Scialla J, et al.; Chronic Renal Insufficiency Cohort (CRIC) Study Group. Fibroblast growth factor 23 and risks of mortality and endstage renal disease in patients with chronic kidney disease. JAMA. 2011;305:2432-39.
27. Patil VC, Patil HV, Shah KB, Vasani JD, Shetty P. Diastolic dysfunction in asymptomatic type 2 diabetes mellitus with normal systolic function. J Cardiovasc Dis Res. 2011;2(4):213-22.
28. Ernande L, Bergerot C, Girerd N, Thibault H, Davidsen ES, Gautier Pignon-Blanc P, et al. Longitudinal myocardial strain alteration is associated with left ventricular remodeling in asymptomatic patients with type 2 diabetes mellitus. J Am Soc Echocardiogr. 2014;27(5):479-88.
29. Caliskan M, Turan Y, Caliskan Z, Gullu H, Ciftci FC, Avci E, et al. Previous gestational diabetes history is associated with impaired coronary flow reserve. Ann Med. 2015;47(7):615-23.
30. Garland JS, Holden RM, Ross R, Adams MA, Nolan RL, Hopman WM, et al. Insulin resistance is associated with Fibroblast Growth Factor-23 in stage 3–5 chronic kidney disease patients. J Diabetes Complications. 2014;28(1):61-5.
31. Holecki M, Chudek J, Owczarek A, Olszanecka-Glinianowicz M, Bożentowicz-Wikarek M, Duława J, et al. Inflammation but not obesity or insulin resistance is associated with increased plasma fibroblast growth factor 23 concentration in the elderly. Clin Endocrinol (Oxf). 2015;82(6):900-9.
32. Hanks LJ, Casazza K, Judd SE, Jenny NS, Gutiérrez OM. Associations of fibroblast growth factor-23 with markers of inflammation, insulin resistance and obesity in adults. PLoS One. 2015;10(3):e0122885.

The effect of levothyroxine treatment on left ventricular function in subclinical hypothyroidism

Valentina Velkoska Nakova[1], Brankica Krstevska[2], Elizabeta Srbinovska Kostovska[3], Olivija Vaskova[4], Ljubica Georgievska Ismail[5]

[1] University "Goce Delchev", Faculty of Medical Science, Clinical Hospital, Shtip, R. Macedonia
[2] University Clinic of Endocrinology, Diabetes and Metabolic Disorders, Medical Faculty, Skopje, R. Macedonia
[3] University Clinic of Cardiology, Medical Faculty, Skopje, R. Macedonia
[4] Institute of Patophysiology and Nuclear Medicine, Medical Faculty, Skopje, R. Macedonia
[5] University Clinic of Cardiology, Medical Faculty, Skopje, R. Macedonia

Correspondence to:
valentina.velkoska@yahoo.com

ABSTRACT

Objective: Treatment of subclinical hypothyroidism (ScH), especially the mild form of ScH, is controversial because thyroid hormones influence cardiac function. We investigate left ventricular systolic and diastolic function in ScH and evaluate the effect of 5-month levothyroxine treatment. Subjects and methods: Fifty-four patients with newly diagnosed mild ScH (4.2 <TSH < 10.0 mU/L) and 30 euthyroid subjects matched by age were analysed. Laboratory analyses and an echocardiography study were done at the first visit and after 5 months in euthyroid stage in patients with ScH. Results: Compared to healthy controls, patients with ScH had a lower E/A ratio (1.03 ± 0.29 vs. 1.26 ± 0.36, p < 0.01), higher E/e' sep. ratio (7.62 ± 2.29 vs. 6.04 ± 1.64, p < 0.01), higher myocardial performance index (MPI) (0.47 ± 0.08 vs. 0.43 ± 0.07, p < 0.05), lower global longitudinal strain (GLS) (-19.5 ± 2.3 vs. -20.9 ± 1.7%, p < 0.05), and lower S wave derived by tissue Doppler imaging (0.077 ± 0.013 vs. 0.092 ± 0.011 m/s, p < 0.01). Levothyroxine treatment in patients with ScH contributed to higher EF (62.9 ± 3.9 vs. 61.6 ± 4.4%, p < 0.05), lower E/e' sep. ratio (6.60 ± 2.06 vs. 7.62 ± 2.29, p < 0.01), lower MPI (0.43 ± 0.07 vs. 0.47 ± 0.08%, p < 0.01), and improved GLS (-20.07 ± 2.7 vs. -19.55 ± 2.3%, p < 0.05) compared to values in ScH patients at baseline. Furthermore, in all study populations (ScH patients before and after levothyroxine therapy and controls), TSH levels significantly negatively correlated with EF (r = -0.15, p < 0.05), E/A (r = -0.14, p < 0.05), GLS (r = -0.26, p < 0.001), and S/TDI (r = -0.22, p < 0.01) and positively correlated with E/e' sep. (r = 0.14, p < 0.05). Conclusion: Patients with subclinical hypothyroidism versus healthy individuals had subtle changes in certain parameters that indicate involvement of systolic and diastolic function of the left ventricle. Although the values of the parameters were in normal range, they were significantly different compared to ScH and the control group at baseline, as well as to the ScH groups before and after treatment. The results of our study suggest that patients with ScH must be followed up during treatment to assess improvement of the disease. Some of the echocardiography obtained parameters were reversible after levothyroxine therapy. Arch Endocrinol Metab. 2018;62(4):392-8

Keywords

Subclinical hypothyroidism; thyroid replacement therapy; systolic function; diastolic function

INTRODUCTION

Subclinical hypothyroidism (ScH) is defined as a condition with a slight increase in serum concentration of thyrotropin (TSH) with normal values of circulating thyroid hormones, free thyroxine (FT4) and triiodothyronine (FT3).

The upper limit of TSH from which thyroid replacement therapy should start is still a topic of debate (1,2). Treatment is generally recommended in severe ScH (TSH value above 10 mU/L) (2-6). When the TSH value is less than 10 mU/L, treatment may be indicated in relation to age, presence of goiter, or antithyroid antibodies. One meta-analysis (7) proposed starting with thyroid replacement therapy when TSH levels are above 7 mU/L. Previous research (8) showed increased risk of atherosclerosis in patients with ScH at levels above 7 mU/L.

Thyroid hormones influence cardiac function (9,10). They regulate the transcription of structural and regulatory proteins in the cardiovascular system (11), predispose chronic inflammation and tissue changes (collagen alteration, dehydration), and also cause hemodynamic changes through their effect on smooth muscles in the arterial wall (10,12). All these can alter cardiac function and together with atherosclerosis increase the risk of cardiovascular manifestations.

Research has revealed that substitution therapy with levothyroxine in ScH with TSH values above 10 mU/L could improve left ventricular (LV) function (13-16). Whether the same is true for mild ScH (TSH values less than 10 mU/L) is unknown.

The aim of the study was to evaluate the effect of levothyroxine therapy on LV systolic and diastolic function in patients with a mild form of ScH (4.2 < TSH < 10.0 mU/L) and after 5 months in euthyroid stage, using two-dimensional echocardiography, pulse Doppler, tissue Doppler, and two-dimensional speckle tracking imaging. An additional aim of the study was to predict which parameters derived by echocardiography can be used to monitor patients with ScH.

SUBJECTS AND METHODS

Patients

The prospective study was conducted at the University Clinic of Endocrinology and the University Clinic of Cardiology in Skopje, R. Macedonia. The study included a control group and patients with a newly diagnosed mild form of ScH. The control group consisted of 30 healthy euthyroid patients (normal FT4, FT3, and TSH of 0.2–4.2 mU/L). The criteria for a diagnosis of mild ScH were 4.2 mU/L < TSH < 10.0 mU/L with normal serum FT4 10.3–24.45 pmol/L and FT3 4.2–8.1 pmol/L. According to the recommendations of the British Thyroid Association, patients with ScH were placed on thyroid replacement therapy if one of the following criteria were present: at least three signs or symptoms of hypothyroidism, positive anti-TPO antibodies and positive anti-Tg antibodies, positive family history of thyroid disease, and thyroid enlargement or goiter on ultrasonography (17). The starting dose of L-thyroxine was 25 µg. TSH was measured every 8 weeks for dose adjustment. After 5 months in continuous euthyroid state, echocardiography was repeated. The euthyroid state was achieved with a mean dose of 60.8 ± 19 µg in mean duration of 7.5 ± 2.2 months. During a period of three years, 54 consecutive patients were included in the ScH group.

The control group was included to compare echocardiography parameters from the mild form of SCH at baseline.

Exclusion criteria

Patients with a previous history of thyroid disease receiving therapy for thyroid or cardiovascular function were not included. Patients who were cigarette smokers or who had cardiovascular disease, hypertension, hypothalamic-pituitary disease, depression, psychosis, bipolar disorders, diabetes, chronic pancreatitis, hepatic or renal disease, ovulatory dysfunction, infertility, or pregnancy were also not included.

Ethical aspects

All patients gave informed consent to participate in the study after careful explanation of the testing protocol. The study was conducted in accordance with the Declaration of Helsinki and approved by the Ethics Committee at the Medical Faculty in Skopje, R. Macedonia.

METHODS

At the first visit to the University Clinic of Endocrinology, blood samples for TSH, FT4, and FT3 were taken from all patients. At the same time, at the Outpatient Department of Cardiology Clinic, transthoracic echocardiography was done. Two-dimensional (2D) echocardiography, pulsed wave (PW) Doppler, tissue Doppler imaging (TDI), and 2D speckle tracking echocardiography were used to assess left ventricular systolic and diastolic function.

Laboratory tests

All blood samples for thyroid hormones were collected from the antecubital vein between 08.00 and 09.00 a.m. TSH, FT4, and FT3 were determined by the super-sensitive chemiluminescent immunoassay (Immulite 2000, Siemens Medical Solutions Diagnostics, Los Angeles, CA, USA). The functional sensitivity for TSH was 0.004 µIU/mL, for FT4 0.3 ng/dL, and FT3 0.4 ng/dL.

Echocardiographic measurements

Standard assessments of LV dimensions and wall thickness were performed in standard views on commercially available equipment (Vivid 7, GE) according to the joint recommendations of the American Society of Echocardiography and the European Association of Cardiovascular Imaging (18). LV volume and ejection fraction were calculated using the biplane method of disks (modified Simpson's rule). Left atrial volume was derived by the biapical area-length method and indexed to body surface area (LAVI) (18). Diastolic parameters were obtained by pulsed Doppler by placing a sample volume at the point of touching the mitral leaflets: early mitral flow (E wave, in m/s) and late mitral flow (A wave, m/s), their ratio (E/A, m/s), and deceleration time (DT, msec). Pulmonary venous flow was analysed using PW Doppler. We estimate peak systolic flow (S wave, m/s), early diastolic flow (d wave, m/s), s/d ratio, and atrial reversal flow (Ar, m/s), including Ar-A duration (msec) difference (19). PW TDI was performed in the apical 4-chamber view to assess annular early and late diastolic velocities (19). The recording was performed at a sweep speed of 100 mm/s at end-expiratory apnea. The septal, lateral, and average early diastolic velocities were measured, then the ratio of mitral flow E wave and TDI e' wave (E/e') for each of these annular velocities was calculated. By TDI we also estimate S wave like a maximal systolic velocity (m/sec) which is a parameter for evaluation of longitudinal systolic function (20). With the values of isovolumetric contractile time (IVCT, msec), isovolumetric relaxation time (IVRT, msec), and ejection time (ET, msec) derived by TDI, we calculated the myocardial performance index (MPI), which is a parameter for global left systolic function. We use the formula MPI = IVCT + IVRT / ET. The average of three consecutive cardiac cycles was taken for measurement of each echocardiographic index.

Global and regional peak systolic longitudinal strain was assessed from apical 2-chamber, 4-chamber, and long-axis views using speckle tracking analysis (21). Recordings were processed using an acoustic tracking software (EchoPac, GE, USA), allowing offline semiautomated analysis of speckle-based strain. All images were recorded with a high frame rate (> 50 frames/s). A semiautomatic myocardial tracking system was used, with manual correction of the endocardial border in end-systole and manual adjustment of the region of interest, if needed. The end of systole was defined as the point of aortic valve closure. The software automatically detected the frame-to-frame movement of the natural ultrasound reflecting markers (speckles) on standard ultrasonic images in two dimensions. The LV was divided into 17 segments, and each segment was analysed individually. Only myocardial segments considered to be of adequate quality by both the automatic system and the operator were included in the analysis. Global longitudinal strain for the LV was automatically provided as the average value of the regional peak systolic longitudinal strain of the three apical views by the software.

Statistical analysis

Categorical parameters were summarized as percentages and continuous parameters as mean ± SD. The normal distribution of variables was verified with the Shapiro-Wilk test. As the distribution was normal, Student's independent *t*-test was used for the comparison of the quantitative data between the control group and the ScH group at baseline. Student's paired t-test was used for the comparison of the quantitative data before and after the levothyroxine therapy in the ScH group. For the comparison of categorical variables the chi-square test, Yates correction was used. The correlation between the tested parameters was determined using the Pearson correlation. All data analysis was performed using SPSS version 14.0 (IBM SPSS, Inc., Chicago, Illinois) and p value ≤ 0.05 was considered significant.

RESULTS

Patients and normal controls were well matched for age, sex, BMI, and BSA. Heart rate was similar in both groups, but significantly increased in the ScH group after the levothyroxine treatment. The systolic blood pressure was significantly higher in the ScH group at baseline than in the control group, but the treatment with levothyroxine didn't make any changes. The diastolic blood pressure was similar in both groups, without difference after levothyroxine treatment. As expected, TSH levels were significantly higher in the ScH group than in the control group. FT4 and FT3 levels, although in the reference range, were significantly lower in the ScH group at baseline than in the control group. Interestingly, after the thyroid substitution therapy, FT4 and FT3 levels significantly increased in the ScH group (Table 1).

The LV diameters and volumes were similar in both groups, ScH at baseline and control groups. Overall, only EF (although in referent range in all analysed groups) statistically significantly increased in the ScH group after the levothyroxine therapy (Table 2).

The results from echocardiography (systolic and diastolic parameters) in all analysed groups were in normal range, but some of them were statistically different compared to ScH and the control group at baseline, as well as to the ScH groups before and after treatment. The transmitral E/A ratio was lower and E/e' sep. ratio was higher in the ScH group at baseline than in the control group. The E/e' sep. ratio significantly decreased in the ScH group after levothyroxine therapy. The MPI was higher in the ScH group at baseline than in the control group and significantly decreased after levothyroxine therapy. The GLS was significantly reduced in the ScH group at baseline in comparison to the control group and significantly improved after levothyroxine therapy. The S wave estimated from TDI was significantly lower in the ScH group at baseline

Table 1. Demographic, clinical, and hormonal parameters of study population

	Control group (n = 30)	Baseline ScH (n = 54)	ScH after 5 months (n = 54)	Statistical significance
Age (years)	39.3 ± 11.7	43.1±12.4		NS
Sex (m:f)	3 : 27 (10%)	2.52 (3.7%)		NS
BMI (kg/m²)	24.3 ± 3.0	26.7 ± 4.2	25.7 ± 4.2	NS
BSA (m²)	1.78 ± 0.15	1.79 ± 0.17	1.78 ± 0.16	NS
HR (bpm)	76.4 ± 9.1	73.4 ± 9.8	77.1 ± 9.9	$p < 0.05^{b}$
Systolic BP (mmHg)	107.3 ± 28.4	123.3 ± 16.4	122.1 ± 14.2	$p < 0.05^{a,c}$
Diastolic BP (mmHg)	77 ± 13.4	80.0 ± 9.3	79.2 ± 8.4	NS
TSH mU/L	1.7 ± 1.05	8.1 ± 1.3	2.8 ± 2.6	$p< 0.001^{a,b}$
FT4 pmol/L	15.4 ± 2.2	12.3 ± 2.0	15.2 ± 2.6	$p < 0.01^{a,b}$
FT3 pmol/L	5.2 ± 2.1	4.5 ± 1.1	6.4 ± 3.3	$p < 0.05^{a,b}$

Displayed results are average ± std deviation and percentages. Comparisons between the groups were performed by Student's *t*-test (independent and dependent) for continuous variables and $\chi 2$ test for categorical variables.

[a] Statistical significance for controls *vs.* baseline ScH; [b] statistical significance for baseline ScH *vs.* ScH after 5 months; [c] statistical significance for controls *vs.* ScH after 5 months.

BMI: body mass index; BSA: body surface area; HR: heart rate; BP: blood pressure; NS: no significance.

Table 2. Echocardiographic parameters of left ventricular function in the study population

	Control group (n = 30)	Baseline ScH (n = 54)	ScH after 5 months (n = 54)	Statistical significance
LA (mm)	31.7 ± 3.1	31.3 ± 3.9	31.7 ± 3.9	NS
LAVI (ml/m²)	24.4 ± 4.31	21.9 ± 5.77	20.7 ± 5.43	NS
LVEDD (mm)	46.0 ± 4.8	46.4 ± 4.3	45.6 ± 4.1	NS
LVED vol (mL³)	79.1 ± 11.9	81.7 ± 18.4	79.0 ± 18.6	NS
LVES vol (mL³)	31.3 ± 7.0	31.6 ± 7.8	30.6 ± 6.5	NS
EF (%)	62.8 ± 2.3	61.6 ± 4.4	62.9 ± 3.9	$p < 0.05^{b}$
IVS (mm)	10.4 ± 1.1	10.8 ± 0.9	10.8 ± 1.0	NS
PW (mm)	8.7 ± 1.2	8.7 ± 1.2	8.7 ± 1.1	NS
E/A (m/sec)	1.26 ± 0.36	1.03 ± 0.29	1.09 ± 0.34	$p < 0.01^{a,c}$
DT(msec)	156.8 ± 29.7	167.9 ± 38.6	158.5 ± 32.2	NS
E/e' sep.	6.04 ± 1.64	7.62 ± 2.29	6.60 ± 2.06	$p < 0.01^{a,b}$
E/e' lat.	6.08 ± 1.24	6.35 ± 1.62	6.03 ± 1.74	NS
E/e' average	6.06 ± 1.24	6.98 ± 1.9	6.74 ± 1.7	NS
IVCT (msec)	60.04 ± 10.9	64.14 ± 13.4	60.29 ± 12.7	NS
IVRT (msec)	66.39 ± 8.3	67.27 ± 13.7	65.0 ± 12.8	NS
MPI	0.43 ± 0.07	0.47 ± 0.08	0.43 ± 0.07	$p < 0.05^{a}$; $p < 0.01^{b}$
s/d	1.26 ± 0.11	1.26 ± 0.16	1.25 ± 0.22	NS
GLS (%)	-20.9 ± 1.7	-19.55 ± 2.3	-20.07 ± 2.7	$p < 0.001^{a}$; $p < 0.05^{b}$
S/TDI (m/sec)	0.092 ± 0.011	0.077 ± 0.013	0.078 ± 0.01	$p < 0.01^{a,c}$
Ar-A	-18.87 ± 10.78	-25.2 ± 16.1	-23.4 ± 9.1	NS

Displayed results are average ± std deviation and percentages. Comparisons between the groups were performed by Student's *t*-test (independent and dependent) for continuous variables and χ^2 test for categorical variables.

[a] Statistical significance for controls *vs.* baseline ScH; [b] Statistical significance for baseline ScH *vs.* ScH after 5 months; [c] statistical significance for controls *vs.* ScH after 5 months.

LA: left atrial systolic diameter; LAVI: left atrial volume index; LVEDD: end-diastolic diameters; PW: the left ventricular posterior wall; IVS: interventricular septum thickness; LVESV: left ventricular end-systolic volume; LVEDV: left ventricular end-diastolic volume; EF: ejection fraction; E/A: ratio between transmitral early and late diastolic peak flow velocities; A dur: duration of the atrial contraction; DT: time between E velocity deceleration time to the baseline; S wave obtained by TDI, maximal systolic flow velocity; IVCT: isovolumetric contraction time; IVRT: isovolumetric relaxation time; MPI: myocardial performance index; s: systolic velocity of the pulmonary veins; d: diastolic velocity of the pulmonary veins; their ratio (s/d); Ar: retrograde pulmonary venous flow during the atrial contraction–atrial reversal; A-Ar: difference in time of duration of the A wave from transmitral flow by PW and duration of the Ar wave from pulmonary vein flow; GLS: global longitudinal strain.

than in the control group, without changes after the levothyroxine therapy (Table 2). Analysing how many patients had diastolic dysfunction, according to new guidelines for the evaluation of diastolic function by echocardiography, showed that there were only three patients with ScH (22). In all three patients diastolic dysfunction was reversible after thyroid replacement therapy.

Considering the entire study population, the TSH levels (before and after levothyroxine therapy) significantly negatively correlated with EF ($r = -0.15$, $p < 0.05$), E/A ratio ($r = -0.14$, $p < 0.05$), GLS ($r = -0.26$, $p < 0.001$), and S/TDI ($r = -0.22$, $p < 0.01$) and positively correlated with E/e' sep. ($r = 0.14$, $p < 0.05$).

DISCUSSION

The results of the study presented subtle changes in the LV systolic and diastolic function which were reversible after thyroid replacement therapy. Although the values of the echocardiography parameters were in normal range in all analysed groups (control, ScH at baseline, and SCH after treatment), there were statistically significant differences between some parameters compared to the control and ScH group at baseline, as well as to the ScH group before and after treatment.

Our results show that the ScH group at baseline had statistically significantly higher values for systolic blood pressure. This result is similar to the results in one meta-analysis published in 2014. The study includes the analysis of 20 studies and found a slight increase in systolic blood pressure in patients with ScH versus the control group (23). Systolic blood pressure did not decrease significantly after the levothyroxine treatment. The average value for systolic blood pressure in the ScH group at baseline was normal (123.3 ± 16.4 mmHg), so the thyroid replacement therapy probably had no clinical significance in reducing its value. Thus, we can conclude that ScH had no significant impact on the arterial blood pressure, in contrast to what is already known about clinical hypothyroidism. Therefore, we do not expect the thyroid replacement therapy to significantly decrease the already normal values for systolic blood pressure.

Heart rate statistically significantly increased after thyroid replacement therapy. These changes are consistent with the known mechanism of action of thyroid hormones. From a clinical point of view, the increase in heart rate after treatment was still in the normal range (77.1 ± 9.9 minute), but there was statistical significance. None of the patients after treatment had tachycardia or arrhythmia.

At baseline, echocardiographic parameters of LV function were not significantly different between the control and the ScH group, which were similar with results from other studies (15,24-28). Five months of levothyroxine therapy statistically significantly increased the EF. Only a small (1.3%) increase in EF was sufficient to make EF equal to the value (62.9 ± 3.9%) as in the control group. In the study of Ilic and cols. (29), one-year therapy with levothyroxine showed results similar to ours. It is important to mention that all studies (including ours) that analyse the EF in patients with ScH have normal values for EF.

The parameter S derived from TDI, which is a parameter to assess systolic function of LV, was statistically significantly lower in the ScH group compared to the control group. This proves the abnormal longitudinal systolic function of LV in ScH, which is first affected in LV systolic dysfunction (30,31). The parameter S/TDI did not recover after treatment, but there was statistically significant correlation between TSH and S/TDI. More aggressive treatment for lowering TSH value may result in statistically significant changes in S/TDI. Completely identical results were shown in the study of Ilic and cols. (29). The average age in the study of Ilic and cols. (29) is similar to ours, but they analysed only women aged less than 45 years. Probably studies with a large number of patients involving only women in reproductive age are needed to confirm the impact of ScH on S wave derived from TDI.

Results for MPI showed deterioration in global systolic and diastolic function of the LV in ScH, and its reversibility after thyroid replacement therapy. Our results were consistent with those from other clinical studies (24,25,29). The average values of TSH in those studies are similar to this study. There was no statistically significant correlation between TSH and MPI. The lack of correlation between TSH and MPI may be due to small changes in the value of MPI that occur at higher values of TSH.

Global longitudinal strain is considered more sensitive than EF in assessing LV global systolic function, especially when the EF is normal, in favour of subclinical LV dysfunction. Values of GLS in the control group and ScH group at baseline were within the normal range, but still with statistically significantly different values in the ScH group. GLS significantly improved after the levothyroxine therapy. TSH significantly negatively correlated with GLS. Two studies examined GLS in ScH, and both of them showed results similar to ours (29,32).

The results from Doppler transmitral flow and velocities estimated by TDI showed changes in some parameters which are defined as parameters for diastolic function assessment. Although the values of some parameters were in the normal range, there is a statistically significant difference between the values of the control and ScH groups. This is shown by statistically significantly lower E/A ratio, and higher E/e' sep. ratio in the ScH group compared to the control group.

After 5 months of euthyroid state, the E/A ratio did not increase significantly. In a study by Yazici and cols. (25) the E/A ratio was statistically significantly lower in patients with ScH compared to the control group. In the same study, the ratio increased significantly after 6 months of euthyroid state and continued to increase after 12 months of euthyroid state. A study by Erkan and cols. (33) showed results similar to ours. Therefore, a longer euthyroid state or more aggressive treatment for lowering TSH may be required to achieve a statistically significant increase in the E/A ratio, after treatment. At the end of the study the average TSH value was 2.8 ± 2.6 mU/L. In the assessment of diastolic function the E/e' sep. ratio is a more sensitive parameter than the E/e' lat. ratio. A statistically significant difference in the E/e' sep. ratio, but not in the E/e' lat. Ratio, was found in other studies (24,28). Three patients in the ScH group had diastolic dysfunction, which was reversible after thyroid replacement therapy. Diastolic dysfunction is mainly attributed to ScH because other potential causes of diastolic dysfunction (hypertension, diabetes mellitus) were excluded in this study. Parameters which measured diastolic dysfunction can be applied to all patients with ScH and also to follow them during treatment.

Statistically significant correlations between TSH and analysed parameters were weak ($r < 0.5$). The weak correlation coefficient may be due to higher TSH values at the end of the study. The r values were lower for correlations with diastolic parameters. Probably systolic parameters are more sensitive on L-T4 treatment, and diastolic parameters need a longer period of treatment.

Summarizing the results, ScH did not cause cardiac failure by itself, but thyroid substitution therapy improves some parameters of LV function. We analysed only patients with mild ScH, which means rapid detection of thyroid dysfunction. If ScH is detected later, according to the correlations, we expected worsening of LV parameters.

There are some limitations in this study. The design is not that of a blind or double-blind study which includes L-thyroxine and placebo. We followed the parameters of systolic and diastolic function, but we did not directly observe cardiovascular morbidity and mortality, which requires very long-term monitoring of patients.

The advantages of the study compared to previous similar studies are the inclusion of young people with no risk factors for cardiovascular disease which can influence systolic and diastolic parameters, and the inclusion of patients with mild ScH. Thus, this study confirmed the benefit of levothyroxine treatment in patients with ScH with lower values of TSH. Today, when there is a lack of recommendations for treatment of mild ScH, this study moves the limits for initiation with treatment from the lower values of TSH.

In conclusion, patients with ScH versus healthy individuals had subtle changes in certain parameters that indicate involvement of systolic and diastolic function of the LV in ScH. Although the values of the parameters were in normal range, they were significantly different compared to ScH and the control group at baseline, as well as to the ScH groups before and after treatment. The results of our study suggest that the patients with ScH deserve to be followed up during treatment.

REFERENCES

1. UK guidelines for the use of thyroid function tests. 2006. Available from: www.british-thyroid-association.org/TFT_guideline_final_version_July_2006.pdf. Accessed on: Jul 10, 2009.
2. Garber JR, Cobin RH, Gharib H, Hennessey JV, Klein I, Mechanick JI, et al.; American Association of Clinical Endocrinologists and American Thyroid Association Taskforce on Hypothyroidism in Adults. Clinical practice guidelines for hypothyroidism in adults: cosponsored by the American Association of Clinical Endocrinologists and the American Thyroid Association. Endocr Pract. 2012;18(6):988-1028.
3. Cooper DS. Clinical practice. Subclinical hypothyroidism. N Engl J Med. 2001;345(4):260-5.
4. Chu JW, Crapo LM. The treatment of subclinical hypothyroidism is seldom necessary. J Clin Endocrinol Metab. 2001;86(10):4591-9.
5. McDermott MT, Ridgway EC. Subclinical hypothyroidism is mild thyroidfailure and should be treated. J Clin Endocrinol Metab. 2001;86(10):4585-90.

6. Garber JR, Cobin RH, Gharib H, Hennessey JV, Klein I, Mechanick JI, et al.; American Association of Clinical Endocrinologists and American Thyroid Association Taskforce on Hypothyroidism in Adults. Clinical practice guidelines for hypothyroidism in adults: cosponsored by the American Association of Clinical Endocrinologists and the American Thyroid Association. Thyroid. Thyroid. 2012;22:1200-35.
7. Rodondi N, den Elzen WPJ, Bauer DC, Cappola AR, Razvi S, Walsh JP, et al.; Thyroid Studies Collaboration. Subclinical hypothyroidism and the risk of coronary heart disease and mortality. JAMA. 2010;304(12):1365-74.
8. Velkoska Nakova V, Bosevski M, Dimitrovski Ch, Krstevska B. Subclinical hypothyroidism and risk to carotid atherosclerosis. Arq Bras Endocrinol Metab. 2011;55(7):475-80.
9. Kahaly GJ. Cardiovascular and atherogenic aspects of subclinical hypothyroidism. Thyroid. 2000;10(8):665-79.
10. Biondi B, Palmieri EA, Lombardi G, Fazio S. Subclinical hypothyroidism and cardiac function. Thyroid. 2002;12(6):505-10.
11. Aksoy D, Cinar N, Harmanci A, Karakaya A, OkanYildiz B, Usman A, et al. Serum resistin and high sensitive CRP levels in patients with subclinical hypothyroidism before and after L-thyroxine therapy. Med Sci Monit. 2013;19:210-5.
12. Klein I. Thyroid hormone and the cardiovascular system. Am J Med. 1990;88(6):631-7.
13. Biondi B, Fazio S, Palmieri EA, Carella C, Panza N, Cittadini A, et al. Left ventricular diastolic dysfunction in patients with subclinical hypothyroidism. J Clin Endocrinol Metab. 1999;84(6):2064-7.
14. Monzani F, DiBello V, Caraccio N, Bertini A, Giorgi D, Giusti C, et al. Effect of levothyroxine on cardiac function and structure in subclinical hypothyroidism: a double blind, placebo-controlled study. J Clin Endocrinol Metab. 2001;86(3):1110-5.
15. Vitale G, Galderisi M, Lupoli GA, Celentano A, Pietropaolo I, Parenti N, et al. Left ventricular myocardial impairment in subclinical hypothyroidism assessed by a new ultrasound tool: pulsed tissue Doppler. J Clin Endocrinol Metab. 2002;87(9):4350-5.
16. Brenta G, Mutti LA, Schnitman M, Fretes O, Perrone A, Matute ML. Assessment of left ventricular diastolic function by radionuclide ventriculography at rest and exercise in subclinical hypothyroidism, and its response to L-thyroxine therapy. Am J Cardiol. 2003;91(11):1327-30.
17. British Ministry of Health – recommendations. Available from: http://www.bcguidelines.ca/guideline_thyroid.html. Accessed on: Feb. 23, 2012.
18. Lang RM, Badano LP, Mor-Avi V, Afilalo J, Armstrong A, Ernande L, et al. Recommendations for Cardiac Chamber Quantification by Echocardiography in Adults: An Update from the American Society of Echocardiography and the European Association of Cardiovascular Imaging. Eur Heart J Cardiovasc Imaging. 2015;16(3):233-71.
19. Nagueh SF, Appleton CP, Gillebert TC, Marino PN, Oh JK, Smiseth OA, et al. Recommendations for the evaluation of left ventricular diastolic function by echocardiography. Eur J Echocardiogr. 2009;10(2):165-93.
20. Chaha NS, Lim TK, Jain P, Chambers JC, Kooner JS, Senior R. Normative reference values for the tissue Doppler imaging parameters of left ventricular function: a population-based study. Eur J Echocardiogr. 2010;11(1):51-6.
21. Mor-Avi V, Lang RM, Badano LP, Belohlavek M, Cardim NM, Derumeaux G, et al. Current and evolving echocardiographic techniques for the quantitative evaluation of cardiac mechanics: ASE/EAE consensus statement on methodology and indications endorsed by the Japanese Society of Echocardiography. J Am Soc Echocardiogr. 2011;24(3):277-313.
22. Naguch SE, Smiseth OA, Appleton CP, Byrd BF, Dokainish H, Edvardsen T, et al.: Recommendations for the Evaluation of Left Ventricular Diastolic Function by Echocardiography: An Update from the American Society of Echocardiography and the European Association of Cardiovascular Imaging. J Am Soc Echocardiogr. 2016;29(4):277-314.
23. Ye Y, Xie H, Zeng Y, Zhao X, Tian Z, Zhang S. Association between subclinical hypothyroidism and blood pressure--a meta-analysis of observational studies. Endocr Pract. 2014;20(2):150-8.
24. Öner FA, Yurdakul S, Öner E, Arslanta□ MK, Usta M, Ergüney M. Evaluation of ventricular functions using tissue Doppler echocardiography in patients with subclinical hypothyroidism. Turk Kardiyol Dern Ars. 2011;39(2):129-36.
25. Yazici M, Gorgulu S, Sertbas Y, Erbilen E, Albayrak S, Yildiz O, et al. Effects of thyroxin therapy on cardiac function in patients with subclinical hypothyroidism: index of myocardial performance in the evaluation of left ventricular function. Int J Cardiol. 2004;95(2-3):135-43.
26. Franzonia F, Galettaa F, Fallahia P, Tocchini L, Merico G, Braccini L, et al. Effect of L-thyroxine treatment on left ventricular function in subclinical hypothyroidism. Biomed Pharmacother. 2006;60(8):431-6.
27. Oztutk S, Alcelik A, Ozyasar M, Dikbas O, Ayhan S, Ozlu F, at al. Evaluation of left ventricular systolic asynchrony in patients with subclinical hypothyroidism. Cardiol J. 2012;19(4):374-80.
28. Ozturk S, Dikbas O, Baltaci D, Ozyasar M, Erdem A, Eyhan SS, et al. Evaulation of atrial conduction abnormalities and left atrial mechanical functions in patients with subclinical thyroid disorders. Endokrynol Pol. 2012;63(4):286-93.
29. Ilic S, Tadic M, Ivanovic B, Caparevic Z, Trbojevic B, Celic V. Left and right ventricular structure and function in subclinical hypothyroidism: the effects of one-year levothyroxine treatment. Med Sci Monit. 2013 Nov 10;19:960-8.
30. Ho CY, Solomon SD. A clinician's guide to tissue Doppler imaging. Circulation. 2006;113(10):e396-8.
31. Gillam L, Otto CM. Advanced approaches in echocardiography. Rio de Janeiro: Elsevier. 2012.
32. Sunbul M, Durmus E, Kivrak T, Yildiz H, Kanar BG, Ozben B, et al. Left ventricular strain and strain rate by two-dimensional speckle tracking echocardiography in patients with subclinical hypothyroidism. Eur Rev Med Pharmacol Sci. 2013;17(24):3323-8.
33. Erkan G, Erkan AF, Cemri M, Karaahmetoglu S, Cesur M, Cengel A. The evaluation of diastolic dysfunction with tissue Doppler echocardiography in women with subclinical hypothyroidism and the effect of L-thyroxine treatment on diastolic dysfunction: a pilot study. J Thyroid Res. 2011;2011:654304.

Combination therapy of curcumin and alendronate modulates bone turnover markers and enhances bone mineral density in postmenopausal women with osteoporosis

Fatemeh Khanizadeh[1], Asghar Rahmani[2], Khairollah Asadollahi[3], Mohammad Reza Hafezi Ahmadi[4]

[1] Obstetrician/Gynecology, Shahid Beheshti University of Medical Science, Tehran, Iran
[2] Ilam University of Medical Science, Ilam, Iran
[3] Clinical epidemiology, Departament of Social Medicine, Faculty of Medicine, Ilam University of Medical Sciences, Ilam, Iran
[4] Department of Pathology, Ilam University of Medical Science, Ilam, Iran

Correspondence to:
Khairollah Asadollahi,
Departament Social Medicine,
Faculty of Medicine,
Ilam University of Medical Sciences, Ilam, Iran
Masoud_1241@yahoo.co.uk

ABSTRACT

Objective: This study evaluated the effects of combination therapy of curcumin and alendronate on BMD and bone turnover markers in postmenopausal women with osteoporosis. Subjects and methods: In a randomized, double-blind trial study, 60 postmenopausal women were divided into three groups: control, alendronate, and alendronate + curcumin. Each group included 20 patients. Total body, total hip, lumbar spine and femoral neck BMDs were measured by dual-energy X-ray absorptiometry (DXA) at baseline and after 12 months of therapy. Bone turnover markers such as bone-specific alkaline phosphatase (BALP), osteocalcin and C-terminal cross-linking telopeptide of type I collagen (CTx) were measured at the outset and 6 months later. Results: Patients in the control group suffered a significant decrease in BMD and increased bone turnover markers at the end of study. The group treated with only alendronate showed significantly decreased levels of BALP and CTx and increased levels of osteocalcin compared to the control group. The alendronate group also showed significant increases in the total body, total hip, lumbar spine and femoral neck BMDs at the end of study compared to the control group. In the curcumin + alendronate group, BALP and CTx levels decreased and osteocalcin levels increased significantly at the end of study compared to the control and alendronate groups. BMD indexes also increased in four areas significantly at the end of study compared to the control and alendronate groups. Conclusion: The combination of curcumin and alendronate has beneficial effects on BMD and bone turnover markers among postmenopausal women with osteoporosis. Arch Endocrinol Metab. 2018;62(4):438-45

Keywords
Post menopause; osteoporosis; alendronate; curcumin; bone mineral density

INTRODUCTION

One of the main health problems for postmenopausal women is a progressive loss of bone density and, possibly, osteoporosis (1). Studies have shown that half of these patients suffer from osteoporosis and its associated complications, such as bone fractures. Studies have demonstrated that most changes of bone density in postmenopausal women are due to the hormonal changes associated with ovarian function after menopause (2). Despite a growing trend of osteoporosis in postmenopausal women, effective therapeutic and preventive measures have yet to be developed.

Bisphosphonates and hormone replacement therapy (HRT) are two main methods to prevent or treat osteoporotic women's postmenopausal problems. The use of HRT is limited due to its cardiovascular complications, increased risk of breast cancer and vaginal bleeding (3). Long-term bisphosphonates application raises concerns about microdamage accumulation and excessive acceleration of mineralization, osteonecrosis of the jaw and atypical insufficiency fractures in the skeleton system (4). These disadvantages explain why so many studies focus on finding new anti-osteoporotic treatments.

Natural substances can be complementary or alternative means to prevent and treat osteoporosis (5). Curcumin, derived from the turmeric plant (*Curcumin longa* L.), has been shown in laboratory studies to have anti-inflammatory, antioxidant, antifungal and chemopreventive effects (6). Recently, the effects of curcumin on bone remolding and metabolism have been reported in animal studies (7). The anti-osteoporotic effects of curcumin include inhibiting osteoclastogenesis by activating NF-kB ligand (8), inhibiting osteoclasts proliferation, and increasing osteoclasts apoptosis (9). Curcumin's protective effect against the bone deteriorations, induced by glucocorticoids through the activation of microRNA-365 via the suppression of matrix metalloproteinase-9 (MMP-9), has also been reported (10). Studies have also reported that curcumin produces beneficial changes in bone turnover and bone strength (11).

Despite the beneficial effects of curcumin on bone metabolism, the anti-osteoporotic effects of curcumin have not been studied comprehensively in postmenopausal women with osteoporosis. An experimental study reported that the combination of alendronate and curcumin had beneficial effects on bone remodeling and bone mechanical strength in ovariectomized rats (12). Another study showed significant changes in bone turnover and bone strength in a rat model of postmenopausal osteoporosis reported for curcumin (13). Randomized clinical trial (RCT) study reported that treatment of postmenopausal women with alendronate suppressed bone turnover and increased the BMD (14,15). Also, alendronate can reduce the incidence of vertebral fractures in these patients (16). The safety and efficacy have been reported in long term (10-year) treatment with alendronate in RCTs (17). Despite the inhibitory effects of curcumin on the osteoporotic process in various conditions, the effects of curcumin have not been investigated in the treatment or prevention of osteoporosis in postmenopausal women. The current study investigated the combined effects of curcumin and alendronate on bone turnover markers and bone densitometric features related to osteoporosis in postmenopausal women.

SUBJECTS AND METHODS

Patient selection and study design

This randomized, double-blind clinical trial study was conducted in an outpatient clinic, specialized in osteoporosis treatment. The study's participants were among healthy postmenopausal women, 55 to 65 years of age, who had at least 5 years since their last menstrual period. In the present study osteoporosis was diagnosed by bone mineral densitometry that was defined by both WHO and applied protocol by previous studies (18). Bone density which was 2.5 SD or more below the young normal mean (T score <-2.5) was classified as showing osteoporosis, while a BMD T score between –1 and –2.5 was classified as showing osteopenia. The WHO definition is applied to postmenopausal women using DXA measurement at the spine, hip or forearm. The aims and scope of the study were orally explained to all subjects, and written informed consent was obtained from all participants. The study was confirmed by the ethics committee of Ilam University of Medical Sciences according to the ethical issues of clinical trials (code no: Ir.medilam.rec.1394.184). The study was registered with the Iranian registry of clinical trials (code no: IRCT2016030424308N1) and the study duration was 12 months. All subjects were identified as new cases of osteoporosis and had not yet received any associated treatment. Exclusion criteria in the current study were as follows: history of bone metabolic diseases; application of drugs affecting bone and metabolism such as bisphosphonates, calcium, and vitamin D, current or past vitamin D deficiency; hormonal problems and HRT; coagulopathy and thromboembolic diseases; cardiovascular and cereberovascular diseases; history of drug abuse, smoking or alcohol use and any unwanted reaction or drug side effect during study. Those who could not continue until the end of study were also excluded. Sixty qualified patients were randomly divided into 3 equal groups of control, alendronate, and alendronate + curcumin (the eligible patients entered into the 3 mentioned groups one by one respectively). The alendronate was administered by 5 mg/day dose, determined from a previously study (15), and the curcumin was administered by 110 mg/day dose (11); both were given for 12 months. All subjects also received calcium supplements (1,000–1,500 mg/day) of calcium carbonate. The control group only received calcium supplements as described above. The drugs dosages applied in this study were the same as used by previous studies in which the effectiveness and safety of the drugs were confirmed. Patients were advised to report any unwanted reaction or drug side effects promptly and in case of need refer to our clinic or emergency department. One of the excluding criteria for participants was any unwanted reaction or drug side effect during drug application. All participants completed the study period without dropping out.

BMD measurement

BMDs of the lumbar spine (L1–L4), femoral neck, total hip and total body were determined by dual-energy X-ray absorptiometry (DXA) at the beginning of the study and after 6 months using equipment manufactured by a single supplier (Hologic, Waltham, MA). The raw BMD data from all subjects were pooled for analyses. The study defined osteoporosis according to World Health Organization (WHO) criteria (19).

Bone turnover markers assay

To evaluate the biomarkers, fasting blood samples were obtained from all subjects at the beginning and end of study. The obtained blood samples were centrifuged (1,000 rpm for 10 min) and stored –at -70°C to measure the biomarkers. All assessments were performed in a central laboratory. For the bone formation assay, this study measured the level of BALP (Hybritech, San Diego, CA) and osteocalcin (CIS Biointernational, France) using the radioimmunoassay systems method (18). For the bone resorption marker, this study analyzed the level of urine C-terminal cross-linking telopeptide of type I collagen (Crosslaps, Osteometer A/S and Copenhagen, Denmark) (18).

Statistical analysis

The quantitative and qualitative data are presented as the mean ± standard deviation (SD) and frequency, respectively. T test, Chi-square and ANOVA were applied for comparison of the results appropriately. Statistical analysis of data was performed by SPSS 19 (SPSS Inc, Chicago, USA) software. A p value < 0.05 was considered significant.

RESULTS

Patients' data

The mean ± SD years of postmenopausal state in patients treated with alendronate (10.40 ± 1.50 years) and alendronate + curcumin (9.85 ± 1.89 years) did not statistically differ from the control group (10.45 ± 1.90 years, p = 0.669). The mean ± SD of estradiol levels among alendronate (23.64 ± 10.61) and alendronate + curcumin (26.53 ± 9.11) groups also did not show any significant difference to the control group (25.63 ± 9.54, p = 0.531). The mean ± SD of the follicle stimulating hormone (FSH) levels were not significantly different between groups (p = 0.874). The levels of markers related to bone metabolism and osteoporosis (such as calcium, ALP and phosphorus) also did not differ significantly among the three groups (p = 0.459, p = 0.621 and p = 0.341) (Table 1).

Effect of alendronate and curcumin on bone turnover markers

The mean ± SD of bone turnover markers among differennt groups is shown by Figure 1. Figure 1A shows that by the end of study, the BALP of patients in the control group (13.96 ± 1.1 µg/L, 95% CI: 12.03-15.1) slightly increased compared to the baseline (13.29 ± 1.5 µg/L, 95% CI: 12.65-14.3) (p = 0.432). However, in both groups of alendronate alone and in combination with curcumin, the BALP level at the end of study decreased compared to the beginning (11.04 ± 0.9 µg/L, 95% CI: 9.02-13.1 vs. 13.54 ± 1.6 µg/L, 95% CI: 11.6-15.1, p = 0.023 and 13.16 ± 1.3 µg/L, 95%CI: 10.05-14.6, vs. 10.2 ± 1.2 µg/L, 95%CI: 9.02-12.4, p = 0.012 respectively). The BALP level of the alendronate group was also significantly lower than the BALP level of the control group by the end of study (p = 0.030). Also, the BALP level at the end of study in the alendronate + curcumin group differed significantly from the alendronate only and control groups at the end of study (p = 0.020, p = 0.035, respectively).

Table 1. Basic information of participants

Variables	Control	Alendronate	Alendronate+Cur	P value
Age (year)	58.55 ± 12.45	60.50 ± 11.95	58.00 ± 10.78	0.772
BMI (kg/m^2)	24.95 ± 3.14	24.55 ± 3.60	24.50 ± 5.70	0.840
Postmenopausal duration (year)	10.45 ± 1.90	10.40 ± 1.50	9.85 ± 1.89	0.669
Estradiol (pg/mL)	25.63 ± 9.54	23.64 ± 10.61	26.53 ± 9.11	0.531
FSH (mIU/mL)	87.43 ± 16.43	79.13 ± 21.43	83.54 ± 18.43	0.874
ALP (IU/L)	126.32 ± 42	129.43 ± 37	122.24 ± 27	0.621
Calcium (mg/dL)	9.32 ± 0.34	9.04 ± 0.51	9.21 ± 0.63	0.459
Phosphorus (mg/dL)	4.3 ± 1.3	4.76 ± 0.76	4.7 ± 0.61	0.341
Total number	20	20	20	

BMI: body mass index; FSH: follicle-stimulating hormone.

Figure 1B shows the osteocalcin results for the three groups. The mean ± SD of osteocalcin increased at the end of study compared with the baseline in the control group, although this increase was not statistically significant (19.37 ± 1.7 μg/L, 95%CI: 19.07-20.05 vs. 18.95 ± 1.3 μg/L, 95%CI: 18.87-20.01, $p = 0.432$). In the alendronate group, the level of osteocalcin at the end of study decreased compared to the baseline (19.45 ± 1.2 μg/L, 95%CI: 19.02-21.3 vs. 19.75 ± 1.4 μg/L, 95%CI: 19.12-21.6, $p = 0.620$). Similarly, the mean ± SD of osteocalcin in the alendronate + curcumin group level at the end of study decreased compared to baseline. This decrease was not statistically significant (19.02 ± 1.1 μg/L, 95%CI: 17.06-22.14 vs. 20.3 ± 1.3 μg/L, 95%CI: 18.4-23.1, $p = 0.231$).

CTx changes are shown in Figure 1C. At the end of study, the levels of CTx marker in the control group significantly increased compared to the baseline (0.326 ± 0.027 μg/L, 95%CI: 0.12-0.48 vs. 0.317 ± 0.033 μg/L, 95%CI: 0.22-0.53, $p = 0.020$). Unlike the control group, the CTx levels in the alendronate group, at the end of study showed a significant reduction compared to the baseline (0.318 ± 0.012 μg/L, 95%CI: 0.19-0.44 vs. 0.323 ± 0.011 μg/L, 95%CI: 0.25-0.46, $p = 0.043$). Levels of CTx in alendronate + curcumin group showed a significant reduction at the end of study compared to the baseline (0.301 ± 0.017 μg/L, 95%CI: 0.27-0.42 vs. 0.318 ± 0.033 μg/L, 95%CI: 0.23-0.35, $p = 0.013$). The mean serum level of CTx in the alendronate + curcumin group was also significantly

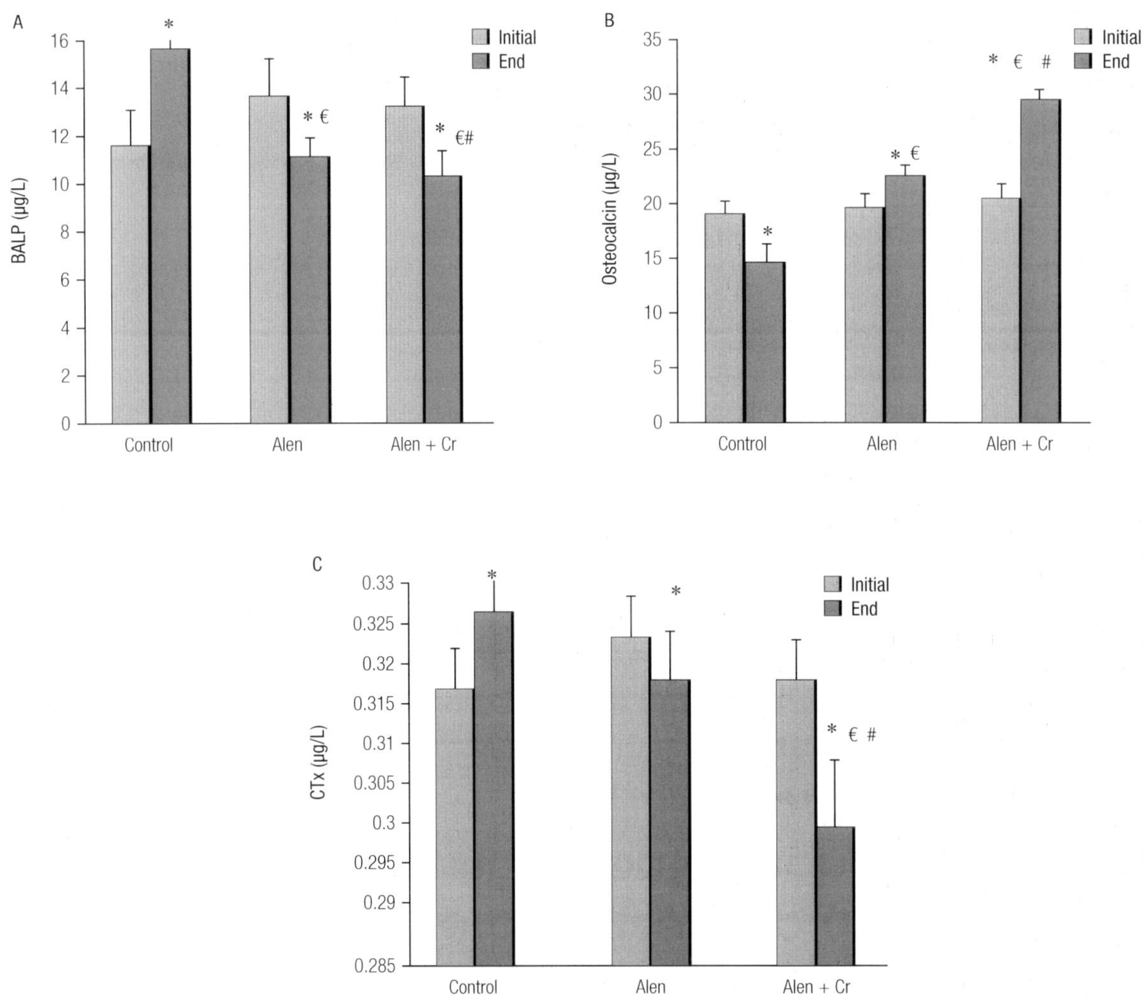

Figure 1. Effect of different drug groups on bone turnover markers in postmenopausal women with osteoporosis.

* = p < 0.05: end level compared with initial of study in control group. € = p < 0.05: end level compared with initial of study in alendronate. # = p < 0.05: end level compared with end of study in alendronate + curcumin group.

BALP: bone-specific alkaline phosphatase, CTx: C-terminal cross-linking telopeptide of type I collagen.

less than its level in the alendronate alone and control groups ($p = 0.020$, $p = 0.037$, respectively).

Effect of alendronate and curcumin on bone densitometry

Densitometric changes of the total hip BMD are shown by Figure 2A. The mean ± SD of BMD decreased significantly at the end of study compared to the baseline (0.796 ± 0.003, 95%CI: 0.74-0.82 vs. 0.807 ± 0.007, 95%CI: 0.78-0.83, $p = 0.031$). In the alendronate alone and alendronate + curcumin groups, the mean ± SD of BMD showed a significant increase at the end of study compared to the baseline (0.817 ± 0.007, 95%CI: 0.77-0.84 vs. 0.806 ± 0.009, 95%CI: 0.76-0.83, $p = 0.001$ and 0.829 ± 0.002, 95%CI: 0.76-0.84 vs. 0.812 ± 0.006, 95%CI: 0.75-0.83, $p = 0.01$, respectively). Changes in the total hip BMD (Figure 2B) in the alendronate alone and alendronate + curcumin groups significantly increased compared to the control group at the end of study ($p = 0.035$, $p = 0.046$, respectively). The total hip BMD level in the alendronate + curcumin group showed a significant increase compared to the BMD level in the alendronate group ($p = 0.044$).

Changes in the femoral neck BMD (Figure 2C) were almost similar to the total hip BMD results; the mean ± SD of the BMD in the control group was significantly lower at the end of study than the baseline (0.712 ± 0.002, 95%CI: 0.69-0.74 vs. 0.718 ± 0.008, 95%CI: 0.70-0.73, $p = 0.024$). In the alendronate group, the mean ± SD of the femoral neck BMD at the end of study also increased compared to the baseline (0.720 ± 0.002, 95%CI: 0.66-0.78 vs. 0.718 ± 0.003, 95%CI: 0.67-0.79, $p = 0.56$). The alendronate + curcumin group also showed increased levels in the femoral neck BMD at the end of study compared to the baseline (0.718 ± 0.001, 95%CI: 0.67-0.78 vs. 0.715 ± 0.002, 95%CI: 0.63-0.75, $p = 0.063$). Changes in the BMD in both alendronate and alendronate + curcumin groups compared to the control group were statistically significant ($p = 0.025$, $p = 0.030$, respectively).

Changes in the total body BMD are shown in Figure 2D. Like the other variables, the mean ± SD values of BMD in the control group decreased significantly at the end of study compared to the baseline (0.985 ± 0.006,

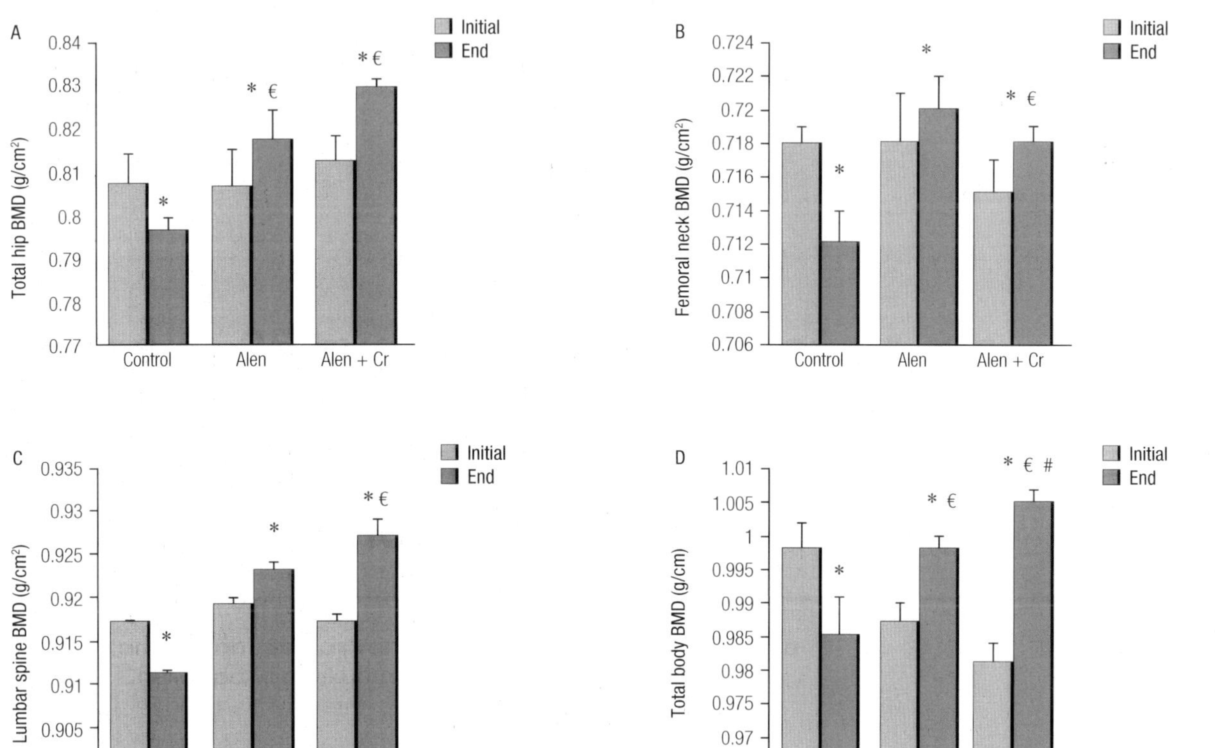

Figure 2. Effect of different drug groups on bone mineral density (BMD) in postmenopausal women with osteoporosis.

* = $p < 0.05$: end level compared with initial of study in control group. € = $p < 0.05$: end level compared with initial of study in alendronate. # = $p < 0.05$: end level compared with end of study in alendronate + curcumin group.

95%CI: 0.91-1.2 vs. 0.998 ± 0.004, 95%CI: 0.95-1.3, $p = 0.024$). The mean ± SD values of total body BMD among alendronate and alendronate + curcumin groups increased significantly at the end of study compared to the baseline (0.998 ± 0.002, 95%CI: 0.97-1.34 vs. 0.987 ± 0.003, 95%CI: 0.94-1.42, $p = 0.022$ and 1.005 ± 0.002, 95%CI: 0.98-1.45 vs. 0.981 ± 0.003, 95%CI: 0.93-1.33, $p = 0.020$). The mean ± SD values of BMD in the alendronate and alendronate + curcumin groups also significantly increased compared to the control group ($p = 0.034$ and $p = 0.014$, respectively).

DISCUSSION

Postmenopausal women are commonly at risk of a progressive loss of bone density and, possibly, osteoporosis. The aim of this study was to evaluate the combined effects of curcumin and alendronate on BMD and bone turnover markers in postmenopausal women with osteoporosis. Studies have shown that aging is associated with reduced BMD and bone tissue microarchitecture destruction and that these changes increase bone fragility (20). These destructive and progressive changes occur more rapidly in postmenopausal women. Postmenopausal women, due to hormonal deficiencies, fail to achieve peak bone mass or bone mass is more readily destroyed (21). The results of this study showed that markers related to bone turnover (such as BALP and CTx) increased significantly among postmenopausal women in the control group at the end of study compared to other groups, while osteocalcin decreased in this group. Similarly, the densitometric results showed that BMD indices in postmenopausal women at the end of study significantly decreased compared to other groups. The mechanism driving these changes indicated various factors and showed that estrogen deficiency in postmenopausal women leads to decreased BMD through the thinning of bone trabeculae. Thus, when estrogen decreased, differentiation and proliferation of osteoclasts dramatically increased (22). According to this mechanism, one means of preventing osteoporosis in postmenopausal women is HRT and in this field, bisphosphonates are the most important and well-known drugs. This study's results showed that alendronate effectively reduced the levels of BALP and CTx and increased osteocalcin by the end of study. When compared to the values at the study's onset, these changes were significantly different for the BALP and osteocalcin markers but were not significantly different for the CTx. The results showed that the mean level of BALP and CTx in the alendronate group decreased significantly after one year. The osteocalcin levels in the alendronate group also increased significantly compared to the control group. These results mean that alendronate could effectively decrease bone turnover markers in postmenopausal women. A densitometric study also showed that the alendronate group exhibited a significantly increase in total body, waist, hip and lumbar spine BMDs at the end of study compared to the onset. This outcome revealed that alendronate is beneficial to preventing the development of osteoporosis in postmenopausal women. Previous clinical and laboratory studies support this study's finding. For example, a study by Iwamoto et al demonstrated that treating women, with and without type 2 diabetes, with alendronate reduced the level of alkaline phosphatase (ALP) and increased lumbar spine BMD compared to control group (23). That study also examined the possible side effects of alendronate and did not observe any instances of complications such as atrial fibrillation, atypical diaphyseal femoral fracture or jaw osteonecrosis. Another study by Iwamoto showed that alendronate significantly decreased the average levels of ALP and NTX and increased lumbar spine BMD in postmenopausal women after one year. That study also showed that alendronate reduced the incidence of vertebral and non-vertebral fractures (24). Correspondingly, the present study's results showed that treatment with alendronate for one year reduced bone turnover markers and increased the BMD values of the total body, waist, hip, and lumbar spine. Experimental investigations have reported evidences supporting the assertion that alendronate inhibits osteoporosis. Lindtner and cols. examined the osteoanabolic effects of alendronate and zoledronate on the process of human bone marrow stromal cells (hBMSCs) osteogenesis in women with osteoporosis and that these compounds could increase the differentiation of hBMSC classes. That study also reported that these compounds could reduce the osteopontin marker levels in hBMSCs lines (25). While most studies on the effects of alendronate on osteoporosis in postmenopausal women utilized monotherapy, Hejdova and cols. examined the beneficial effects of combining alendronate and calcitonin on BMD in postmenopausal women (26). Although several studies have reported alendronate's antiresorptive properties and it has been used as a first-line treatment for osteoporosis, possible side effects have raised concerns about the benefits and harms of bisphosphonates. In fact, studies have shown that long-term use of BPs was associated with an increased risk of stroke and deep vein thrombosis (DVT); this effect is probably caused by an estrogen-induced effect due to release of clotting factors (27-29). As for these concerns the current study aimed to combine alendronate with curcumin, which has reportedly shown beneficial effects on osteoporosis in clinical and *in vitro* investigations and can inhibit alendronate's side effects through its antioxidant properties (30). For example, studies have shown that curcumin can inhibit the activity of the tissue factor involved in thrombotic disorders and decrease platelet activity or inhibit platelet aggregation (31). In addition to curcumin's advantage in reducing the side effects of BPs, several studies have reported curcumin's beneficial effects in preventing osteoporosis in experimental and clinical models (32). The present study's results clearly showed the efficacy of curcumin in combination with alendronate on bone turnover markers and densitometric indices. The results showed that curcumin in combination with alendronate significantly decreased BALP and sCTx markers at the end of study compared to the control group. The present study also found that curcumin in combination with alendronate significantly increased BMD compared to the alendronate and control groups alone. This study's results are the first to report the beneficial effects of a therapy combining curcumin with a BP in postmenopausal women with osteoporosis. To date, no study had been conducted with this type of combination therapy. Most studies had been carried out as monotherapy and administered curcumin or alendronate separately. Similar results were observed in Cho and cols.'s study, which showed that eight weeks application of high doses of curcumin decreased the ALP, telopeptide-C, and osteocalcin markers in ovariectomized rats compared to the control group. That study also showed that curcumin could reveal a dose-dependent increase in BMD compared with the control group (33). Another study by Cho and cols. showed that curcumin in combination with alendronate reduced the bone turnover markers (ALP and CTX) compared with a control group in ovariectomized rats. In another study by Kim and cols, models of ovariectomized rats demonstrated that curcumin inhibited osteoclastogenesis by increasing the activity of a receptor-mediated of NF-kB (34). While previous clinical trial studies have reported some beneficial effects of curcumin on other musculoskeletal problems such as osteoarthritis, cartilage disease (Cartilaginous), and sarcoma pathology of skeletal muscle (35), our study is the first to report the effects of a combination therapy on osteoporosis among postmenopausal women. The exact mechanisms through which curcumin significantly inhibits osteoporosis have not been determined, but evidences suggest that curcumin inhibits the process of osteoporosis by a series of multi-stage activities. The stages of this process include inhibiting NF-kB and RANKL signaling, inhibiting the production of nitric oxide and reactive oxygen species (ROS) and synthesizing inflammatory cytokines. Curcumin also may inhibit the differentiation and proliferation of osteoclasts (5). This study revealed that both curcumin and alendronate improved the densitometric status and bone remodeling markers of postmenopausal women; however, these findings were significantly higher among those who received curcumin and alendronate as combined compared to the groups receiving these medications lonely. This result indicated that combined application of curcumin and alendronate may be a useful option for prevention and treatment of osteoporosis among postmenopausal women. This study had some limitations such as: groups treated with curcumin alone and the effects of curcumin were not revealed because of limited screening and patient numbers as well as patients' incompatibility. The study also did not examine the fracture risk of women in the study and only examined bone turnover markers and BMD. It is hoped that these points will be examined in future clinical trial studies.

Authors' contributions: Khanizadeh F and Hafezi Ahmadi MR participated in data collection, data analysis, and interpretation of the results and drafted the manuscript. Asadollahi K and Rahmani A participated in manuscript preparation and critical review. All authors have read and approved the article for publication.

Acknowledgements: we thank our colleagues in the Faculty of Medicine, Ilam University of Medical Sciences, participants, coordinators and data reviewers who assisted in this study.

Funding/Support: Ilam University of Medical Sciences, Ilam, Iran, supported this study.

REFERENCES

1. Chesnut CH, Silverman S, Andriano K, Genant H, Gimona A, Harris S, et al. A randomized trial of nasal spray salmon calcitonin in postmenopausal women with established osteoporosis: the prevent recurrence of osteoporotic fractures study. PROOF Study Group. Am J Med. 2000;109(4):267-76.
2. Briot K, Cortet B, Thomas T, Audran M, Blain H, Breuil V, et al. 2012 update of French guidelines for the pharmacological treatment of postmenopausal osteoporosis. Joint Bone Spine. 2012;79(3):304-13.
3. Writing Group for the Women's Health Initiative Investigators. Risks and benefits of estrogen plus progestin in healthy postmenopausal women: principal results from the Women's Health Initiative randomized controlled trial. JAMA. 2002;288(3):321-33.
4. Whyte MP, Wenkert D, Clements KL, McAlister WH, Mumm S. Bisphosp honate-induced osteoporosis. N Engl J Med. 2003;31:349(5):457-63.
5. Yang MW, Wang TH, Yan PP, Chu LW, Yu J, Gao ZD, et al. Curcumin improves bone microarchitecture and enhances mineral density in APP/PS1 transgenic mice. Phytomedicine. 2011;18(2-3):205-13.
6. Joe B, Vijaykumar M, Lokesh BR. Biological properties of curcumin-cellular and molecular mechanisms of action. Crit Rev Food Sci Nutr. 2004;44(2):97-111.
7. Ozaki K, Kawata Y, Amano S, Hanazawa S. Stimulatory effect of curcumin on osteoclast apoptosis. Biochem Pharmacol. 2000;59(12):1577-81.
8. Bharti AC, Takada Y, Aggarwal BB. Curcumin (diferuloylmethane) inhibits receptor activator of NF-kappa B ligand-induced NF-kappa B activation in osteoclast precursors and suppresses osteoclastogenesis. J Immunol. 2004;172(10):5940-7.
9. Bell NH. RANK ligand an d the regulation of skeletal remodeling. J Clin Invest. 2003;111(8):1120-2.
10. Li G, Bu J, Zhu Y, Xiao X, Liang Z, Zhang R. Curcumin improves bone microarchitecture in glucocorticoid-induced secondary osteoporosis mice through the activation of microRNA-365 via regulating MMP-9. Int J Clin Exp Pathol. 2015;8(12):15684-95.
11. Taty Anna K, Elvy Suhana MR, Das S, Faizah O, Hamzaini AH. Anti-inflammatory effect of Curcuma longa (turmeric) on collagen-induced arthritis: an anatomico-radiological study. Clin Ter. 2011;162(3):201-7.
12. Cho DC, Kim KT, Jeon Y, Sung JK. A synergistic bone sparing effect of curcumin and alendronate in ovariectomized rat. Acta Neurochir (Wien). 2012;154(12):2215-23.
13. French DL, Muir JM, Webber CE. The ovariectomized, mature rat model of postmenopausal osteoporosis: an assessment of the bone sparing effects of curcumin. Phytomedicine. 2008;15(12):1069-78.
14. Kushida K, Shiraki M, Nakamura T, Kishimoto H, Morii H, Yamamoto K, et al. The efficacy of alendronate in reducing the risk of vertebral fracture in Japanese patients with osteoporosis: a randomized, double-blind, active-controlled double-dummy trial. Curr Ther Res Clin Exp. 2002;63(9):606-20.
15. Iwamoto J, Sato Y, Uzawa M, Takeda T, Matsumoto H. Seven years' experience with alendronate in postmenopausal Japanese women with osteoporosis. Ther Clin Risk Manag. 2010;6:201-6.
16. Lo JC, O'Ryan FS, Gordon NP, Yang J, Hui RL, Martin D, et al.; Predicting Risk of Osteonecrosis of the Jaw with Oral Bisphosphonate Exposure (PROBE) Investigators. Prevalence of osteonecrosis of the jaw in patients with oral bisphosphonate exposure. J Oral Maxillofac Surg. 2010;68(2):243-53.
17. Bone HG, Hosking D, Devogelaer JP, Tucci JR, Emkey RD, Tonino RP, et al.; Alendronate Phase III Osteoporosis Treatment Study Group. Ten years' experience with alendronate for osteoporosis in postmenopausal women. N Engl J Med. 2004;350(12):1189-99.
18. Weinstein RS, Parfitt AM, Marcus R, Greenwald M, Crans G, Muchmore DB. Effects of raloxifene, hormone replacement therapy, and placebo on bone turnover in postmenopausal women. Osteoporos Int. 2003;14(10):814-22.
19. Gifre L, Vidal J, Carrasco JL, Muxi A, Portell E, Monegal A, et al. Risk factors for the development of osteoporosis after spinal cord injury. A 12-month follow-up study. Osteoporos Int. 2015;26(9):2273-80.
20. Canpolat S, Tug N, Seyran AD, Kumru S, Yilmaz B. Effects of raloxifene and estradiol on bone turnover parameters in intact and ovariectomized rats. J Physiol Biochem. 2010;66(1):23-8.
21. Riggs BL, Khosla S, Melton LJ. 3rd Sex steroids and the construction and conservation of the adult skeleton. Endocr Rev. 2002;23(3):279-302.
22. Parhami F. Possible role of oxidized lipids in osteoporosis: could hyperlipidemia be a risk factor? Prostaglandins Leukot Essent Fatty Acids. 2003;68(6):373-8.
23. Iwamoto J, Takeda T, Sato Y, Uzawa M. Comparison of the effect of alendronate on lumbar bone mineral density and bone turnover in men and postmenopausal women with osteoporosis. Clin Rheumatol. 2007;26(2):161-7.
24. Iwamoto J, Sato Y, Uzawa M, Takeda T, Matsumoto H. Three-year experience with alendronate treatment in postmenopausal osteoporotic Japanese women with or without type 2 diabetes. Diabetes Res Clin Pract. 2011;93(2):166-73.
25. Lindtner RA, Tiaden AN, Genelin K, Ebner HL, Manzl C, Klawitter M, et al. Osteoanabolic effect of alendronate and zoledronate on bone marrow stromal cells (BMSCs) isolated from aged female osteoporotic patients and its implications for their mode of action in the treatment of age-related bone loss. Osteoporos Int. 2014;25(3):1151-61.
26. Hejdova M, Palicka V, Kucera Z, Vlcek J. Effects of alendronate and calcitonin on bone mineral density in postmenopausal osteoporotic women. An observational study. Pharm World Sci. 2005;27(3):149-53.
27. Shiraishi A, Miyabe S, Nakano T, Umakoshi Y, Ito M, Mihara M. The combination therapy with alfacalcidol and risedronate improves the mechanical property in lumbar spine by affecting the material properties in an ovariectomized rat model of osteoporosis. BMC Musculoskelet Disord. 2009;10:66.
28. Yang KY, Lin LC, Tseng TY, Wang SC, Tsai TH. Oral bioavailability of curcumin in rat and the herbal analysis from Curcuma longa by LC-MS/MS. J Chromatogr B Analyt Technol Biomed Life Sci. 2007;853(1-2):183-9.
29. Carroll CE, Benakanakere I, Besch-Williford C, Ellersieck MR, Hyder SM. Curcumin delays development of medroxyprogesterone acetate-accelerated 7,12-dimethylbenz[a]anthracene-induced mammary tumors. Menopause. 2010;17(1):178-84.
30. Hussan F, Ibraheem NG, Kamarudin TA, Shuid AN, Soelaiman IN, Othman F. Curcumin Protects against Ovariectomy-Induced Bone Changes in Rat Model. Evid Based Complement Alternat Med. 2012;2012:174916.
31. Pan CJ, Tang JJ, Shao ZY, Wang J, Huang N. Improved blood compatibility of rapamycin-eluting stent by incorporating curcumin. Colloids Surf B Biointerfaces. 2007;59(1):105-11.
32. Mawani Y, Orvig C. Improved separation of the curcuminoids, syntheses of their rare earth complexes, and studies of potential antiosteoporotic activity. J Inorg Biochem. 2014;132:52-8.
33. Cho DC, Jung HS, Kim KT, Jeon Y, Sung JK, Hwang JH. Therapeutic advantages of treatment of high-dose curcumin in the ovariectomized rat. J Korean Neurosurg Soc. 2013;54(6):461-6.
34. Kim WK, Ke K, Sul OJ, Kim HJ, Kim SH, Lee MH, et al. Curcumin protects against ovariectomy-induced bone loss and decreases osteoclastogenesis. J Cell Biochem. 2011;112(11):3159-66.
35. Peddada KV, Peddada KV, Shukla SK, Mishra A, Verma V. Role of Curcumin in Common Musculoskeletal Disorders: a Review of Current Laboratory, Translational, and Clinical Data. Orthop Surg. 2015;7(3):222-31.

Low serum 25-hydroxy vitamin D levels are associated with aggressive breast cancer variants and poor prognostic factors in patients with breast carcinoma

Arunkumar Karthikayan[1], Sathasivam Sureshkumar[1], Dharanipragada Kadambari[1], Chellappa Vijayakumar[1]

[1] Department of Surgery, Jawaharlal Institute of Postgraduate Medical Education and Research (JIPMER), Pondicherry, India

Correspondence to:
Sathasivam Sureshkumar
Jawaharlal Institute of Postgraduate Medical Education and Research
605006 – Pondicherry, India
drsureshkumar08@yahoo.com

Dharanipragada Kadambari
Jawaharlal Institute of Postgraduate Medical Education and Research
605006 – Pondicherry, India
kadambari1901@gmail.com

ABSTRACT

Objective: This study was conducted to assess the serum 25-hydroxy (OH) vitamin D levels in patients with breast cancer compared to healthy controls and to identify its association with aggressive breast cancer phenotypes. Materials and methods: Serum 25-OH vitamin D levels of 78 breast cancer patients and 78 matched healthy controls were estimated using ELISA. The cases and controls were matched with respect to age, menopausal status, parity, weight, height and co-morbidities. Prognostic factors like grade of tumour, hormone receptor status, *HER2 neu* status and lymphovascular invasion were compared with 25-OH vitamin D levels. Results: The mean serum 25-OH vitamin D levels of cases were significantly lower compared to the controls (22.33 ± 8.19 vs. 37.41 ± 12.9 ng/mL; $p = 0.0001$). Patients with higher grades of tumour, non-luminal types of breast cancer and breast cancers with estrogen receptor negativity had significantly lower serum 25-OH vitamin D levels than their opposing groups. Patients with excellent and good Nottingham's prognostic Index (NPI) had significantly higher serum 25-OH vitamin D levels than the moderate and poor NPI groups. Conclusion: Newly diagnosed breast cancer patients have significantly lower serum 25-OH vitamin D levels than healthy controls. Lower level of serum 25-OH vitamin D correlates with aggressive breast cancer phenotypes. Arch Endocrinol Metab. 2018;62(4):452-9

Keywords

25-hydroxy vitamin D; carcinoma breast; prognostic factors; vitamin D metabolism; cancer prophylaxis

INTRODUCTION

Breast cancer is the commonest malignancy among women worldwide (1). Vitamin D has a wide range of immunogenic and anti-proliferative action throughout the body, in addition to its well-known endocrine actions. Vitamin D deficiency has been correlated with increased incidence of malignancies of breast, prostate, and colon (2). Suboptimal vitamin D levels are hypothesized to lead to unhindered cellular proliferation, angiogenesis, and metastasis (3). Suboptimal vitamin D levels in women diagnosed with breast cancer have been shown to correlate with poor overall survival and decreased distant disease free survival (4).

Though Western literature shows a correlative relationship between vitamin D status and increased incidence of breast cancer, its impact in the Indian population is of questionable value because India is a tropical country with abundant sunshine throughout the year. This study might form part of the missing links in the vitamin D and breast cancer scenario in India. The Indian and white European populations vary significantly in their characteristics, and a positive correlation in this study as in its Western counterparts might pave the way for larger observational studies defining the level of vitamin D deficiency in Asian Indians (5). If large-scale studies show a significant correlation, it might pave the way for better understanding in the management of breast cancer.

MATERIALS AND METHODS

Study design

This study was a hospital-based case control study conducted over a period of 2 years. All the newly diagnosed breast cancer patients presenting to a tertiary care center in South India were included in the study. The study was evaluated by the institute's ethics committee and a formal clearance was obtained (JIP/IEC/2012/26/324). The nature, methodology, and risks involved in the study were explained to the patients and informed consent was obtained. All the information collected was kept confidential and patients were given full freedom to withdraw at any point during the study. All provisions of the Declaration of Helsinki were followed in this study.

Cases and controls

Newly diagnosed breast cancer patients not on any vitamin D supplementation for the past 6 months were included in the study. Patients who were diagnosed elsewhere or partially treated at outside hospitals and who had taken vitamin D supplementation in the previous 6 months were excluded from the study. Details regarding demographic parameters, parity, menopausal status, co-morbidities, family history of breast cancer, clinical features, height, weight, examination findings pertaining to breast carcinoma, and baseline laboratory parameters were collected.

The controls were selected from apparently healthy women volunteers accompanying the patients attending this institute after due informed written consent. The cases and controls were matched with respect to age, menopausal status, parity, weight, height, co-morbidities and renal function test, so that the confounding factors affecting the serum 25-OH vitamin D levels are avoided.

All the participants included were the residents of Tamil Nadu and Pondicherry states in South India with latitude of 11.1271° N- 11.9139° N, 78.6569° E- 79.8145° E. The climate in this part of country is classified as tropical wet and dry (megathermal) by the Köppen-Geiger system where the population gets sun exposure in most parts of the year. Additionally, the clothing habit of women in this part of the country enables them to get adequate sun exposure.

Serum 25-OH vitamin D level estimation

The serum 25-OH vitamin D levels were estimated with DIA Source immunoassay KAP 1971 25-OH vitamin D Total ELISA Kits. The assay was calibrated to the ID-LC/MS-MS reference method. 25-OH vitamin D level ≥ 30 ng/mL was considered sufficiency. Ten to < 30 ng/mL was taken as 25-OH vitamin D insufficiency and 0 to < 10 ng/mL as deficiency. The above cut-off values were selected based on the recommendation of Endocrine Society practice guidelines (6).

Outcome parameters studied

The bold sample for serum 25-OH vitamin D level estimation was taken at the time of diagnosis confirmation by core needle biopsy. The blood sample was collected from the healthy female volunteers after matching at the outpatient department. The demographic characteristics were recorded including age, BMI, height, weight, and Hb. Status of menopause was recorded in both the groups. Details of all the breast cancer patients were discussed in the tumor board for making informed decisions regarding the treatment plans. The breast cancer patients' biopsy reports were followed up after surgery. Details like grade of the tumor, hormone receptor status, *HER2 neu* status, lymphovascular invasion, and Nottingham's prognostic index (NPI) were collected and studied to compare the level of vitamin D and its association with the above parameters.

Statistical analyses

The distribution of data on 25-OH vitamin D levels will be assessed by using the Kolmogorov-Smirnov test and accordingly expressed as the mean with standard deviation. Data were analyzed using SPSS software version 17. The 25-OH vitamin D levels between the two groups were compared by using chi-square test, and the mean 25-OH vitamin D level was compared using Student's t-test. Association between serum 25-OH vitamin D levels and various breast cancer prognostic parameters such as tumor stage, grade, histological type receptor status, etc., was analyzed using ANOVA and Student's t-test. A p value of < 0.05 was considered as statistically significant.

RESULTS

All the newly diagnosed patients attending the breast cancer clinic were screened for inclusion in the study. Seventy-eight cases over a period of 2 years were included after satisfying the inclusion/exclusion criteria. Seventy-eight controls were studied after necessary matching as mentioned in the cases and control definition.

Demographic parameters like age, height, and weight in both control and breast cancer groups were comparable. The BMI was the same in both groups and fell within the normal range for all of the subjects and controls (Table 1).

Table 1. Comparison of baseline characteristics between cases and controls

Parameters	Controls (n = 78) (Mean ± SD)	Cases (n = 78) (Mean ± SD)	*p* value (Student *t* test)
Age (years)	45.8 ± 10.1	47.1 ± 10.7	0.439
BMI (kg/m²)	22 ± 2.3	22 ± 2.2	0.940
Height (cm)	162.6 ± 2.6	161.9 ± 2.7	0.133
Weight (kg)	58.2 ± 5.8	57.8 ± 5.4	0.660
Hemoglobin (g/dL)	12 ± 0.8	11.8 ± 0.8	0.184

Base line vitamin D levels

Around 4% of the women in the breast cancer group were vitamin D deficient, whereas in the control group no women had vitamin D deficiency. Of the breast cancer patients, 82% had vitamin D insufficiency, in contrast to 35% in the control group ($p < 0.001$). Only 14% of patients had sufficient vitamin D levels compared to 65% of controls who had sufficient vitamin D levels (Table 2).

Vitamin D levels versus breast cancer prognostic parameters

An equal number of premenopausal and postmenopausal women were in the two groups. No significant difference was observed between serum 25-OH vitamin D levels in postmenopausal women and premenopausal women (20.13 ± 8.51 ng/mL vs. 23.7 ± 7.77 ng/mL; $p = 0.06$). Women who did not fall into the clear-cut category of premenopausal or postmenopausal were classified into the perimenopausal group, and seven of such women were not included in the analysis. No patients presented in stages I and IV. The clinical stage of a tumor did not bear any statistically significant relationship with the serum 25-OH vitamin D levels in this study. A statistically significant association ($p = 0.001$) was observed between serum 25-OH vitamin D levels and histological grades of breast cancer. Patients with poorly differentiated (grade 3) breast cancer had lower 25-OH vitamin D levels than patients with moderately (grade 2) and well-differentiated (grade 1) tumors (Table 3).

Table 2. Comparison of serum 25-OH vitamin D levels in cases and controls

25-OH vitamin D levels	Controls		Cases		*p* valuex
	N (%)	25(OH) vitamin D Level (ng mL) Mean ± SD	N (%)	25(OH) Vitamin D Level (ng/mL) Mean ± SD	
Deficiency	0	NA	3 (3.9%)	8.5 ± 1.5	NA
Insufficiency	27 (34.6%)	26 ± 2.8	64 (82%)	20.3 ± 4.7	**< 0.001***
Sufficiency	51 (65.4%)	43.5 ± 10.8	11 (14.1)	38.1 ± 4.8	0.112*
Mean serum 25(OH) vitamin D level	78	37.4 ± 12.2	78	22.3 ± 8.2	**0.0001****

* Chi-square test, ** Student *t* test.

Table 3. Association between serum 25-OH vitamin D levels and breast cancer prognostic parameters

Breast cancer prognostic parameters		Serum 25(OH) vitamin D level (ng/mL)	*p* value
Menopausal status	Premenopausal (n = 48)	23.7 ± 7.8	0.060*
	Postmenopausal (n = 23)	20.1 ± 8.5	
Stage of tumour	Stage I (n = 0)	0	0.598**
	Stage II A (n = 9)	24.8 ± 7.7	
	Stage IIB (n = 40)	21.3 ± 8	
	Stage IIIA (n = 25)	23.4 ± 9.2	
	Stage III B (n = 4)	21.1 ± 4.1	
Grade of tumour	Grade 1 (n = 16)	29.5 ± 10.4	**0.001****
	Grade 2 (n = 53)	21.7 ± 6	
	Grade 3 (n = 9)	13.4 ± 3.7	

*Student's *t* test, **ANOVA.

Vitamin D levels versus NPI

NPI was used as a surrogate indicator for aggressiveness of a tumor. On analyzing the association with the individual prognostic category, 25-OH vitamin D levels did not show a significant association with the NPI. However, when the NPI was grouped to include various prognostic categories into two groups – Group I (index ≤ 3.4) consisting of the excellent (index ≤ 2.4) and good prognostic categories (index ≤ 2.4-3.4) and Group II (index > 3.4) consisting of the moderate I (index 3.41-4.40), moderate II (index 4.41-5.4), and poor (index ≥ 5.41) prognostic categories – serum 25-OH vitamin D in Group II showed significantly lower mean concentration than in Group I (25.48 ± 8.86 ng/mL vs. 20.46 ± 7.24 ng/ml; p = 0.008) (Table 4).

Table 4. Association between serum 25-OH vitamin D levels and Nottingham's prognostic index (NPI)

Prognostic category	NPI Score	Serum 25 (OH) Vitamin D levels (ng/mL) Mean ± SD	*p* value
Excellent (n = 7)	≤ 2.4	28.6 ± 10.3	
Good (n = 22)	2.4 – 3.4	24.5 ± 8.4	
Moderate I (n = 21)	3.4 – 4.4	20.6 ± 7.5	0.075*
Moderate II (n = 19)	4.4 – 5.4	19.9 ± 8.4	
Poor (n = 9)	> 5.4	21.3 ± 3.6	
Group I (n = 29) (Excellent, good)	≤ 3.4	25.5 ± 8.9	**0.008****
Group II (n = 49) (Moderate I & II, Poor)	> 3.4	20.5 ± 7.2	

* ANOVA, ** Student's *t* Test.

Vitamin D levels versus IHC molecular phenotypes

The molecular phenotypes of breast cancer were segregated using IHC status as surrogate markers. On analyzing the individual molecular phenotype, the vitamin D levels did not yield any significant association with any of the luminal A, luminal B, *HER2*, and basal phenotypes of the tumors. However, when the phenotypes were categorized into a non-luminal group (*HER2* and basal) and a luminal group (luminal A and luminal B), the non-luminal group had a significantly lower mean serum 25-OH vitamin D level as opposed to the luminal group (20.6 ± 8.1 vs. 24.3 ± 8 ng/mL; p = 0.045) (Table 5).

Table 5. Association between serum 25-OH vitamin D levels and molecular phenotypes of breast cancer

Molecular Phenotypes	Serum 25 (OH) Vitamin D Levels (ng/mL) Mean ± SD	p value
Luminal (n = 37)	24.3 ± 8	**0.045***
Non-luminal (n = 41)	20.6 ± 8.1	
Luminal A (n = 25)	23.6 ± 7.4	0.206**
Luminal B (n = 12)	25.7 ± 9.4	
Her 2 (n = 15)	21 ± 9.1	
Basal (n = 26)	20.3 ± 7.6	

* Student's *t* Test, ** ANOVA.

Vitamin D levels versus lymphovascular invasion and estrogen receptors

The group of patients with lymphovascular invasion in breast cancer had no significant association with lower mean vitamin D value compared to the group without lymphovascular invasion (p = 0.360). Patients with estrogen receptor positivity had significantly higher serum 25-OH vitamin D levels compared to the patients with negative estrogen receptors (24.28 ± 7.99 vs. 20.57 ± 8.08; p = 0.045) (Table 6).

Table 6. Association between serum 25-OH vitamin D Levels with histopathology parameters

Histopathology parameters		Serum 25 (OH) Vitamin D levels (ng/mL)	p value (Student *t* test)
Lymphovascular Invasion	Present (n = 17)	20.7 ± 7.2	0.360
	Absent (n = 61)	22.8 ± 8.5	
Estrogen Receptor	Present (n = 37)	24.3 ± 8	**0.045**
	Absent (n = 41)	20.6 ± 8.1	

DISCUSSION

Multiple studies have shown associations between adequate vitamin D, circulating vitamin D levels, and a decreased incidence of malignancies of colon, breast, ovary, prostate, kidney, pancreas, etc. (3,4). It has been shown that a mean vitamin D level of 40 to 60 ng/mL will be able to prevent about three-fourths of the deaths from breast and colon cancer in the United States and Canada (2). Multiple laboratory tests on tissue cultures have shown that the malignant cell growth is inhibited by vitamin D metabolites, and there has been re-differentiation in some instances (3,4,7). The proposed mechanisms for the said action includes up-regulation of adherence and signaling between epithelial cells, contact inhibition of proliferation, differentiation, cell cycle stabilization, promotion of apoptosis, anti-neoangiogenesis, and down-regulation of glycogen synthase kinase 3 (GSK-3) that decreases the in-vitro proliferation of colorectal, pancreatic, prostate, and other cancer cells (7).

According to Garland's DINOMIT model of carcinogenesis, vitamin D deficiency plays a role in arresting carcinogenesis at various levels. This finding could pave the way for including vitamin D in the adjuvant treatment regime of epithelial cancers (2). Vitamin D and its metabolites, if linked with specific cancer types, can be used as nonspecific markers of aggressiveness. Adequate vitamin D levels are beneficial not only to decreasing the incidence of malignancy but also in a multitude of various health conditions, autoimmune conditions, infections, and chronic medical disorders. Food fortification with vitamin D could be considered if future large-scale studies show a similar picture.

In the current study, vitamin D insufficiency in the control group was around 35%, which was much lower than the range reported in Indian literature (5). Large-scale population-based studies have shown that serum 25-OH vitamin D levels are inversely associated with breast cancer risk in a concentration-dependent fashion (7). Garland and cols. reviewed around 3000 articles investigating the association of vitamin D and its metabolites with cancer (2). Imtiaz and cols., in their study on Pakistani women, found that 95.6% of women with breast cancer and 77% of healthy women were deficient in vitamin D, which was statistically significant ($p < 0.001$) (3). Harinarayan and cols. in their study found that 70% of South Indian women are deficient in vitamin D, 29% have insufficient levels, and only 1% has sufficient vitamin D levels (5).

Previous studies have shown a correlation between high BMI and low vitamin D levels (8). Since the BMI of the patients and controls were matched in the present study, the effect of BMI as a confounding variable has been suppressed to prevent a spurious association of vitamin D insufficiency with cases. In the current study, the postmenopausal women in the cases had low mean serum 25-OH vitamin D levels compared to the premenopausal group; however, the difference was not statistically significant. Using a statistical adjustment for menopausal status is advocated if the difference in the mean 25-OH vitamin D levels significantly differ in both the groups. Earlier studies have shown that postmenopausal women may have a relatively low 25-OH vitamin D concentration (9).

Association of 25-OH vitamin D levels with breast cancer patients

The clinical stages of tumors did not bear any statistically significant relationship with the serum 25-OH vitamin D levels in this study. A similar finding was obtained in the study by Imtiaz and cols. on Pakistani women (3). The commonest presentation of breast cancer is a painless breast lump. Most of the people in rural India tend to neglect these symptoms. As a result, patients with advanced clinical stage at presentation are a common occurrence in the Indian setting. Because patients' health-seeking behavior is a confounding factor in assessing the clinical staging at presentation, it may not be expected to show any association with vitamin D levels (10).

Patients with poorly differentiated breast cancer had lower vitamin D levels than patients with moderately and well-differentiated tumors. The above finding has been explained by previous studies in which it was demonstrated that vitamin D metabolites inhibit proliferation and promote apoptosis and differentiation (11).

Chollet and cols. showed that NPI, which was used to prognosticate primarily operable breast cancer in the adjuvant setting, retains its prognostic value in the neo-adjuvant setting also (12). When the NPI prognostic groups were reorganized to form two groups – namely Group I (excellent and good prognosis) and Group II (moderate I, moderate II, and poor prognosis) – it was found that Group I had statistically significant higher serum 25-OH vitamin D levels than Group II ($p = 0.008$).

NPI is directly proportional to tumor grade. In the present study, the serum 25-OH vitamin D levels of the patients at diagnosis have a statistically significant association with tumor grade. Hence, the relationship of serum 25-OH vitamin D levels with various grades of tumors might contribute to its association with NPI. Because NPI has been used as a marker for prognosis, it could be assumed that a low serum 25-OH vitamin D level is one of the markers of poor prognosis.

Gene expression profiling in breast cancer has resulted in the identification of several major breast cancer subtypes. The best characterized of these subtypes are luminal A, luminal B, *HER2*, and basal-like carcinoma. Immuno-phenotyping with ER, PR, and *HER2* biomarkers can be used as a surrogate for molecular category of breast cancer (13-15). Luminal sub-group constitutes approximately 70% of invasive breast cancers. It is characterized by high expression of hormone receptors that are found more in luminal A. Luminal B tends to be at a higher histological grade than luminal A. Luminal B, sometimes called triple positive breast cancer, is more likely to have lymph node metastasis and may respond more to chemotherapy. Some luminal B tumors over-express *HER2*. These tumors are slow growing, respond well to hormone therapy and usually has a better prognosis (14,15,20). *HER2* constitutes around 15% of invasive breast cancers which are characterized by *HER2* over-expression, gene amplification and low expression of hormone receptors. These tumors have relatively poorer prognosis. Basal tumors are subgroup of the so-called triple-negative breast cancers. It is characterized by low expression of hormone receptors and *HER2* genes. Basal epithelial genes and basal cytokeratins (EGFR, CK 5/6) are highly expressed. The BRCA-associated breast cancers fall in this group. It has a poorer prognosis (15).

Using IHC findings as surrogate markers, luminal A and luminal B were grouped as luminal type breast cancer. *HER2 neu* and basal-like groups were classified as non-luminal breast cancer. Like other study results, patients with luminal types of breast cancer had higher serum 25-OH vitamin D levels than patients with the non-luminal types (14-16). The presence of lymphovascular invasion in the pathology specimen is a marker of poor prognosis. In the current study, the difference between serum 25-OH vitamin D levels among tumors with and without lymphovascular invasion was not statistically significant ($p = 0.360$). A similar observation was reported in the study by Imtiaz and cols. (3). Because the presence of tumor emboli within vascular spaces within the realm of a tumor is a common finding, rigorous sampling techniques are required to prevent this finding from being mistaken for the presence of true lymphovascular invasion (15).

Estrogen receptor negativity is one of the poor prognostic indicators in breast cancer (13). The anti-proliferative action of vitamin D in breast cancer could partly be mediated by its role in down-regulating estrogen receptor abundance in breast cancer (7,11). Because estrogen causes increased growth of breast cancer, this anti-estrogenic effect of vitamin D is of much interest. Vitamin D induces estrogen receptor expression in ER-negative breast cancers, thereby restoring their response to anti-estrogens, according to Santos-Martinez and cols. (16). The above-mentioned fact could form the way for a possible new therapeutic approach of adding vitamin D to potentiate adjuvant hormonal therapy in the future. Imtiaz and cols. could not demonstrate a correlation of vitamin D levels with parameters like histological grade of a tumor and estrogen receptor status (3). The present study, however, was able to document a statistically significant correlation between grade of a tumor ($p = 0.001$), estrogen receptor status ($p = 0.045$), luminal and non-luminal breast cancer ($p = 0.045$), and serum 25-OH vitamin D levels.

A unique feature of this study is that the study population was from the southern part of India, where studies comparing breast cancer and serum 25-OH vitamin D levels are scarce in this population. The study and control groups were matched meticulously in various aspects like age, BMI, menstrual status, parity, and co-morbidities like diabetes and hypertension. According to Chollet and cols., NPI also retains its prognostic value in the post-chemotherapy setting (12). In the present study, NPI had been used as an indicator of poor prognosis.

Robsahm and cols. analyzed the published literature on the inverse association of vitamin D on cancer survival and evaluated the possible reverse causation (17). It has been shown that the duration of the cancer, chemotherapy, and other modalities of cancer treatment may have an adverse effect on vitamin D levels. It is plausible that the inverse association of lower vitamin D levels and cancer could be due to the adverse effect of cancer treatment on vitamin D levels with a potential reverse causation. Because the duration and severity of cancer, various cancer treatments, and time of serum sample collection play a vital role in establishing the temporal association, the present study excluded patients who were diagnosed elsewhere or partially treated at outside hospitals. To avoid the possible adverse effect of chemotherapy and hormonal therapy on vitamin D levels, only newly diagnosed breast cancer patients were included in the present study.

Despite the different stages of cancer, one's population group and different sites of cancer may have an effect on vitamin D levels. Robsahm and cols. concluded that the association of lower vitamin D levels and inferior cancer survival is consistent even after adjusting for these confounders. Because a possibility of introducing vitamin D supplementation for the general population exists when extrapolating the study results, until strong evidence to prove the inverse association of vitamin D levels and breast cancer is available from the carefully structured prospective trials, the potential reverse causation should be considered when discussing this important subject. Results from the VITamin D and OmegA-3 TriaL (VITAL) on the efficacy of vitamin D supplementation in the prevention of cancer are much awaited and could possibly answer the above unsolved issue (18).

A limitation of this study was that patients who attended the hospital were selected based on convenient sampling. The current study was not a community-based one and patients were not followed up. Because it was a one-time estimate of vitamin D levels, it cannot be taken as an indicator of the duration of exposure to low serum levels of vitamin D that may have contributed to the increased risk for breast cancer. The sample size included in the present study is relatively small due to limited resources. A population-based study with a larger sample may provide better insight into this important subject.

Future studies may also include detailed assessment of nutritional status and quantification of sunlight exposure (time of exposure, duration) and skin color that would enable examination of the association of the above factors with serum 25-OH vitamin D levels. Large-scale studies that measured serum parathormone, serum calcium, bone mineral density, and serum 25-OH vitamin D levels in the Indian setting will help in defining a vitamin D classification in the Indian setting. The response to chemotherapy in patients in the neoadjuvant setting and its correlation, if any, with the vitamin D values could be studied. If a positive correlation were found, then it would pave the way for using vitamin D levels as a prognostic marker for assessing the response to chemotherapy (19).

In conclusion, higher grades of tumors had lower serum 25-OH vitamin D levels than lower grades. Luminal types of breast cancer had higher serum 25-OH vitamin D levels than the non-luminal types. Patients with estrogen receptor positivity had higher serum 25-OH vitamin D levels than those with absence of estrogen receptor. It was found that patients with excellent and good NPI prognoses had statistically significant higher serum 25-OH vitamin D levels than the moderate and poor NPI prognoses groups, whereas menopausal status, the clinical stage at presentation, and lymphovascular invasion did not show a statistically significant correlation with serum 25-OH vitamin D.

Funding: there was no fund/financial grant obtained for this study.

REFERENCES

1. Estimated cancer incidence, mortality and prevalence worldwide in 2012. Globocan 2012. Available from: http://globocan.iarc.fr/Pages/fact_sheets_population.aspx. Accessed on: Nov 28, 2017.
2. Garland CF, Gorham ED, Mohr SB, Garland FC. Vitamin D for cancer prevention: global perspective. Ann Epidemiol. 2009;19(7):468-83.
3. Imtiaz S, Siddiqui N, Raza SA, Loya A, Muhammad A. Vitamin D deficiency in newly diagnosed breast cancer patients. Indian J Endocrinol Metab. 2012;16(3):409-13.
4. Vrieling A, Hein R, Abbas S, Schneeweiss A, Flesch-Janys D, Chang-Claude J. Serum 25-hydroxyvitamin D and postmenopausal breast cancer survival: a prospective patient cohort study. Breast Cancer Res. 2011;13(4):R74.
5. Harinarayan CV, Ramalakshmi T, Venkataprasad U. High prevalence of low dietary calcium and low vitamin D status in healthy south Indians. Asia Pac J Clin Nutr. 2004;13(4):359-64.
6. Holick MF, Binkley NC, Bischoff-Ferrari HA, Gordon CM, Hanley DA, Heaney RP, et al. Evaluation, treatment, and prevention of vitamin D deficiency: an Endocrine Society clinical practice guideline. J Clin Endocrinol Metab. 2011;96(7):1911-30.
7. Crew KD, Gammon MD, Steck SE, Hershman DL, Cremers S, Dworakowski E, et al. Association between plasma 25-hydroxyvitamin D and breast cancer risk. Cancer PrevRes (Phila). 2009;2(6):598-604.
8. Holick MF, Chen TC. Vitamin D deficiency: a worldwide problem with health consequences. Am J Clin Nutr. 2008;87(4):1080S-6S.
9. Aggarwal S, Nityanand. Calcium and vitamin D in post menopausal women. Indian J EndocrinolMetab2013; 17(Suppl 3): S618-20.
10. Subramanian P, Oranye NO, Masri AM,Taib NA, Ahmad N. Breast cancer knowledge and screening behavior among women with a positive family history: a cross sectional study. Asian Pac J Cancer Prev. 2013;14(11):6783-90.
11. James SY, Mackay AG, Colston KW. Effects of 1, 25dihydroxyvitamin D3 and its analogues on induction of apoptosis in breast cancer cells. J Steroid Biochem Mol Biol. 1996;58(4):395-401.
12. Chollet P, Amat S, Belembaogo E, Cure H, de LM, Dauplat J, et al. Is nottingham prognostic index useful after induction chemotherapy in operable breast cancer? Br J Cancer. 2003;89(7):1185-91.
13. Manjunath S, Prabhu JS, Kaluve R, Correa M, Sridhar TS. Estrogen Receptor Negative Breast Cancer in India: Do We Really Have Higher Burden of this Subtype? Indian J Surg Oncol. 2011;2(2):122-5.
14. Lips EH, Mulder L, de Ronde JJ, Mandjes IA, Koolen BB, Wessels LF, et al. Breast cancer subtyping by immunohistochemistry and histological grade outperforms breast cancer intrinsic subtypes in predicting neoadjuvant chemotherapy response. Breast Cancer ResTreat. 2013;140(1):63-71.
15. Sanati S, Hameed O, Warrick JI, Allred C. Breast Pathology. In: Humphrey PA, Dehner LP, Pfeifer JD, editors. The Washington

Manual of Surgical Pathology. 2nd ed. Washington; Lippincott Williams & Wilkins; 2012. p. 298-328.

16. Santos-Martinez N, Diaz L, Ordaz-Rosado D, Garcia-Quiroz J, Barrera D, Avila E, et al. Calcitriol restores antiestrogen responsiveness in estrogen receptor negative breast cancer cells: a potential new therapeutic approach. BMC Cancer. 2014;14:230.
17. Robsahm TE, Schwartz GG, Tretli S. The inverse relationship between 25-hydroxyvitamin D and cancer survival: discussion of causation. Cancers. 2013;5(4):1439-55.
18. Manson JE, Bassuk SS, Lee IM, Cook NR, Albert MA, Gordon D, et al. The VITamin D and OmegA-3 TriaL (VITAL): rationale and design of a large randomized controlled trial of vitamin D and marine omega-3 fatty acid supplements for the primary prevention of cancer and cardiovascular disease. Contemp Clin Trials. 2012;33(1):159-71.
19. Goodwin PJ, Ennis M, Pritchard KI, Koo J, Hood N. Prognostic effects of 25-hydroxyvitamin D levels in early breast cancer. J Clin Oncol. 2009;27(23):3757-63.

Importance of abdominal circumference and body mass index values in predicting male hypogonadism – A practical approach

Paulo Eduardo Dietrich Jaworski[1], Anderson Ramos[1], Arthur Radaelli Nicoleit[1], Luis Fernando de Almeida Bacarin[2], Pedro Olivo Neto[2]

[1] Departamento de Urologia, Hospital Universitário Evangélico de Curitiba, Curitiba, PR, Brasil
[2] Faculdade de Medicina, Faculdade Evangélica do Paraná (Fepar), Curitiba, PR, Brasil

Correspondence to:
Paulo Eduardo Dietrich Jaworski
Hospital Universitário Evangélico de Curitiba, Departamento de Urologia
Alameda Augusto Stellfeld, 1980, 5° andar
pj@paulojaworski.com.br

ABSTRACT

Objective: The objective of this study was to correlate the values of abdominal circumference (AC) and body mass index (BMI) with the levels of total testosterone (TT), free testosterone (FT) and sexual hormone binding globulin (SHBG). We aimed to analyze the association between the anthropometric values and variations in the hormonal levels. **Subjects and methods:** A transversal prospective study was conducted. A total of 159 patients were included in the study. **Results:** BMI was inversely correlated with TT and SHBG ($p = 0.02$ and $p = 0.006$, respectively). AC was also inversely correlated with TT and SHBG ($p = 0.006$ and $p < 0.0001$, respectively). However, BMI did not correlate signicantly with these hormonal levels after adjusting for age. **Conclusion:** This finding led to the conclusion that AC had a stronger inverse correlation than BMI with TT and SHBG. Our data suggested that AC alone can be used as an anthropometric parameter to help simplify the identification of men with low serum TT levels. Arch Endocrinol Metab. 2017;61(1):76-80

Keywords
Abdominal; circumference; obesity; testosterone

INTRODUCTION

Population aging has widespread consequences on all sections of organized civil society. From a medical perspective, clinicians are called upon to address the prevention, treatment and even retardation of the consequences of aging. Aging women experience a decrease in estrogen which invariably evolves into menopause, a very well-known condition that is often discussed by doctors and patients. Aging men usually develop a decrease in androgen levels (1). These biochemical findings and the associated specific symptoms are known as Androgen Deficiency of the Aging Male (ADAM). The array of associated symptoms include decreased libido, erectile dysfunction, decreased ejaculate volume, hair loss, weakness, and anemia (2). Low testosterone levels can also lead to decreased bone mineral density and lean mass, increased fat mass, and increased cardiovascular risk including atherosclerosis and the metabolic syndrome (3-6).

Despite being the subject of many studies, male hypogonadism and ADAM are not easily identified during office consultations, due to cultural and even social characteristics of Brazilian males, particularly among the elderly. A method to effectively identify these patients is necessary in order to expand the multidisciplinary treatment of the aging male population, with the aim to improve their global quality of life.

The objective of this study was to analyze two anthropometric values, abdominal circumference (AC) and body mass index (BMI), and compare them to serum levels of total testosterone (TT), free testosterone (FT) and sexual hormone binding globulin (SHBG). We aimed to identify the best anthropometric-hormonal correlation that could help identify patients with a potential diagnosis of ADAM.

SUBJECTS AND METHODS

A transversal prospective study was conducted. We included male outpatients in our service who were greater than 40 years old in a random manner, without distinction by race or ethnicity. Patients were excluded if any other possible cause of hypogonadism was identified during the consultation (*e.g.*, use of medication, testis affections, hyperprolactinemia). All of the subjects signed an informed consent form. A total of 159 men agreed to participate in the study. The institutional Ethics Committee approved the study.

The data collection took place over 4 months, between April and August of 2013. The anthropometric data (height, weight and abdominal circumference) and age were measured in a preliminary interview. Each subject had a fasting blood sample drawn between 8:00 h and 10:00 h. Serum levels of total testosterone, free testosterone and SHBG were analyzed.

The total testosterone and SHBG levels were measured using chemiluminescence immunoassay (CLIA) kits, and the free testosterone was calculated according to Vermeulen's Formula (http://www.issam.ch/freetesto.htm). Height was measured in meters (m) and weight in kilograms (kg), and both measurements were obtained with the subject barefoot and wearing only underpants. The AC was measured in centimeters (cm), using the landmark of the average point between the 10th rib and the iliac crest at the axillary line. The subjects were divided into two groups, patients with an AC higher than 102 cm and patients with an AC lower than 102 cm, based on the AC criteria for patients at high risk for metabolic disease (7). The BMI was calculated and patients were also divided in two groups, patients with a BMI higher than 30 and patients with a BMI lower than 30, based on the World Health Organization criteria for obesity classification (8). The data were organized in a frequency and contingency table. The Kolmogorov-Smirnov test was used to determine the sample distribution. The central tendency was displayed as the average and standard deviation for parametric data, whereas the median and interquartile intervals were used for non-parametric data.

The AC and BMI were individually correlated with TT, FT and SHBG levels using the Spearman test. Multiple linear regression was used to analyze independent variables and to correlate age, BMI and AC. The ANCOVA was used to analyze correlations between hormonal values and the 4 groups of subjects, according to their BMI (higher than 30, lower than 30) and AC (higher than 102 cm, lower than 102 cm).

All the statistical tests were deemed significant at a p-value lower than 0.05. The analytical software utilized was MedCalc v.10.0.

RESULTS

The demographic data are displayed in Table 1. The median age was 66.7 years. The average BMI was 28.1 kg/m^2 and the average AC was 98.7 cm.

Table 1. Demographic and hormonal data

N	**159**
Age	66.7 (58.4 – 71.9)*
BMI	28.1 (± 4.3)#
AC	98.7 (±11.46)#
Total testosterone	369 (291 – 423.6)*
Free testosterone	6.66 (5.17 – 8.28)*
SHBG	39.1 (30.8 – 50.8)*

* Median (inter-quartile interval); # Average (standard deviation).

BMI was inversely correlated with TT and SHBG, both significantly, but the correlation between BMI and FT was not significant. AC was also inversely correlated with TT and SHBG and these results were with statistically significant. The data are shown in Table 2.

Table 2. Anthropometric measurements and hormonal correlations*

	FT	**TT**	**SHBG**
BMI	0.809	0.03	0.006
AC	0.895	0.006	< 0.001

* Spearman's p-value.

An age-adjusted linear regression analysis demonstrated correlation between the anthropometric parameters and hormonal levels, and the results are shown in Table 3. We tried to refine our analysis, knowing that the age range could bias the results. Again, we confirmed that BMI and AC both correlated with TT and SHBG.

Table 3. Adjusted partial correlation* between anthropometric measurements and FT, TT and SHBG

	Abdominal circumference (AC)	**Body mass index (BMI)**
Free testosterone		
Age adjustment	P = 0.419	P = 0.459
AC adjustment	-	P = 0.669
Age and BMI adjustment	P = 0.59	-
Total testosterone		
Age adjustment	P = 0.002	P = 0.025
Age and AC adjustment	-	P = 0.306
Age and BMI adjustment	P = 0.019	-
SHBG		
Age adjustment	P < 0.001	P = 0.015
AC adjustment	-	P = 0.681
Age and BMI adjustment	P < 0.001	-

* Multiple linear regression p-value (CI = 95%).

Table 4. Mean free testosterone, total testosterone and SHBG in different anthropometric subgroups

	AC < 102 cm			AC > 102 cm			p-value*
	N	Mean	SD	N	Mean	SD	
Free testosterone	101	7.35	0.31	58	6.96	0.41	0.324
SHBG	101	44.61	1.47	58	37.29	1.94	0.001
Total testosterone	101	394.69	13.7	58	342.74	18.2	0.007
	BMI < 30			BMI > 30			p-value*
	N	Mean	SD	N	Mean	SD	
Free testosterone	47	7.51	0.22	112	6.88	32.17	0.753
SHBG	47	48.08	1.35	112	37	0.67	0.004
Total testosterone	47	411.4	8.87	112	360	2.36	0.09

* ANCOVA's p-value.

The group analysis, displayed in Table 4, revealed that men with an AC lower than 102 cm had significantly lower TT and SHBG levels than men with an AC higher than 102 cm. When the BMI groups were compared, we found that men with a BMI lower than 30 had significantly higher SHBG levels than men with a BMI higher than 30. No significant differences were observed between the groups when TT and FT were analyzed.

DISCUSSION

Men's testosterone synthesis decreases with age, whereas central obesity tends to increase (1,9). Many authors have demonstrated the existence of an inverse correlation between total testosterone and central obesity when they are analyzed in the same subject (10-12). The proposed pathophysiology is that visceral fat is associated with lower plasmatic SHBG concentration (13,14), which results in more testosterone in a free form, resulting in negative feedback to the pituitary gland, which inhibits the production luteinizing hormone and lowers its level. Therefore, the low SHBG levels decrease testosterone production (14). Moreover, abundant cytokine production within the fat tissue also inhibits testosterone production through intracellular mechanisms. Alpha tumor necrosis factor (α-TNF), for instance, inhibits steroid production inside Leydig cells, at the intracellular transcription level, whereas interleukine-1 (IL-1) inhibits the cholesterol side-chain cleavage by the p450 cytochrome inside the Leydig cells (15).

Central obesity and increased abdominal circumference are conditions that correlate to each other. Increased abdominal circumference has been described as the best indicator of central obesity (14), total body fat (16) and visceral fat (17,18), particularly in men who are more than 40 years of age. When the production of androgenic hormones in these groups of patients was examined, Svartberg and cols. concluded in the Tromsø study that abdominal circumference values were inversely associated with serum levels of TT, FT and SHBG (11). In addition, they reported a higher strength of association between abdominal circumference and TT, FT and SHBG when compared to the association between BMI and TT, FT and SHBG. The investigators proposed that, within that patient population, the simple measurement of AC could be useful to anticipate levels of serum testosterone (19). Similarly, Seidell and cols. have shown that men with higher visceral fat values have lower total and free testosterone serum levels (10).

Multiple transversal and longitudinal studies (11,20,21) have shown that aging men experience progressive declines in their TT and FT levels. This down variation is physiological (11,20), and it is caused by a reduction in testicular function associated with a reduction in the activity of the hypothalamic-pituitary axis (22,23). By adjusting our data for age, we reduced the chance of an eventual distortion in the comparison of the variables and men in different ages. We found that, even after this adjustment, our results remained consistent and statistically significant.

There is controversy in the literature about the cause and effect theory of low androgen levels and obesity. Some authors have suggested that obesity has a causal role in the decline of androgen levels. They state that weight loss can partially reverse low TT and SHBG levels (24-26). However, Khaw and Barrett-Connor showed that TT and SHBG were inversely correlated with visceral fat and age, suggesting that testosterone can mobilize abdominal fat deposits (13). During the 15 observation years of The Massachusetts Male Aging Study (27), there was evidence that low testosterone and SHBG levels could predict the incidence of the metabolic syndrome. Ding and cols. concluded that low SHBG levels can predict the risk of developing type 2 diabetes mellitus (28).

Within our pool of subjects, AC was inversely correlated with TT and SHBG levels. Moreover, AC correlated in a stronger and more consistent manner with TT and SHBG than BMI. Because we recruited a considerable number of men with a heterogeneous age profile and preformed their serum sample analysis in the same laboratory and during the same time interval of 2 hours in the morning, we eliminated diurnal variability in the testosterone levels and provided reliability to our data and results. The limitations of this study include the different sizes of the AC and BMI groups, the limited number of participants and the fact that all of the subjects were recruited from a tertiary urology outpatient clinic, so our findings may not be generalizable to other patient populations.

In conclusion, in this study we found that abdominal circumference had a stronger inverse correlation with TT and SHBG than body mass index. A measured abdominal circumference of greater than 102 cm can be used as anthropometric data to predict low TT and SHBG levels in patients evaluated in a medical office. This simple information can contribute to the correct identification of androgen deficiency symptoms in aging men.

Funding: the authors state no financial interest of any kind.

REFERENCES

1. Vermeulen A, Goemaere S, Kaufman JM. Testosterone, body composition and aging. J Endocrinol Invest. 1999;22(5 Suppl):110-6.
2. Petak SM, Nankin HR, Spark RF, Swerdloff RS, Rodriguez-Rigau LJ; American Association of Clinical Endocrinologists. American Association of Clinical Endocrinologists Medical Guidelines for clinical practice for the evaluation and treatment of hypogonadism in adult male patients--2002 update. Endocr Pract. 2002;8(6):440-56.
3. Barrett-Connor EL.Testosterone and risk factors for cardiovascular disease in men. Diabete Metab. 1995;21(3):156-61.
4. Simon D, Charles MA, Nahoul K, Orssaud G, Kremski J, Hully V, et al. Association between plasma total testosterone and cardiovascular risk factors in healthy adult men: The Telecom Study. J Clin Endocrinol Metab. 1997;82(2):682-5.
5. Zmuda JM, Cauley JA, Kriska A, Glynn NW, Gutai JP, Kuller LH. Longitudinal relation between endogenous testosterone and cardiovascular disease risk factors in middle-aged men. A 13-year follow-up of former Multiple Risk Factor Intervention Trial participants. Am J Epidemiol. 1997;146(8):609-17.
6. Hak AE, Witteman JC, de Jong FH, Geerlings MI, Hofman A, Pols HA. Low levels of endogenous androgens increase the risk of atherosclerosis in elderly men: the Rotterdam study. J Clin Endocrinol Metab. 2002;87(8):3632-9.
7. Grundy SM, Cleeman JI, Daniels SR, Donato KA, Eckel RH, Franklin BA, et al.; American Heart Association; National Heart, Lung, and Blood Institute. Diagnosis and management of the metabolic syndrome: an American Heart Association/National Heart, Lung, and Blood Institute Scientific Statement. Circulation. 2005;112(17):2735-52.
8. Clinical Guidelines on the Identification, Evaluation, and Treatment of Overweight and Obesity in Adults--The Evidence Report. National Institutes of Health. Obes Res. 1998 Sep;6 Suppl 2:51S-209S.
9. Lahti-Koski M, Pietinen P, Männistö S, Vartiainen E. Trends in waist-to-hip ratio and its determinants in adults in Finland from 1987 to 1997. Am J Clin Nutr. 2000;72(6):1436-44.
10. Seidell JC, Björntorp P, Sjöström L, Kvist H, Sannerstedt R. Visceral fat accumulation in men is positively associated with insulin, glucose, and C-peptide levels, but negatively with testosterone levels. Metabolism. 1990;39(9):897-901.
11. Svartberg J, von Mühlen D, Sundsfjord J, Jorde R. Waist circumference and testosterone levels in community dwelling men. The Tromsø study. Eur J Epidemiol. 2004;19(7):657-63.
12. Chen RY, Wittert GA, Andrews GR. Relative androgen deficiency in relation to obesity and metabolic status in older men. Diabetes Obes Metab. 2006;8(4):429-35.
13. Khaw KT, Barrett-Connor E. Lower endogenous androgens predict central adiposity in men. Ann Epidemiol. 1992;2(5):675-82.
14. Haffner SM, Valdez RA, Stern MP, Katz MS. Obesity, body fat distribution and sex hormones in men. Int J Obes Relat Metab Disord. 1993;17(11):643-9.
15. Lin T, Wang D, Stocco DM. Interleukin-1 inhibits Leydig cell steroidogenesis without affecting steroidogenic acute regulatory protein messenger ribonucleic acid or protein levels. J Endocrinol. 1998;156(3):461-7.
16. Lean ME, Han TS, Deurenberg P. Predicting body composition by densitometry from simple anthropometric measurements. Am J Clin Nutr. 1996;63(1):4-14.
17. Lemieux S, Prud'homme D, Bouchard C, Tremblay A, Després JP. A single threshold value of waist girth identifies normal-weight and overweight subjects with excess visceral adipose tissue. Am J Clin Nutr. 1996;64(5):685-93.
18. Han TS, McNeill G, Seidell JC, Lean ME. Predicting intra-abdominal fatness from anthropometric measures: the influence of stature. Int J Obes Relat Metab Disord. 1997;21(7):587-93.
19. Svartberg J, Midtby M, Bønaa KH, Sundsfjord J, Joakimsen RM, Jorde R. The associations of age, lifestyle factors and chronic disease with testosterone in men: the Tromsø Study. Eur J Endocrinol. 2003;149(2):145-52.
20. Harman SM, Metter EJ, Tobin JD, Pearson J, Blackman MR; Baltimore Longitudinal Study of Aging. Longitudinal effects of aging on serum total and free testosterone levels in healthy men. Baltimore Longitudinal Study of Aging. J Clin Endocrinol Metab. 2001;86(2):724-31.

21. Feldman HA, Longcope C, Derby CA, Johannes CB, Araujo AB, Coviello AD, et al. Age trends in the level of serum testosterone and other hormones in middle-aged men: longitudinal results from the Massachusetts male aging study. J Clin Endocrinol Metab. 2002;87(2):589-98.
22. Winters SJ, Troen P. Episodic luteinizing hormone (LH) secretion and the response of LH and follicle-stimulating hormone to LH-releasing hormone in aged men: evidence for coexistent primary testicular insufficiency and an impairment in gonadotropin secretion. J Clin Endocrinol Metab. 1982;55(3):560-5.
23. Deslypere JP, Kaufman JM, Vermeulen T, Vogelaers D, Vandalem JL, Vermeulen A. Influence of age on pulsatile luteinizing hormone release and responsiveness of the gonadotrophs to sex hormone feedback in men. J Clin Endocrinol Metab. 1987;64(1):68-73.
24. Vermeulen A, Kaufman JM, Deslypere JP, Thomas G. Attenuated luteinizing hormone (LH) pulse amplitude but normal LH pulse frequency, and its relation to plasma androgens in hypogonadism of obese men. J Clin Endocrinol Metab. 1993;76(5):1140-6.
25. Pasquali R, Vicennati V, Scopinaro N, Marinari G, Simonelli A, Flamia R, et al. Achievement of near-normal body weight as the prerequisite to normalize sex hormone-binding globulin concentrations in massively obese men. Int J Obes Relat Metab Disord. 1997;21(1):1-5.
26. Bhasin S, Jasjua GK, Pencina M, D'Agostino R Sr, Coviello AD, Vasan RS, et al. Sex hormone-binding globulin, but not testosterone, is associated prospectively and independently with incident metabolic syndrome in men: the framingham heart study. Diabetes Care. 2011;34(11):2464-70.
27. O'Donnell AB, Araujo AB, McKinlay JB. The health of normally aging men: The Massachusetts Male Aging Study (1987-2004). Exp Gerontol. 2004;39(7):975-84.
28. Ding EL, Song Y, Manson JE, Hunter DJ, Lee CC, Rifai N, et al. Sex hormone-binding globulin and risk of type 2 diabetes in women and men. N Engl J Med. 2009;361(12):1152-63.

Impact of an inpatient multidisciplinary glucose control management program

Denise P. Momesso[1], Rubens Carmo Costa Filho[1], João Luiz Ferreira Costa[1], Felipe Saddy[1], Ayla Mesquita[1], Marcela Calomeni[1], Claudia dos Santos Silva[1], Jacqueline Farret[1], Mariana Leon Vasques[1], Aline G. Santos[1], Ana Paula Vieira Cabral[1], Dayane Ribeiro[1], Luciana Reis[1], Maria de Fátima M. Muino[1], Roberta Santiago Vitorino[1], Claudio Amorim Monteiro[1], Evandro Tinoco[1], Andre Volschan[1]

[1] Hospital Pró-Cardíaco, Rio de Janeiro, RJ, Brasil

Correspondence to:
Denise Momesso
Rua General Polidoro, 192
22280-003 – Rio de Janeiro, RJ, Brazil
endocrinologia@denisemomesso.com.br

ABSTRACT

Objective: Glycemic control has been increasingly recognized as a critical element in inpatient care, but optimal management of blood glucose in the hospital setting remains challenging. The aims of this study were to describe and evaluate the impact of the implementation of an inpatient multidisciplinary glucose control management program on glucose control in hospitalized patients. Materials and methods: Retrospective analysis of medical records and glucose monitoring data obtained by point-of-care testing (POCT) in hospitalized patients before (May 2014) and after (June 2015 and May 2017) the implementation of the program. Results: We analyzed 6888, 7290, and 7669 POCTs from 389, 545, and 475 patients in May 2014, June 2015, and May 2017, respectively. Hyperglycemia (≥ 180 mg/dL) occurred in 23.5%, 19.6%, and 19.3% POCTs in May 2014, June 2015, and May/2017, respectively ($p < 0.001$), while severe hyperglycemia (≥ 300 mg/dL) was observed in 2.5%, 2.2%, and 1.8% of them, respectively ($p = 0.003$). Hyperglycemia (≥ 180 mg/dL) reduced significantly from May 2014 to June 2015 (16.3%, $p < 0.001$) and from May 2014 to May 2017 (17.8%, $p < 0.001$). No significant changes occurred in hypoglycemic parameters. Conclusions: The implementation of an inpatient multidisciplinary glucose control management program led to significant reductions in hyperglycemic events. The key elements for this achievement were the development of institutional inpatient glycemic control protocols, establishment of a multidisciplinary team, and continuing educational programs for hospital personnel. Altogether, these actions resulted in improvements in care processes, patient safety, and clinical outcomes of hospitalized patients. Arch Endocrinol Metab. 2018;62(5):514-22

Keywords
Hyperglycemia; hypoglycemia; inpatient glucose control; diabetes mellitus; systems, point-of-care

INTRODUCTION

Glycemic control has been increasingly recognized as a critical element in inpatient care (1-7). Several lines of evidence corroborate the concept that both hyperglycemia and hypoglycemia are associated with adverse outcomes to the patient. Hyperglycemia may occur in hospitalized patients with known diabetes or acutely ill individuals with previously normal glucose tolerance ("stress hyperglycemia") due to increased circulating counterregulatory hormones in response to stress. Irrespective of the cause, hyperglycemia on an inpatient setting is an independent marker of increased morbidity and mortality. During treatment of hyperglycemia, a major concern is the occurrence of hypoglycemia, which is also an independent risk factor for poor clinical outcomes (8-15). Therefore, great emphasis has been placed on optimizing the treatment of hospitalized patients with diabetes and hyperglycemia.

Based on data from multiples studies and clinical trials, the management of hyperglycemia in a hospital setting has recently evolved (16-23). Current consensus statements from the American Diabetes Association, American Association of Clinical Endocrinologists, Endocrine Society, and Brazilian Diabetes Association have recommended therapy of critically ill patients with persistent hyperglycemia, starting at a blood glucose level of 180 mg/dL; once insulin is started, the therapeutic glucose target should be within the 140-180 mg/dL range (1-6). In noncritical care patients, the recommended values are < 140 mg/dL for fasting glucose and < 180 mg/dL for random glucose, and the preferable regimen is the use of a basal insulin along with premeal and supplemental insulin, instead of sliding scale insulin. Optimal glycemic control also includes the prevention of hypoglycemia (1-6,24-26). Reducing the variability in glucose levels may also be important in improving outcomes (27,28).

Despite existing evidence, the optimal glucose management in a hospital setting remains challenging, as the achievement of improved glycemic control in a hospital setting meets numerous obstacles. In this scenario, the American College of Endocrinology, the American Diabetes Association, and the Brazilian Diabetes Society have released calls to action outlining strategies for a successful implementation of inpatient glucose control management programs (2,5,7). System-based key issues outlined included the need for the development and evaluation of: 1) clinical protocols to guide management, clinical decisions, and prescriptions; 2) multidisciplinary glucose control management teams; and 3) provider-delivered educational programs to improve knowledge and address barriers to achieving glycemic control (2,5,7,29,30).

The aims of this study were to describe and evaluate the impact of the implementation of a multidisciplinary glucose control management program for hospitalized patients. The study was conducted to determine if such program would improve inpatient safety by reducing the number of hyperglycemic events.

MATERIALS AND METHODS

The study was conducted at the *Pró-Cardíaco Hospital*, a 99-bed, tertiary-care, medical and surgical center located in Rio de Janeiro, Brazil. The medical center comprises an emergency room, two adult intensive care units (ICU), one coronary care unit, one surgical intensive care unit, one surgical semi-intensive care unit, three clinical semi-intensive units, one oncology care unit, and one day clinic. The hospital has an extensive referral network and includes outpatient specialty treatment and imaging centers, clinics, and rehabilitation centers.

Since 2001, the ICUs of the hospital have developed a protocol of insulin treatment for critically ill patients. In 2012, we introduced a hospital-wide inpatient multidisciplinary glucose control management program (MGCP) to facilitate the development of uniform glucose management policies and staff education based on current clinical practice guidelines. The main hallmarks of this program were the development of an Institutional inpatient glycemic control protocols in January 2012, and the establishment of a multidisciplinary glycemic control team in June 2014.

Institutional inpatient glycemic control protocols

In 2012, institutional glycemic control protocols were developed in an effort to improve and standardize the glycemic control of hospitalized patients. These protocols are aligned with international and local recommendations (2-6) and are frequently revised and updated based on these recommendations and local assistance requirements.

According to the institutional protocol, blood glucose levels of all critical and noncritical care patients admitted to the hospital are monitored using point-of-care testing (POCT). Glucose monitoring may be suspended 72 hours after admission of noncritically ill patients and in those without diabetes or current illness, or not using medications associated with hyperglycemia or hypoglycemia. Monitoring may also be suspended in patients whose blood glucose measurements have been within the normal range for 72 hours. All results obtained by POCT are downloaded directly from the glucometer (Precision®, Abbott Diabetes Care Inc., Alameda, CA, USA) to the patient's electronic medical records. In case of glucose measurements ≤ 40 mg/dL or ≥ 300 mg/dL, a direct notification is sent via e-mail from the medical record to the endocrinologist in charge of the patient.

Insulin therapy is the method of choice for glycemic control in hospitalized patients with hyperglycemia. The institutional protocol recommends the discontinuation of antidiabetic drugs for most patients upon hospital admission for acute illness. Patients with type 1 or 2 diabetes receiving insulin as multiple daily injections require treatment with basal-bolus insulin regimens, and their insulin doses are modified according to the patient's clinical status.

In noncritical care patients, the glycemic targets set by the institutional protocol are < 140 mg/dL before meals and < 180 mg/dL for random glucose measurements. In patients with terminal illness and/or limited life expectancy, the glycemic target is < 180 mg/dL. In noncritical care patients, POCTs are performed based on the timing of the meals: before meals in patients receiving an oral diet, every 6 hours in those with continuous enteral or parenteral nutrition, and every 4 hours in patients not receiving diet. Patients with hyperglycemia (glucose level ≥ 200 mg/dL) undergo more frequent glucose measurements for detection and treatment of hyperglycemia, prevention of hypoglycemia following supplemental insulin administration, and prevention of glycemic variability. The protocol recommends a basal-bolus insulin regimen, including a basal component with a long-acting insulin analogue (glargine or detemir) or intermediate-acting insulin (NPH) once or twice daily, and a bolus component with ultra-rapid-acting insulin (lispro) administered according to meals and supplemental doses according to glycemic levels. Ultra-rapid insulin analogues are the insulin of choice for the bolus component of the regimen at our institution, based on evidence in the literature showing better glycemic control in hospitalized patients with this type of insulin when compared with regular insulin, with a lower number of hypoglycemic episodes (24). The total dose of insulin administered is individualized and based on the patient's previous insulin regimen, glycemic levels, total body weight, clinical status, and nutritional therapy. Basal insulin is administered to all patients with previous insulin regimens and in those with sustained hyperglycemia. In insulin-naïve patients, the recommended initial total daily insulin dose is 0.2-0.5 U/kg/day, with approximately 50% of the dose administered as basal insulin (preferably glargine) and the remainder as bolus insulin. Bolus insulin contemplates the patient's diet and carbohydrate intake, as follows: bolus insulin before meals in patients on an oral diet, every 6 hours in those on continuous enteral or parenteral nutrition therapy, and 3 to 4 times a day before meals in patients receiving cyclic enteral nutrition. The supplemental component of bolus insulin is administered according to the patient's glucose level. Our institution has five different supplemental insulin regimens: (i) usual insulin dose; (ii) reduced insulin dose, recommended for patients at risk for hypoglycemia; (iii) increased insulin dose, recommended for patients with insulin resistance; (iv) a regimen for patients with terminal illness and/or limited life expectancy; and (v) a regimen for patients with no oral or enteral nutritional therapy (fasting).

For critical care patients, blood glucose levels are measured at one-hour intervals. Insulin therapy is started in critically ill patients with sustained hyperglycemia, defined as at least two glucose measurements ≥ 180 mg/dL, using continuous intravenous regular insulin infusion. In patients with continuous intravenous insulin infusion, the glycemic targets are 140-180 mg/dL, and glucose levels < 100 mg/dL should be avoided. Insulin infusion is adjusted every hour according to glucose levels. The continuous intravenous insulin infusion protocol used at the institution was adapted from the Yale Insulin Infusion Protocol for critically ill patients, as previously described (23).

Multidisciplinary glycemic control team

A multidisciplinary glycemic control team was created at our institution in June 2014. The main goal of its implementation was to develop a centralized multidisciplinary team to address barriers to achieving glycemic control in the hospital setting. The team is chaired by an endocrinologist and includes physicians (endocrinologist, intensivists, hospitalists, and house staff), nurse practitioners, pharmacists, dietitians, and POCT/laboratory medicine specialists. The team aims at promoting the correct implementation of protocols for management of hyperglycemia and hypoglycemia, educating physicians and nurses on the proper use of these protocols, performing continuous education of health care professionals, promoting clinical decision aids, and surveilling performance measures for quality improvement. The members of the team deliberate on regular monthly meetings and on a daily basis during continuous patient care.

Education programs for hospital personnel

The educational programs for hospital personnel are delivered on a regular basis and include the participation of nurses, house staff, physicians, pharmacists, and dietitians. Educational sessions are often offered in the hospital at different time periods to ensure delivery to as many staff members as possible. All staff members (physicians, nurses, pharmacists, and dietitians) are exposed to the educational program upon joining the hospital staff. Regular educational sessions are delivered at different hospital units (a total of 10 units) at a maximum interval of 6 months. Once weekly, the endocrinologist in charge delivers educational orientation to staff members during patient care (on-site training).

The main aspects outlined in these educational programs include the impact of inpatient glycemic control on patient care, introduction and reinforcement of protocols for management of hyperglycemia and hypoglycemia, information about patients at risk for hypoglycemia and hyperglycemia, identification of signs of hypoglycemia, characteristics of the different types of insulin and administration routes (intravenous or subcutaneous for basal insulin administration, prandial or correction doses), a review of insulin requirements during health and illness, inpatient use of antihyperglycemic agents, the influence of diet, the importance of respecting the appropriate time of glucose measurement, and proper documentation of patient treatment.

Glucose monitoring by point-of-care testing

Glucose monitoring by POCT was performed with the glucometers Precision Xceed Pro (PXP)® and FreeStyle Precision Pro (FSPP)® (Abbott Diabetes Care Inc., Alameda, CA, USA). In noncritical patients, glycemic measurements with POCT used capillary blood samples obtained by fingertip puncture after local hygiene, while in critical patients, venous or arterial blood samples were used instead. The same type of blood source was used in each patient according to his or her clinical status. Areas with edema, lesions, hypoperfusion, and/or venous infusion routes with continuous infusion of solutions were avoided during blood drawing.

The glucometers underwent continuous quality control. All devices were calibrated every 24 hours with high and low glucose control samples; when calibration was not performed in 24 hours, the glucometer was automatically blocked from use or for POCT. All glucometers underwent a harmonization process every 6 months, consisting on a comparison of the results obtained by POCT with those obtained by the laboratory (Dimension®, Siemens Healthcare Diagnostics, Deerfield, IL, USA). During the study, the variation coefficient between the results obtained by the POCT and those by the laboratory was < 10.78% in all glucometers, which is aligned with standards of care (31).

Glycemic control quality indicators

Since the MGCP implementation, quality indicators of glycemic control, hypoglycemia, and hyperglycemia were monthly assessed using data from the POCTs. All results obtained by POCT were electronically downloaded directly from Abbott's Precision® glucometer to the software using the Abbott Precision Web System (Abbott Diabetes Care Inc., Alameda, CA, USA) and to the patient's electronic medical records, providing accurate data for the indicators. Calculation of the rates of hyperglycemia and hypoglycemia were as follows: (i) hyperglycemia (≥ 180 mg/dL) as the number of glucose measurements by POCT ≥ 180 mg/dL (numerator) divided by the total number of glucose measurements by POCT performed in that given period (denominator), (ii) severe hyperglycemia (≥ 300 mg/dL) as the number of glucose measurements by POCT ≥ 300 mg/dL (numerator) divided by the total number of glucose measurements by POCT performed in the period (denominator), (iii) hypoglycemia (≤ 70 mg/dL) as the number of glycemic measurement by POCT ≤ 70 mg/dL (numerator) divided by the total number of glycemic measurement by POCT performed in the period (denominator), (iv) severe hypoglycemia (≤ 40 mg/dL) as the number of glycemic measurement by POCT ≤ 40 mg/dL (numerator) divided by the total number of glycemic measurement by POCT performed in the period (denominator).

Adherence to the institutional inpatient glycemic protocols was measured regularly by a revision of the patient's prescriptions and medical records.

Data collection

We performed a retrospective analysis of the medical records of the patients admitted to the hospital. We analyzed the data obtained in May 2014, before the MGCP implementation, and in June 2015 and May 2017, after the MGCP implementation.

The inclusion criteria were all critical and noncritical patients admitted to the hospital, aged ≥ 18 years, who had blood glucose measured by POCT by Abbott's Precision® glucometer according to the institutional protocol, and a length of stay ≥ 2 days. The exclusion criteria were age < 18 years, length of stay shorter than 2 days, and admissions limited to the emergency room or to the day-clinic unit. We also excluded the results of POCT glucose monitoring obtained during surgical procedures.

We analyzed the quality indicators of glycemic control and the results of glucose monitoring obtained by POCT before the implementation of the MGCP in May 2014 and after the implementation of the MGCP in June 2015 and May 2017. Based on blood glucose levels, the patients were characterized as having hyperglycemia (≥ 180 mg/dL), severe hyperglycemia (≥ 300 mg/dL), hypoglycemia (≤ 70 mg/dL), or severe hypoglycemia (≤ 40 mg/dL). The rates of hyperglycemia (≥ 180 mg/dL), severe hyperglycemia

(≥ 300 mg/dL), hypoglycemia (≤ 70 mg/dL), and severe hypoglycemia (≤ 40 mg/dL) were calculated as described above.

Adherence to the institutional inpatient glycemic protocols was also analyzed by a revision of the patients' prescriptions and medical records in May 2014, June 2015, and May 2017. A prescription was considered to be not compliant to the institutional protocols if inadequate to the diet or clinical scenario. Inadequacy with the diet was present when the prescription was not conformed with the type of diet (*i.e.*, oral, enteral, and parenteral diets, or fasting), not coordinated with the POCT, or when insulin was not administered around mealtime. Inadequacy with the clinical scenario occurred when the insulin prescribed was not suitable for the patient's clinical status according to the institutional protocol (*i.e.*, intravenous insulin for critical patients, subcutaneous insulin for noncritical patients, basal-bolus insulin regimen for noncritical patients with sustained hyperglycemia and/or previous use of a basal-bolus insulin regimen, or supplemental subcutaneous insulin for noncritical patients in accordance to patients characteristics (usual insulin dose, risk of hypoglycemia, insulin resistance, terminal illness, and/or limited life expectancy).

The local institutional ethics committee approved the study.

Statistical analysis

Continuous data are presented as mean and standard deviation values or median values and range. Comparisons of categorical variables were performed with the Fisher's exact or chi-square test, while continuous variables were compared using Student's t test.

The statistical analyses were performed with the software programs SPSS, version 20 (SPSS Inc., Chicago, IL, USA), Minitab 16, and Excel Office 2010. Statistical significance was set at $p < 0.05$.

RESULTS

The clinical characteristics of the hospitalized patients undergoing glucose monitoring in May 2014, June 2015, and May 2017 are described in Table 1. The groups had comparable baseline clinical characteristics except for age, which differed among the groups.

We analyzed 6888, 7290, and 7669 POCTs from 389, 545, and 475 patients in May 2014, June 2015, and May 2017, respectively. The mean number of glucose measurements per patient was 2.39 ± 1.96, 2.39 ± 2.26, and 3.64 ± 2.76 in May 2014, June 2015, and May 2017, respectively. There was a significant increase in glucose monitoring from May 2014 to May 2017 ($p = 0.007$), but no differences between May 2014 and June 2015 ($p = 0.99$).

Table 2 describes the quality indicators of inpatient glycemic control. In May 2014, June 2015, and May 2017, the rates were 23.5%, 19.6%, and 19.3%, respectively, for hyperglycemia (≥ 180 mg/dL; $p < 0.001$), and 2.5%, 2.2%, and 1.8%, respectively, for severe hyperglycemia (≥ 300 mg/dL; $p = 0.003$).

Table 1. Baseline clinical characteristics of hospitalized patients with glucose measured by point-of-care testing (POCT)

	May 2014	June 2015	May 2017	p value
Number of patients undergoing POCT	389	545	475	
Age (years)	72.7 ± 16.6	73.0 ± 16.2	75.6 ± 14.6	0.04*
Admission				
Clinical patients	80.8%	83.9%	78.5%	0.086
Surgical patients	19.2%	16.1%	21.5%	
Patients' characteristics at admission				
Critical care	10.4%	13.4%	9.7%	0.141
Noncritical care	89.6%	86.6%	90.3%	
Diabetes mellitus	33.7%	30.4%	35.1%	0.176
Rate of hyperglycemia (≥ 180 mg/dL) on admission	22.1%	18.9%	19.6%	0.465
Length of stay (days)	5 (2-919)	5 (2-919)	5 (2-967)	0.98
Intravenous insulin protocol	7.3%	8.8%	6.5%	0.371

Data are expressed as mean ± standard deviation, mean (range), or percentage. * Statistically significant ($p < 0.05$).

The rates of hyperglycemia (≥ 180 mg/dL) reduced significantly from May 2014 to June 2015 (16.3%, $p < 0.001$) and from May 2014 to May 2017 (17.8%, $p < 0.001$). Similarly, the rates of severe hyperglycemia (≥ 300 mg/dL) reduced statistically significantly from May 2014 to May 2017 (28.5%, $p = 0.003$), but were non-statistically significant between May 2014 and June 2015 (13.6%, $p = 0.175$) (Figures 1 and 2).

There was no statistically significant change in hypoglycemic parameters over time (Table 2). Rates of hypoglycemia (≤ 70 mg/dL) were 0.9%, 1.8%, and 1.0% in May 2014, June 2015, and May 2017, respectively ($p = 0.710$), while the rates of severe hypoglycemia (≤ 40 mg/dL) showed a non-statistically significant decrease of 34.3% from May 2014 to May 2017 ($p = 0.336$).

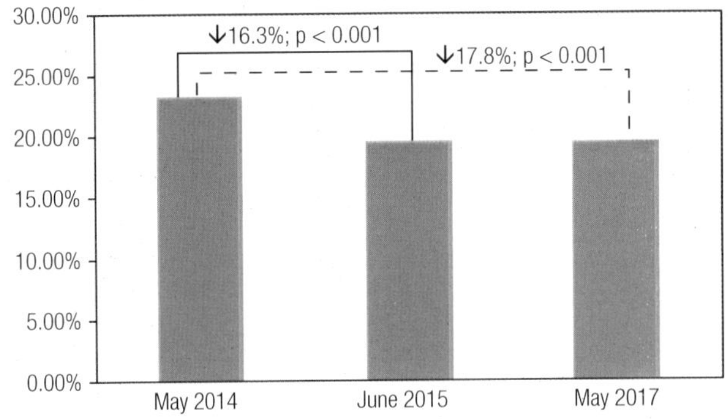

Figure 1. Rates of hyperglycemia (≥ 180 mg/dL) in hospitalized patients in May 2014, June 2015, and May 2017.

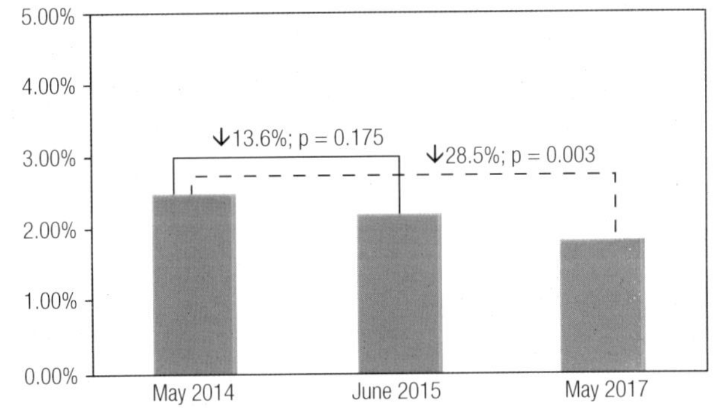

Figure 2. Rates of severe hyperglycemia (≥ 300 mg/dL) among hospitalized patients in May 2014, June 2015, and May 2017.

Table 3 describes the rates of adherence to the institutional inpatient glycemic protocols. Adherence to the protocol improved over time. The proportion of prescriptions not compliant with the institutional protocols decreased from 34.2% in May 2014 to 10.1% in June 2015, and 7.5% in May 2017 ($p < 0.001$). We found significant decreases in diet and clinical scenario inadequacies over time from May 2014 to May 2017.

DISCUSSION

The implementation of an inpatient multidisciplinary glucose control management program (MGCP) had a positive impact on glycemic control in hospitalized patients at our center. We observed that the key elements for this achievement were the implementation

Table 3. Rates of adherence to the institutional inpatient glycemic protocols

	May 2014	June 2015	May 2017	p value
Prescriptions not compliant with the institutional protocols	34.2%	10.1%	7.5%	< 0.001*
Noncompliance with clinical scenario	20.0%	6.3%	5.2%	0.026*
Noncompliance with diet	17.4%	3.8%	2.5%	0.006*

Data are expressed as percentage. * Statistically significant ($p < 0.05$).

Table 2. Quality indicators of inpatient glycemic control

	May 2014	June 2015	May 2017	p value
Number of patients undergoing POCT	389	545	475	-
Number of glucose readings with POCT	6888	7290	7669	-
Glucose level – mean (SD) (mg/dL)	158.9 ± 60.7	150.5 ± 59.1	150.3 ± 57.8	< 0.001*
Glucose level – median (IQR) (mg/dL)	147.0 (118-188)	138.0 (1120-177)	137.0 (109-178)	< 0.001*
Rate of severe hypoglycemia (≤ 40 mg/dL)	0.2% (n = 12)	0.1% (n = 7)	0.1% (n = 9)	0.336
Rate of hypoglycemia (≤ 70 mg/dL)	0.9% (n = 65)	1.8% (n = 129)	1.0% (n = 79)	0.710
Rate of hyperglycemia (≥ 180 mg/dL)	23.5% (n = 1620)	19.6% (n = 1428)	19.3% (n = 1521)	< 0.001*
Rate of severe hyperglycemia (≥ 300 mg/dL)	2.5% (n = 175)	2.2% (n = 160)	1.8% (n = 143)	0.003*

SD: standard deviation; IQR: interquartile range; POCT: point-of-care testing. * Statistically significant ($p < 0.05$).

of institutional inpatient glycemic control protocols, establishment of a multidisciplinary glycemic control team, and continuous educational programs for hospital personnel. Altogether, these actions resulted in a significant reduction in hyperglycemic events and improved safety among inpatients.

The development of institutional inpatient glycemic control protocols was important in guiding initial management, clinical decisions, and prescriptions at our center. With the protocols, we were able to standardize our policies and the patients' glycemic control. Since the implementation of the institutional protocols, different educational programs were delivered for hospital staff training. These protocols need to be constantly reevaluated and updated based on newly available evidence in the literature and on local demands of patient care. Other centers have described similar improvements in clinical outcomes with the adoption of insulin protocols for glucose management in critical and noncritical patients (17,18,23,29,30,31-33).

Considered alone, the implementation of the institutional inpatient glycemic control was probably not enough to improve the process of care. The protocol was implemented in January 2012, and in May 2014, we observed that a great proportion of the prescriptions were still not compliant to the protocol. We then hypothesized that the staff education programs should be optimized and further actions should be taken, including the implementation of a multidisciplinary glycemic control team and the dissemination of quality indicators of glucose control. Indeed, we found that the implementation of hospital-wide glucose policies was best facilitated by targeted educational programs and clinical decision support infrastructure to facilitate acceptance by the hospital personnel. We then observed a significantly increased adherence to the institutional inpatient glycemic control protocols over time, accompanied by improved quality indicators of glycemic control in June 2015 and May 2017.

The establishment of a centralized multidisciplinary glycemic control team was a core and critical element in the development of our inpatient glucose management program. Through regularly scheduled monthly meetings and a culture of collaboration and teamwork, the members of the team promoted the implementation of protocols, education interventions, clinical decision aids, performance measures, and quality indicators of glycemic control across continuous inpatient care. In fact, we observed significant reductions of 17.8% in the rate of hyperglycemia (≥ 180 mg/dL) and 28.5% in the rate of severe hyperglycemia (≥ 300 mg/dL) from May 2014 to May 2017, before and after the implementation of the multidisciplinary glycemic control team, respectively. These reductions in hyperglycemic events were already observed one year before (in June 2015), and improved even further in May 2017, suggesting a continuous improvement in patient care and quality outcomes.

Our educational programs focused on the major challenges to optimal glucose management. Similar to other centers, the main obstacles we encountered included unanticipated nutritional changes, poor coordination of the POCT with the administration of insulin around mealtime, unanticipated changes in clinical status or medications, use of medications associated with increased insulin resistance (such as glucocorticoids, often in variable and changing doses), failure by clinicians of making adjustments in glycemic therapy based on daily blood glucose patterns, prolonged use of sliding scale insulin as monotherapy, multiple system/organizational barriers such as lack of communication and/or deficient knowledge of diabetes management among providers and caregivers (7,29,30,32,33). Notably, we demonstrated that a collaborative work of the nurses, dietitians, and physicians reduced the inadequacy of the prescription with the type of diet and improved the coordination of POCT and administration of insulin around mealtime.

The impact of the MGCP on hypoglycemic events in inpatients was less established. We observed a nonsignificant 34.3% reduction in the rate of severe hypoglycemia (≤ 40 mg/dL), which might be due to the low rate of such event at our center. The rates of hypoglycemia (≤ 70 mg/dL) were similar over time. Hypoglycemia is a possible unwanted consequence of improved control of hyperglycemia and may be associated with increased morbidity (3-5,21). Therefore, our results of reduced hyperglycemia without increased hypoglycemic events demonstrate that our institutional protocols were safe. Indeed, it has been demonstrated that the implementation of standardized insulin order sets with less strict glycemic targets and frequent glucose monitorization are associated with better glycemic control and produce expected benefits in terms of patient safety across different hospitals (18,23,25,29,30,32,33).

Our study has limitations inherent to its retrospective, nonrandomized design and the absence of a concurrent control group. This study was intended to evaluate intermediary outcomes as a quality improvement for hospitalized patients, and we did not evaluate morbidity, mortality, or other important clinical outcome data other than the rates of hyperglycemia and hypoglycemia. Another limitation regarding the analysis of the glycemic data was the potential for an increased type I error (*i.e.*, a false-positive result) due to clustering of POCT values within patients and increased monitoring frequency upon observation of a hyperglycemic event. Indeed, the number of glucose monitoring tests among patients with normal glucose values may affect the proportion of abnormal values. Nevertheless, according to our institutional protocol, patients with hyperglycemia have more frequent POCT than those with normal glucose values.

Finally, despite the decrease in hyperglycemia rates, they still require further reduction, and efforts will be made for this purpose. Despite the fact that our quality indicators of glycemic control seem to be aligned with those of other hospitals, hyperglycemia in hospitalized patients is still frequently observed (34). The creation of a national benchmarking process would be important for the development of best practices and improved management of inpatient hyperglycemia (35).

In conclusion, the implementation of an inpatient multidisciplinary glucose control management program at our center was associated with improved care process and clinical outcomes, demonstrated by continued reductions in rates of hyperglycemic events. The key elements for these achievements were the development of institutional inpatient glycemic control protocols, establishment of a multidisciplinary team, and continuing educational programs for hospital personnel. Therefore, our results suggest that an inpatient multidisciplinary glucose control management program increased the awareness of the value of treating hyperglycemia in hospitalized patients, representing an important feature for inpatient safety and quality improvement.

Acknowledgments: the authors are grateful to Antonio Sérgio Cordeiro da Rocha, Plinio Nascimento Gomes, Graziela Mendonça, Robertta Mendonça Macedo Pinheiro, Tatiana de Jesus Pereira, Monica Cabral, and Andrea Medeiros for their important assistance and skillful advice.

REFERENCES

1. Inzucchi SE. Management of hyperglycemia in the hospital setting. N Engl J Med. 2006;355:1903-11.
2. ACE/ADA Task Force on Inpatient Diabetes. American College of Endocrinology and American Diabetes Association consensus statement on inpatient diabetes and glycemic control. Endocr Pract. 2006;12:458-68.
3. Moghissi ES, Korytkowski MT, DiNardo M, Einhorn D, Hellman R, Hirsch IB, et al. American Association of Clinical Endocrinologists; American Diabetes Association. American Association of Clinical Endocrinologists and American Diabetes Association consensus statement on inpatient glycemic control. Diabetes Care. 2009;32:1119-31.
4. Umpierrez GE, Hellman R, Korytkowski MT, Kosiborod M, Maynard GA, Montori VM, et al. Management of hyperglycemia in hospitalized patients in non- critical care setting: an Endocrine Society Clinical Practice Guideline. J Clin Endocrinol Metab. 2012;97:16-38.
5. Controle da glicemia no paciente hospitalizado. Posicionamento oficial da Sociedade Brasileira de Diabetes n° 3/2015. Available from: www.diabetes.org.br/profissionais.
6. Standards of Medical Care in Diabetes 2018. American Diabetes Association. Available from: http://care.diabetesjournals.org/content/41/Supplement_1.
7. Draznin B, Gilden J, Golden SH, Inzucchi SE; PRIDE investigators, Baldwin D, et al. Pathways to quality inpatient management of hyperglycemia and diabetes: a call to action. Diabetes Care. 2013;36:1807-14.
8. Krinsley JS. Association between hyperglycemia and increased hospital mortality in a heterogeneous population of critically ill patients. Mayo Clin Proc. 2003;78:1471-8.
9. Lipton JA, Barendse RJ, Van Domburg RT, Schinkel AF, Boersma H, Simoons MI, et al. Hyperglycemia at admission and during hospital stay are independent risk factors for mortality in high risk cardiac patients admitted to an intensive cardiac care unit. Eur Heart J Acute Cardiovasc Care. 2013;2:306-13.
10. Fuentes B, Castillo J, San José B, Leira R, Serena J, Vivancos J, et al.; Stroke Project of the Cerebrovascular Diseases Study Group, Spanish Society of Neurology. The prognostic value of capillary glucose levels in acute stroke: the Glycemia in Acute Stroke (GLIAS) study. Stroke. 2009;40:562-8.
11. Capes SE, Hunt D, Malmberg K, Gerstein HC. Stress hyperglycaemia and increased risk of death after myocardial infarction in patients with and without diabetes: a systematic overview. Lancet. 2000;355:773-8.
12. McAlister FA, Majumdar SR, Blitz S, Rowe BH, Romney J, Marrie TJ. The relation between hyperglycemia and outcomes in 2,471 patients admitted to the hospital with community-acquired pneumonia. Diabetes Care. 2005;28:810-5.
13. Egi M, Bellomo R, Stachowski E, French CJ, Hart G. Variability of blood glucose concentration and short-term mortality in critically ill patients. Anesthesiology. 2006;105:244-52.
14. Krinsley JS. Glycemic variability and mortality in critically ill patients: the impact of diabetes. J Diabetes Sci Technol. 2009;3:1292-301.
15. Malmberg K, Norhammar A, Wedel H, Ryden L. Glycometabolic state at admission: important risk marker of mortality in conventionally treated patients with diabetes mellitus and acute myocardial infarction: long-term results from the Diabetes and Insulin-Glucose Infusion in Acute Myocardial Infarction (DIGAMI) study. Circulation. 1999;99:2626-32.
16. Furnary AP, Zerr KJ, Grunkemeier GL, Starr A. Continuous intravenous insulin infusion reduces the incidence of deep sternal wound infection in diabetic patients after cardiac surgical procedures. Ann Thorac Surg. 1999;67:352-60.
17. van den Berghe G, Wouters P, Weekers F, Verwaest C, Bruyninckx F, Schetz M, et al. Intensive insulin therapy in critically ill patients. N Engl J Med. 2001;345:1359-67.
18. Krinsley JS. Effect of an intensive glucose management protocol on the mortality of critically ill patients. Mayo Clinic Proc. 2004;79: 992-1000.

19. Malmberg K, Rydén L, Wedel H, Birkeland K, Bootsma A, Dickstein K, et al. Intense metabolic control by means of insulin in patients with diabetes mellitus and acute myocardial infarction (DIGAMI 2): effects on mortality and morbidity. Eur Heart J. 2005;26:650-61.
20. Van den Berghe G, Wilmer A, Hermans G, Meersseman W, Wouters PJ, Milants I, et al. Intensive insulin therapy in the medical ICU. N Engl J Med. 2006;354:449-61.
21. The NICE-SUGAR Study Investigators. Intensive versus Conventional Glucose Control in Critically Ill Patients. N Engl J Med. 2009;360:1283-97.
22. Griesdale DE, de Souza RJ, van Dam RM, Heyland DK, Cook DJ, Malhotra A, et al. Intensive insulin therapy and mortality among critically ill patients: a meta-analysis including NICE-SUGAR study. CMJA. 2009;180:821-7.
23. Shetty S, Inzucchi SE, Goldberg PA, Cooper D, Siegel MD, Honiden S. Adapting to the new consensus guidelines for managing hyperglycemia during critical illness: the updated Yale insulin infusion protocol. Endocr Pract. 2012;18:363-70.
24. Ko KJ, Tomor V, Nathanson BH, Bouchard JR, Aagren M, Dubois RW. Does type of bolus insulin matter in the hospital? Retrospective cohort analysis of outcomes between patients receiving analogue versus human insulin. Clin Ther. 2010;32:1954-66.
25. Umpierrez GE, Smiley D, Zisman A, Prieto LM, Palacio A, Ceron M, et al. Randomized study of basal-bolus insulin therapy in the inpatient management of patients with type 2 diabetes (RABBIT 2 trial). Diabetes Care. 2007;30:2181-6.
26. Hirsch IB. Sliding Scale Insulin, Time to stop sliding. JAMA. 2009;301:213-4.
27. Egi M, Bellomo R. Reducing glycemic variability in intensive care unite patients: a new therapeutic target? J Diabetes Sci Tecnol. 2009;3:1302-8.
28. Krinsley S. Glycemic variability and mortality in critically ill patients: the impact of diabetes. J Diabetes Sci Technol. 2009;3(6):1292-301.
29. Maynard GA, Holdych J, Kendall H, Harrison K, Montgomery PA, Kulasa K. Improving glycemic control safely in critical care patients: a collaborative systems approach in nine hospitals. Endocr Pract. 2017;23:583-93.
30. Maynard GA, Childers D, Holdych J, Kendall H, Hoag T, Harrison K. Improving Glycemic Control Safely in Non-Critical Care Patients: A Collaborative Systems Approach in Nine Hospitals. Jt Comm J Qual Patient Saf 2017;43:179-88.
31. Diretrizes para a gestão e garantia de qualidade dos testes laboratoriais remotos da Sociedade Brasileira de Patologia Clínica/Medicina Laboratorial (SBPC/ML) 2a edição; 2016; Editora Manole Ltda.
32. Munoz M, Pronovost P, Dintzis J, Kemmerer T, Wang NY, Chang YT, et al. Implementing and evaluating a multicomponent inpatient diabetes management program. Jt Comm J Qual Patient Saf. 2012;38:195-206.
33. Hermayer KL, Cawley P, Arnold P, Sutton A, Crudup J, Kozlowski L, et al. Impact of improvement efforts on glycemic control and hypoglycemia at a university medical center. J Hosp Med. 2009;4:331-9.
34. Cook CB, Kongable GL, Potter DJ, Abad VJ, Leija DE, Anderson M, et al. Inpatient glucose control: a glycemic survey of 126 US hospitals. J Hosp Med. 2009;4:E7-E14.
35. Goldberg PA, Bozzo JE, Thomas PG, Mesmer MM, Sakharova OV, Radford MJ, et al. "Glucometrics": assessing the quality of inpatient glucose management. Diabetes Technol Ther. 2006;8:560-9.

Association between undercarboxylated osteocalcin, bone mineral density, and metabolic parameters in postmenopausal women

Leila C. B. Zanatta[1], Cesar L. Boguszewski[1], Victoria Z. C. Borba[1], Carolina A. Moreira[1,2]

[1] Divisão de Endocrinologia (SEMPR), Departamento de Medicina Interna, Universidade Federal do Paraná (UFPR), Curitiba, PR, Brasil
[2] Laboratório PRO, Seção de Histomorfometria Óssea, Fundação Pró-Renal, Curitiba, PR, Brasil

Correspondence to:
Carolina Aguiar Moreira
Medicina Interna,
Universidade Federal do Paraná
Av. Agostinho Leao Junior, 285
80030-110 – Curitiba, PR, Brasil
carolina.aguiar.moreira@gmail.com

ABSTRACT

Objective: Osteocalcin has been associated with several effects on energy and glucose metabolism. However, the physiological role of undercarboxylated osteocalcin (U-osc; the hormonally active isoform of osteocalcin) is still controversial. To correlate the serum levels of U-osc with bone mineral density (BMD) values and metabolic parameters in postmenopausal women. Subjects and methods: Cross-sectional study including 105 postmenopausal women (age 56.5 ± 6.1 years, body mass index [BMI] 28.2 ± 4.9 kg/m^2) grouped based on the presence of three or less, four, or five criteria of metabolic syndrome according to the International Diabetes Federation (IDF). The subjects underwent dual-energy x-ray absorptiometry (DXA) for the assessment of body composition and BMD and blood tests for the measurement of U-osc and bone-specific alkaline phosphatase (BSAP) levels. Results: The mean U-osc level was 3.1 ± 3.4 ng/mL (median 2.3 ng/mL, range 0.0-18.4 ng/mL) and the mean BSAP level was 12.9 ± 4.0 ng/mL (median 12.1 ng/mL, range 7.3-24.4 ng/mL). There were no associations between U-osc and BSAP levels with serum metabolic parameters. Lower fasting glucose levels were observed in participants with increased values of U-osc/femoral BMD ratio (3.61 ± 4 ng/mL versus 10.2 ± 1.6 ng/mL, $p = 0.036$). When the participants were stratified into tertiles according to the U-osc/femoral BMD and U-osc/lumbar BMD ratios, lower fasting glucose levels correlated with increased ratios ($p = 0.029$ and $p = 0.042$, respectively). Conclusion: Based on the ratio of U-osc to BMD, our study demonstrated an association between U-osc and glucose metabolism. However, no association was observed between U-osc and metabolic parameters. The U-osc/BMD ratio is an innovative way to correct the U-osc value for bone mass. Arch Endocrinol Metab. 2018;62(4):446-51

Keywords
Undercarboxylated osteocalcin; metabolic syndrome; glucose; energy metabolism; diabetes mellitus; bone mineral density

INTRODUCTION

Some studies over the past decade have shown that bone is associated with important physiologic mechanisms involving the control of energy metabolism and glucose homeostasis, attracting great interest in the understanding of the role of bone as an endocrine organ (1-9).

Osteocalcin is a protein produced by osteoblasts and present in two forms, carboxylated and undercarboxylated (U-osc). The carboxylated form is synthesized and stored in the mineral matrix, while U-osc is produced from the degradation of bone matrix and released into the circulation as a hormonally active isoform (2). U-osc has been shown to stimulate cell proliferation and increase insulin production. In addition, U-osc stimulates adiponectin expression in adipose cells, which in turn increases insulin sensitivity and energy metabolism (10). Insulin has direct participation in the process of decarboxylation of osteocalcin, allowing the formation and release of metabolically active U-osc (11). These actions together reveal a positive feedback mechanism involving pancreatic beta cells, adipose tissue, and bone.

Some epidemiological studies have supported the hypothesis of a positive effect of osteocalcin on glucose and energy metabolism (12-23). However, the association of these metabolic parameters with U-osc, in particular, remains elusive (24-36). Based on these facts, the aim of the present study was to correlate serum levels of U-osc and bone mineral density (BMD) with metabolic parameters in a group of healthy, postmenopausal women.

SUBJECTS AND METHODS

The recruitment for the study occurred between February 2012 and March 2013. The inclusion criteria comprised female gender, postmenopausal status (amenorrhea for more than 1 year), and age below 70 years. The exclusion criteria included diabetes mellitus; renal, hepatic or cardiac dysfunction; bone disease or secondary osteoporosis; cancer; and use of hypoglycemic agents, glucocorticoids, anticonvulsants or antiresorptive drugs.

A total of 180 women were evaluated. Of these, 35 were excluded due to a diagnosis of osteoporosis based on densitometric values and use of antiresorptive medications, 36 due to a diagnosis of diabetes, and 4 due to a diagnosis of cancer (Figure 1).

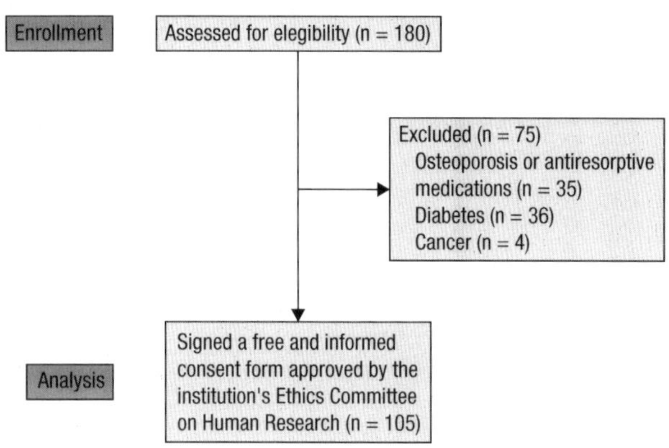

Figure 1. Study Flowchart.

All participants signed a consent form approved by the institution's Ethics Committee on Human Research.

The participants underwent a clinical evaluation and were classified according to clinical parameters, including body mass index (BMI), waist circumference, and blood pressure, which followed the 2005 classification of the International Diabetes Federation (IDF 2005) (37). Values of BMI were considered normal if between 18.5–24.99 kg/m^2, overweight if 25–29.99 kg/m^2, class I obese if 30-34.99 kg/m^2, class II obese if 35-39.99 kg/m^2, and class III obese if greater than 40 kg/m^2.

Blood samples were collected between 8:00 and 9:00 am after an 8-hour overnight fast. Levels of U-osc were measured with the Glu-OC EIA Kit (Takara Bio Inc., Otsu, Japan; reference values 0.25-8 ng/mL, intra-assay and interassay variations 4.4% and 5.67%, respectively). For this measurement, blood was collected in ice-cold tubes and immediately centrifuged in a cold centrifuge, and the serum was stored in cryotubes at -80°C. Levels of bone-specific alkaline phosphatase (BSAP, a specific marker of bone formation) were determined with the LIAISON® BAP OSTASE® assay (normal range 15-120 μg/dL, intra-assay variation 4.5%) simultaneously to those of U-osc in order to better evaluate the hormonal action of osteocalcin on bone metabolism.

Glucose was measured by a hexokinase/glucose-6-phosphate dehydrogenase method (normal values < 99 mg/dL) and insulin by chemiluminescence (normal values 2.5-30 μUI/mL). The homeostasis model assessment of insulin resistance (HOMA-IR) was used to measure insulin sensitivity using the following formula: (fasting glucose in mg/dL X fasting insulin in UI/mL) / 405 (38). The methods used to measure the remaining variables and their respective normal values are as follows: C-reactive protein (CRP) – turbidimetry (normal values < 0.5 mg/dL); high-density lipoprotein (HDL)-cholesterol – direct, homogeneous method (low values ≤ 40 mg/dL and high values ≥ 60 mg/dL); triglycerides (TG) – glycerol phosphate oxidase (optimal values < 150 mg/dL, borderline values 150-200 mg/dL, increased values > 200 mg/dL); creatinine – alkaline picrate method (normal values 0.57-1.11 mg/dL); calcium – Arsenazo III (normal values 8.6-10.3 mg/dL); phosphorus – UV phosphomolybdate (normal values 2.3-4.7 mg/dL); PTH – chemiluminescence (normal values 11.7-61.1 pg/mL); 25-hydrox yvitamin D3 – CLIA (normal values 30-100 ng/mL); alanine aminotransferase (ALT) and aspartate aminotransferase (AST) – colorimetric method (normal values 0-55 IU/L and 5-34 IU/L, respectively).

All patients were evaluated in regards to the presence of criteria for metabolic syndrome and grouped according to the number of criteria present as (A) three or fewer, (B) four, or (C) five. According to the IDF 2005 recommendations, the participants were deemed as having a normal waist circumference when this measurement was below 80 cm, and normal blood pressure when the values were below 130/85 mmHg. The finding of serum glucose levels below 100 mg/dL, TG below 150 mg/dL, and HDL-cholesterol above 50 mg/dL was also considered normal.

The participants were also evaluated and categorized according to parameters of body composition.

Measurements of lumbar spine (L1 to L4) and total femoral BMD, as well as those of body composition (percentage total fat), were performed with a properly calibrated Lunar Prodigy Advance (GE Healthcare, Madison, WI, USA), with a coefficient of variation of 2% and by the same examiner.

The ratios U-osc/lumbar BMD and U-osc/femoral BMD were calculated using absolute U-osc (ng/mL) values divided by the BMD observed in the lumbar and total femoral regions (g/m^2), respectively.

Statistical analysis

Serum U-osc and BSAP levels, as well as the ratios U-osc/femoral BMD and U-osc/lumbar BMD were compared with the following metabolic parameters: BMI, waist circumference, systolic and diastolic blood pressure, and total fat percentage assessed by dual-energy x-ray absorptiometry (DXA; total fat), TG, HDL-cholesterol, fasting glucose, insulin, HOMA-IR, and CRP. Levels of PTH, 25-hydroxyvitamin D3, calcium, inorganic phosphorus, albumin, AST, ALT, and creatinine were measured to exclude bone, kidney, and liver disease.

The data are described as mean and standard deviation values unless otherwise stated. The Mann-Whitney and Kruskal-Wallis tests were used for comparisons between groups. The chi-square test was used to estimate the association between U-osc categorized into tertiles and parameters of metabolic syndrome. Correlations between U-osc and the ratios U-osc/lumbar BMD and U-osc/femoral BMD with values of metabolic variables and BMD were estimated using Spearman's rank correlation coefficient. A p value below 0.05 was considered significant.

Table 1. Clinical characteristics and results of biochemical tests of 105 postmenopausal women included in the study

Variable	Mean	Median	SD	Range
Age (years)	56.5	56.0	6.1	43.0 - 70.0
BMI (kg/m²)	28.2	27.4	4.9	19.7 - 41.1
Waist circumference (cm)	91.7	90.0	11.3	66.0 - 122.0
Total body fat (%)	41.2	41.7	6.6	23.7 - 54.9
SBP (mmHg)	127.4	120	11.26	90 - 190
DPB (mmHg)	78.8	80	19.57	60 - 110
Triglycerides (mg/dL)	126.7	107.5	58.0	43.0 - 319.0
HDL-cholesterol (mg/dL)	47.8	46.0	12.3	29.0 - 100.0
Blood glucose (mg/dL)	92.7	91.0	10.6	65.0 - 126.0
Insulin (µUI/mL)	10.5	9.1	5.9	2.9 - 33.0
HOMA-IR	2.5	2.0	1.6	0.6 - 9.0
CRP (mg/dL)	0.53	0.33	0.71	0.33 - 6.73
25-hydroxyvitamin D3 (ng/mL)	21.1	20.7	7.0	7.5 - 55.0
U-Osc (ng/mL)	3.1	2.3	3.4	0.0 - 18.4
BSAP (µg/dL)	12.9	12.1	4.0	7.3 - 24.4

SD: standard deviation; BMI: body mass index; SBP: systolic blood pressure; DBP: diastolic blood pressure; HDL-cholesterol: high-density lipoprotein cholesterol; HOMA-IR: homeostasis model assessment of insulin resistance; CRP: C-reactive protein; U-Osc: undercarboxylated osteocalcin; BDAP: bone-specific alkaline phosphatase.

RESULTS

The clinical characteristics and results of biochemical tests of the study participants are summarized in Table 1. A total of 76 women (72.4%) presented three or fewer criteria for metabolic syndrome, while 18 (17.1%) had four criteria, and 11 (10.5%) had all five criteria for the syndrome. Osteopenia was observed in 57 (54%) participants, while osteoporosis was observed in 21 (20%) of them. When the participants were categorized according to BMI values, 26 (25%) had normal weight, 44 (42%) had overweight, 22 (21%) had class I obesity, and 13 (12%) had class II or III obesity. There were no significant correlations observed between U-osc levels and metabolic parameters, percent total fat, or CRP levels.

The median values of the ratio U-osc/femoral BMD were significantly different in participants with normal (< 99 mg/dL) compared with those with increased (≥ 100 mg/dL) blood glucose levels (2.6 mg/dL and 1.4 mg/dL, respectively, $p = 0.036$), as demonstrated in Figure 2.

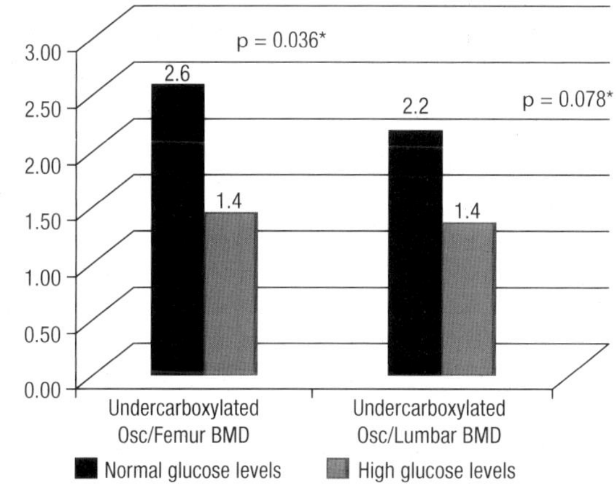

Figure 2. Relationship between the median values of the ratio undercarboxylated osteocalcin (U-osc)/lumbar body mineral density (BMD) and U-osc/femoral BMD with glucose levels in postmenopausal women.

Normal glucose values = below 99 mg/dL; high glucose values = equal to or above 100 mg/dL.

* Mann-Whitney test; $p < 0.05$.

When the ratios U-osc/lumbar BMD and U-osc/femoral BMD were categorized into tertiles, participants in the upper tertiles of both ratios had lower fasting glucose levels. Among participants with lumbar ratio values above 2.985 (ng.mL)/(g/m^2), only 12% presented increased glucose levels (p = 0.042) (Figure 3), while for those with femoral ratio values equal to or greater than 3.31 (ng/mL)/(g/m^2), only 10% had increased glucose levels (p = 0.029) (Figure 4).

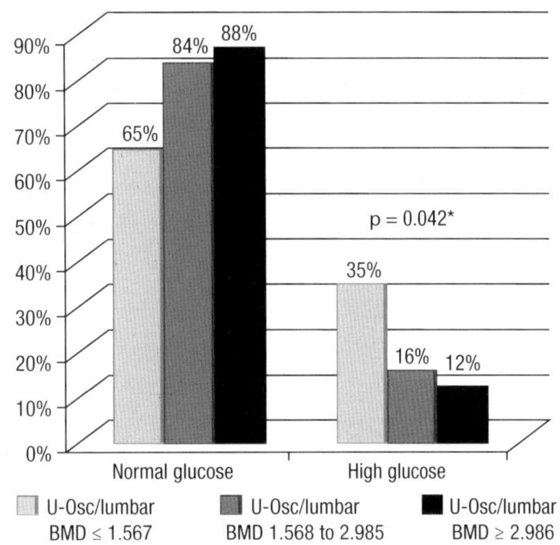

Figure 3. Percentage of women with ratios of undercarboxylated osteocalcin (U-osc)/lumbar body mineral density (BMD), categorized into tertiles according to blood glucose levels.

* Chi-square test; $p < 0.05$.

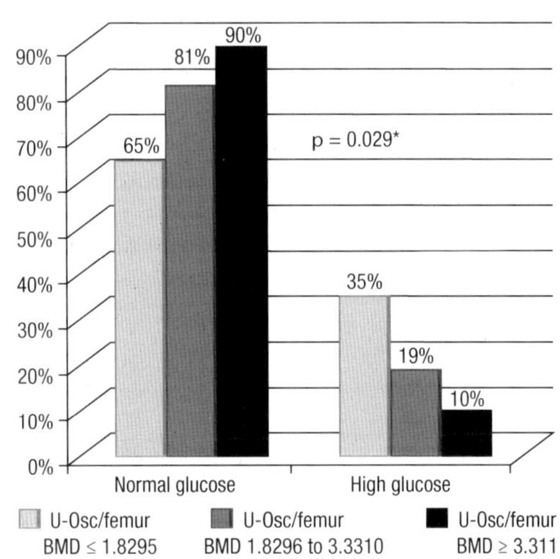

Figure 4. Percentage of women with ratios of undercarboxylated osteocalcin (U-osc)/femoral body mineral density (BMD) categorized into tertiles according to blood glucose levels.

* Chi-square test; $p < 0.05$.

No correlation was observed between U-osc and femoral or lumbar BMD values (r = 0.122, p = 0.218 and r = 0.058, p = 0.560, respectively). Similarly, the correlation between fasting glucose levels with femoral and lumbar BMD was not significant (r = 0131, p = 0.186 and r = 0.033, p = 0.737, respectively).

Levels of BSAP were not significantly associated with BMD values or metabolic parameters.

DISCUSSION

The results of this cross-sectional study show an inverse association between the ratio U-osc/femoral BMD with blood glucose levels, which was demonstrated by greater ratio values in the subgroup of patients with normal glucose levels. Similarly, when the ratios (lumbar and femoral) were stratified into tertiles, there was an inverse association of both ratios with blood glucose levels. The U-osc/BMD ratio is an innovative way to correct t U-osc values according to the patient's bone mass and was applied in this study in a similar way that leptin/fatty tissue ratio was applied in a study by Paz-Filho and cols. (39). Since osteocalcin is a specific bone protein that is increased in postmenopausal, resorptive conditions, we believe that the correction of osteocalcin values by the patient's BMD yields a more adjusted parameter of the involvement of bone on energy and glucose metabolism.

Similar results were not observed for BSAP, a marker exclusively related to bone and without metabolic effects. Additionally, no correlation of BMD values and U-osc or glucose alone was observed, which allows us to infer that these independent variables had no influence on osteocalcin values.

Similarly to our findings, Shea and cols. and Mori and cols. found no association between U-osc and indices of insulin resistance (30,31). Additionally, Kanazawa and cols. evaluated women with diabetes and found no association between U-osc and blood glucose parameters (25).

Another group of researchers found no association between metabolic syndrome and U-osc (32). Schafer and cols. reported that anabolic treatment for osteoporosis with PTH(1-84) increased U-osc levels, but showed no correlation with increased leptin levels (33).

It is important to point out that the studies focused on U-osc differ from those assessing total osteocalcin, which has been associated with metabolic and atherosclerotic parameters in diabetic and nondiabetic populations of both genders (12-23). An important limitation of studies with U-osc is a lack of homogeneity and specificity of commercially available assays to detect this specific osteocalcin isoform (34-36).

In contrast to our findings, Hwang and cols. found that tertiles of U-osc values had a significant inverse correlation with blood glucose levels and insulin sensitivity (24). Other authors have also shown an inverse association between U-osc levels and fasting glucose, HbA1c, total body, and visceral fat in 180 diabetic men (25). Diaz-Lopez and cols. found that lower levels of total osteocalcin and U-osc were independently associated with a higher risk of diabetes mellitus in individuals with increased cardiovascular risk (26). Pollock and cols. evaluated 140 children with and without prediabetes and observed that children with prediabetes had lower total osteocalcin and U-osc levels, along with worst indices of insulin secretion (27,28). Yeap and cols. showed that increased U-osc level was both a marker of bone turnover and an independent predictor of reduced diabetes risk. Additionally, the increased rate of bone remodeling in senescence could be associated with a reduced risk of diabetes mellitus (29).

The limitations of the present study include the small number of women with increased blood glucose levels (only 24 of the 105 participants), class II and III obesity (only 13 participants), and of those with all criteria for metabolic syndrome (11 participants). Physical activity (resistive or aerobic), which could influence U-osc levels and BMD values (42,43), was not considered in the statistical models. The oral glucose tolerance test and the hyperinsulinemic-euglycemic clamp, which are superior tests in evaluating insulin resistance compared with the HOMA-IR index, were not performed. The cross-sectional evaluation of this study does not allow us to infer a causal relationship between U-osc levels and metabolic parameters.

In conclusion, the results of this study show that the ratios U-osc/lumbar BMD and U-osc/femoral BMD had a significant inverse association with blood glucose levels in a group of nondiabetic, postmenopausal women. This finding reinforces the link between glucose and bone metabolism.

Acknowledgment: we thank SEMPR (Endocrinology Department) for excellent assistance during the studies. The authors wrote the manuscript and are responsible for its final content. All authors read and approved the final version of the manuscript.

REFERENCES

1. Clemens TL, Karsenty G. The osteoblast: an insulin target cell controlling glucose homeostasis. J Bone Miner Res. 2011;26(4): 677-80.
2. Lee NK, Sowa H, Hinoi E, Ferron M, Ahn JD, Confavreux C, et al. Endocrine regulation of energy metabolism by the skeleton. Cell. 2007;130(3):456-69.
3. Ducy P. The role of osteocalcin in the endocrine cross-talk between bone remodelling and energy metabolism. Diabetologia. 2011;54(6):1291-7.
4. Zanatta LC, Boguszewski CL, Borba VZ, Kulak CA. Osteocalcin, energy and glucose metabolism. Arq Bras Endocrinol Metabol. 2014l;58(5):444-51.
5. Crier PE. Glicemic and hipoglicemic homeostasis. In: Kronenberg HM, Melmed S, Polonsky KS, Larsen PR. Williams Textbook of Endocrinology, 11th ed. 2009. p. 1190-6.
6. Galic S, Oakhill JS, Steinberg GR. Adipose tissue as an endocrine organ. Mol Cell Endocrinol. 2010;316(2):129-39.
7. Ducy P, Amling M, Takeda S, Priemel M, Schilling AF, Beil FT, et al. Leptin inhibits bone formation through a hypothalamic relay: a central control of bone mass. Cell. 2000;100(2):197-207.
8. Cohen B, Novick D, Rubinstein M. Modulation of insulin activities by leptin. Science. 1996;274(5290):1185-8.
9. Ducy P, Desbois C, Boyce B, Pinero G, Story B, Dunstan C, et al. Increased bone formation in osteocalcin-deficient mice. Nature. 1996;382(6590):448-52.
10. Karsenty G, Oury F. The central regulation of bone mass, the first link between bone remodeling and energy metabolism. J Clin Endocrinol Metab. 2010;95(11):4795-801.
11. Lee NK, Karsenty G. Reciprocal regulation of bone and energy metabolism. Trends Endocrinol Metab. 2008;19(5):161-6.
12. Im JA, Yu BP, Jeon JY, Kim SH. Relationship between osteocalcin and glucose metabolism in postmenopausal women. Clin Chim Acta. 2008;396(1-2):66-9.
13. Kindblom JM, Ohlsson C, Ljunggren O, Karlsson MK, Tivesten A, Smith U. Plasma osteocalcin is inversely related to fat mass and plasma glucose in elderly Swedish men. J Bone Miner Res. 2009;24(5):785-91.
14. Pittas AG, Harris SS, Eliades M, Stark P, Dawson-Hughes B. Association between serum osteocalcin and markers of metabolic phenotype. J Clin Endocrinol Metab. 2009;94(3):827-32.
15. Yeap BB, Chubb SA, Flicker L, McCaul KA, Ebeling PR, Beilby JP, et al. Reduced serum total osteocalcin is associated with metabolic syndrome in older men via waist circumference, hyperglycemia, and triglyceride levels. Eur J Endocrinol. 2010;163(2):265-72.
16. Kanazawa I, Yamaguchi T, Yamamoto M, Yamauchi M, Kurioka S, Yano S, et al. Serum osteocalcin level is associated with glucose metabolism and atherosclerosis parameters in type 2 diabetes mellitus. J Clin Endocrinol Metab. 2009;94(1):45-9.
17. Goliasch G, Blessberger H, Azar D, Heinze G, Wojta J, Bieglmayer C, et al. Markers of bone metabolism in premature myocardial infarction (≤ 40 years of age). Bone. 2011;48(3):622-6.
18. Zhou M, Ma X, Li H, Pan X, Tang J, Gao Y, et al. Serum osteocalcin concentration in relation to glucose and lipid metabolism in Chinese individual. Eur J Endocrinol. 2009;161(5):723-9.
19. García-Martín A, Cortés-Berdonces M, Luque-Fernández I, Rozas-Moreno P, Quesada-Charneco M, Muñoz-Torres M. Osteocalcin as a marker of metabolic risk in healthy postmenopausal women. Menopause. 2011;18(5):537-41.
20. Fernández-Real JM, Izquierdo M, Ortega F, Gorostiaga E, Gómez-Ambrosi J, Moreno-Navarrete JM, et al. The relationship of serum osteocalcin concentration to insulin secretion, sensitivity,

and disposal with hypocaloric diet and resistance training. J Clin Endocrinol Metab. 2009;94(1):237-45.

21. Saleem U, Mosley Jr TH, Kullo IJ. Serum osteocalcin is associated with measures of insulin resistance, adipokine levels, and the presence of metabolic syndrome. Arterioscler Thromb Vasc Biol. 2010;30(7):1474-8.
22. Bao Y, Ma X, Yang R, Wang F, Hao Y, Dou J, et al. Inverse relationship between serum osteocalcin levels and visceral fat area in Chinese men. J Clin Endocrinol Metab. 2013;98(1):345-51.
23. Winhofer Y, Handisurya A, Tura A, Bittighofer C, Klein K, Schneider B, et al. Osteocalcin is related to enhanced insulin secretion in gestational diabetes mellitus. Diabetes Care. 2010;33(1):139-43.
24. Hwang Y-C, Jeong I-K, Ahn KJ, Chung HY. The uncarboxylated form of osteocalcin is associated with improved glucose tolerance and enhanced beta-cell function in middle-aged male subjects. Diabetes Metab Res Rev. 2009;25(8):768-72.
25. Kanazawa I, Yamaguchi T, Yamauchi M, Yamamoto M, Kurioka S, Yano S, et al. Serum undercarboxylated osteocalcin was inversely associated with plasma glucose level and fat mass in type 2 diabetes mellitus. Osteoporos Int. 2011;22(1):187-94.
26. Diaz-Lopez A, Bullo M, Juanola-Falgarona M, Martinez-Gonzalez MA, Estruch R, Covas M-I, et al. Reduced serum concentrations of carboxylated and undercarboxylated osteocalcin are associated with risk of developing type 2 diabetes mellitus in a high cardiovascular risk population: a nested case-control study. J Clin Endocrinol Metab. 2013;98(11):4524-31.
27. Pollock NK, Bernard PJ, Gower BA, Gundberg CM, Wenger K, Misra S. Lower uncarboxylated osteocalcin concentrations in children with prediabetes is associated with beta-cell function. J Clin Endocrinol Metab. 2011;96(7):E1092-9.
28. Reinehr T, Roth CL. A new link between skeleton, obesity and insulin resistance: relationships between osteocalcin, leptin and insulin resistance in obese children before and after weight loss. Int J Obes (Lond). 2010;34(5):852-8.
29. Yeap BB, Alfonso H, Chubb SA, Gauci R, Byrnes E, Beilby JP, et al. Higher serum undercarboxylated osteocalcin and other bone turnover markers are associated with reduced diabetes risk and lower estradiol concentrations in older men. J Clin Endocrinol Metab. 2015;100(1):63-71.
30. Shea MK, Gundberg CM, Meigs JB, Dallal GE, Saltzman E, Yoshida M, Jacques PF, Booth SL. Gamma-carboxylation of osteocalcin and insulin resistance in older men and women. Am J Clin Nutr. 2009;90(5):1230-5.
31. Mori K, Emoto M, Motoyama K, Lee E, Yamada S, Morioka T, et al. Undercarboxylated osteocalcin does not correlate with insulin resistance as assessed by euglycemic hyperinsulinemic clamp technique in patients with type 2 diabetes mellitus. Diabetol Metab Syndr. 2012;4(1):53.
32. Fodor D, Vesa S, Albu A, Simon S, Craciun A, Muntean L. The relationship between the metabolic syndrome and its components and bone status in postmenopausal women. Acta Physiol Hung. 2014;101(2):216-27.
33. Schafer AL, Sellmeyer DE, Schwartz AV, Rosen CJ, Vittinghoff E, Palermo L, et al. Change in undercarboxylated osteocalcin is associated with changes in body weight, fat mass, and adiponectin: parathyroid hormone (1-84) or alendronate therapy in postmenopausal women with osteoporosis (the PaTH study). J Clin Endocrinol Metab. 2011;96(12):E1982-9.
34. Vergnaud P, Garnero P, Meunier PJ, Bréart G, Kamihagi K, Delmas PD. Undercarboxylated osteocalcin measured with a specific immunoassay predicts hip fracture in elderly women: the EPIDOS Study. J Clin Endocrinol Metab. 1997;82(3):719-24.
35. Nimptsch K, Hailer S, Rohrmann S, Gedrich K, Wolfram G, Linseisen J. Determinants and correlates of serum undercarboxylated osteocalcin. Ann Nutr Metab. 2007;51(6):563-70.
36. Aonuma H, Miyakoshi N, Hongo M, Kasukawa Y, Shimada Y. Low serum levels of undercarboxylated osteocalcin in postmenopausal osteoporotic women receiving an inhibitor of bone resorption. Tohoku J Exp Med. 2009;218(3):201-5.
37. Alberti KG, Zimmet P, Shaw J; IDF Epidemiology Task Force Consensus Group. The metabolic syndrome – a new worldwide definition. Lancet. 2005;366(9491):1059-62.
38. Matthews DR, Hosker JP, Rudenski AS, Naylor BA, Treacher DF, Turner RC. Homeostasis model assessment: insulin resistance and beta-cell function from fasting plasma glucose and insulin concentrations in man. Diabetologia. 1985 Jul;28(7):412-9.
39. Paz-Filho GJ, Volaco A, Suplicy HL, Radominski RB, Boguszewski CL. Decrease in leptin production by the adipose tissue in obesity associated with severe metabolic syndrome. Arq Bras Endocrinol Metabol. 2009;53(9):1088-95.
40. Miura M. Biochemical markers of bone turnover. New aspect. An automated assay for measuring bone turnover markers. Clin Calcium. 2009;19(8):1160-9.
41. Szulc P, Chapuy MC, Meunier PJ, Delmas PD. Serum undercarboxylated osteocalcin is a marker of the risk of hip fracture in elderly women. J Clin Invest. 1993;91(4):1769-74.
42. Levinger I, Zebaze R, Jerums G, Hare DL, Selig S, Seeman E. The effect of acute exercise on undercarboxylated osteocalcin in obese men. Osteoporos Int. 2011;22(5):1621-6.
43. Pollock NK, Bernard PJ, Wenger K, Misra S, Gower BA, Allison JD, et al. Lower bone mass in prepubertal overweight children with prediabetes. J Bone Miner Res. 2010;25(12):2484-93.

Exercise training improves quality of life in women with subclinical hypothyroidism: a randomized clinical trial

Francisco Zacaron Werneck[1], Emerson Filipino Coelho[1], Saulo Peters Almas[2], Marília Mendes do Nascimento Garcia[3], Heloina Lamha Machado Bonfante[4], Jorge Roberto Perrout de Lima[3], Patrícia dos Santos Vigário[5], Míriam Raquel Meira Mainenti[6], Patrícia de Fátima dos Santos Teixeira[2], Mário Vaisman[2]

[1] Universaidade Federal de Ouro Preto (UFOP), Ouro Preto, MG, Brasil
[2] Universidade Federal do Rio de Janeiro (UFRJ), Rio de Janeiro, RJ, Brasil
[3] Universidade Federal de Juiz de Fora (UFJF), Juiz de Fora, MG, Brasil
[4] Faculdade de Ciências Médicas e da Saúde de Juiz de Fora (Suprema), Juiz de Fora, MG, Brasil
[5] Centro Universitário Augusto Motta (Unisuam), Rio de Janeiro, RJ, Brasil
[6] Escola de Educação Física do Exército (EsEFEx), Rio de Janeiro, RJ, Brasil

Correspondence to:
Francisco Zacaron Werneck
Rua Dr. Idolindo Daibert, 155/401
36037-320 – Juiz de Fora, MG, Brazil
fzacaron@oi.com.br

ABSTRACT

Objective: The aim was to evaluate the quality of life (HRQoL) in women with subclinical hypothyroidism (sHT) after 16 weeks of endurance training. Subjects and methods: In the first phase, a cross-sectional study was conducted in which 22 women with sHT (median age: 41.5 (interquartile range: 17.5) years, body mass index: 26.2 (8.7) kg/m^2, thyroid stimulating hormone > 4.94 mIU/L and free thyroxine between 0.8 and 1.3 ng/dL were compared to a group of 33 euthyroid women concerned to HRQoL. In the second phase, a randomized clinical trial was conducted where only women with sHT were randomly divided into two groups: sHT-Tr (n = 10) – participants that performed an exercise program – and sHT-Sed (n = 10) – controls. Exercise training consisted of 60 minutes of aerobic activities (bike and treadmill), three times a week, for 16 weeks. The HRQoL was assessed by the SF-36 questionnaire in the early and at the end of four months. Results: Women with sHT had lower scores on functional capacity domain in relation to the euthyroid ones (77.0 ± 23.0 *vs.* 88.8 ± 14.6; p = 0.020). The sHT-Tr group improved functional capacity, general health, emotional aspects, mental and physical component of HRQoL after training period, while the sHT-Sed group showed no significant changes. Conclusion: After 16 weeks of aerobic exercise training, there were remarkable improvements in HRQoL in women with sHT. Arch Endocrinol Metab. 2018;62(5):530-6

Keywords
Hypothyroidism; quality of life; exercise training; functional capacity

INTRODUCTION

Thyroid hormones (T_3 and T_4) act on most body cells, and changes in serum concentrations of these hormones cause impact on health of people (1). When thyroid hormones are normal and thyroid stimulating hormone (TSH) is above the reference values, subclinical hypothyroidism (sHT) is characterized (2). It is estimated that the prevalence of sHT in the general population is around 4% to 10%, which is higher among women (3).

The sHT patients may present signs and characteristic symptoms of hypothyroidism such as: fatigue, weight gain, dyslipidemia, psychological disorders, cardiovascular disorders, and increased risk of coronary artery disease and mortality (3,4). The effects of hypothyroidism on health related quality of life (HRQoL) are well established (5-7), but the results are controversial in sHT (3,4).

There is evidence that sHT is associated to worse scores in HRQoL domains such as: functional capacity, health perception, vitality and emotional aspects (6-8). In contrast, some studies do not support these findings (9-11). In part, the divergence of results can be explained by the degree of change in TSH levels. It seems that worse HRQoL are observed in patients with TSH higher than 10 mIU/L (2,6), although recent cross-sectional study has not confirmed this hypothesis (11).

Conventional treatment of sHT is done through hormone replacement with levothyroxine (**L-T_4**) that is associated with decreased clinical manifestations in various organs and systems (4,12). It is emphasized, however, that it has produced conflicting results in the improvement of HRQoL and at the symptoms of patients in different studies (8,13).

Exercise is associated to a better HRQoL in different populations (14,15). However, few studies have investigated the effects of exercise on HRQoL of patients with sHT (16). Thus, this study aimed at evaluating if exercise improves HRQoL in women with sHT. According to previous studies with subclinical disorders (16,17), exercise is taken as hypothesis that also improve HRQoL in sHT.

SUBJECTS AND METHODS

Subjects

A total of 55 female participants were included, aged 20-60 years old, which composed two study groups: sHT group is consisted of 22 women recruited in the Endocrinology Service of Hospital and Maternity Terezinha de Jesus of *Faculdade de Ciências Médicas e da Saúde de Juiz de Fora*, Brazil. The inclusion criteria for the sHT group were: show two doses, with a minimum interval of four weeks of serum TSH above the adopted reference upper limit (4.94 mIU/L) and level of T_{4L} within the reference range (0.70 to 1.48 ng/dL). The control group consisted of 33 euthyroid women with normal values of serum TSH, anti-TPO (anti-thyroid peroxidase antibody) and free T4 within the reference ranges for the used kits and absence of thyroid disease history. Others criteria adopted for both groups were: absence of comorbidities and no physical exercise program for at least three months. Patients with sHT or euthyroid participants with any chronic and/or cardiovascular disease, smokers, those who were using drugs or substances that could interfere in thyroid function, in heart rate or blood pressure, as well as those with musculoskeletal inability toperform physical exercises were excluded from the study. The study was approved by the local ethics committee (no. 0164/10), and all participating groups signed free informed term of consent prior to participation in the study.

Study design

Initially a cross sectional study comparing patients with sHT and euthyroid women concerned to signs and symptoms of hypothyroidism and HRQoL was performed. Subsequently, only sHT patients were randomized to participate or not in the exercise program. The patients were followed in both prospective study groups without masking. A resting echocardiography and exercise cardiopulmonary test were performed for clinical assessment of cardiac structure and cardiorespiratory function before the prospective phase. Two patients with severe changes in blood pressure and heart rate during the exercise test were excluded from randomization. Patients who participated in exercise training (n = 10) were denominated sHT-Tr, while those who did not participate in exercise training (n = 10) were denominated sHT-Sed. Exercise training consisted of aerobic activities, three times a week, for 16 weeks, supervised by the authors. The sHT-Sed patients were instructed for maintaining their usual daily life activities. After four months of intervention or observation, the tests conducted at the beginning of the study were repeated.

Hormonal measures, level of physical activity and anthropometric measures

The TSH, T_4L and anti-TPO levels were measured by third generation chemiluminescenceimmunometric assay (BeckmanCoulter®, Access2®). The reference values for TSH and free T_4 were 0.35 to 4.94 mUI/mL and 0.70 to 1.48 ng/dL, respectively. The anti-TPO levels > 35 UI/mL were considered positive. The level of physical activity was assessed using the Baecke's Habitual Physical Activity Questionnaire, in its translated version and validated for Portuguese (18). In anthropometric assessment, body mass and height (Filizola scale with 0.1 kg and 10 mm precision, respectively), in order to calculate the Body Mass Index (BMI; kg/m^2) were measured.

Signs and symptoms of hypothyroidism – Clinical score

The specific signals and symptoms of hypothyroidism were evaluated by Billewicz scale modified (19). The scale consists of 12 clinical signals and symptoms of hypothyroidism: dry skin, rough skin, decreased sweating, weight gain, paresthesia, hoarseness, decreased hearing, constipation, periorbital edema, slow movements, cold skin, and slow Achilles reflex. A point (1) was assigned when the presence of signal or symptoms or zero (0) in his absence was found.

The maximum scale score is 12 points; scores lower than 3 are expected in euthyroid women; among 3 and 5, in sHT; and higher than 5 in hypothyroidism.

Measure of health related quality of life

The SF-36 (Medical Outcomes Study 36 – Item Short-Form Health Survey) was used to assess the HRQoL of participants in their translated version and validated for Portuguese (20). The SF-36 is consisted of 36 items distributed in eight dimensions: functional capacity, physical aspects, pain, general health, vitality, social aspects, emotional aspects and mental health. The answers are presented in likert scale. The score of each domain ranges from 0 to 100 points and higher the score, higher HRQoL. The physical component was calculated by the average of the following scales: functional capacity, physical aspects, pain and general health; and the mental component: vitality, social aspects, emotional aspects and mental health.

Exercise program

The exercise program consisted of aerobic activities with supervision of a physical education professional, involved in the study. The frequency of training was three times a week for 16 weeks. Each aerobic exercise session consisted of 60 minutes, divided into four phases: heating (5 minutes), ergometric bicycle (25 minutes), treadmill (25 minutes) and resting (5 minutes). The training was individually prescribed based on exercise cardiopulmonary test and maximum heart rate estimated by age (HR_{max} = 220 - age). The training intensity was controlled by HR between 65 and 75% of HR_{max}. The training was continuous and participants could walk, walk with inclination or run in treadmill. The HR was monitored during training sessions by HR monitor (Polar®). Blood pressure and rate of perceived exertion were measured every 10 minutes. After exercise session, stretching exercises were performed by participants and also stimulated to drink fluids.

Statistical analysis

Descriptive analysis was presented as mean ± standard deviation or median (1st quartile, 3rd quartile). In the cross sectional study, comparisons between patients and euthyroid women were measured using Student's t tests or Mann-Whitney test. A two way repeated measures analysis of variance (ANOVA) (2X2) was performed to determine if significance differences between groups and time. If significant main effects or interactions were present a Bonferroni post hoc analysis was conducted. For the analysis of qualitative variables, Fisher's Exact Test was used. Relationship among quantitative variables was performed using Pearson's correlation test. As clinically relevant differences was considered the differences of at least 10 points on the scale of 0 to 100 (21). To assess the internal consistency of SF-36, the alpha Cronbach was used. All analyzes were carried out by using the statistical package SPSS 24.0 (IBM Corp., Armonk, NY). The significance level was set at $P < 0.05$.

RESULTS

Cross sectional study

The general characteristics and LQRH scores of women with sHT and euthyroid are shown in Table 1. In the sHT group, a total of 41% showed positive anti-TPO, while all euthyroid presented anti-TPO negative. There were no significant differences among groups regarding

Table 1. General characteristics and quality life scores of women with subclinical hypothyroidism (sHT) and euthyroid

	sHT (n = 22)	Euthyroid (n = 33)
Age (years)	39.4 ± 10.6	38.8 ± 8.7
TSH (mU/L)	5.58 (5.16–7.53)	2.10 (1.94–2.53)*
T_4 (ng/dL)	0.95 (0.85–1.03)	0.98 (0.94–1.00)
Body mass (kg)	69.3 ± 17.0	69.8 ± 11.8
BMI (kg/m²)	26.4 ± 5.5	26.3 ± 5.0
Level of physical activity	7.1 ± 0.9	8.3 ± 1.3*
Signals and symptoms	3.5 ± 1.6	2.5 ± 1.0*
Domains and scores of SF-36		
Functional capacity	77.0 ± 23.0	88.8 ± 14.6*
Limitation by physical aspects	67.0 ± 40.4	81.1 ± 33.1
Pain	68.0 ± 26.6	68.4 ± 23.7
General health	71.1 ± 16.3	72.5 ± 19.2
Vitality	53.6 ± 23.0	58.0 ± 24.5
Social aspects	73.3 ± 29.2	70.1 ± 27.0
Limitation by emotional aspects	56.1 ± 45.3	57.6 ± 44.3
Mental health	66.4 ± 20.9	65.3 ± 24.5
Physical component	70.8 ± 20.3	77.7 ± 18.0
Mental component	62.3 ± 26.3	62.8 ± 25.4

Values: Mean ± SD and Median (Interquartile Range).
TSH: thyrotropin; T_4: free thyroxine; BMI: body mass index; Level of physical activity measured by Baecke test; Signals and Symptoms of hypothyroidism measured by Zulewski test.
* Patients with sHT versus controls, significant difference $p < 0.05$.

the variable potentials of confounding age ($p = 0.85$), body mass ($p = 0.91$), BMI ($p = 0.94$) and menopause status ($p = 0.28$). The sHT patients showed lower levels of physical activity ($p < 0.001$) and higher number of signals and symptoms ($p = 0.02$). Regarding LQRH, sHT patients showed lower scores on "functional capacity" domain ($p = 0.02$) compared to euthyroid. In other domains there were no significant differences observed between groups, however women with sHT showed consistently lower scores, except in "social aspects". No relationship was found between TSH, signals and symptoms and life quality ($p > 0.05$). The internal consistency of 36 questions of SF-36 was satisfactory (Cronbach's alpha = 0.92). All domains also showed satisfactory coefficients (0.70 to 0.90). This means that the investigated sample reported high level of consistency in the answers to the survey questions.

Randomized clinical trial

After randomization, there were no significant differences between the sHT-Tr and sHT-Sed groups related to age ($p = 0.25$), TSH ($p = 0.85$), T4 ($p = 0.74$), body mass ($p = 0.35$), BMI ($p = 0.35$), level of physical activity ($p = 0.11$), signals and symptoms ($p = 0.53$), menopause and all domains of life quality life ($p > 0.05$).

Analyses revealed a significant (group x time) interaction effect concerned functional capacity, general health, emotional aspects, psychological component, and physical component (Table 2). The sHT-Tr group showed improvement in these domains. On the other hand, the sHT-Sed group after four months of observation, showed no significant changes in all domains assessed by SF-36. Both groups showed no significant changes in signals and symptoms number ($p > 0.05$).

DISCUSSION

This study compared the HRQoL of women with sHT and the euthyroid and assessed the impact of physical exercise on this outcome. The main findings were: 1) sHT is associated to a worse perception of HRQoL; 2) Women with sHT showed improvements in multiple assessed domains of HRQoL after aerobic exercise training during four months.

In the cross sectional study, it was found that patients with sHT showed more signals and symptoms and lower functional capacity compared to control euthyroid group, what has been mentioned previously in other studies (6-8). Besides that, in our study, there was a greater presence of signs and symptoms in sHT patients compared to the control group. Similar results were beforehand observed (13). Previously, a study reported that the presence of signals and symptoms of thyroid dysfunction may be related to decreased quality

Table 2. General characteristics and quality life scores of patients with subclinical hypothyroidism before and after 4 months of exercise training (sHT-Tr) or observation (sHT-Sed)

	sHT-Tr (n = 10)		sHT-Sed (n = 10)		Group effect	Time effect	Interaction
	Baseline	4 months	Baseline	4 months			
Signals and symptoms	3.8 ± 2.0	3.3 ± 1.6	3.1 ± 1.4	3.1 ± 2.0	0.53	0.50	0.50
Domains and components of SF-36							
Functional capacity	73.0 ± 26.4	86.5 ± 9.4	85.0 ± 11.5	82.0 ± 17.7	0.58	0.21	0.049*
Limitation by physical aspects	65.0 ± 42.8	92.5 ± 12.1	75.0 ± 37.3	67.5 ± 44.2	0.55	0.37	0.12
Pain	67.7 ± 29.3	71.7 ± 17.6	72.7 ± 24.7	68.8 ± 24.3	0.92	0.99	0.36
General health	68.1 ± 17.4	83.0 ± 13.9	75.0 ± 16.2	69.5 ± 18.0	0.61	0.22	0.01*
Vitality	53.0 ± 30.7	70.0 ± 19.4	56.0 ± 16.3	56.5 ± 22.0	0.57	0.07	0.08
Social aspects	75.0 ± 27.0	87.5 ± 14.4	80.0 ± 28.4	77.5 ± 25.5	0.80	0.30	0.13
Limitation by emotional aspects	43.3 ± 49.8	90.0 ± 22.5	76.7 ± 35.3	63.3 ± 39.9	0.81	0.12	0.01*
Mental health	64.4 ± 26.5	76.4 ± 17.4	68.8 ± 17.1	68.0 ± 22.4	0.82	0.13	0.08
Physical component	68.5 ± 25.7	83.4 ± 6.6	76.9 ± 12.9	72.0 ± 20.2	0.82	0.29	0.04*
Mental component	59.0 ± 30.6	81.0 ± 14.4	70.4 ± 20.9	66.4 ± 24.3	0.86	0.09	0.02*

Values: Mean ± SD.
TSH: thyrotropin; T_4: free thyroxine; BMI: body mass index; Level of physical activity measured by Baecke test; Signals and symptoms of hypothyroidism measured by Zulewski test.
* Significant difference $p < 0.05$, ANOVA 2x2.

of life (11). But it is difficult to distinguish sHT from the euthyroid only by signals and symptoms (22). This could explain the lack of difference in quality of life comparing these two groups in some studies (11).

Regarding the quality of life, there is controversy concerned to the results of studies involving patients with sHT (3). In our study, a worse quality of life in women with sHT was observed, mainly through the reduction of functional capacity compared to the euthyroid ones. Corroborating our results, there are studies that observed lower scores of functional capacity in women with sHT, associated with the worst perceptions of health, vitality and emotional aspects (6-8).

An earlier research found that patients with sHT showed lower scores in physical and psychological aspects and greater complaints related to fatigue, which cause damage to their daily activities (5). According to these authors, the decreased quality of life negatively influences mood and enhance anxiety and depression rates in sHT. In addition, studies showed lower functional capacity, general health and physical aspect (6) and worst health perception by patients with sHT, especially in the vitality factor, related to the psychological aspect (8). However, studies on Italy (9), Australia (10) and Netherlands (11) populations prove no worsening in quality of life in patients with sHT.

Studies have earlier identified worst quality of life in sHT (9,11). The results could be related not for disease diagnosis itself, but by the fact that patients are labeled as "sick" or their conscience are sick. Quality of life is a multidimensional and subjective construct, difficult for defining and systematization, which makes complex its operationalization (23). This, in part, could explain the divergent results reported in previous studies. Furthermore, another explanation would be no standardization of the criteria for assessing quality of life (24).

In the follow-up study, exercise training improves HRQoL after four months of intervention. There were increased domain scores for functional capacity, general aspects of health, emotional aspects and psychological and physical component. After 4 months of training, the patients had functional capacity values, general health, emotional aspects and higher mental and physical component of the normative values of Brazilian healthy women of the same age (25). Similar benefits were observed by other researchers (16), who conducted a study which evaluates the influence of a medium impact exercise program in relation to quality of life and cardiorespiratory fitness of women with sHT. Participants were subjected to a program that consisted of activity for 3 weekly sessions of 60 minutes during 12 weeks. After 12 weeks of intervention, women showed improvement in quality of life, through a higher score in most domains of SF-36, especially in relation to vitality, general health, social aspects of health and mental health. Furthermore, participants who were subjected to exercise program increased their cardiovascular fitness. In patients with subclinical hyperthyroidism it was found improvement in relation to the disease symptoms, especially in the perception of fatigue after 12 weeks of aerobic training (17).

It is unknown the actual mechanism responsible for the psychological effects of physical exercise, although it is recognized that it is an interaction of psychophysiological factors. In patients with coronary artery disease, for example, poor quality of life is associated to reduced exercise ability (14,15) and more tendency to fatigue (15). It is known that physical exercise is the main intervention used for physical fitness improvement and that it is positively related to quality of life (14,15,23,26). A systematic review to assess the association between physical activity and quality of life found that, in cross-sectional and longitudinal studies, the highest level of physical activity was related to a better perception of quality of life in apparently healthy adults or in different conditions of disease, regardless of sex (23). Moreover, a meta-analysis concluded that individuals with chronic diseases who received intervention to increase the level of physical activity improved their quality of life and that those who received supervised interventions showed the best result (24).

In clinical practice, the decision for whether or not treating the patient with sHT is connected to observed signals and symptoms, including patient complaints (3). Treatment with levothyroxine is generally associated with reduced pain, improvements in overall health and physical aspects (13), but not necessarily with better quality of life (27,28). In the present study, from the clinical point of view, the improvement observed in the quality of life of patients after physical training was moderate to high magnitude (> 10 points in SF-36 scales) (21). Thus, it is plausible to speculate that the improvement in the quality life of patients with sHT may be due to increased level of physical activity, physical fitness improvement and reduced signals and symptoms. Therefore, physical activity can be used as a strategy to improve health perception of these patients and should be encouraged by doctors and stimulate as a key element for the adoption of a healthy lifestyle for patients with sHT. Furthermore, the assessment of quality of life should be used in the diagnostic of these patients.

It is known that most patients with sHT tend to normalize spontaneously the TSH, especially those with TSH < 10 mIU/l. This normalization has no a well – defined pattern, although most patients may normalize their TSH levels between 6 and 18 months (29). In this same study, more than half of the patients had negative anti-TPO, and the changes in TSH were not correlated to the presence of anti-TPO (27). In this study, all patients practically showed TSH < 10 mIU/l. The effects of physical training on thyroid hormones are still a matter of debate in the literature and should be investigated in further studies. As limitations of the study, include the small sample size and the performed research only with women, not allowing, thus, expanding the results for male individuals.

In conclusion, the results suggest that women with subclinical hypothyroidism tend to have consistently lower scores on domains of quality of life compared to euthyroid women. However, physical exercise has been able to adjust these losses and therefore, should be encouraged in this group of patients. Further studies are necessary to better understand the optimal dose and the type of exercise would be more efficient to improve quality of life in women with sHT.

Acknowledgements: this study was funded by *Coordenação de Aperfeiçoamento de Pessoal de Nível Superior* (CAPES) and *Universidade Federal de Ouro Preto* (UFOP).

REFERENCES

1. Hoermann R, Midgley JEM, Larisch R, Dietrich JW. Recent advances in thyroid hormone regulation: toward a new paradigm for optimal diagnosis and treatment. Front Endocrinol (Lausanne). 2017;8:364.
2. Surks MI1, Ortiz E, Daniels GH, Sawin CT, Col NF, Cobin RH, et al. Subclinical thyroid disease: scientific review and guidelines for diagnosis and management. JAMA. 2004;291(2):228-38.
3. Sgarbi JA, Teixeira PFS, Maciel LMZ, Mazeto GMFS, Vaisman M, Montenegro Junior RM, et al. Consenso brasileiro para a abordagem clínica e tratamento do hipotireoidismo subclínico em adultos: recomendações do Departamento de Tireoide da Sociedade Brasileira de Endocrinologia e Metabologia. Arq Bras Endocrinol Metabol. 2013;57(3):166-83.
4. Cooper DS, Biondi B. Subclinical thyroid disease. Lancet. 2012;379(9821):1142-54.
5. Gulseren S, Gulseren L, Hekimsoy Z, Cetinay P, Ozen C, Tokatlioglu B. Depression, anxiety, health-related quality of life, and disability in patients with overt and subclinical thyroid dysfunction. Arch Med Res. 2006;37(1):133-9.
6. Vigário P, Teixeira P, Reuters V, Almeida C, Maia M, Silva M, et al. Perceived health status of women with overt and subclinical hypothyroidism. Med Princ Pract. 2009;18(4):317-22.
7. Vigário Pdos S, Vaisman F, Coeli CM, Ward L, Graf H, Carvalho G, et al. Inadequate levothyroxine replacement for primary hypothyroidism is associated with poor health-related quality of life-a Brazilian multicentre study. Endocrine. 2013;44(2):434-40.
8. Razvi S, McMillan CV, Weaver JU. Instruments used in measuring symptoms, health status and quality of life in hypothyroidism: a systematic qualitative review. Clin Endocrinol (Oxf). 2005;63(6):617-24.
9. Bianchi GP, Zaccheroni V, Solaroli E, Vescini F, Cerutti R, Zoli M, et al. Health-related quality of life in patients with thyroid disorders. Qual Life Res. 2004;13(1):45-54.
10. Bell RJ, Rivera-Woll L, Davison SL, Topliss DJ, Donath S, Davis SR. Well-being, health-related quality of life and cardiovascular disease risk profile in women with subclinical thyroid disease – a community-based study. Clin Endocrinol (Oxf). 2007;66(4):548-56.
11. Klaver EI, van Loon HC, Stienstra R, Links TP, Keers JC, Kema IP, et al. Thyroid hormone status and health-related quality of life in the LifeLines Cohort Study. Thyroid. 2013;23(9):1066-73.
12. Razvi S, Shakoor A, Vanderpump M, Weaver JU, Pearce SH. The influence of age on the relationship between subclinical hypothyroidism and ischemic heart disease: a metaanalysis. J Clin Endocrinol Metab. 2008;93(8):2998-3007.
13. Reuters VS, Almeida Cde P, Teixeira Pde F, Vigário Pdos S, Ferreira MM, Castro CL, et al. Effects of subclinical hypothyroidism treatment on psychiatric symptoms, muscular complaints, and quality of life. Arq Bras Endocrinol Metabol. 2012;56(2):128-36.
14. Imayama I, Alfano CM, Mason CE, Wang C, Xiao L, Duggan C, et al. Exercise adherence, cardiopulmonary fitness and anthropometric changes improve exercise self-efficacy and health-related quality of life. J Phys Act Health. 2013;10(5):676-89.
15. Staniute M, Bunevicius A, Brozaitiene J, Bunevicius R. Relationship of health-related quality of life with fatigue and exercise capacity in patients with coronary artery disease. Eur J Cardiovasc Nurs. 2014;13(4):338-44.
16. Garces-Arteaga A, Nieto-Garcia N, Suarez-Sanchez F, Triana-Reina HR, Ramírez-Vélez R. Influence of a medium-impact exercise program on health-related quality of life and cardiorespiratory fitness in females with subclinical hypothyroidism: an open-label pilot study. J Thyroid Res. 2013;2013:592801.
17. Vigário Pdos S, Chachamovitz DS, Cordeiro MF, Teixeira Pde F, de Castro CL, de Oliveira FP, et al. Effects of physical activity on body composition and fatigue perception in patients on thyrotropin-suppressive therapy for differentiated thyroid carcinoma. Thyroid. 2011;21(7):695-700.
18. Florindo A, Latorre M. Validação do questionário de Baecke de avaliação da atividade física habitual em homens adultos. Rev Bras Med Esporte. 2003;9:121-8.
19. Zulewski H, Müller B, Exer P, Miserez AR, Staub JJ. Estimation of tissue hypothyroidism by a new clinical score: evaluation of patients with various grades of hypothyroidism and controls. J Clin Endocrinol Metab. 1997;82(3):771-6.
20. Ciconelli RM, Ferraz MB, Santos W, Meinão I, Quaresma MR. Tradução para a língua portuguesa e validação do questionário genérico de avaliação de qualidade de vida SF-36 (Brasil SF-36). Rev Bras Reumatol. 1999;39(3):143-50.

21. Osoba D, Rodrigues G, Myles J, Zee B, Pater J. Interpreting the significance of changes in health-related quality-of-life scores. J Clin Oncol. 1998;16(1):139-44.
22. Biondi B, Cooper DS. The clinical significance of subclinical thyroid dysfunction. Endocr Rev. 2008;29(1):76-131.
23. Pucci GCMF, Rech CR, Fermino RC, Reis RS. Associação entre atividade física e qualidade de vida em adultos. Rev Saude Publica. 2012;46(1):166-79.
24. Conn VS, Hafdahl AR, Brown LM. Meta-analysis of quality-of-life outcomes from physical activity interventions. Nurs Res. 2009;58(3):175-83.
25. Laguardia J, Campos MR, Travassos C, Najar AL, Anjos LA, Vasconcelos MM. Dados normativos brasileiros do questionário Short Form-36 versão 2. Rev Bras Epidemiol. 2013;16(4):889-97.
26. Gillison FB, Skevington SM, Sato A, Standage M, Evangelidou S. The effects of exercise interventions on quality of life in clinical and healthy populations; a meta-analysis. Soc Sci Med. 2009;68(9):1700-10.
27. Burns RB, Bates CK, Hartzband P, Smetana GW. Should We Treat for Subclinical Hypothyroidism?: Grand Rounds Discussion From Beth Israel Deaconess Medical Center. Ann Intern Med. 2016;164(11):764-70.
28. Rugge JB, Bougatsos C, Chou R. Screening and treatment of thyroid dysfunction: an evidence review for the U.S. Preventive Services Task Force. Ann Intern Med. 2015;162(1):35-45.
29. Díez JJ, Iglesias P, Burman KD. Spontaneous normalization of thyrotropin concentrations in patients with subclinical hypothyroidism. J Clin Endocrinol Metab. 2005;90(7):4124-7.

Association of serum thyrotropin levels with coronary artery disease documented by quantitative coronary angiography: a transversal study

Pedro D. Ortolani Jr.[1], João H. Romaldini[1], Ricardo A. Guerra[1], Evandro S. Portes[1], George C. X. Meireles[2], João Pimenta[2]

[1] Serviço de Endocrinologia, Hospital do Servidor Público Estadual de São Paulo, Instituto de Assistência Médica ao Servidor Público Estadual (HSPE-IAMSPE), São Paulo, SP, Brasil
[2] Serviço de Cardiologia, Hospital do Servidor Público Estadual de São Paulo, Instituto de Assistência Médica ao Servidor Público Estadual (HSPE-IAMSPE), São Paulo, SP, Brasil

Correspondence to:
Pedro Dirceu Ortolani Júnior
Serviço de Endocrinologia,
Hospital do Servidor Público Estadual
Rua Pedro de Toledo, 1.800
04039-000 – São Paulo, SP, Brasil
pdojr@terra.com.br

ABSTRACT

Objective: The association between coronary artery disease (CAD) and thyroid function remains controversial. We evaluated the thyroid function and graduated well-defined CAD as confirmed by quantitative coronary angiography (CA). Subjects and methods: We evaluated the serum TSH, free thyroxine, free triiodothyronine and thyroid antibody levels in 300 consecutive patients (age 61.6 ± 9.9 years and 54% were male) undergoing CAD diagnosis as confirmed by CA. Plaques with ≥ 50% stenosis being indicative of obstructive CAD, and patients were divided into groups according to main epicardial coronary arteries with plaques (0, 1, 2, 3). Lipid profiles and a homeostasis model assessment (HOMA-IR) were determined. Results: Serum median (25% and 75% percentile) TSH levels in patients with group 2 and 3 (2.25; 1.66-3.12 mU/L and 4.99; 4.38-23.60 mU/L, respectively) had significantly higher TSH concentrations (p < 0.0001) than the group 0 (1.82; 1.35-2.51 mU/L). Furthermore, patients of group 3 had higher TSH concentration (p < 0.0001) than those of group 1 (1.60; 0.89-2.68 mU/L). Group 3 were older (64 ± 8.5 vs. 59 ± 9.5, p = 0.001), had more patients with dyslipidemia (84% versus 58%, p < 0.001), male (54% versus 44%, p = 0.01), hypertension (100% versus 86%, p < 0.001), and smoking (61% versus 33%, p < 0.001) than group 0. Multivariate stepwise logistic analysis showed TSH, age, HbA1c, and HOMA-IR were the CAD associated variables. Conclusions: In this cohort, elevated TSH levels in the high normal range or above are associated with the presence and severity of CAD besides may represent a weak CAD risk factor. Arch Endocrinol Metab. 2018;62(4):410-5

Keywords
TSH; coronary artery disease; coronary angiography

INTRODUCTION

Hypothyroidism is typically associated with elevated endothelial dysfunction and increased all-cause mortality in addition to cardiac death and/or hospitalization (1-3). Several studies have shown that coronary atherosclerosis in subjects with hypothyroidism is more frequent and severe than in normal subjects (4). In addition, there is some evidence that an elevated serum TSH in association with serum thyroid peroxidase antibody (TPOAb) may alter the traditional risk factors for coronary arterial disease (CAD), perhaps because of the accumulation of circulating levels of atherogenic total cholesterol (TC) and low-density lipoprotein (LDL) cholesterol particles (5-9). Consequently, the relation between thyroid dysfunction and CAD remains questionable (10), however, some authors have found a positive correlation between serum TSH levels and the presence and severity of coronary stenosis (6,11-14); other authors have found no correlation between these two parameters (15,16). In contrast, Coceani and cols. observed a negative correlation with serum FT3 (but not with FT4 levels) and CAD (17). On the other hand, Miura and cols. found that independent of conventional cardiovascular risk factors, thyroid hormones (FT3 and FT4) inversely correlated with coronary artery disease, especially men (18,19). A meta-analysis demonstrated that high TSH values were associated with cardiovascular risk in patients < 65 years old, whereas another study reported that in patients > 85 years old, increased serum TSH values played a protective role against the development of CAD (20,21). Furthermore, it remains to be determined whether serum TSH, FT4, FT3, TPOAb or thyroglobulin antibody (TgAb) levels are associated with CAD development. The aim of this study was to yield greater insight into the assessment of thyroid function parameters and lipid concentrations in consecutive patients undergoing quantitative coronary angiography (CA).

SUBJECTS AND METHODS

Patients

Data were obtained from 343 consecutive patients in the Cardiology Outpatient Unit, *Hospital do Servidor Público Estadual de São Paulo, Instituto de Assistência Médica ao Servidor Público Estadual* (HSPE-IAMSPE) in Brazil that were referred for CA because of signs or symptoms relevant to CAD. All of the patients satisfied two inclusion criteria: 1) characteristic signs of myocardial ischemia on non-invasive tests and 2) clinical recommendation for further assessment. We used a questionnaire to assess classical risk factors for CAD such as diabetes, hypertension, dyslipidemia, smoking, and a family history of premature CAD (defined as ≤ 55 years old for males and ≤ 65 years old for females). Patients were excluded in cases with a history of thyroid diseases, documented CAD, acute CAD, or ischemic equivalent (such as dyspnea, sickness, confusion, stroke or pulmonary edema, compatible electrocardiographic signs, or increased creatine kinase-MB [CK-MB)] and/or troponin levels) (22). We excluded patients who were using amiodarone, levothyroxine, or antithyroid drugs (such as methimazole or propylthiouracil). Forty-three patients were excluded, and the remaining 300 patients were enrolled in the study. All of the patients included in the study received an explanation of the purpose of the study and signed a consent form. This work was submitted to the Research Ethics Committee of IAMSPE and approved without restrictions.

Assessment of CA

All of the patients were assessed via CA and further analyzed by an independent observer who was not involved in patients medical care. The quantification of the CA was performed manually. The CA was carried out using a femoral approach and a 6- or 7-F guiding catheter. Right and left CAs were performed in multiple projections using standard techniques and used to evaluate coronary artery stenosis (23). CAD was defined according to CA results, and significant stenosis was defined as a decrease in internal diameter of ≥ 50%, which could affect one or more of the main epicardial coronary arteries (such as the right coronary, left anterior descending, or circumflex arteries) and classified as group 1, 2, or 3 according the number of vessels with significant stenosis (24). Patients were classified as group 0 if they had no CAD or when the main epicardial coronary arteries were < 50% of the internal diameter.

Biochemical analysis

Blood samples were drawn after overnight fasting prior to the CA. For the hormone assessment, patient samples were stored at -20°C until the time of measurement and analyzed in our laboratory. Blood glucose levels were estimated using the glucose oxidase method. Hemoglobin A1c (HbA1c), CK-MB, and cardiac troponin levels were determined by HPLC, electrochemiluminescent immunoassay, and two-site enzyme-linked immunosorbent assay methods, respectively. Serum TC, triglycerides (TG), and high-density lipoprotein (HDL) cholesterol levels were measured enzymatically. To determine LDL-cholesterol levels, the formula from Friedewald and cols. was used (25). Serum creatinine level was analyzed using a colorimetric method, and hepatic enzyme levels were determined enzymatically.

Hormonal analysis

Serum TSH, FT4, and FT3 levels were measured using direct chemiluminescent technology (Advia Centaur XP Immunoassay System; Siemens Healthcare Diagnostics, Deerfield, IL, USA) using reference values ranging from 0.3–4.1 mU/L for TSH, 0.8–2.0 ng/dL for FT4, and 1.6–4.1 pg/mL for FT3. The mean interassay CV was 3.1, 11.0, and 8.9 % for TSH, FT4, and FT3, respectively. TPOAb and TgAb serum concentrations were determined via a chemiluminescent immunometric assay (Diagnostic Products Co., Los Angeles, CA, USA), and values > 35 IU/L were considered to be positive. Serum insulin was analyzed using a chemiluminescent immunometric assay (Diagnostic Products Co.). The homeostasis model assessment of insulin resistance (HOMA-IR) index was determined using serum glucose and insulin values: fasting insulin (mU/mL)×fasting blood glucose (mg/dL)/405. Body mass index (BMI) was expressed as kg/m^2.

Statistical analysis

Differences between the groups were verified by the Kruskal-Wallis in conjunction with the Dunn's multiple comparison tests, and thereafter they were compared two-by-two using the Mann-Whitney rank test. Chi-square or Fischer's exact tests were used to compare proportions Univariate and multivariate analyses with multinomial logistic regression analysis were used to evaluate the risks associated with CA results. For univariate analysis a less-restrictive alpha level with a 0.1 was used, and so a broad range of variables are considered for inclusion in the model. Thereafter, a backward stepwise multiple regression analysis was employed using CAD as dependent variable. A beta coefficient, standard error of beta coefficient (SE), and 95% confidence interval were obtained. SAS software version 9.4 (SAS Institute Inc., Cary, NC) was used for all analyses.

RESULTS

Characteristics of patients that were analyzed and patient demographics are reported in Table 1. All enrolled patients underwent all tests according to schedule. The mean age was of 61.6 ± 9.9, > 90% of patients had hypertension, 72% had dyslipidemia, and almost half of them were smokers. Mean serum TSH levels were 3.0 ± 2.7 (SD) mU/L, and 11% of patients had positive thyroid antibodies. Significant stenosis (≥ 50% in one or more main epicardial vessels)

Table 1. Baseline characteristics of 300 patients participants in the study

Variables	Number (%) or mean ± SD
Age, years	61.6 ± 9.9
Male	162 (54)
Diabetes mellitus	107 (36)
Hypertension	275 (92)
Smoking	147 (49)
Family history of CAD[a]	70 (23)
Dyslipidemia	215 (72)
BMI, kg/m^2	28.2 ± 4.5
Total cholesterolemia, mg/dL	178.7 ± 37.9
HDL-cholesterolemia, mg/dL	49.1 ± 14.1
Trygliceridemia, mg/dL	134 ± 73.1
HbA1c, %	6.3 ± 1.4
LDL-cholesterolemia, mg/dL	101 ± 31.9
Thyroid antibodies[b]	34 (11)
TSH, mU/L	3.0 ± 2.7
FT4, ng/dL	1.2 ± 0.4
FT3, ng/dL	2.9 ± 0.6

SD: standard deviation.

[a] CAD coronary artery disease. [b] Presence of serum thyroglobulin antibody and thyroid peroxidase antibody.

was observed in 62% (185) of patients. Arterial vessel stenosis was observed in 60 patients (group 1), 64 patients had two stenosed vessels (group 2), and 61 patients had three stenosed vessels (group 3). Figure 1 shows the results of serum TSH concentration in patients undergoing CA examination. Serum median and a 25% and 75% percentile of TSH levels in patients of group 2 (2.25; 1.66-3.12 mU/L) and group 3 (4.99; 4.38-23.60 mU/L) had significantly higher TSH concentrations ($p < 0.0001$) than the group 0 (1.82; 1.35-2.51 mU/L). Furthermore, patients of group 3 had higher TSH concentration ($p < 0.0001$) than those of group1 (1.60; 0.89-2.68 mU/L) as shown Figure 1. Moreover, group 3 had significant more patients with dyslipidemia, hypertension and smoking than group 0 patients. In group 3, the mean HbA1c levels were higher than other groups, and were older as shown Table 2. The group 2 had similar figure; had more male, smoking and diabetes patients as well as high HbA1c level, and older than group 0. Univariate logistical regression analysis revealed that male sex, diabetes mellitus, hypertension, dyslipidemia, smoking, older age and TSH were significant risk factors for CAD (Table 3). Thereafter, as shown in Table 4, the stepwise backward multiple regression model of CAD identified TSH, older age, HbA1c, and HOMA-IR as CAD risk factors ($R^2 = 0.377$; Adjusted $R^2 = 0.369$; SE = 0.922 F = 42.526; p-value = 0.0001).

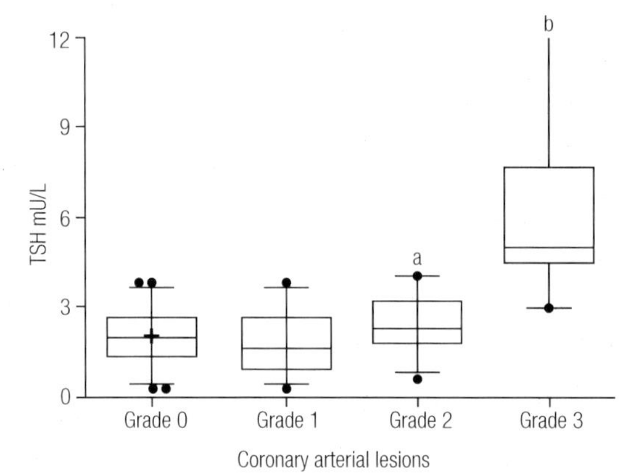

Figure 1. Box-and-whisker plot of the differences in the serum TSH median observed between patients undergoing the coronary angiography. Group 0; absence of coronary artery disease (when the vessels were < 50% of the internal diameter). Group 1, 2, and 3; according to the number of vessels with significant stenosis. The median is the center line, the ends of the box represent the 25th and 75th percentiles, and the ends of the lines extend to the 2.5th and 97.5th percentiles.

Differences between the groups were analyzed by the Kruskal-Wallis test. (H = 203.5; $p < 0.0001$).

[a] $p < 0.02$ vs. group 0; [b] $p < 0.0001$ vs. group 0, 1 and 2 (Verified by the Mann-Whitney test was used).

Table 2. Characteristics of patients according to the coronary artery angiography

Variables	Group 0[a]	Group 1	Group 2	p[b]	Group 3	p[c]
number	115	60	64		61	
Age, mean ± SD	59 ± 9.5	61.4 ± 10.1	63.8 ± 10.6	0.002	64.7 ± 8.5	0.001
Male, n (%)	51 (44)	31 (52)	36 (56)	0.015	33 (54)	0.01
Diabetes mellitus, n (%)	31 (27)	19 (32)	25 (39)	0.0001	33 (54)	0.107
Hypertension, n (%)	99 (86)	55 (92)	60 (94)	0.142	61 (100)	0.0001
Smoking, n (%)	38 (33)	32 (53)	39 (65)	0.001	37 (61)	0.0007
Familiar history of CAD	24 (21)	17 (28)	13 (20)	1.001	17 (28)	0.259
Dyslipidemia, n (%)	67 (58)	44 (73)	54 (84)	0.142	51 (84)	0.0001
BMI, Kg/m², mean ± SD	29.0 ± 4.9	27.2 ± 4.0	27.5 ± 4.3	0.059	28.3 ± 3.9	0.097
Total cholesterolemia, mg/dL	185.2 ± 35.2	174.7 ± 39.1	174.4 ± 39.2	0.610	175.3 ± 38.9	0.088
HDL-cholesterolemia, mg/dL	50.3 ± 11.7	49.7 ± 12.4	48.0 ± 15.7	0.210	47.4 ± 12.7	0.130
Trygliceridemia, mg/dL	131 ± 70.6	136.3 ± 83.2	133.3 ± 65.4	0.450	137.6 ± 76.2	0.213
LDL-cholesterolemia, mg/dL	108 ± 32.5	97.7 ± 33.7	99.5 ± 29.8	0.750	100.5 ± 33.1	0.923
HbA1c, %, mean ± SD	6.0 ± 1.2	6.1 ± 1.3	6.5 ± 1.4	0.002	6.7 ± 1.8	0.018
Thyroid antibodies[d], n (%)	12 (10)	9 (15)	7 (10.9)	0.607	7 (11.4)	0.596
TSH, mU/L	2.7 ± 2.1	3.1 ± 2.6	2.9 ± 2.1	0.025	3.5 ± 3.8	0.0001
FT4, ng/dL	1.1 ± 0.2	1.1 ± 0.2	1.2 ± 0.2	0.139	1.1 ± 0.2	0.758
FT3, ng/dL	2.9 ± 0.5	2.9 ± 0.6	3.0 ± 0.5	0.254	2.9 ± 0.5	0.800

SD: standard deviation.

[a] Group was classified as the number of main epicardial vessels with stenosis: Group 0 when vessels without lesion or less than 50% of the internal diameter, Group 1 when one vessel with lesion equal or more than 50% of the internal diameter, Group 2 when two vessels with lesion equal or more than 50% of the internal diameter, Group 3 when three vessels with lesion equal or more than 50% of the internal diameter.

[b] p-values significant between patients with Group 0 and Group-2, and no significant with Group 1.

[c] p-values significant between patients with Group 0 and Group 3, and no significant with Group 1 and Group 2.

[d] Presence of serum thyroglobulin antibody and thyroid peroxidase antibody Kruskal-Wallis was used ($H = 7357.8$; $p < 0.00010$. Mann-Whitney test was used for continuous variables between the groups, and the Chi-Square or Fischer's exact test was used for categorical variables.

Table 3. Risk factors associated with coronary arterial disease in patients undergoing coronary angiography by univariate logistic regression analysis

Variable	Adjusted odds ratio	95% Confidence Interval	p
Age, years	1.05	1.02–1.07	< 0.01
Male	1.93	1.27–2.93	< 0.01
Diabetes mellitus	1.17	1.41–3.34	< 0.01
Hypertension	3.55	1.53–8.24	< 0.01
Dyslipidemia	2.74	1.70–4.42	< 0.01
Smoking	2.35	1.54–3.57	< 0.01
HOMA-IR	1.12	1.05–1.20	< 0.01
HbA1c	1.32	1.13–1.54	< 0.01
TSH	1.07	0.99–1.16	= 0.08

Variables such as familiar history of CAD ($p = 0.45$), BMI ($p = 0.21$), thyroid antibodies ($p = 0.78$), FT4 ($p = 0.58$) and FT3 were not independent risk associated with CAD.

Table 4. Result from stepwise backward regression analysis for presence of coronary arterial disease in patients undergoing coronary angiography

Variables	Coefficients	SE[a]	Beta	*t*	p
TSH	0.238544459	0.021348719	0.52981	11.173	0.0008
Age	0.018485266	0.005520596	0.159255363	3.348	0.0009
HbA1c[b]	0.454384746	0.121113561	0.17814673	3.752	0.0002
HOMA-IR[c]	0,026698419	0.11200489	0.112782451	2.38	0.017

[a] SE, the estimated standard deviation of the error in the model.

[b] Hemoglobin A1c.

[c] The homeostasis model assessment of insulin resistance.

Independent variables such as sex ($p = 0.31$), diabetes mellitus ($p = 0.27$), hypertension ($p = 0.33$), dyslipidemia (0.25) and smoking ($p = 0.94$) were not included in the model.

DISCUSSION

In this study, we have demonstrated that within our study population, patients with two or three stenosed arterial vessels at the CA assessment had higher serum TSH levels than patients with no stenosis. This study shown that serum TSH level was associated with risk of stenosis, detected during the CA, especially for patients with older age, higher levels of HbA1c and presence of insulin resistance. Serum FT4 or FT3 levels had no effect on the presence of stenosis. Recent meta-analysis provided some important information about the role of thyroid autoimmunity as a possible risk factor for CAD and suggested that biomarkers of thyroid autoimmunity do not add independent prognostic information for CAD outcomes (26). In the present study population, there was no association between significant stenosis seen on the CA and the presence of circulating TPOAb or TgAb. Although our findings using stepwise backward multiple regression model of CAD identified TSH, older age, HbA1c, and HOMA-IR as CAD predictors besides TSH were a weak independent risk factor for CAD. These data are consistent with the hypothesis that serum TSH values, even within in the upper normal reference range, are associated with the presence of stenosis (10). Endothelial dysfunction has been detected in hypothyroid patients, and it has been shown to be associated with low-intensity chronic inflammation, arterial vasodilatation reduction, and the presence of circulating TPOAb or TgAb (27,28). A limitation of our study was the small number of enrolled patients, which reduced the strength of the reported associations. Furthermore, in an attempt to decrease the influence of acute coronary syndrome, we included only select patients without clinical symptoms of cardiac disease such as chest pain or patients with manifestations of ischemic heart disease. On the other hand, it seems that there was no clear agreement on the association of serum TSH, FT4, and FT3 values with CAD. A multicenter prospective study, including 55,000 patients, revealed that elevated serum TSH levels (particularly levels > 10 mU/L) were associated with an increased risk of cardiac events and mortality due to CAD, and Chaker and cols. found that high levels of TSH might increase the risk of stroke in patients < 65 years old (29,30). Auer and cols. identified a positive correlation between serum TSH levels and the presence and severity of CAD without excluding patients with previous thyroid disease (31). Miura and cols. studied angina patients found in CAD patients lower FT4 and FT3 levels as compared to patients without coronary stenosis (18). On the contrary, Coceani and cols. assessed approximately 1,000 patients (excluding individuals with acute myocardial infarction) and found no correlation between serum TSH or FT4 levels and CAD and observed a negative correlation only with serum FT3 levels (17). We did not find any association between serum FT4 and/or FT3 levels and CAD. A direct correlation between TC and LDL cholesterol is well-known, even when serum TSH values are within the reference range, and is usually associated with insulin resistance and in smokers (8,32). Among the many factors associated with CAD, Tatar and cols. reported a direct effect of serum TSH in the upper normal reference range on an increase in arterial stiffness in dialysis patients with euthyroidism (33). On the other hand, serum TSH also increased inflammatory molecules and inhibited nitric oxide production due to oxidative stress as demonstrated by Desideri and cols. and Dardano and cols. (34,35). We were unable to find any evidence for an association between lipid profiles and serum TSH levels, most likely due to the fact that the majority of patients were taking dyslipidemia drugs. Despite the elevated frequency of hypertensive patients in our study population, no association with serum TSH values was noted.

Some paper found results similar to ours study: Yun and cols. used a serum TSH cutoff point of 2.1 mU/L; observed a significant correlation between serum TSH levels and coronary artery lesions in patients with unstable angina (36). Furthermore, using the median serum TSH value (1.73 mU/L) as a cutoff value, Yang and cols. studied the hospital-based diagnoses of myocardial infarction in 318 patients and found an association between elevated serum TSH values (still within the reference range) and CAD (37). Daswani and cols. found lower FT3 levels in patients with three stenosed vessels were more affected in CAD than in normal patients (38). Finally, the possibility that serum TSH levels is a cardiovascular risk factor has been a subject of debate, and a broad studies are needed for answer this point. In summary, our study suggests that in a population with multiple risk factors for CAD development, there is an association with high serum TSH, even in the upper normal range, with presence and severity of CAD as detected with CA. Furthermore, elevated serum TSH may represent a weak CAD risk factor.

REFERENCES

1. Sara JD, Zhang M, Gharib H, Lerman LO, Lerman A. Hypothyroidism is associated with coronary endothelial dysfunction in women. J Am Heart Assoc. 2015;4(8):e002225.
2. Ning N, Gao D, Triggiani V, Iacoviello M, Mitchell JE, Ma R, et al. Prognostic role of hypothyroidism in heart failure: A Meta-Analysis. Medicine (Baltimore). 2015;94(30):e1159.
3. Cappola AR, Ladenson PW. Hypothyroidism and atherosclerosis. J Clin Endocrinol Metab. 2003;88(6):2438-44.
4. Cappola AR, Fried LP, Arnold AM, Danese MD, Kuller LH, Burke GL, et al. Thyroid status, cardiovascular risk, and mortality in older adults. JAMA. 2006;295(9):1033-41.
5. Hollowell JG, Staehling NW, Flanders WD, Hannon WH, Gunter EW, Spencer CA, et al. Serum TSH, T(4), and thyroid antibodies in the United States population (1988 to 1994): National Health and Nutrition Examination Survey (NHANES III). J Clin Endocrinol Metab. 2002;87(2):489-99.
6. Walsh JP, Bremner AP, Bulsara MK, O'Leary P, Leedman PJ, Feddema P, et al. Subclinical thyroid dysfunction as a risk factor for cardiovascular disease. Arch Intern Med. 2005;165(21):2467-72.
7. Biondi B. Heart failure and thyroid dysfunction. Eur J Endocrinol. 2012;167(5):609-18.
8. Canaris GJ, Manowitz NR, Mayor G, Ridgway EC. The Colorado thyroid prevalence study. Arch Intern Med. 2000;160(4):526-34.
9. Ochs N, Auer R, Bauer DC, Nanchen D, Gussekloo J, Cornuz J, et al. Meta-analysis: subclinical thyroid dysfunction and the risk for coronary heart disease and mortality. Ann Intern Med. 2008;148(11):832-45.
10. Rodondi N, Bauer DC. Subclinical hypothyroidism and cardiovascular risk: how to end the controversy. J Clin Endocrinol Metab. 2013;98(6):2267-9.
11. Iervasi G, Molinaro S, Landi P, Taddei MC, Galli E, Mariani F, et al. Association between increased mortality and mild thyroid dysfunction in cardiac patients. Arch Intern Med. 2007;167(14):1526-32.
12. Tseng FY, Lin WY, Lin CC, Lee LT, Li TC, Sung PK, et al. Subclinical hypothyroidism is associated with increased risk for all-cause and cardiovascular mortality in adults. J Am Coll Cardiol. 2012;60(8):730-7.
13. Hak AE, Pols HA, Visser TJ, Drexhage HA, Hofman A, Witteman JC. Subclinical hypothyroidism is an independent risk factor for atherosclerosis and myocardial infarction in elderly women: the Rotterdam Study. Ann Intern Med. 2000;132(4):270-8.
14. Imaizumi M, Akahoshi M, Ichimaru S, Nakashima E, Hida A, Soda M, et al. Risk of ischemic heart disease and all-cause mortality in subclinical hypothyroidism. J Clin Endocrinol Metab. 2004;89(7):3365-70.
15. Rodondi N, Newman AB, Vittinghoff E, de Rekeneire N, Satterfield S, Harris TB, et al. Subclinical hypothyroidism and the risk of heart failure, other cardiovascular events and death. Arch Intern Med. 2005;165(21):2460-6.
16. Asvold BO, Bjøro T, Platou C, Vatten LJ. Thyroid function and the risk of coronary heart disease: 12-year follow-up of the HUNT Study in Norway. Clin Endocrinol (Oxf). 2012;77(6):911-7.
17. Coceani M, Iervasi G, Pingitore A, Carpeggiani C, L'Abbate A. Thyroid hormone and coronary artery disease: from clinical correlations to prognostic implications. Clin Cardiol. 2009;32(7):380-5.
18. Miura S, Iitaka M, Suzuki S, Fukasawa N, Kitahama S, Kawakami Y, et al. Decrease in serum levels of thyroid hormone in patients with coronary heart disease. Endocr J. 1996;43(6):657-63.
19. Kim ES, Shin JA, Shin JY, Lim DJ, Moon SD, Son HY, et al. Association between low serum free thyroxine concentrations and coronary artery calcification in healthy euthyroid subjects. Thyroid. 2012;22(9):870-6.
20. Razvi S, Shakoor A, Vanderpump M, Weaver JU, Pearce SH. The influence of age on the relationship between subclinical hypothyroidism in ischemic heart disease: a metaanalysis. J Clin Endocrinol Metab. 2008;93(8):2998-3007.
21. Gussekloo J, van Exel E, de Craen AJ, Meinders AE, Frölich M, Westendorp RG. Thyroid status, disability and cognitive function, and survival in old age. JAMA. 2004;292(21):2591-9.
22. Cohn PF, Fox KM, Daly C. Silent ischemia. Circulation. 2003;108(10):1263-77.
23. Williams DO, Gruntzig A, Kent KM et al. Guidelines for the performance of percutaneous transluminal coronary angioplasty. Circulation. 1982;66(4):693-4.
24. Brown BG, Bolson E, Frimer M, Dodge HT. Quantitative coronary arteriography: estimation of dimensions, hemodynamic resistance, and atheroma mass of coronary artery lesions using the arteriogram and digital computation. Circulation. 1977;55(2):329-37.
25. Friedewald WT, Levy RI, Fredrickson DS. Estimation of the concentration of low-density lipoprotein cholesterol in plasma, without the use of preparative centrifuge. Clin Chem. 1972;18(6):499-502.
26. Collet TH, Bauer DC, Cappola AR, Asvold BO, Weiler S, Vittinghoff E, et al. Thyroid antibody status, subclinical hypothyroidism, and the risk of coronary heart disease: an individual participant data analysis. J Clin Endocrinol Metab. 2014;99(9):3356-62.
27. Taddei S, Caraccio N, Virdis A, Dardano A, Versari D, Ghiadoni L, et al. Low-grade systemic inflammation causes endothelial dysfunction in patients with Hashimoto's thyroiditis. J Clin Endocrinol Metab. 2006;91(12):5076-82.
28. Xiang GD, He YS, Zhao LS, Hou J, Yue L, Xiang HJ. Impairment of endothelium-dependent arterial dilation in Hashimoto's thyroiditis patients with euthyroidism. Clin Endocrinol (Oxf). 2006;64(6):698-702.
29. Rodondi N, den Elzen WP, Bauer DC, Cappola AR, Razvi S, Walsh JP, et al. Thyroid Studies Collaboration: Subclinical hypothyroidism and the risk of coronary heart disease and mortality. JAMA. 2010;304(12):1365-74.
30. Chaker L, Baumgartner C, den Elzen WP, Collet TH, Ikram MA, Blum MR, et al.; Thyroid Studies Collaboration. Thyroid function within the reference range and the risk of stroke: An individual participant data analysis. J Clin Endocrinol Metab. 2016 Nov;101(11):4270-82.
31. Auer J, Berent R, Weber T, Lassnig E, Eber B. Thyroid function is associated with the presence and severity of coronary atherosclerosis. Clin Cardiol. 2003;26(12):569-73.
32. Bakker SJ, ter Maaten JC, Popp-Snijders C, Slaets JP, Heine RJ, Gans RO. The relationship between thyrotropin and low density lipoprotein cholesterol is modified by insulin sensitivity in healthy euthyroid subjects. J Clin Endocrinol Metab. 2001;86(6):1206-11.
33. Tatar E, Sezis Demirci M, Kircelli F, Gungor O, Yaprak M, Asci G, et al. The association between thyroid hormones and arterial stiffness in peritoneal dialysis patients. Int Urol Nephrol. 2012;44(2):601-6.
34. Desideri G, Bocale R, Milardi D, Ghiadoni L, Grassi D, Necozione S, et al. Enhanced proatherogenic inflammation after recombinant human TSH administration in patients monitored for thyroid cancer remnant. Clin Endocrinol. 2009;71(3):429-33.
35. Dardano A, Ghiadoni L, Plantinga Y, Caraccio N, Bemi A, Duranti E, et al. Recombinant Human Thyrotropin Reduces Endothelium-Dependent Vasodilation in Patients Monitored for Differentiated Thyroid Carcinoma. J Clin Endocrinol Metab. 2006;91(10):4175-78.
36. Yun KH, Jeong MH, Oh SK, Lee EM, Lee J, Rhee SJ, et al. Relationship of thyroid stimulating hormone with coronary atherosclerosis in angina patients. Int J Cardiol. 2007;122(1):56-60.
37. Yang L, Zou J, Zhang M, Xu H, Qi W, Gao L, et al. The relationship between thyroid-stimulating hormone within the reference range and coronary artery disease: impact of age. Endocr J. 2013;60(6):773-9.
38. Daswani R, Jayaprakash B, Shetty R, Rau NR. Association of thyroid function with severity of coronary artery disease in euthyroid patients. J Clin Diag Res. 2015;9(6):10-3.

Body composition, resting energy expenditure and inflammatory markers: impact in users of depot medroxyprogesterone acetate after 12 months follow-up

Gisele Almeida Batista[1], Aglécio Luiz de Souza[1], Daniela Miguel Marin[1], Marina Sider[1], Vaneska Carvalho Melhado[1], Arlete Maria Fernandes[1], Sarah Monte Alegre[1]

[1] Faculdade de Ciências Médicas, Universidade Estadual de Campinas (FCM-Unicamp), Campinas, SP, Brasil

Correspondence to:
Sarah Monte Alegre
Rua Tessália Viera de Camargo, 126
Cidade Universitária Zeferino Vaz
13083-887 – Campinas, SP, Brasil
salegre@fcm.unicamp.br

ABSTRACT

Objective: The aim of this study was to evaluate for 12 months the changes of body weight using Depot Medroxyprogesterone Acetate (DMPA) and if these changes are related to inflammatory markers. **Subjects and methods:** Twenty women of childbearing age who chose the DMPA, without previous use of this method, BMI < 30 kg/m², and 17 women using IUD TCu 380A, participated in the study. At the baseline and after one year, changes in weight gain, body composition by the bioimpedance electric method, resting energy expenditure (REE) by the indirect calorimetry method, inflammatory markers and HOMA-IR were assessed. **Results:** After 12 months of evaluation, we could observe a significant increase in the DMPA group in weight (3,01 kg) and BMI, while the IUD group's only significant increase was observed in the BMI. Relative to REE there was an increase of basal metabolic rate (BMR) in both groups after one year. The sub-group DMPA that gained < 3 kg had increased significant weight, BMI and body surface (BS) with respiratory quotient (RQ) reduction, while the sub-group that gained ≥ 3 kg had a significant increase in weight, BMI, BS, fat-free mass, fat mass, BMR, Leptin, HOMA-IR and waist circumference, with RQ significantly reduced. **Conclusion:** Our study found significant changes in weight, body composition and metabolic profile of the population studied in the first 12 months of contraceptive use. These changes mainly increased body weight, leptin levels and HOMA-IR which can contribute to the development of some chronic complications, including obesity, insulin resistance and diabetes mellitus. Arch Endocrinol Metab. 2017;61(1):70-5

Keywords
Obesity; body composition; resting energy expenditure; depot medroxyprogesterone acetate; leptin

INTRODUCTION

Obesity is considered a serious public health problem that affects developed countries as well as developing ones. Globally, there are an estimated 1.5 billion overweight adults, of which approximately 500 million are obese (1). In Brazil, 50.8% of the population over 18 years old are overweight and 17.5% are obese (2). This complex and chronic disorder of multifactorial etiology is the result of positive energy balance, and genetic and environmental factors are involved in developing this metabolic disorder (3,4). In women, the use of hormonal contraceptives has been associated with weight gain and changes in body composition.

Depot medroxyprogesterone acetate (DMPA) is an injectable contraceptive method and in its formulation contains 150 mg of DMPA administered every 3 months intramuscularly at a plasma concentration of approximately 1 ng/mL (5). According to the characteristics of contraceptive efficacy, safety and low cost, and ease of access due to its ready availability from public health systems in several countries, including Brazil, millions of women choose to use this method (6). Despite having a potential negative effect on bones, the most common reason for discontinuing use of DMPA is increased body weight (7). Most prospective studies that have assessed the body composition of these progestin users, with at least 30 months of use, show a weight gain associated with an increase in body fat deposits (8,9).

In a study with HIV-infected women was evaluated the association between DMPA use with inflammatory markers (10). However, no studies in healthy women linking weight gain after using DMPA with inflammatory markers. Therefore, the aim of this study was to evaluate for 12 months the changes of body weight using DMPA and if these changes are related to inflammatory markers.

SUBJECTS AND METHODS

Subjects

This was a prospective cohort study with women attending the family planning clinic at the Gynecology and Obstetrics Department, University of Campinas (Unicamp), Brazil. Sample size was calculated from the demand for women seen in the clinic who opted for the contraceptive DMPA method and the percentage of women who have segment to method use for at least 12 months. The women were selected from February 2011 to March 2012.

Women of childbearing age who chose the injectable contraceptive DMPA without previous use of this method, body mass index (BMI) < 30 kg/m^2, and women using the non-hormonal contraception copper intrauterine device (TCu 380A IUD), were invited to participate in the study. The participants were aged between 18 and 40 years. The groups were paired at baseline, becoming a homogeneous group in relation to age (± 1 year), and BMI (± 1 kg/m^2).

After signing an informed consent form, they were interviewed to collect data and personal medical and family history. An administration every three months of 150 mg of DMPA was given and follow-up was maintained for one year. The women in the control group, TCu 380A IUD users, underwent the same procedures provided for inclusion into the DMPA group.

Exclusion criteria were: women with diabetes mellitus (DM) type 1 or 2; those with a family history of diabetes; those who had fasting glucose > 100 mg/dL after 8 hours of fasting or after a 120 minute oral glucose tolerance test had 75 g glucose blood glucose > 140 mg/dL; women breast-feeding; those with co-morbidities that contribute to the variation in body weight such as hyper- and hypothyroidism; chronic renal failure and transplant of any organ; use of medications that may be related to weight gain and/or development of insulin resistance such as the chronic use of corticosteroids, antipsychotics, diuretics and statins. Patients with hirsutism and/or hyperandrogenism and polycystic ovary syndrome were also excluded.

Initially, 49 women were evaluated. Throughout the monitoring period, 11 volunteers were excluded either for not returning for follow-up or because they became pregnant. One participant was excluded from the group by initiating physical activity after use of DMPA. At the end of the study we evaluated 37 women, 20 from the DMPA group and 17 from the IUD group (Figure 1).

This study was approved by the Ethics Committee of the Faculty of Medical Sciences – Unicamp, and all the volunteers who agreed to participate signed a consent form.

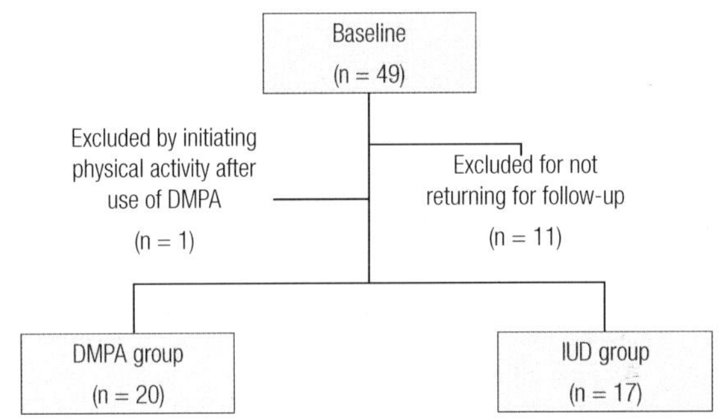

Figure 1. Flow chart of the study.

Anthropometric measurements and body composition

Anthropometric assessment was performed by a single examiner. Weight (kg) and height (m) were measured using a Welmy mechanical scale with 100 g precision and capacity of 200 kg. Height was measured by a stadiometer coupled to the scale with a precision of 0.5 cm. Waist circumference (WC) was measured with an inelastic 2 m tape dimension. The anatomical point used was the midpoint between the last rib and the iliac crest.

Nutritional status was assessed by calculating the BMI, recommended by the World Health Organization 1995 and 1997 (11).

The percent body fat (% fat), weight, fat mass (FM) and fat-free mass (FFM) were assessed by Bioimpedance Electric (BIA) using the equipment Biodynamics – Bioimpedance Analiser model 310.

Resting energy expenditure

The resting energy expenditure (REE), basal metabolic rate (BMR) and substrate used to obtain energy were assessed by the indirect calorimetry method. For this, a Vmax Encore 29 device coupled to a canopy gas exchange was used.

The consumption of oxygen (O_2) and the elimination of carbon dioxide (CO_2) in liters per minute as well as tidal volume were reported in this procedure. From these primary measures, the values of energy expenditure in kilocalories per day were obtained along with the respiratory quotient (RQ). The mean values obtained in steady state, prefixed as smaller variations than 5% in RQ and 10% in CO_2 were considered.

Biochemical assays

Serum adiponectin, interleukin (IL) – 6, visfatin, leptin, tumor necrosis factor-α (TNF-α), insulin and glucose were performed at baseline and after one year of using the method. The blood samples were centrifuged, and serum was immediately stored in small aliquots in a freezer at -80°C. Dosages of adipocytokines and insulin were performed in serum by enzyme immunoassay in duplicate by enzyme-linked immunosorbent assay (ELISA) using commercial kits with high sensitivity and specificity.

Insulin resistance

Homeostasis model assessment of insulin resistance (HOMA-IR) was calculated according to the formula: fasting insulin (μU/L) x fasting glucose (nmol/L)/22.5. Those considered normal values are < 2.7 (12).

Statistical analysis

All results are expressed as mean ±SD. The Mann-Whitney test was used to compare the variables between two groups. The Wilcoxon test was used for comparison of group time fixing. For comparison of numerical measurements between times and groups ANOVA was used for repeated measurements with transformation stations. The significance level for statistical tests was 5% ($P < 0.05$). The SAS program for Windows version 9.2 was used to perform the analyses.

RESULTS

After 12 months of evaluation, we could observe a significant increase in the DMPA group in weight (61.95 kg ± 9.69 x 64.96 kg ± 9.40, $p = 0.0007$), BMI (23.74 kg/m² ± 3.47 x 24.88 kg/m² ± 3.43, $p = 0.0007$) and body surface (BS) (1.65 ± 0.14 x 1.69 ± 0.13 $p = 0.0148$), while the IUD group's only significant increase was observed in the BMI variable (24.26 kg/m² ± 2.67 x 24.56 kg/m² ± 2.84, $p = 0.0007$) (Table 1).

Relative to REE and RQ, there was an increase of BMR in both groups after one year (DMPA group: 1087.05 kcal/d ± 252.06 x 1319.30 kcal/d ± 133.53, $p = 0.0027$, IUD group: 1187.59 kcal/d ± 246.23 x 1303.18 kcal/d ± 104.02, $p = 0.0027$). The RQ was significantly reduced after 12 months of study in groups DMPA (0.91 x 0.77, $p < 0.0001$) and IUD (0.87 x 0.78, $p < 0.0001$) (Table 2).

Table 3 shows the subdivision of the DMPA group for weight gain after 12 months follow-up. The sub-group that gained < 3 kg had a significant increase in weight (61.24 kg ± 10.38 x 62.51 kg ± 9.95, $p = 0.0156$), BMI (23.44 kg/m² ± 4.25 x 23.93 kg/m² ± 4.15, $p = 0.0313$) and BS (1.64 ± 0.12 x 1.66 ± 0.12 $p = 0.0313$) with RQ reduction (0.87 ± 0.09 x 0.77 ± 0.03, $p = 0.0313$), while the sub-group that gained ≥ 3 kg had a significant increase in weight (61.1 kg ± 8.63 x 66.63 kg ± 8.48, $p = 0.002$), BMI (23.47 kg/m² ± 3.50 x 25.55 kg/m² ± 3.46, $p = 0.002$), BS (1.64 ± 0.11 x 1.71 ± 0.11, $p = 0.002$), FFM (42.01 kg ± 4.18 x 45.19 kg ± 4.74, $p = 0.0059$), FM (19.14 kg ± 5.26 x 21.44 kg ± 5.82, $p = 0.0273$), BMR (997.70 kcal/d ± 202.72 x 1318.20 kcal/d ± 157.58, $p = 0.0117$), Leptin (78.05 ± 76.25 x 236.86 ± 214.93, $p = 0.0195$), HOMA-IR (0.70 ± 0.41 x 1.92 ± 1.41, $p = 0.0059$) and WC (75.90 cm ± 7.52 x 79.49 cm ± 7.75, $p = 0.002$), with RQ significantly reduced (0.95 ± 0.12 x 0.77 ± 0.04, $p = 0.002$).

Table 1. Characteristics of the DMPA and DIU groups

Variable	Baseline			12 months		
	DMPA (n = 20)) Mean ± SD	IUD (n = 17) Mean ± SD	¥ P value	DMPA (n = 20) Mean ± SD	IUD (n = 17) Mean ± SD	¥ P value
Age (years)	29,7 ± 6,2	28,4 ± 5,8	0,4682	–	–	
Weight (kg)	61,95 ± 9,69	61,24 ± 6,98	0,5449	64,96* ± 9,40	61,76 ± 7,53	0,0007
BMI (kg/m²)	23,74 ± 3,47	24,26 ± 2,67	0,911	24,88* ± 3,43	24,56** ± 2,84	0,0007
BS	1,65 ± 0,14	1,62 ± 0,09	0,4127	1,69* ± 0,13	1,63 ± 0,10	0,0148
WC (cm)	75,47 ±7,28	77,61 ± 7,88	0,0178	76,74 ± 6,27	75,38 ± 5,66	0,1834

¥: Mann-Whitney test. Statistical significance: p < 0,05. * Depo group difference between baseline and after 12 months. ** DIU group difference between baseline and after 12 months. BS: body surface; WC: waist circumference; BMI: body mass index.

Table 2. Resting energy expenditure and respiratory quotient baseline and after 12 months

Variable	Baseline			12 months		
	DMPA (n = 20) Mean ± SD	IUD (n = 17) Mean ± SD	¥ P value	DMPA (n = 20) Mean ± SD	IUD (n = 17) Mean ± SD	¥ P value
BMR (kcal/d)	1087,05 ± 252,06	1187,59 ± 246,23	0,3674	1319,30* ± 133,53	1303,18** ± 104,02	0,0027
RQ	0,91 ± 0,11	0,87 ± 0,09	0,8134	0,77* ± 0,03	0,78** ± 0,03	< 0,0001

¥: Mann-Whitney test. Statistical significance: $p < 0,05$. * Difference Depo group between baseline and after 12 months. ** Difference IUD group between baseline and after 12 months. RQ: respiratory quotient; BMR: basal metabolic rate.

Table 3. Characteristics of DMPA group subdivided by weight gain after12 months

	Baseline	12 months		Baseline	12 months	
	< 3 kg (n = 7)		+ P value	> 3 kg (n = 10)		+ P value
	Mean ± SD	Mean ± SD		Mean ± SD	Mean ± SD	
Weight	61,24 ± 10,38	62,51[c] ± 9,95	0,0156	61,1 ± 8,63	66,63[d] ±8,48	0,002
BMI	23,44 ± 4,25	23,93[c] ± 4,15	0,0313	23,47 ± 3,50	25,55[d] ± 3,46	0,002
BS	1,64 ± 0,12	1,66[c] ± 0,12	0,0313	1,64 ± 0,11	1,71[d] ± 0,11	0,002
% Fat	30,70 ± 5,58	29,30 ± 6,99	0,5625	30,87 ± 4,58	31,76 ± 6,12	0,7891
FFM	42,51 ± 5,32	43,94 ± 6,50	0,1406	42,01 ± 4,18	45,19[d] ± 4,74	0,0059
FM	19,44 ± 6,07	18,57 ± 6,20	0,7813	19,14 ± 5,26	21,44[d] ± 5,82	0,0273
BMR	1224,43 ±2 66,82	1334,29 ± 125,04	0,1563	997,70 ± 202,72	1318,20[d] ± 157,58	0,0117
RQ	0,87 ± 0,09	0,77[c] ± 0,03	0,0313	0,95 ± 0,12	0,77[d] ± 0,04	0,002
Adiponectin	10,20 ± 3,21	8,60 ± 4,82	0,375	5,89 ± 1,90	5,96 ± 2,80	0,8457
Leptin	133,53 ± 156,77	174,20 ± 184,10	0,2969	78,05 ± 76,25	236,86[d] ± 214,93	0,0195
Visfatin	44,78 ± 10,82	45,76 ± 21,36	0,8125	50,68 ± 31,83	43,81 ± 16,23	0,4316
IL-6	1,30 ± 0,42	1,91 ± 1,80	1	1,12 ± 0,77	2,02 ± 2,71	1
TNF-α	4,70 ± 2,11	4,28 ± 3,33	0,2969	4,31 ± 1,98	3,62 ± 1,67	0,1934
HOMA-IR	1,25 ± 1,44	1,15 ± 0,84	0,5781	0,70 ± 0,41	1,92[d] ± 1,41	0,0059
WC	74,14 ± 8,35	75,67 ± 8,97	0,125	75,90 ± 7,52	79,49[d] ± 7,75	0,002

+: Wilcoxon test. Statistical significance: $p < 0,05$. c: Difference sub-group weight gain < 3 kg comparing baseline and after 12 months. d: Difference sub-group weight gain > 3 kg comparing baseline and after 12 months.

FFM: free fat mass; FM: fat mass; BMR: basal metabolic rate.

DISCUSSION

We can consider that our population has a differential in relation to other studies evaluating the effect of DMPA, considering that our group was paired with the control group at baseline for BMI (± 1 kg/m^2) and age (± 1 year), becoming a homogeneous group. Our study found that after 12 months of follow-up the injectable DMPA users had significant weight gain (3.01 kg). As most prospective studies evaluating the effect of DMPA were for at least 30 months (6,8,9), we can consider that the follow-up period of our study is short compared to the others, but we can already observe significant changes in important variables studied.

To better assess changes in weight and body composition, we made a subdivision of the DMPA group for weight gain (< 3 kg and > 3 kg), and observed significant changes in weight and body composition in both groups, but the group which gained > 3 kg had the more pronounced changes. This group had a mean gain of 5.53 kg, increased fat mass (2.3 kg) and fat-free mass (3.18 kg) after 12 months follow-up. The increase in fat-free mass in users of DMPA may be explained by the androgenic effect of this contraceptive method (13).

Berenson and Rahman (9), to compare changes in weight and body composition between different contraceptive methods, observed at 24 months of follow-up an increase of 4.4 kg and after 36 months a gain of 5.1 kg in the DMPA group. Of the 5.1 kg that the volunteers put on after 36 months, 4.1 kg were of fat mass. Moreover, a significant increase in total body lean mass after 30 months of follow-up was observed.

The main contributing factor to the increase in body weight after use of DMPA reported in most studies is the increase in fat deposits. After 30 months of follow-up of users of medroxyprogesterone, Clark and cols. (8) observed a gain of 6.1 kg, which is fully represented by increased fat mass. There are two other possible mechanisms that might explain the weight gain associated with DMPA use: the first is its glucocorticoid-like activity, which appears to be associated with increased fat, including visceral fat (14). However, secondly, it is also possible that the state of hypoestrogenism induced by the injectable may be another factor responsible for the increase in weight and body fat (15).

In our study, the subgroup that gained more weight at the end of the study also had a significant increase in waist circumference and HOMA-IR. Increased waist circumference is indicative of an increase in subcutaneous and visceral adipose tissue. HOMA-IR, although not yet characterized as insulin resistance (HOMA-IR > 2.7) in our group, indicates a probable trend for the development of insulin resistance with increased exposure time for the contraceptive method. Accumulation of excess fat can be a critical modulation factor for insulin sensitivity, since it promotes the release of free fatty acids into the adipocyte circulation (16,17). In addition, excess adiposity and adipocyte dysfunction result in dysregulation of adipokines, which may contribute to the development of various metabolic complications through altered glucose and lipid homeostasis as well as inflammatory responses (18,19).

In relation to changes in inflammatory markers, we observed a slight decrease in adiponectin levels, although it was not significant in the DMPA group. A greater reduction in the levels of this marker associated with weight gain and increased body fat can contribute to the development of insulin resistance. Moreover, there was a significant increase in leptin levels in the group with greater weight gain. Leptin is directly related to body fat in both experimental models and in humans (20,21), and is also related to food intake (22). These alterations relative to subclinical inflammation agree with those present in situations of obesity. The adipose tissue contributes to inflammation in both obese vascular and non-vascular tissues (23). Abnormal levels of fatty acids, lipids, cytokines and activate monocytes adipose tissue, increased secretion of inflammatory cytokines such as TNF-α, leptin, interleukin (IL)-1, IL-6, visfatin and reduced the secretion of anti-inflammatory cytokine adiponectin (24).

This study also has the important evaluation point of resting energy expenditure and respiratory quotient, given that data on basal metabolism with DMPA use are scarce, only two studies have assessed the resting energy expenditure in healthy women using DMPA (25,26). The basal metabolic rate increased significantly in the DMPA group and control. However, a more significant increase in this variable in subgroup DMPA, which gained more weight (> 3 kg), can be seen. This increase is mainly explained by an increase in fat mass and fat-free mass as well. In obese, the resting energy expenditure can be influenced mainly by fat-free mass, which is the largest contributing factor of variance of the basal metabolic rate (50-60%), and fat mass which represents (5-6%) of influence on the variation basal metabolic rate (27). The respiratory quotient of the two groups decreased after 12 months follow-up, indicating a change in metabolism of energy substrates. The volunteers at baseline had a characteristic respiratory quotient of high sugar metabolism but by the end of the study the profile changed with lipids starting to metabolize.

This study had the limitation of a small number of patients; including more patients could strengthen our results. Also we did not evaluate the lipid profile of the volunteers.

In conclusion, our study found significant changes in weight, body composition and metabolic profile of the population studied in the first 12 months of contraceptive use. These changes mainly increased body weight, leptin levels and HOMA-IR which can contribute to the development of some chronic complications, including obesity, insulin resistance and diabetes mellitus. According to the changes observed in our study, we suggest a more careful assessment of women who will start using the method as well as those who are already using this method of contraception. The exposure time method is considered the most important factor for the development of these changes.

Acknowledgements: we thank Fapesp for funding this research, Cleide Silva for their assistance in the analysis and statistical interpretation and to all the volunteers of this research.

REFERENCES

1. Finucane MM, Stevens GA, Cowan MJ, Danaei G, Lin JK, Paciorek CJ, et al.; Global Burden of Metabolic Risk Factors of

Chronic Diseases Collaborating Group (Body Mass Index). National, regional, and global trends in body-mass index since 1980: systematic analysis of health examination surveys and epidemiological studies with 960 country-years and 9·1 million participants. Lancet. 2011;377(9765):557-67.

2. Ministério da Saúde, Secretaria de Vigilância em Saúde: Vigitel Brasil: vigilância de fatores de risco e proteção para doenças crônicas por inquérito telefônico. Brasília; 2012.
3. Aoi N, Soma M, Nakayama T, Rahmutula D, Kosuge K, Izumi Y, et al. Variable number of tandem repeat of the 5'-flanking region of type-C human natriuretic peptide receptor gene influences blood pressure levels in obesity-associated hypertension. Hypertens Res. 2004;27(10):711-6.
4. Kosuge K, Soma M, Nakayama T, Aoi N, Sato M, Haketa A, et al. Human uncoupling protein 2 and 3 genes are associated with obesity in Japanese. Endocrine. 2008;34(1-3):87-95.
5. Kahn HS, Curtis KM, Marchbanks PA. Effects of injectable or implantable progestin-only contraceptives on insulin-glucose metabolism and diabetes risk. Diabetes Care. 2003;26(1):216-25.
6. Pantoja M, Medeiros T, Baccarin MC, Morais SS, Bahamondes L, Fernandes AM. Variations in body mass index of users of depot-medroxyprogesterone acetate as a contraceptive. Contraception. 2010;81(2):107-11.
7. Bakry S, Abdullah A. Effect of depot medroxyprogesterone (DMPA) on body weight and serum lipid profile in adult female rats. Egypt J Biochem Molec Biol. 2008;2(1):17-30.
8. Clark MK, Dillon JS, Sowers M, Nichols S. Weight, fat mass, and central distribution of fat increase when women use depot-medroxyprogesterone acetate for contraception. Int J Obes (Lond). 2005;29(10):1252-8.
9. Berenson AB, Rahman M. Changes in weight, total fat, percent body fat, and central-to-peripheral fat ratio associated with injectable and oral contraceptive use. Am J Obstet Gynecol. 2009;200(3):329.e1-8.
10. Weinberg A, Park JG, Bosch R, Cho A, Livingston E, Aweeka F, et al. Effect of Depot Medoxyprogesterone Acetate on Immune Functions and Inflammatory Markers of HIV-Infected Women. J Acquir Immune Defic Syndr. 2016;71(2):137-45.
11. WHO. Obesity: preventing and managing the global epidemic. Genebra; 1997.
12. Geloneze B, Vasques AC, Stabe CF, Pareja JC, Rosado LE, Queiroz EC, et al. HOMA1-IR and HOMA2-IR indexes in identifying insulin resistance and metabolic syndrome: Brazilian Metabolic Syndrome Study (BRAMS). Arq Bras Endocrinol Metabol. 2009;53(2):281-7.
13. Camargos AF, Melo VH, Carneiro MM, Reis FM. Ginecologia ambulatorial baseada em evidências científicas. 2. ed. Belo Horizonte: Coopmed; 2008. p. 288-90.
14. Harte C, Henry MT, Murphy KD, Mitchell TH. Progestogens and Cushing's syndrome. Ir J Med Sci. 1995;164(4):274-5.
15. Toth MJ, Tchernof A, Sites CK, Poehlman ET. Effect of menopausal status on body composition and abdominal fat distribution. Int J Obes Relat Metab Disord. 2000;24(2):226-31.
16. Perseghin G, Ghosh S, Gerow K, Shulman GI. Metabolic defects in lean nondiabetic offspring of NIDDM parents: a cross-sectional study. Diabetes. 1997;46(6):1001-9.
17. Boden G. Obesity and free fatty acids. Endocrinol Metab Clin North Am. 2008;37(3):635-46, viii-ix.
18. Hauner H. Secretory factors from human adipose tissue and their functional role. Proc Nutr Soc. 2005;64(2):163-9.
19. Halberg N, Wernstedt-Asterholm I, Scherer PE. The adipocyte as an endocrine cell. Endocrinol Metab Clin North Am. 2008;37(3):753-68, x-xi.
20. Pratley RE, Nicolson M, Bogardus C, Ravussin E. Plasma leptin responses to fasting in Pima Indians. Am J Physiol. 1997;273(3 Pt 1):E644-9.
21. Considine RV, Sinha MK, Heiman ML, Kriauciunas A, Stephens TW, Nyce MR, et al. Serum immunoreactive-leptin concentrations in normal-weight and obese humans. N Engl J Med. 1996;334(5):292-5.
22. Weigle DS, Duell PB, Connor WE, Steiner RA, Soules MR, Kuijper JL. Effect of fasting, refeeding, and dietary fat restriction on plasma leptin levels. J Clin Endocrinol Metab. 1997;82(2):561-5.
23. Rajala MW, Scherer PE. Minireview: The adipocyte--at the crossroads of energy homeostasis, inflammation, and atherosclerosis. Endocrinology. 2003;144(9):3765-73.
24. Wang Z, Nakayama T. Inflammation, a link between obesity and cardiovascular disease. Mediators Inflamm. 2010;2010:535918.
25. Pelkman CL, Chow M, Heinbach RA, Rolls BJ. Short-term effects of a progestational contraceptive drug on food intake, resting energy expenditure, and body weight in young women. Am J Clin Nutr. 2001;73(1):19-26.
26. Steward RG, Bateman LA, Slentz C, Stanczyk FZ, Price TM. The impact of short-term depot-medroxyprogesterone acetate treatment on resting metabolic rate. Contraception. 2016;93(4):317-22.
27. Johnstone AM, Murison SD, Duncan JS, Rance KA, Speakman JR. Factors influencing variation in basal metabolic rate include fat-free mass, fat mass, age, and circulating thyroxine but not sex, circulating leptin, or triiodothyronine. Am J Clin Nutr. 2005;82(5):941-8.

Lipid disorders among Black Africans non-users of lipid-lowering medication

Mariana Veronez Borgo[1], Marcelo Perim Baldo[2,3], Rafael de Oliveira Alvim[1], Divanei Zaniqueli[3], Daniel Pires Capingana[5], Pedro Magalhães[5], Amilcar Bernardo da Silva[5], Polyana Romano Oliosa[4], Carmem Luiza Sartório[3], José Geraldo Mill[1,3]

[1] Programa de Pós-Graduação em Saúde Coletiva, Universidade Federal do Espírito Santo (UFES), Vitória, ES, Brasil
[2] Departamento de Fisiopatologia, Universidade Estadual de Montes Claros (Unimontes), Montes Claros, MG, Brasil
[3] Programa de Pós-Graduação em Ciências Fisiológicas, Universidade Federal do Espírito Santo (UFES), Vitória, ES, Brasil
[4] Programa de Pós-Graduação em Nutrição e Saúde, Universidade Federal do Espírito Santo (UFES), Vitória, ES, Brasil
[5] Departamento de Ciências Fisiológicas, Escola de Medicina, Universidade Agostinho Neto (UAN), Luanda, Angola

Correspondence to:
Divanei Zaniqueli
Programa de Pós-Graduação em Ciências Fisiológicas, Universidade Federal do Espírito Santo
Av. Marechal Campos, 1468, Maruípe
29042-755 – Vitória, ES, Brasil
divozaniqueli@hotmail.com

ABSTRACT

Objective: Angola is a sub-Saharan African country where the population has scarce access to lipid-lowering medication. We sought to determine the frequency of lipid disorders among Angolan non-users of lipid-lowering medication. Material and methods: A cross-sectional descriptive study was carried out in a sample of 604 workers from the public sector. Blood pressure and anthropometric data were measured along with biochemical parameters including total cholesterol (TC), triglycerides (TG), low-density lipoprotein cholesterol (LDL-C) and high-density lipoprotein cholesterol (HDL-C). LDL-C to HDL-C ratio (LDL-C/HDL-C) was obtained from LDL-C and HDL-C levels. Results: High frequencies of elevated blood pressure (44.8%), metabolic syndrome (20.2%), increased TC (39.2%) and increased LDL-C (19.3%) were found. Low HDL-C was more frequent in women (62.4% *vs.* 36.1%, $p < 0.001$). Isolated hypercholesterolemia was more frequent in men (9.6% *vs.* 2.5%, $p < 0.001$). Among men TC, TG, LDL-C and LDL-C/HDL-C ratio were higher and HDL-C was lower in obese than in low-weight and normal-weight participants. Among women TC, TG, LDL-C and LDL-C/HDL-C ratio were higher in obese than in normal-weight participants. Significant linear trend of increasing TC and LDL-C levels as age increased was detected for both genders (p for trend < 0.05). Conclusion: The results of our study showed a high frequency of lipid disorders in Angolan non-users of lipid-lowering medication. Arch Endocrinol Metab. 2018;62(5):552-9

Keywords
Lipid disorders; Black Africans; lipid-lowering medication

INTRODUCTION

Dyslipidemia is a multifactorial lipid disorder that is dependent on genetic, environmental and lifestyle factors and is described as one of the most relevant risk factors for cardiovascular diseases (1). Indeed, dyslipidemia has been identified as one of the major modifiable risk factors for ischemic heart disease among young adults (2).

The definition of dyslipidemia is the presence of abnormal blood lipid levels, encompassing increased plasma levels of total cholesterol (TC), low-density lipoprotein (LDL-C) and triglycerides (TG), as well as decreased levels of high-density lipoprotein (HDL-C) (3).

In sub-Saharan Africa, the majority of countries is experiencing a rapid demographic and epidemiological transition (4,5). Several studies have reported the prevalence of cardiovascular risk factors in sub-Saharan African populations (6-8), but these data are limited to a few countries (9,10).

Angola is a sub-Saharan African country where in the last few years, significant economic growth and increased urbanization has occurred (11). These changes may imply an increasing prevalence of diverse cardiovascular risk factors such as obesity, insufficient physical activity, high blood pressure and dyslipidemia.

The Angolan population has scarce access to lipid-lowering pharmacological therapy, which offers an ideal opportunity to analyze the lipid profile in a large sample with minimal interfering factors. Therefore, in this study, we sought to determine the frequency of lipid disorders in an Angolan population consisting of non-users of lipid-lowering medication.

MATERIAL AND METHODS

Study design

This cross-sectional descriptive study was carried out in a sample consisting of civil servants working at Agostinho Neto University (UAN) in Luanda, Angola. The survey was conducted in the Department of Physiology from the Faculty of Medicine. All data were collected from 2009 to 2010, and details of the study design were described elsewhere (12,13). The project was approved by the Independent Ethics Committee on Research of the Faculty of Medicine of Agostinho Neto University following the standard procedures in human research in accordance with the Declaration of Helsinki.

Subjects ≥ 20 years of age working at UAN were invited to participate in a survey of cardiovascular risk factors. From the eligible sample comprising 1,458 staff members, 614 (42%) responded to the invitation. Only nine subjects (1.4%) were excluded from the present analysis due to use of lipid-lowering medication.

Demographics including socioeconomic class, educational level and medical history were collected during an interview using a structured questionnaire, as previously reported (14). Participants were classified as non-smokers (never and former smokers) and current smokers (daily and occasional smokers).

Socioeconomic classes were categorized into quartiles according to average monthly household income: first quartile (low class), second quartile (middle class), third quartile (upper middle class) and fourth quartile (upper class). Education levels were classified into three categories based on the number of years of education: low (≤ four years of education), middle (five to 12 years of education) and high (≥ 13 years of education) (13).

Biochemical analyses

Participants reported to the Faculty of Medicine after 12h of fasting. They were asked to refrain from smoking, physical exercise and caffeinated beverages for at least 12 hours before the visit. Clinical exams were performed in a temperature-controlled room (22°C – 23°C) between 8 a.m. and noon. For determination of serum levels of TC, TG, HDL-C and glucose, venous blood was obtained by standard *forearm venipuncture* and processed immediately using commercially available kits (Biosystems S.A. Costa Brava 30, Barcelona, Spain).

All biochemical parameters were analyzed by enzymatic methods with a spectrophotometer (Biosystems BTS 310, Barcelona, Spain). LDL-C was calculated as previously described (15), and very low-density lipoprotein cholesterol (VLDL-C) was calculated as triglycerides/5 for those participants with TG < 400 mg/dL according to the Third Report of the National Cholesterol Education Program Expert Panel on detection, evaluation and treatment of high blood cholesterol in adults (NCEP-ATP III) (16). The LDL-C to HDL-C ratio (LDL-C/HDL-C) was obtained from LDL-C and HDL-C levels.

Diabetes mellitus was defined as fasting glucose ≥ 126 mg/dL or the use of antidiabetic drugs (17).

Dyslipidemia was classified into four phenotypes in accordance with V Brazilian Guidelines on Dyslipidemia and Atherosclerosis: isolated hypertriglyceridemia (TG ≥ 150 mg/dL), isolated hypercholesterolemia (LDL ≥ 160 mg/dL), mixed hyperlipidemia (TG > 150 and TC ≥ 200 mg/dL) and low HDL-C (isolated reduction of HDL-C, men < 40 mg/dL and women < 50 mg/dL or combined with either increased LDL-C or increased TG) (18).

Metabolic syndrome was defined based on the presence of three or more of the following conditions: waist circumference (WC) > 102 cm (men) or > 88 cm (women), systolic blood pressure (SBP) ≥ 130 mmHg and/or diastolic blood pressure (DBP) ≥ 85 mmHg and/or BP-lowering treatment, fasting triglyceride levels ≥ 150 mg/dL (1.70 mmol/l) or treatment for hypertriglyceridemia, HDL-C < 40 mg/dL (1.04 mmol/l) (men) or < 50 mg/dL (1.30 mmol/l) (women), treatment for dyslipidemia, fasting glucose level ≥ 110 mg/dL or use of anti-diabetic medication (16).

Anthropometric measurements

Anthropometric measures of weight, height, WC and hip circumference (HC) were obtained with participants barefoot and wearing only underwear. Weight was measured to the nearest 0.1 kg using a previously calibrated mechanical scale (SECA GmbH & Co, Germany). A stadiometer fixed to the scale was used to measure body height to the nearest 0.5 cm.

WC and HC were measured twice using an inextensible 1-cm-wide tape measure. WC was measured at the end of a normal expiration at the midpoint between the lower border of the rib cage and the top of the iliac crest (19). The waist-to-hip ratio (WHR) was calculated from the WC and HC.

BMI was calculated as the weight in kilograms divided by height in meters squared (kg/m^2). According to the BMI values, the participants were classified as low weight ($< 18.5\ kg/m^2$), normal weight (18.5–24.9 kg/m^2), overweight (25.0–29.9 kg/m^2) and obese ($\geq 30.0\ kg/m^2$) (20).

Hemodynamic measurements

Blood pressure measurement was performed after a five-minute rest in triplicate in the non-dominant arm with the arm at the level of the heart. Systolic blood pressure (SBP), diastolic blood pressure (DBP) and HR were obtained using a validated, automated digital oscillometric sphygmomanometer (Omron 705CP, Tokyo, Japan). The readings were repeated at three-minute intervals. The mean of the last two readings was recorded. Elevated blood pressure was defined as SBP ≥ 140 mmHg and/or DBP ≥ 90 mmHg and/or the use of antihypertensive drugs.

Statistical analysis

Statistical analysis was performed using SPSS software, version 20.0 (SPSS Inc., Chicago, IL, USA). The data's normality was examined using the Kolmogorov-Smirnov test. Continuous variables were reported as mean ± standard deviation (SD) or as proportions.

Student's t test was used to compare the means of two groups. Linear association between lipid fractions and categories of nutritional status was tested with ANCOVA. The chi-squared test was used to compare proportions. A test for linear trends (Jonckheere-Terpstra test) was performed to test the linear association between the age range as the independent variable and lipid fractions as the dependent variable. Normal distribution curves of total cholesterol and triglycerides were drawn separately for gender and median (P^{50th}) with corresponding interquartile intervals ($P^{25th} - P^{75th}$) provided. The level of significance was set at $p < 0.05$.

RESULTS

Demographic data are summarized in Table 1. As expected, the sample comprised predominantly black individuals. Regarding educational level and socioeconomic status, approximately 60% had at least five years of formal education, and almost 68% were classified as members of the middle/upper socioeconomic class.

Table 1. Demographic characteristics of sample

	N	%
Gender		
Male	291	48
Female	314	52
Total	605	100
Age range (years)		
22-31	88	14.5
32-41	137	22.6
42-51	207	34.2
52-61	149	24.6
62-72	24	4.0
Race/ethnicity		
White	5	0.8
Black	577	95.4
Mulattos	23	3.8
Education level		
Low	243	40.2
Medium	150	24.8
High	212	35.0
Socioeconomic Class		
Low	191	31.6
Middle	203	33.6
Upper	209	34.5
MS	2	0.3

MS: missing data.

Table 2 shows the sample's general characteristics, emphasizing the comparison between genders. The age was similar between genders, but higher BMI and WC were observed in women than in men. A significant gender difference was not detected for SBP and DBP. Moreover, lipid profile was similar between genders, but HDL-C was higher in women than in men ($p < 0.001$).

Overall, a high frequency of elevated blood pressure (44.8%), metabolic syndrome (20.2%), increased TC (39.2%) and increased LDL-C (19.3%) was found. Moreover, gender interfered with the frequency of some risk factors. Obesity, metabolic syndrome and low HDL-C were more frequent in women than in men. On the other hand, smoking and isolated hypercholesterolemia were more frequent in men than in women (Table 3).

Table 4 shows the association between lipid fraction and nutritional status for both genders. Among men, TC, TG, LDL-C and the LDL-C/HDL-C ratio were higher, and HDL-C was lower in obese participants than in low-weight and normal-weight participants.

Table 2. Anthropometric and biochemical characteristics of sample stratified by gender

	Male	Female	*p value*
Age (years)	45.1 ± 11.1	43.8 ± 10.0	0.18
Weight (kg)	67.7 ± 4.7	69.1 ± 15.7	0.33
Height (cm)	167 ± 7.0	159.5 ± 6.6	< 0.001
BMI (kg/m²)	24.0 ± 4.2	27.1 ± 5.8	< 0.001
WC (cm)	79.9 ± 12.8	83.7 ± 13.5	< 0.001
HC (cm)	91.4 ± 9.4	99.5 ± 1.5	< 0.001
WHR	0.87 ± 0.08	0.84 ± 0.09	< 0.001
SBP (mmHg)	137 ± 23	133 ± 27	0.09
DBP (mmHg)	83 ± 14	82 ± 14	0.86
Heart rate (bpm)	67 ± 10	69 ± 10	0.003
Glucose (mg/dL)	95 ± 20	92 ± 19	0.31
TC (mg/dL)	190 ± 42	192 ± 36	0.24
LDL-C (mg/dL)	125 ± 41	125 ± 38	0.79
HDL-C (mg/dL)	44 ± 10	48 ± 11	< 0.001
TG (mg/dL)	101 ± 42	99 ± 38	0.34
VLDL-C (mg/dL)	20± 8	20 ± 7	0.34

BMI: body mass index; WC: waist circumference; HC: hip circumference; WHR: waist-to hip ratio; SBP: systolic blood pressure; DBP: diastolic blood pressure; TC: total cholesterol; LDL-C: low-density lipoprotein cholesterol; HDL-C: high-density lipoprotein cholesterol; VLDL-C: very low-density lipoprotein cholesterol; TG: triglycerides.

Table 3. Risk factors in the sample and stratified by gender

	All	Male	Female	*p value*
Elevated blood pressure	44.8	46.0	43.6	0.30
Diabetes	5.1	5.2	5.1	0.56
Obesity	19.2	8.9	28.7	< 0.001
Metabolic Syndrome	20.2	16.2	23.9	0.01
Smoking	6.1	8.2	4.1	0.03
TC ≥ 200	39.2	38.8	39.5	0.47
Isolated hypercholesterolemia	6.0	9.6	2.5	< 0.001
LDL-C ≥ 160 mg/dL	19.3	20.6	18.2	0.25
Isolated hypertriglyceridemia	4.6	6.2	3.2	0.06
TG ≥ 150 mg/dL	10.7	12.4	9.2	0.13
Mixed hyperlipidemia	1.7	1.7	1.6	0.903
Low-HDL-C	49.8	36.1	62.4	< 0.001

Data are presented as proportions (%). Elevated blood pressure: SBP ≥ 140 mmHg and/or DBP ≥ 90 mmHg or normotensive on antihypertensive medication. Diabetes: fasting glucose ≥ 126 mg/dL or on medication. TC, total cholesterol; LDL-c, low-density lipoprotein cholesterol; HDL-c, high density lipoprotein cholesterol; TG, triglycerides. Isolated hypercholesterolemia: isolated elevation of LDL-C (≥ 160 mg/dL); Isolated hypertriglyceridemia: isolated elevation of TGs (≥ 150 mg/dL); Mixed hyperlipidemia: Increased LDL-C (≥ 160 mg/dL) combined with increased TG (≥ 150 mg/dL). Low HDL-C: isolated reduction of HDL-C (Men < 40 mg/dL, Women < 50 mg/dL) or in association with elevated LDL-C and TG.

A similar difference was found in overweight participants compared with low-weight participants, but in TG levels, such a difference was not detected

Table 4. Association between lipid fraction and weight status

	Low weight	Normal weight	Overweight	Obese
Male				
n (%)	16 (5.6)	168 (58.3)	78 (27.1)	26 (9.0)
TC (mg/dL)	168 ± 26	184 ± 39	199 ± 46*†	214 ± 33*†
TG (mg/dL)	78 ± 34	98 ± 36	108 ± 49†	123 ± 46*†
LDL-C (mg/dL)	104 ± 25	119 ± 39	135 ± 46*†	149 ± 36*†
HDL-C (mg/dL)	48 ± 14	46 ± 10	42 ± 10*†	40 ± 8*†
LDL-C/HDL-C	2.4 ± 1.0	2.8 ± 1.3	3.4 ± 1.4*†	3.9 ± 1.5*†
Female				
n (%)	11(3.6)	111(36.4)	93 (30.5)	90 (29.5)
TC (mg/dL)	191± 29	186 ± 35	196 ± 33*	197 ± 39*
TG (mg/dL)	88 ± 37	94 ± 34	97 ± 40	109 ± 41#*
LDL-C (mg/dL)	125 ± 29	118 ± 35	129 ± 34*	129 ± 44*
HDL-C (mg/dL)	48 ± 7	49 ± 11	47 ± 12	46 ± 11
LDL-C/HDL-C	2.7 ± 0.7	2.6 ± 1.1	2.9 ± 1.2	3.1 ± 1.5*

Data are mean ± standard deviation. TC: total cholesterol; TG: triglycerides; LDL-C: low density lipoprotein cholesterol; HDL-C: high density lipoprotein cholesterol; LDL-C/HDL-C: LDL-C to HDL-C ratio. *$p < 0.05$ *vs.* normal weight, #$p < 0.05$ *vs.* overweight, †$p < 0.05$ *vs.* low weight. Comparisons adjusted for age.

between overweight and normal-weight men. On the other hand, among women, TC and LDL-C were higher in obese and overweight participants than in normal-weight participants, and TG was higher in obese participants than in low-weight and normal-weight participants. The LDL-C/HDL-C ratio was higher in obese participants than in normal-weight participants, but HDL-C was not different across the categories of nutritional status.

A significant linear trend of increasing TC, LDL-C and TG levels as well as decreasing HDL-C levels with increasing age was observed among women (p for trend < 0.05) (Figure 1). On the other hand, a significant linear trend of increasing TC and LDL-C levels with increasing age was detected (p for trend < 0.01), but no significant linear trend was detected between age range and HDL-C and TG among men.

Figure 2 shows the distribution curves of TC and TG for women and men. The medians with interquartile intervals for TC were 191 mg/dL (170-215 mg/dL) and 189 mg/dL (159-217 mg/dL) in women and men, respectively. Likewise, the medians with corresponding interquartile intervals for TG were 91 mg/dL (75-118 mg/dL) and 96 mg/dL (74-120 mg/dL), respectively. The areas under the distribution curves provide the proportion of individuals with TC and TG above the 75th percentile.

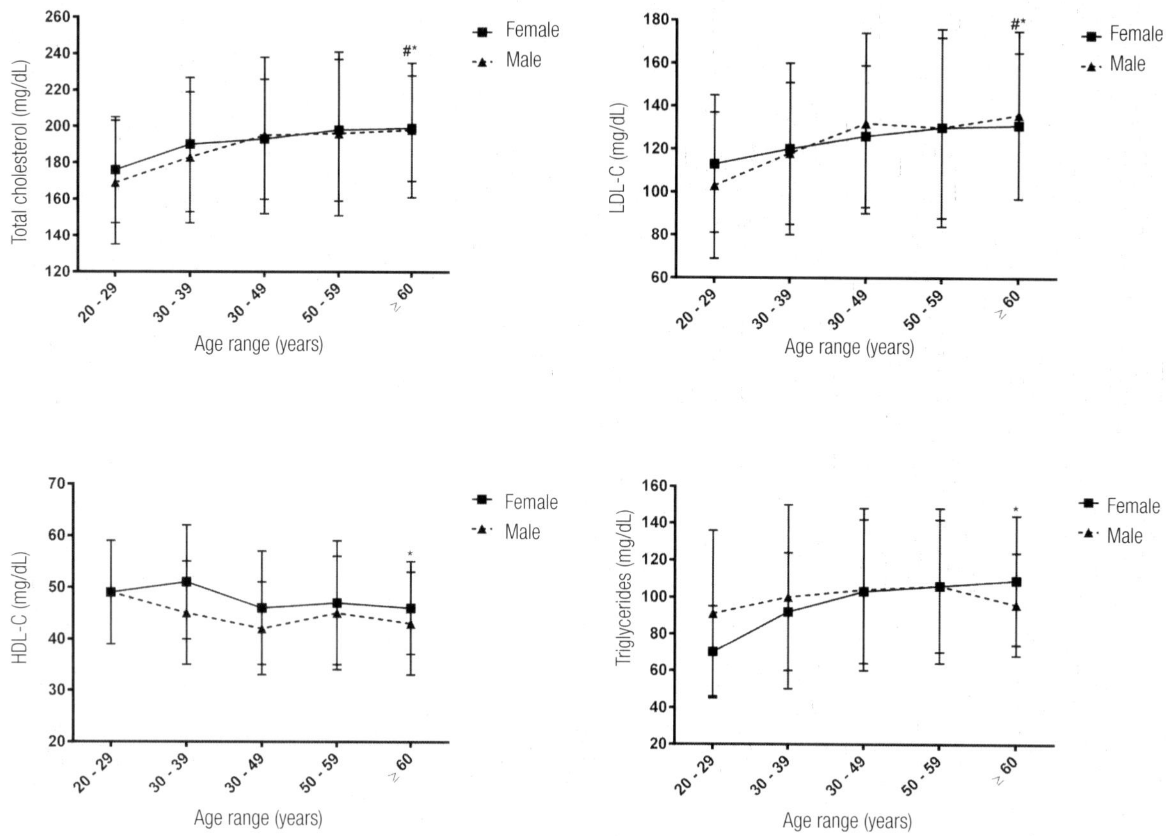

Figure 1. Test for significant linear trend between age range and total cholesterol, LDL-C, HDL-C and triglycerides. # men, p for trend < 0.05 ; *women, p for trend < 0.05.

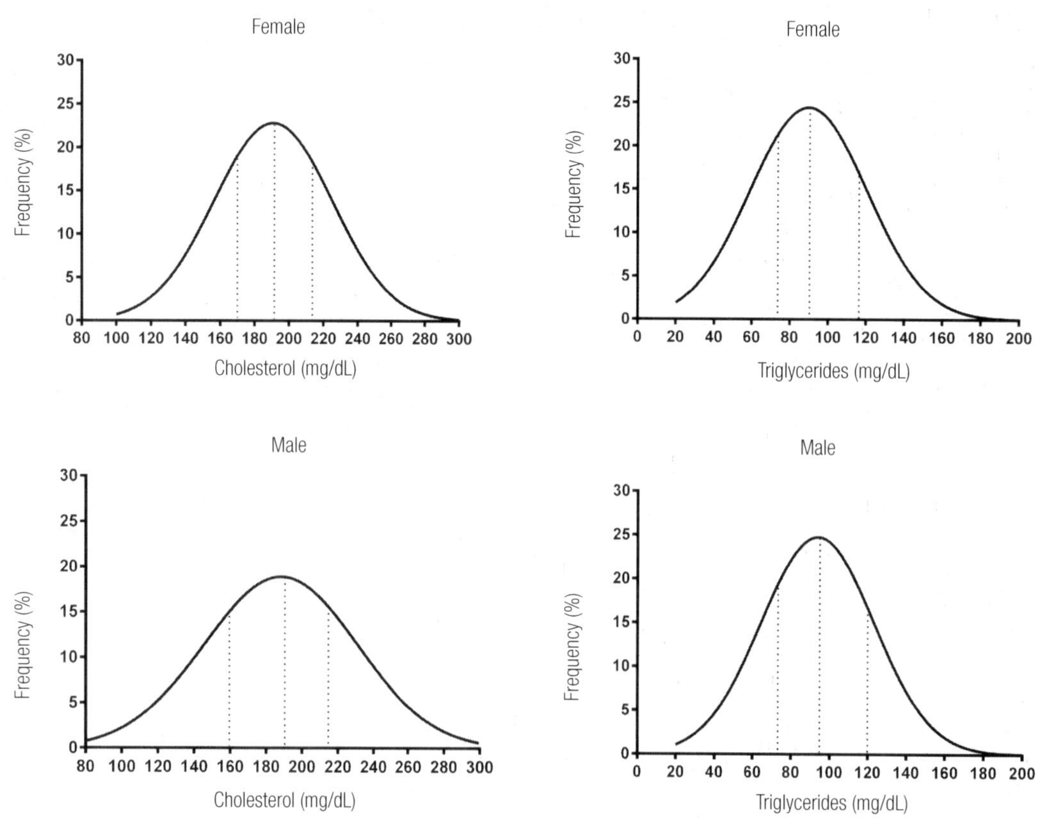

Figure 2. Nornal distribution curves of total cholesterol and triglycerides separately by gender. Dot lines indicate 25th, 50th and 75th percentiles from the left to the right.

DISCUSSION

The present study was carried out in Angolan civil servants, predominantly black and of middle/upper socioeconomic class. Higher frequencies of obesity, metabolic syndrome and low HDL-C were found in women than in men. On the other hand, obesity seems to cause the lipid profile to undergo greater changes in men than in women. Moreover, a significant linear trend of increasing TC and LDL-C levels as age increased was detected for both genders.

Epidemiologic studies have shown that elevated serum levels of cholesterol in the population increases the risk for coronary heart disease (21,22). Moreover, dyslipidemia, among other risk factors, has been implicated in the pathogenesis of stroke (23).

Data from the 2003 through 2006 NHANES survey were analyzed to determine the proportion of the US population with abnormalities in the lipid profile (24). Despite the existence of efficacious and cost-effective treatment guidelines, high prevalence of lipid abnormalities such as high LDL-C (27.0%), elevated TG levels (30.0%) and low HDL-C (23%) was reported. Although the study described here is not a population-based cohort, compared with the US population, Angolan civil servants have a lower proportion of high LDL-C (19.3%) and elevated TG (10.7%) and a much higher proportion of low HDL-C (49.8%), which is in great part affected by the huge proportion of low HDL-C observed in women (62.4%). Indeed, this finding is alarming given the strong association of low HDL-C with atherosclerosis (25).

An expert panel from the American College of Cardiology/American Heart Association recommended that all individuals over 20 years of age with LDL-C levels above 190 mg/dL should be encouraged to either start or continue statin use for prevention of coronary heart disease and stroke (26). However, statins are still widely underused in the clinical setting, and poor adherence to statin therapy has become a major concern for preventive cardiology (27).

Recently, a Finnish population-based study showed the cardiovascular burden of medication non-adherence (28). The rate of adherence to statins was 58% in men and 60% in women, which the authors classified as intermediate. In addition, compared with adherent patients, the adjusted odds ratio for stroke death in non-adherents was 2.04 (CI95% 1.72–2.43) at the year of death or at the end of follow-up.

Regarding African populations, most of the studies dealing with adherence to statin therapy were conducted among people of African descent living outside Africa. One of these studies reported that ethnicity (African American) was among the predictors of non-adherence to statin therapy (29). Moreover, among white and black Medicare beneficiaries discharged from the hospital following an ischemic stroke, the adherence to statin therapy was lower in African Americans than in white subjects (30).

Lack of access to medical care has been considered one of the plausible explanations for the differences in the adherence to statin therapy between black and white subjects. However, a previous study has shown that even without access barriers, African Americans were less adherent to medication therapies, including statins (31).

To our knowledge, the adherence rate to lipid-lowering pharmacological therapy has not been documented in black African countries. Recently, a retrospective longitudinal study among Ghanaian heart failure patients has shown that statin users had a higher survival rate than those non-users who underwent another therapeutic option, but therapy adherence was not within the study's scope (32).

In the current study, around 60% of the volunteers claimed to have a good, or high, education level, and 68.1% comprised the middle or upper socioeconomic class. However, the mean values for the metabolic parameters were similar to those previously reported in the lower socioeconomic strata from black African populations (33). This result reflects the epidemiological transition of the Angolan population because even with enhanced socioeconomic status, the frequency of metabolic syndrome and elevated cholesterol levels remain meaningfully high, and this scenario tends to get worse as age advances.

Because this study was cross-sectional, it is not appropriate to establish a causal relationship between non-adherence to lipid-lowering therapy and cardiovascular risk factors. Indeed, this study was not designed to address this particular issue. In addition, as the sample was composed of public sector workers, the results should not be extrapolated to the whole Angolan population. However, it is worth wondering whether a high frequency of lipid disorders without treatment was observed in a population comprising almost two-thirds of the middle/upper-income segment and what to expect from a representative sample of the population comprising approximately 85% of the low-income class.

In summary, a high frequency of lipid disorders was observed among Angolan non-users of lipid-lowering medication. Longitudinal studies should be conducted to highlight the long-term consequences of non-treated lipid disorders in the Angolan population.

Acknowledgements: we appreciate the cooperation of the public--sector workers at UAN and the great work of the laboratory technicians.

Funding Statement: this work was supported by the Science and Development Foundation of Agostinho Neto University, Angola, Africa.

REFERENCES

1. Musunuru K. Atherogenic dyslipidemia: cardiovascular risk and dietary intervention. Lipids. 2010;45(10):907-14.
2. Faisal AW, Ayub M, Waseem T, Khan RS, Hasnain SS. Risk factors in young patients of acute myocardial infarction. J Ayub Med Coll Abbottabad. 2011;23(3):10-3.
3. Jacobson TA, Maki KC, Orringer CE, Jones PH, Kris-Etherton P, Sikand G, et al.; NLA Expert Panel. National Lipid Association Recommendations for Patient-Centered Management of Dyslipidemia: Part 2. J Clin Lipidol. 2015;9(6 Suppl):S1-122.e1.
4. Yusuf S, Reddy S, Ounpuu S, Anand S. Global burden of cardiovascular diseases: part I: general considerations, the epidemiologic transition, risk factors, and impact of urbanization. Circulation. 2001;104(22):2746-53.
5. National Research Council. The Continuing Epidemiological Transition in sub-Saharan Africa: A Workshop Summary. Thomas J. Plewes and Kevin Kinsella, Rapporteurs. Committee on National Population, Division of Behavioral and Social Sciences and Education. Washington, DC: The National Academies Press; 2012.
6. Henry-Okafor Q, Cowan PA, Wicks MN, Rice M, Husch DS, Khoo MS. Effect of obesity on cardiovascular disease risk factors in African American women. Biol Res Nurs. 2012;14(2):171-9.
7. Hamer M, von Känel R, Reimann M, Malan NT, Schutte AE, Huisman HW, et al. Progression of cardiovascular risk factors in black Africans: 3 year follow up of the SABPA cohort study. Atherosclerosis. 2015;238(1):52-4.
8. Bamimore MA, Zaid A, Banerjee Y, Al-Sarraf A, Abifadel M, Seidah NG, et al. Familial hypercholesterolemia mutations in the Middle Eastern and North African region: a need for a national registry. J Clin Lipidol. 2015;9(2):187-94.
9. Makuyana D, Gomo Z, Munyombwe T, Matenga JA, Hakim JG. Metabolic syndrome disorders in urban black Zimbabweans with type 2 Diabetes mellitus. Cent Afr J Med. 2004;50(3-4):24-9.
10. Kengne AP, Limen SN, Sobngwi E, Djouogo CF, Nouedoui C. Metabolic syndrome in type 2 diabetes: comparative prevalence according to two sets of diagnostic criteria in sub-Saharan Africans. Diabetol Metab Syndr. 2012;4:22.
11. Pinto TN. Growing cities pose challenges for African economies. Geopolitical Intelligence Services. 2016. Available from: https://www.gisreportsonline.com/growing-cities-pose-challenges-for-african-economies,economy,2046,report.html. Access on: Aug. 20 2018.
12. Magalhães P, Capingana DP, Silva AB, Ferreira AV, de Sá Cunha R, Rodrigues SL, et al. Age- and gender-specific reference values of pulse wave velocity for African adults: preliminary results. Age (Dordr). 2013;35(6):2345-55.
13. Capingana DP, Magalhães P, Silva AB, Gonçalves MA, Baldo MP, Rodrigues SL, et al. Prevalence of cardiovascular risk factors and socioeconomic level among public-sector workers in Angola. BMC Public Health. 2013;13:732.
14. Baldo MP, Zaniqueli DA, Magalhães P, Capingana DP, Silva AB, Mill JG. Gender-specific determinants of blood pressure elevation in Angolan adults. Blood Press. 2017;26(1):9-17.
15. Friedewald WT, Levy RI, Fredrickson DS. Estimation of the concentration of low-density lipoprotein cholesterol in plasma, without use of the preparative ultracentrifuge. Clin Chem. 1972;18(6):499-502.
16. National Cholesterol Education Program (NCEP) Expert Panel on Detection, Evaluation, and Treatment of High Blood Cholesterol in Adults (Adult Treatment Panel III). Third Report of the National Cholesterol Education Program (NCEP) Expert Panel on Detection, Evaluation, and Treatment of High Blood Cholesterol in Adults (Adult Treatment Panel III) final report. Circulation. 2002;106(25):3143-421.
17. American Diabetes Association. Diagnosis and classification of diabetes mellitus. Diabetes Care. 2010;33 Suppl 1:S62-9.
18. Xavier HT, Izar MC, Faria Neto JR, Assad MH, Rocha VZ, Sposito AC, et al. [V Brazilian Guidelines on Dyslipidemias and Prevention of Atherosclerosis]. Arq Bras Cardiol. 2013;101(4 Suppl 1):1-20.
19. Lean ME, Han TS, Morrison CE. Waist circumference as a measure for indicating need for weight management. BMJ. 1995;15(6998):158-61.
20. Batsis JA, Nieto-Martinez RE, Lopez-Jimenez F. Metabolic syndrome: from global epidemiology to individualized medicine. Clin Pharmacol Ther. 2007;82(5):509-24.
21. Anderson KM, Castelli WP, Levy D. Cholesterol and mortality. 30 years of follow-up from the Framingham study. JAMA. 1987;257(16):2176-80.
22. Law MR, Wald NJ, Thompson SG. By how much and how quickly does reduction in serum cholesterol concentration lower risk of ischaemic heart disease? BMJ. 1994;308(6925):367-72.
23. Writing Group Members, Mozaffarian D, Benjamin EJ, Go AS, Arnett DK, Blaha MJ, Cushman M, et al.; American Heart Association Statistics Committee; Stroke Statistics Subcommittee. Executive Summary: Heart Disease and Stroke Statistics – 2016 Update: A Report From the American Heart Association. Circulation. 2016;133(4):447-54.
24. Tóth PP, Potter D, Ming EE. Prevalence of lipid abnormalities in the United States: the National Health and Nutrition Examination Survey 2003-2006. J Clin Lipidol. 2012;6(4):325-30.
25. Emerging Risk Factors Collaboration, Di Angelantonio E, Sarwar N, Perry P, Kaptoge S, Ray KK, Thompson A, et al. Major lipids, apolipoproteins, and risk of vascular disease. JAMA. 2009;302(18):1993-2000.
26. Stone NJ, Robinson JG, Lichtenstein AH, Bairey Merz CN, Blum CB, Eckel RH, et al.; American College of Cardiology/American Heart Association Task Force on Practice Guidelines. 2013 ACC/AHA guideline on the treatment of blood cholesterol to reduce atherosclerotic cardiovascular risk in adults: a report of the American College of Cardiology/American Heart Association Task Force on Practice Guidelines. J Am Coll Cardiol. 2014;63(25 Pt B):2889-934.
27. Bates TR, Connaughton VM, Watts GF. Non-adherence to statin therapy: a major challenge for preventive cardiology. Expert Opin Pharmacother. 2009;10(18):2973-85.

28. Herttua K, Martikainen P, Batty GD, Kivimäki M. Poor Adherence to Statin and Antihypertensive Therapies as Risk Factors for Fatal Stroke. J Am Coll Cardiol. 2016;67(13):1507-15.

29. Ellis JJ, Erickson SR, Stevenson JG, Bernstein SJ, Stiles RA, Fendrick AM. Suboptimal statin adherence and discontinuation in primary and secondary prevention populations. J Gen Intern Med. 2004;19(6):638-45.

30. Albright KC, Zhao H, Blackburn J, Limdi NA, Beasley TM, Howard G, et al. Racial differences in statin adherence following hospital discharge for ischemic stroke. Neurology. 2017;88(19):1839-48.

31. Charles H, Good CB, Hanusa BH, Chang CC, Whittle J. Racial differences in adherence to cardiac medications. J Natl Med Assoc. 2003;95(1):17-27.

32. Bonsu KO, Owusu IK, Buabeng KO, Reidpath DD, Kadirvelu A. Statin Treatment and Clinical Outcomes of Heart Failure Among Africans: An Inverse Probability Treatment Weighted Analysis. J Am Heart Assoc. 2017;6(4):pii: e004706.

33. Njelekela MA, Mpembeni R, Muhihi A, Mligiliche NL, Spiegelman D, Hertzmark E, et al. Gender-related differences in the prevalence of cardiovascular disease risk factors and their correlates in urban Tanzania. BMC Cardiovasc Disord. 2009;9:30.

29

Dapagliflozin versus saxagliptin as add-on therapy in patients with type 2 diabetes inadequately controlled with metformin

Julio Rosenstock[1], Chantal Mathieu[2], Hungta Chen[3], Ricardo Garcia-Sanchez[3], Gabriela Luporini Saraiva[3]

[1] Dallas Diabetes Research Center at Medical City, Dallas, TX, USA
[2] UZ Leuven, Leuven, Belgium
[3] AstraZeneca, Gaithersburg, MD, USA

Correspondence to:
Julio Rosenstock
Dallas Diabetes Research Center at Medical City, 7777 Forest Lane C-685
75230 – Dallas, Texas, USA
juliorosenstock@dallasdiabetes.com

ABSTRACT

Objective: This analysis compared the efficacy and safety of the sodium–glucose cotransporter-2 (SGLT2) inhibitor, dapagliflozin, and the dipeptidyl peptidase-4 (DPP4) inhibitor, saxagliptin, both added on to metformin. Materials and methods: This was a post-hoc analysis from a double-blind, randomized, 24-week clinical trial (NCT01606007) of patients with type 2 diabetes (T2D) inadequately controlled with metformin. We compared the dapagliflozin 10 mg (n = 179) and saxagliptin 5 mg (n = 176) treatment arms. Results: Dapagliflozin showed significantly greater mean reductions versus saxagliptin in HbA_{1c} (difference versus saxagliptin [95% CI]: –0.32% [–0.54, –0.10]; p < 0.005), fasting plasma glucose (–0.98 [–1.42, –0.54] mmol/L; p < 0.0001), body weight (–2.39 [–3.08, –1.71] kg; p < 0.0001) and systolic blood pressure (SBP) (–3.89 [–6.15, –1.63] mmHg; p < 0.001). More dapagliflozintreated than saxagliptin-treated patients achieved the composite endpoint of HbA_{1c} reduction ≥ 0.5%, weight loss ≥ 2 kg, SBP reduction ≥ 2 mmHg and no major/minor hypoglycemia (24% versus 7%). No major events of hypoglycemia were reported. More patients on dapagliflozin (6%) versus saxagliptin (0.6%) experienced genital infections. Conclusion: Dapagliflozin demonstrated greater glycemic efficacy than saxagliptin with additional benefits on weight and SBP, and the safety profile was consistent with previous studies. Arch Endocrinol Metab. 2018;62(4):424-30

Keywords
Dapagliflozin; type 2 diabetes; SGLT2 inhibitor

INTRODUCTION

Type 2 diabetes (T2D) is a progressive disease, requiring treatment intensification over time in order to maintain glycemic control. Metformin is the gold standard first-line pharmacological treatment (1), and thereafter as glycemia worsens, sequential add-on treatment decisions are based on a number of variables and usually involve the addition of other oral glucoselowering agents (2). Recommendations from clinical guidelines on the management of T2D vary, with some making no specific recommendations on the choice of add-on agent (1), and others advocating a hierarchical order for add-on therapies (3).

The position statement of the American Diabetes Association (ADA) and European Association for the Study of Diabetes (EASD) recommends the use of one of six commonly used antihyperglycemic agents i.e. 1) a sulfonylurea, 2) a thiazolidinedione, 3) a dipeptidyl peptidase-4 (DPP4) inhibitor, 4) a sodium-glucose cotransporter-2 (SGLT2) inhibitor, 5) a glucagon-like peptide-1 (GLP-1) receptor agonist, or 6) a basal insulin analogue, as an add-on therapy when the individualized HbA_{1c} target is not achieved after ~3 months of treatment with metformin alone (1). The ADA/EASD position statement does not recommend any specific preference for a drug to be used as a dual therapy and instead suggests that the drug choice should be individualized based on patient preferences, hypoglycemia risk, side effect profile, and cost, in addition to other patient and disease characteristics (2). The ADA/EASD position statement further details that other drugs such as α-glucosidase inhibitors, colesevelam, bromocriptine and pramlintide may be used in specific situations but are generally not preferred due to their modest efficacy, side-effect profiles and dosing frequency.

DPP4 inhibitors and SGLT2 inhibitors are widelyused therapies for T2D that are associated with a low incidence of hypoglycemia, with DPP4 inhibitors being body-weight neutral (4) and SGLT2 inhibitors promoting weight loss and also reducing systolic blood pressure (SBP) (5-8). It is worth noting that in the 2017 American Association of Clinical Endocrinologists (AACE)/American College of Endocrinology (ACE) comprehensive glycemic control algorithm, SGLT2 inhibitors have been placed before DPP4 inhibitors in the hierarchical order of recommended use as monotherapy as well as add-on therapy (3).

The SGLT2 inhibitors, canagliflozin and empagliflozin, have both been directly compared with a DPP4 inhibitor in prospective randomized controlled trials (9-12). Long-term treatment with empagliflozin

25 mg showed greater reductions in HbA1c, body weight and SBP in comparison with sitagliptin 100 mg (9,10). Canagliflozin 300 mg as add-on to metformin, or metformin and a sulfonylurea, reduced both HbA_{1c} and weight to a greater extent than sitagliptin 100 mg (11,12).

However, to date, no large randomized controlled trial has directly compared the SGLT2 inhibitor dapagliflozin with a DPP4 inhibitor. One previously published study compared the combination of dapagliflozin plus saxagliptin with either drug individually, as add-on therapy in patients inadequately controlled on metformin (≥ 1500 mg/d) (13). This study was powered at 90% to detect a 0.4% difference in HbA_{1c} between the group receiving dapagliflozin plus saxagliptin and the groups receiving dapagliflozin or saxaglitpin individually, but was not powered for comparison of the groups receiving dapagliflozin or saxaglitpin individually. To provide clinicians with research evidence on the use of dapagliflozin compared with a DPP4 inhibitor to incorporate into their professional judgment and clinical decision making, a *post-hoc* analysis of the aforementioned study was conducted to compare the efficacy and safety of the two agents, dapagliflozin and saxagliptin, individually added on to metformin (14). It should be noted that saxagliptin and sitagliptin have demonstrated similar efficacy and safety profiles in a head-to-head noninferiority trial (15) and a systematic review (16).

MATERIALS AND METHODS

Study design

This was a *post-hoc* analysis of 24-week data from a randomized, three-arm, double-blind, active-controlled Phase 3 study (NCT01606007) (13). Patients with T2D were included in the original study if they were aged ≥ 18 years, had inadequate glycemic control (HbA_{1c} ≥ 8.0% and ≤ 12.0%), were on stable metformin therapy (≥ 1500 mg/day) for ≥ 8 weeks before screening and had a BMI ≤ 45.0 kg/m^2. The exclusion criteria were pregnancy, uncontrolled hypertension (SBP ≥ 160 mmHg and diastolic blood pressure ≥ 10 mmHg), fasting plasma glucose (FPG) ≥ 270 mg/dL during the 4-week lead-in period, cardiovascular disease (CVD) within 3 months of screening, congestive heart failure (New York Heart Association functional class IV), an estimated glomerular filtration rate < 60 mL/min/ 1.73 m^2 or serum creatinine ≥ 1.5 mg/dL in men or ≥ 1.4 mg/dL in women, significant hepatic disease, or having received an antidiabetic medication other, having metformin for more than 14 days during the 12 weeks before screening. Patients initially underwent a 4-week lead-in period during which they received metformin extended release (1500–2000 mg/day) before being randomized 1:1:1 to receive dapagliflozin plus saxagliptin, dapagliflozin plus placebo or saxagliptin plus placebo, in addition to metformin.

Primary and secondary efficacy endpoints were re-analyzed to evaluate the efficacy and safety of dapagliflozin versus saxagliptin as add-on to metformin.

The study was designed and performed in accordance with the ethical principles of Good Clinical Practice as defined by the International Conference on Harmonisation and the Declaration of Helsinki. Institutional review boards or independent ethics committees approved each protocol, and each patient provided written informed consent.

Outcomes measured

The primary endpoint was change from baseline to 24 weeks in HbA_{1c}. Secondary endpoints were changes from baseline to 24 weeks in body weight, FPG levels, and 2-hour postprandial glucose (2-hr PPG) levels (from a liquid meal tolerance test). Composite efficacy endpoints were assessed as (1) HbA1c reduction ≥ 0.5% + body weight reduction ≥ 2 kg; (2) HbA1c reduction ≥ 0.5% + SBP reduction ≥ 2 mmHg; (3) HbA_{1c} reduction ≥ 0.5% + body weight reduction ≥ 2 kg + no major/minor hypoglycemia; and (4) HbA1c reduction ≥ 0.5% + body weight reduction ≥ 2 kg + SBP reduction ≥ 2 mmHg + no major/minor hypoglycemia.

Safety assessments included overall adverse events (AEs), hypoglycemia and AEs of special interest including urinary tract and genital infections. Hypoglycemic episodes were classified as minor (symptomatic or asymptomatic with plasma glucose concentration < 63 mg/dL, regardless of need for external assistance) and major (symptomatic requiring third-party assistance due to severe impairment in consciousness or behavior, with or without plasma glucose concentration, < 54 mg/dL, and prompt recovery after glucose or glucagon administration). Change from baseline to 24 weeks in SBP was recorded as a safety assessment.

Statistical analysis

Statistical methods used in this post-hoc analysis were the same as those used in the primary analysis of the study (13). Adjusted mean change from baseline value and 95% CI were derived using the longitudinal repeated measures mixed model with nominal p-values. Composite endpoints were derived using logistic regression with the adjustment for baseline parameter (as applicable, depending on the outcome included in each individual composite endpoint). AE data were summarized using descriptive statistics.

RESULTS

Patient population

Patient demographics and baseline characteristics were balanced across treatment groups. Full baseline characteristics for the dapagliflozin and saxagliptin dose groups have been published previously (13). In brief, mean age was 54 years and mean duration of T2D was 7.6 years. Mean baseline HbA1c was 8.9% (73 mmol/mol) in the dapagliflozin group and 9.0% (75 mmol/mol) in the saxagliptin group. It should be noted that patients enrolled in this study had a high mean baseline HbA_{1c} (8.9%), with 45% having a baseline HbA_{1c} ≥9.0% (13). Mean baseline BMI was 31.5 kg/m^2 in the dapagliflozin group and 31.8 kg/m^2 in the saxagliptin group.

Efficacy outcomes

As an add-on to metformin, both dapagliflozin and saxagliptin reduced HbA1C over the 24-week treatment period (Figure 1A). Dapagliflozin showed a greater adjusted mean reduction from baseline in HbA_{1c} over the 24-week period (−1.20% [95% CI: −1.35, −1.04]) versus saxagliptin (−0.88% [−1.03, −0.72]), with a significant mean difference of −0.32% [−0.54, −0.10]; p < 0.005). The significant differences in adjusted mean change in HbA_{1c} with dapagliflozin versus saxagliptin were observed as early as Week 6 (−0.83% [−0.94, −0.71] versus −0.57% [−0.68, −0.46], respectively; p < 0.005). At 24 weeks, dapagliflozin reduced FPG (mean difference [95% CI]: −0.98 mmol/L [−1.42, −0.54]; p < 0.0001; Figure 1B), 2-hr PPG (mean difference [95% CI]: −1.94 mmol/L [−2.48, −1.39]; p < 0.0001; Figure 1C), and body weight (mean difference [95% CI]: −2.4 kg [−3.1, −1.7]; p < 0.0001; Figure 1D) to a significantly greater extent than saxagliptin.

After 24 weeks, the adjusted mean (95% CI) % proportion of patients achieving an HbA_{1c} < 7% was 22.2% (16.1%, 28.3%) with dapagliflozin versus 18.3% (13.0%, 23.5%) with saxagliptin (difference: -4.0% [−11.8%, 3.9%]; p = 0.32). A greater proportion of dapagliflozin-treated versus saxagliptin-treated patients achieved the composite endpoint of HbA_{1c} reduction ≥ 0.5%, weight loss ≥ 2 kg, SBP reduction ≥ 2 mmHg and no major/minor hypoglycemic events (Table 1). Likewise, greater proportions of dapagliflozintreated versus saxagliptin-treated patients achieved other composite endpoints (Table 1). Supplementary Table 1 shows the proportion of patients falling into the different categories according to HbA_{1c} decrease of < or ≥ 0.5% and weight loss of < or ≥ 2 kg.

Safety

The incidence of AEs was similar between groups, and was described in detail in the main publication (13). The proportion of patients with ≥ 1 AE was 49% for dapagliflozin and 53% for saxagliptin (Supplementary Table 2). Hypoglycemic event rates were low and similar across treatment groups (2 [1%] patients in each group). No major hypoglycemia events were reported. Higher proportions of patients on dapagliflozin (10 [6%]) versus saxagliptin (1 [0.6%]) experienced genital infections. No cases of diabetic ketoacidosis, postural hypotension, amputation or hospitalization for heart failure were reported in this study.

A statistically significant reduction in SBP from baseline to 24 weeks was observed with dapagliflozin (mean [95% CI]: −3.3 [−5.0, −1.7] mmHg) versus a small numerical increase observed with saxagliptin (mean [95% CI]: +0.5 [−1.1, 2.1] mmHg; p = 0.0008).

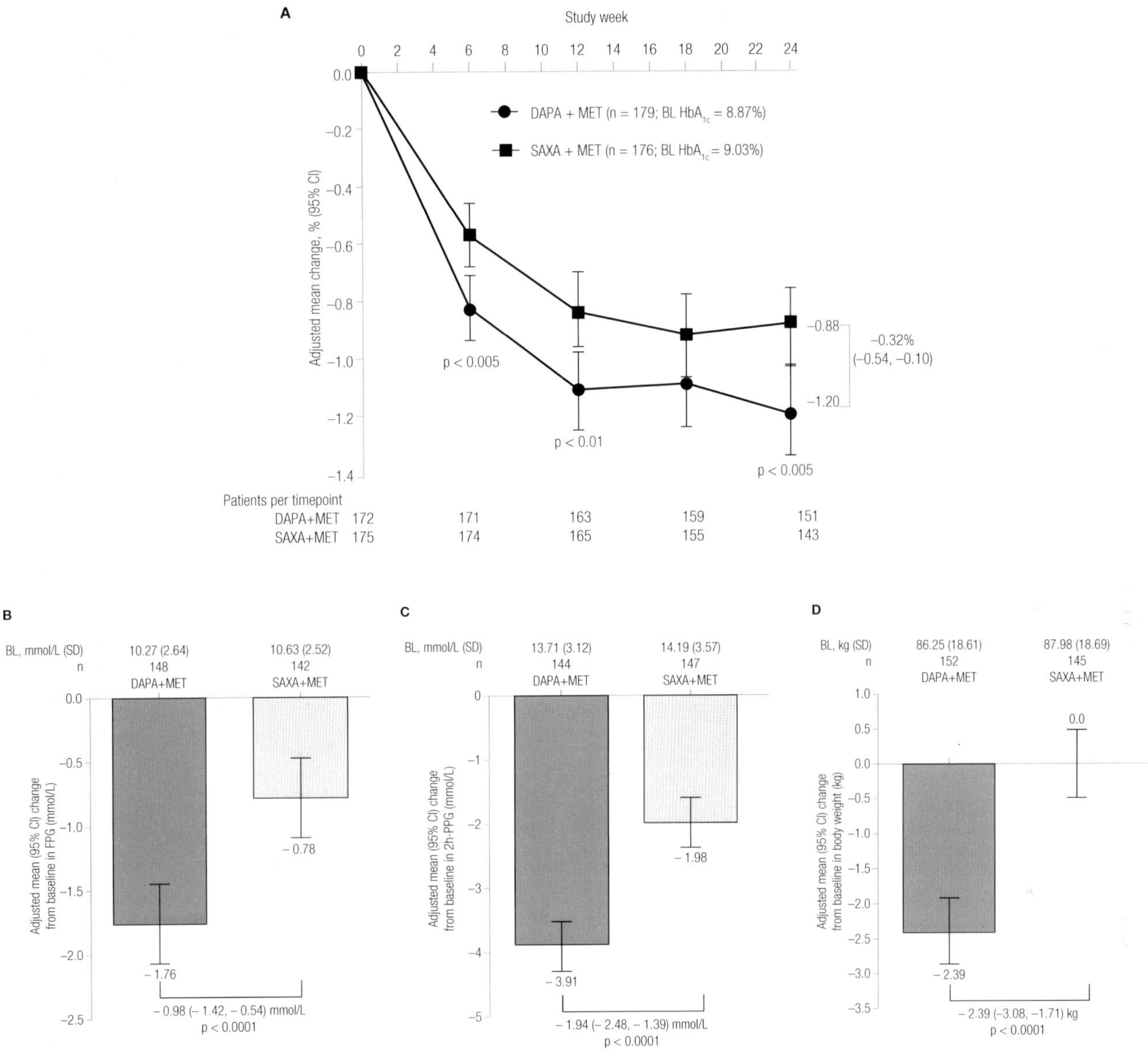

Figure 1. (**A**) Mean change in HbA_{1C} over time in the 24-week treatment period and mean change in (**B**) FPG, (**C**) 2-h PPG, and (**D**) body weight at 24 weeks n is the number of randomized patients with non-missing baseline and Week 24 LOCF values; p-values are for the difference between treatment groups. BL: baseline; DAPA: dapagliflozin; Diff: difference; MET: metformin; SAXA: saxagliptin; CI: confidence interval; FPG: fasting plasma glucose; 2-hr PPG: 2-hour postprandial glucose.

Small increases in total cholesterol of 3.8% (1.5%, 6.3%) and HDL-cholesterol of 7.7% (5.2%, 10.2%) and a non-significant increase in LDL-cholesterol of 1.5% (−3.1%, 6.4%]) were seen in patients receiving dapagliflozin. No significant changes in fasting lipids were seen in patients receiving saxagliptin.

DISCUSSION

Early combination therapy using agents with complementary mechanisms of action is recommended for advancing glucose control (1). Currently, two pharmacologic classes, DPP4 inhibitors and SGLT2 inhibitors, show promise as preferred second-line treatment options given their weight neutral and weight lowering effects, respectively, and low potential for hypoglycemia. Hence, the comparison between dapagliflozin and saxagliptin as add on to metformin is important in this context.

Many patients with T2D are affected by multiple co-morbidities, including obesity, dyslipidemia, and hypertension, all of which are well documented risk

Table 1. Composite efficacy endpoints at 24 weeks

Composite efficacy endpoints	DAPA+MET (n = 179)	SAXA+MET (n = 176)
HbA_{1c} reduction ≥ 0.5% + body wt. reduction ≥ 2 kg + SBP reduction ≥ 2 mmHg + no major/minor hypoglycemia		
Adjusted* % (95% CI)	24.3% (18.0, 30.7)	7.0% (3.3, 10.7)
Adjusted % diff. for SAXA+MET vs DAPA+MET (95% CI for diff.)	17.3% (10.0, 24.7)	
HbA_{1c} reduction ≥ 0.5% + body wt. reduction ≥ 2 kg		
Adjusted* % (95% CI)	38.2% (31.1, 45.4)	11.7% (6.9, 16.4)
Adjusted % diff. for SAXA+MET vs DAPA+MET (95% CI for diff.)	26.6% (18.0, 35.1)	
HbA_{1c} reduction ≥ 0.5% + SBP reduction ≥ 2 mmHg		
Adjusted* % (95% CI)	40.9% (33.7, 48.0)	27.8% (21.4, 34.1)
Adjusted % diff. for SAXA+MET vs DAPA+MET (95% CI for diff.)	13.1% (3.7, 22.5)	
HbA_{1c} reduction ≥ 0.5% + body wt. reduction ≥ 2 kg + no major/minor hypoglycemia		
Adjusted* % (95% CI)	37.7% (30.6, 44.8)	11.7% (6.9, 16.4)
Adjusted % diff. for SAXA+MET vs DAPA+MET (95% CI for diff.)	26.0% (17.5, 34.5)	

n is the number of randomized subjects who received at least one dose of double-blind medication during the treatment period.

* Adjusted for baseline HbA_{1c}.

DAPA: dapagliflozin; diff.: difference; MET: metformin; SAXA: saxagliptin; SBP: systolic blood pressure; wt.: weight.

factors for CVD. In our study, dapagliflozin reduced glycemic parameters including HbA1c, FPG and 2-hr PPG to a significantly greater extent than saxagliptin. Consistent with its glycosuric mechanism, dapagliflozin also reduced body weight and SBP versus saxagliptin. Weight reduction with dapagliflozin may benefit overweight/obese patients with T2D. Reduction in SBP with dapagliflozin is also an added benefit in view of the high prevalence of hypertension in patients with T2D. These results are consistent with other studies of SGLT2 inhibitors versus DPP4 inhibitors (10,11). Such findings may have contributed to the placement of SGLT2 inhibitors in the AACE/ACE comprehensive glycemic control algorithm, suggesting that SGLT2 inhibitors are an important addition for individualizing the treatment of T2D.

The EMPA-REG OUTCOME trial showed that patients with T2D and established CVD disease who received empagliflozin versus placebo, had a lower rate of the primary composite of death from cardiovascular (CV) causes, non-fatal myocardial infarction or nonfatal stroke with substantial reductions in CV mortality when the study drug was added to standard care (17). The results from the CANVAS study further support the effects of SGLT2 inhibitors on CV outcomes, with a significantly lower rate of the composite outcome of death from CV causes, non-fatal myocardial infarction or non-fatal stroke in the canagliflozin group, and also for the exploratory outcomes of hospitalization for heart failure, although canagliflozin did not show a significant reduction on CV mortality (18). More recently, real-world observational evidence has suggested a beneficial class effect of SGLT2 inhibitors (canagliflozin, dapagliflozin and empagliflozin) on CV outcomes (19,20), and findings from the ongoing CV study DECLARE (NCT01730534) may further establish this possible class effect. The CV outcomes trials of DPP4 inhibitors have shown no beneficial effects of DPP4 inhibitors on CV outcomes; however, no increase in the risk of major adverse CV events, such as the combined MACE outcome (CV death, nonfatal myocardial infarction and non-fatal stroke), versus standard care was noted.

As expected, both dapagliflozin and saxagliptin were well tolerated in the current study. Higher proportions of patients on dapagliflozin versus saxagliptin reported genital infections, consistent with previous observations from the dapagliflozin clinical trial program (21). There was a low incidence of hypoglycemia in both treatment groups, which reflects the self-limiting modes of action of these agents, i.e. reduction in the amount of filtered glucose with decreasing blood glucose levels causes a low potential for hypoglycemia with dapagliflozin; and glucose-stimulated insulin secretion decreases in patients treated with saxagliptin as physiological glucose levels are approached, leading to a low risk of hypoglycemia.

A limitation of this study is that it is a *post-hoc* analysis, and should be regarded as hypothesis-generating. These data are still of scientific value as findings from this study are similar to the previously reported data from comparisons between other SGLT2 inhibitors and DPP4 inhibitors in randomized controlled trials (11,12).

In conclusion, in this post-hoc analysis, addition of dapagliflozin or saxagliptin to metformin improved glycemic control in patients poorly controlled with metformin. However, significantly greater glycemic efficacy was observed with dapagliflozin compared with saxagliptin, together with reductions in body weight and blood pressure which may provide additional benefit to many patients with T2D. The safety profiles of both treatments were consistent with previous observations in their respective clinical trials.

Acknowledgements: the authors would like to thank the patients, their families and all investigators involved in this study. They would also like to thank Clifford J Bailey, Aston University, Birmingham, UK, for his contribution in the development of this manuscript. This analysis was supported by AstraZeneca. Editorial support was provided by Shelley Narula of in Science Communications, Springer Healthcare Ltd, London, UK, and was funded by AstraZeneca.

Funding: AstraZeneca.

Disclosure: JR has served on scientific advisory boards and received honoraria or consulting fees from companies involved in development of SGLT2 and DPP4 inhibitors, including Janssen, AstraZeneca, Eli Lilly, Boehringer Ingelheim, Sanofi, and Lexicon; and has also received grants/research support from Pfizer, Merck, Bristol-Myers Squibb, AstraZeneca, Janssen, Eli Lilly, Boehringer Ingelheim, Sanofi and Lexicon. CM serves or has served on the advisory panel for Novo Nordisk, Sanofi, Merck Sharp and Dohme Ltd., Eli Lilly and Company, Novartis, Bristol-Myers Squibb, AstraZeneca, Pfizer, Janssen Pharmaceuticals, Boehringer Ingelheim, Hanmi Pharmaceuticals, Roche Diagnostics, Medtronic, Mannkind, Intrexon and UCB; KU Leuven has received research support for CM from Novo Nordisk, Sanofi, Merck Sharp and Dohme Ltd., Eli Lilly and Company, Roche Diagnostics, Abbott, Intrexon and Novartis; CM serves or has served on the speakers bureau for Novo Nordisk, Sanofi, Merck Sharp and Dohme Ltd, Eli Lilly and Company, Boehringer Ingelheim, Astra Zeneca and Novartis. Hungta Chen, Ricardo Garcia-Sanchez and Gabriela Luporini Saraiva are employees of AstraZeneca

REFERENCES

1. Inzucchi SE, Bergenstal RM, Buse JB, Diamant M, Ferrannini E, Nauck M, et al. Management of hyperglycaemia in type 2 diabetes, 2015: a patient-centred approach. Update to a position statement of the American Diabetes Association and the European Association for the Study of Diabetes. Diabetologia. 2015;58(3):429-42.
2. Ismail-Beigi F, Moghissi E, Tiktin M, Hirsch IB, Inzucchi SE, Genuth S. Individualizing glycemic targets in type 2 diabetes mellitus: implications of recent clinical trials. Ann Intern Med. 2011;154(8):554-9.
3. Garber AJ, Abrahamson MJ, Barzilay JI, Blonde L, Bloomgarden ZT, Bush MA, et al. Consensus Statement by the American Association of Clinical Endocrinologists and American College of Endocrinology on the Comprehensive Type 2 Diabetes Management Algorithm - 2017 Executive Summary. Endocr Pract. 2017;23(2):207-38.
4. Scheen AJ, Van Gaal LF. Combating the dual burden: therapeutic targeting of common pathways in obesity and type 2 diabetes. Lancet Diabetes Endocrinol. 2014;2(11):911-22.
5. Bailey CJ, Gross JL, Hennicken D, Iqbal N, Mansfield TA, List JF. Dapagliflozin add-on to metformin in type 2 diabetes inadequately controlled with metformin: a randomized, double-blind, placebo-controlled 102-week trial. BMC Med. 2013;11:43.
6. Plosker GL. Dapagliflozin: a review of its use in patients with type 2 diabetes. Drugs. 2014;74(18):2191-209.
7. Del Prato S, Nauck M, Duran-Garcia S, Maffei L, Rohwedder K, Theuerkauf A, et al. Long-term glycaemic response and tolerability of dapagliflozin versus a sulphonylurea as add-on therapy to metformin in patients with type 2 diabetes: 4-year data. Diabetes Obes Metab. 2015;17(6):581-90.
8. Johnsson K, Johnsson E, Mansfield TA, Yavin Y, Ptaszynska A, Parikh SJ. Osmotic diuresis with SGLT2 inhibition: analysis of events related to volume reduction in dapagliflozin clinical trials. Postgrad Med. 2016;128(4):346-55.
9. Ferrannini E, Berk A, Hantel S, Pinnetti S, Hach T, Woerle HJ, et al. Long-term safety and efficacy of empagliflozin, sitagliptin, and metformin: an active-controlled, parallel-group, randomized, 78-week open-label extension study in patients with type 2 diabetes. Diabetes Care. 2013;36(12):4015-21.
10. Roden M, Weng J, Eilbracht J, Delafont B, Kim G, Woerle HJ, et al. Empagliflozin monotherapy with sitagliptin as an active comparator in patients with type 2 diabetes: a randomised, double-blind, placebo-controlled, phase 3 trial. Lancet Diabetes Endocrinol. 2013;1(3):208-19.
11. Lavalle-Gonzalez FJ, Januszewicz A, Davidson J, Tong C, Qiu R, Canovatchel W, et al. Efficacy and safety of canagliflozin compared with placebo and sitagliptin in patients with type 2 diabetes on background metformin monotherapy: a randomised trial. Diabetologia. 2013;56(12):2582-92.
12. Schernthaner G, Gross JL, Rosenstock J, Guarisco M, Fu M, Yee J, et al. Canagliflozin compared with sitagliptin for patients with type 2 diabetes who do not have adequate glycemic control with metformin plus sulfonylurea: a 52-week randomized trial. Diabetes Care. 2013;36(9):2508-15.
13. Rosenstock J, Hansen L, Zee P, Li Y, Cook W, Hirshberg B, et al. Dual add-on therapy in type 2 diabetes poorly controlled with metformin monotherapy: a randomized double-blind trial of saxagliptin plus dapagliflozin addition versus single addition of saxagliptin or dapagliflozin to metformin. Diabetes Care. 2015;38(3):376-83.
14. Rosenstock J, Bailey CJ, Mathieu C, Chen H, Garcia-Sanchez R, Saraiva GL. Composite endpoint analysis of dapagliflozin versus saxagliptin as add-on therapy in patients with type 2 diabetes inadequately controlled with metformin. Endocr Pract. 2017;23(1):38A.
15. Scheen AJ, Charpentier G, Ostgren CJ, Hellqvist A, Gause-Nilsson I. Efficacy and safety of saxagliptin in combination with metformin compared with sitagliptin in combination with metformin in adult patients with type 2 diabetes mellitus. Diabetes Metab Res Rev. 2010;26(7):540-9.
16. Craddy P, Palin HJ, Johnson KI. Comparative effectiveness of dipeptidylpeptidase-4 inhibitors in type 2 diabetes: a systematic review and mixed treatment comparison. Diabetes Ther. 2014;5(1):1-41.
17. Zinman B, Wanner C, Lachin JM, Fitchett D, Bluhmki E, Hantel S, et al. Empagliflozin, Cardiovascular Outcomes, and Mortality in Type 2 Diabetes. N Engl J Med. 2015;373(22):2117-28.
18. Neal B, Perkovic V, Mahaffey KW, de Zeeuw D, Fulcher G, Erondu N, et al. Canagliflozin and Cardiovascular and Renal Events in Type 2 Diabetes. N Engl J Med. 2017;377(7):644-57.

19. Nystrom T, Bodegard J, Nathanson D, Thuresson M, Norhammar A, Eriksson JW. Novel oral glucose-lowering drugs are associated with lower risk of all-cause mortality, cardiovascular events and severe hypoglycaemia compared with insulin in patients with type 2 diabetes. Diabetes Obes Metab. 2017;19(6):831-41.
20. Kosiborod M, Cavender MA, Fu AZ, Wilding JP, Khunti K, Holl RW, et al.; CVD-REAL Investigators and Study Group. Lower Risk of Heart Failure and Death in Patients Initiated on Sodium-Glucose Cotransporter-2 Inhibitors Versus Other Glucose-Lowering Drugs: The CVD-REAL Study (Comparative Effectiveness of Cardiovascular Outcomes in New Users of Sodium-Glucose Cotransporter-2 Inhibitors). Circulation. 2017;136(3):249-59.
21. Johnsson KM, Ptaszynska A, Schmitz B, Sugg J, Parikh SJ, List JF. Vulvovaginitis and balanitis in patients with diabetes treated with dapagliflozin. J Diabetes Complications. 2013;27(5):479-84.

Supplementary Table 1. Unadjusted changes in HbA_{1c} and weight at 24 weeks

DAPA + MET	HbA_{1c} decrease of ≥ 0.5%	HbA_{1c} decrease of < 0.5% or HbA1c increase
Weight decrease of ≥ 2 kg	37.6%	9.8%
Weight decrease of < 2 kg or weight increase	34.7%	17.9%
SAXA + MET	HbA_{1c} decrease of ≥ 0.5%	HbA_{1c} decrease of < 0.5% or HbA_{1c} increase
Weight decrease of ≥ 2 kg	12.0%	7.4%
Weight decrease of < 2 kg or weight increase	54.9%	25.7%

Data are proportions of patients (%). DAPA: dapagliflozin; MET: metformin; SAXA: saxagliptin.

Supplementary Table 2. Proportions of patients experiencing adverse events over 24 weeks

n (%)	DAPA + MET (n = 179)	SAXA + MET (n = 176)
≥ 1 Adverse event	87 (49)	93 (53)
≥ 1 Serious adverse event	2 (1)	6 (3)
Adverse events leading to discontinuation	1 (1)	0
Adverse events of special interest		
Hypoglycemia*	2 (1)	2 (1)†
Urinary tract infection	7 (5)	9 (5)
Genital infection	10 (6)	1 (1)
Glomerular filtration rate decrease	0	1 (1)

* Hypoglycemia includes minor and major; † Patients with more than one type of hypoglycemic episode were counted within each category but only once for patients experiencing hypoglycemia; DAPA: dapagliflozin; MET: metformin; SAXA: saxagliptin.

Effects of vitamin D supplementation on pulmonary function in postmenopausal women following an aquatic exercise program

Rodrigo Nolasco[1], Linda D. F. Moreira[1], Danilo S. Bocalini[2], Fernanda C. A. O. Fronza[3], Rosangela Villa Marin[1], Marise Lazaretti-Castro[1]

[1] Departamento de Medicina, Disciplina de Endocrinologia, Faculdade de Medicina, Universidade Federal de São Paulo (Unifesp/EPM), São Paulo, SP, Brasil
[2] Fisiologia Translacional, Programa de Pós-Graduação em Educação Física e Ciências do Envelhecimento, Universidade São Judas Tadeu (USJT), São Paulo, SP, Brasil
[3] Escola de Educação Física e Esporte da Universidade de São Paulo (EEFE/USP), São Paulo, SP, Brasil

Correspondence to:
Rodrigo Nolasco
Ambulatório de Endocrinologia, Universidade Federal de São Paulo
Rua Borges Lagoa, 800
04038-030 – São Paulo, SP, Brasil
rodrigonolasco@yahoo.com.br

ABSTRACT

Objective: This study sought to investigate the effects of vitamin D supplementation and aquatic exercise on pulmonary function in postmenopausal women. **Materials and methods:** This prospective and controlled study included 104 women (62 ± 6.5 years) divided into three groups: a control group lacking vitamin D and calcium supplementation which remained sedentary (CG; n = 17); a control group receiving vitamin D and calcium supplementation which remained sedentary (CDG, n = 33); and a group that completed aquatic exercises three times a week and received vitamin D and calcium supplementation (DTG, n = 54). Data before and after 6 months of the study were analyzed, including serum 25-hydroxyvitamin D (25(OH)D) and calcium concentrations, peak expiratory flow (PEF), forced vital capacity (FVC), and cirtometry. **Results:** We observed significant increases in 25(OH)D concentrations in CDG (52.9 ± 2.4 to 69.1 ± 2.2; nmol/L; p < 0.0001) and DTG groups (55.5 ± 3 to 71.5 ± 3 nmol/L; p < 0.0001). PEF increased by 7 ± 2% (p = 0.0080) in CDG group and 11 ± 2% (p < 0.0001) in DTG group, whereas FVC increased by 7 ± 2% (p = 0.0016) in the CDG group and 10 ± 2% (p < 0.0001) in the DTG group, whereas CG had no changes in any of these parameters. The increment value of cirtometry in DTG group (+43 ± 3%) were significantly (p < 0.0001) higher than those in CG (–4 ± 8%) and CDG (+4 ± 9%) groups. **Conclusion:** Our data suggest that vitamin D supplementation improves pulmonary function parameters in postmenopausal women. Arch Endocrinol Metab. 2017;61(1):28-35

Keywords
Spirometry; cirtometry; cholecalciferol; postmenopause

INTRODUCTION

The large increase in longevity in humans during the last century raised new issues in health care, especially the control of aging-related deterioration (1). Intense efforts have been exerted to obtain new knowledge that can lead to the progression of chronic degenerative diseases and to slow the functional impairment, including deterioration of lung function (2). Vitamin D and calcium are among the potential factors related to maintaining bone and muscle health, and they cannot be separated from osteoporosis prevention in postmenopausal women. Vitamin D produced in the skin via the action of sunlight is converted into calcitriol, a potent hormone, which is important for health. Although its most common effects are on bone metabolism and mineral homeostasis, its receptors have been identified in almost all tissues, suggesting that it might have other roles (3,4).

Lung function also appears to be influenced by vitamin D concentrations, with cross-sectional studies identifying associations of lower plasma concentrations of 25-hydroxyvitamin D (25(OH)D) with worse lung function parameters (5,6). During aging, a gradual decline in the respiratory system occurs, the related factors of which include increased lung compliance, a decreased number of alveoli, and respiratory muscle weakening, as well as rib cage deformities caused by increased thoracic kyphosis because of, among others, vertebral fractures (2).

Different regular physical activities, including water aerobics, have been used to preserve cardiorespiratory and musculoskeletal functions during aging (7). Moreover, research showed that the treatment of vitamin D deficiency in menopausal women can confer musculoskeletal benefits and reduce fall and vertebral fracture rates (8,9). In addition, aquatic exercise studies have also identified beneficial effects on pulmonary function in elderly women (10,11).

While conducting a protocol to test the effects of a differentiated water aerobics program (HydrOS), an opportunity arose to investigate the effects of vitamin D supplementation alone or in combination with high-intensity aquatic exercises on pulmonary function in postmenopausal women.

MATERIAL AND METHODS

Subjects

This was a post hoc analysis of a protocol designed to evaluate the effects of a high-intensity water aerobics program (HydrOS) in postmenopausal women (12). The initial study population consisted of women living in the city of Barueri, São Paulo who were previously sedentary and attending a service center for the elderly (*Parque da Maturidade de Barueri*) and who were selected from volunteers willing to participate in the study according to the following inclusion criteria: postmenopausal for ≥ 5 years, non-institutionalized, and able to understand and respond to commands during the physical and cognitive tests. The exclusion criteria were: any physical conditions that might affect their performance in the physical tests (hypothyroidism, primary hyperparathyroidism, severe osteoarthritis, rheumatic arthritis, edema or ulcer in the lower limbs); chronic kidney disease (serum creatinine > 1.4 mg/dL); diseases that could interfere with bone quality or neuromuscular functions; recent history of hip fracture (< 2 years); thyroid-stimulating hormone level < 0.05 or > 5.5 μIU/mL; dependence on alcohol, tobacco, or illicit drugs; currently receiving treatment with steroids, bisphosphonates, calcitonin, or vitamin D and its metabolites; use of estrogen or selective estrogen receptor modulators; use of drugs that could interfere with postural stability or vitamin D metabolism; uncontrolled high blood pressure; use of a prosthesis; regular physical activity in the last 6 months; serious heart disease; or complications during exercise stress testing that contraindicated physical activity.

The research protocol, as well as the informed consent form, was duly approved by the Ethics Committee of Unifesp (No. 1771/2008). All volunteers who agreed to participate in the study provided written consent.

Design

In this prospective and controlled trial the preselection resulted in a group of 134 previously sedentary women. Of them, 26 were excluded on the basis of the described criteria (Figure 1). The 108 remaining participants (58.8 ± 6.4 years) were randomly divided into two groups. The vitamin D control group (CDG, n = 33) was maintained without regular physical training, and the trained group (DTG, n = 54) participated in the HydrOS protocol over 6 months During the study period, both groups received supplementation with 1000 IU of vitamin D3 and 500 mg of elemental calcium daily. According to the same inclusion and exclusion criteria, a control group of 17 age-matched women with similar clinical characteristics was created. This group did not receive vitamin D nor participate in any physical activity program during the same period. The study design and the flow of subjects can be seen in Figure 1.

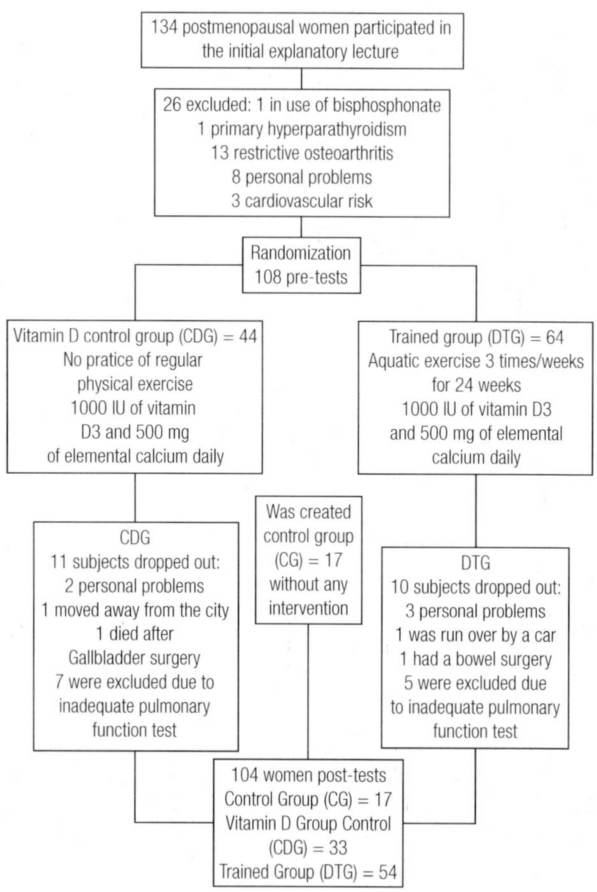

Figure 1. Flow of participants throughout the study.

The post hoc analysis included only patients who completed the study and who met the acceptance criteria of the American Thoracic Society for the analysis of pulmonary function tests (CG, n = 17; CDG, n = 33; and DTG, n = 54).

Supplementation

Prior to the start of the protocol, calcium intake in all groups was evaluated by a nutritionist through 24-h diet recall (13) and the daily calcium intake was similar among the groups. None of the participants received more than 600 mg of calcium daily.

The volunteers in the control group were told to not change their lifestyle or consume any vitamin supplement during the observation period. Under medical supervision, the CDG and DTG groups received one tablet daily containing 1000 IU of cholecalciferol (vitamin D) and 500 mg of elemental calcium (as calcium carbonate) after breakfast. The participants were instructed to maintain their usual diet. During the intervention period with supplementation, the protocol adherence rate was 94% (SD ±3).

Parameters analyzed

The selected subjects were evaluated via anamnesis, functional capacity tests, spirometry, fasting blood collection, and bone densitometry tests to evaluate body composition. Those who did not undergo all procedures and measures or attend at least 85% of the planned sessions were excluded from the study.

Total calcium and 25(OH)D

All volunteers underwent fasting blood collection. A radioimmunoassay method (DiaSorin, Stillwater, MN, USA) was used to determine serum 25(OH)D levels. The intra- and interassay coefficients of variation (CVs) were 5.6 and 10%, respectively. An enzymatic colorimetric method (ADVIA 1650, Bayer Ltd., Tokyo, Japan) was used to measure plasma levels of total calcium (CaT), with intra- and interassay CVs of 1.30 and 1.95%, respectively.

Anamnesis and physical examination

Medical and family history, ethnicity, diet, alcohol intake, smoking, and current medications were searched via anamnesis. The initial physical activity level of each participant was checked using the International Physical Activity Questionnaire, short version, already duly validated (14).

Body composition

Total body mass (kg) and height (cm) were obtained using an analog scale accurate to 0.1 kg (Filizola model 31, Filizola, São Paulo, SP, Brazil). Body composition was examined via whole-body dual energy X-ray absorptiometry (DXA) using a densitometer with a dual emission X-ray source (Hologic Model Discovery A, Waltham, MA, USA). All procedures involving DXA were performed in the Osteometabolic Diseases Clinic of Unifesp Endocrinology Course, and the acquisition of the exams was systematically performed using the same technique and analyzed by the same examiner.

Pulmonary function

Pulmonary function was assessed by spirometry using a digital portable spirometer (One Flow; Clement Clarke International, England). Patients were previously instructed about the testing process. Each individual was positioned sitting while wearing a nose clip with her feet flat on the floor and head in a neutral and raised position. After the explanation, the subject immediately performed a maximal inspiration, followed by forced expiration with the tube placed on the tongue between the teeth and the lips clenched to prevent perioral leaks. At least six full spirometric maneuvers were performed until the difference between the latest maneuvers was < 5%. The best result was employed for the analyses following the American Thoracic Society guidelines and meeting the acceptability and reproducibility criteria (15). The data were automatically transferred to an Amazon PC computer using software provided by the equipment manufacturer (ONE FLOW SOFT; Clement Clarke International, England). The following variables were considered: peak expiratory flow (PEF), forced expiratory volume in the first second of the maneuver (FEV_1), and forced vital capacity (FVC).

The chest expansion evaluation was conducted via dynamic cirtometry at the axillary level using a 1-cm-wide measuring tape in 0.5-cm increments. The test was performed with each participant in a standing position, and the tape was placed at the axillary level around her bare chest. Each participant was instructed to perform a maximum expiration and inspiration, and the difference in centimeters between the two torso circumference values was recorded.

Exercise protocol

The exercise sessions occurred three times a week in in a covered swimming pool with a depth of 1.20–1.40 m and temperature of 29–31°C located in *Parque da Maturidade de Barueri*, São Paulo. During the lessons, we asked the participants to stand in the pool so that the water was near the xiphoid process. To control the training intensity, three heart rate sensors (RS100 BLK; Polar, Finland) were used by three different students in each session so that at the end of 6 months, all participants had already used the heart rate sensor several times. In addition, the participants were taught how to use a Borg CR-10 category scale of perceived exertion (ranging from 0 – nothing at all, to 10 – very, very hard) used along with the measurement of the heart beat rate of the participants during the sessions (12).

During the lessons, we observed that the heart rate shown on the heart rate sensors was equivalent to the grade given by the participants on the Borg CR-10 scale. At every stage of the protocol, various muscle groups (chest and back, biceps and triceps, shoulders, quadriceps and posterior thigh, hip adductors and abductors, and calf and abdominals) were trained. The workout routine was gradually changed from two to five repetition sets of the same exercise, *e.g.*, two sets of 30 s each, then moving on to three sets of 20 s each, followed by four sets of 15 s each, and ending with five sets of 10 s each. For the cardiorespiratory exercises, we used the Borg scale adapted as follows: 60% maximum heart rate (MHR), scale level 6 for 16 minutes of the session; 70% MHR, scale level 7 for 13 minutes of the session; 80% MHR, scale level 8 for 9 minutes of the session; and 90% MHR, scale level 9 for 7 minutes of the session (12). After the 6-month intervention period with a resistance aquatic exercise program, all tests were repeated in the three groups.

Statistical analysis

For all statistical analyses, the results were considered significant at $p < 0.05$. The Kolmogorov-Smirnov test was used to test data normality. The other normally distributed parameters were compared in two manners: intragroup before and after the study using Student's *t*-test for matched samples; and intergroup before and after the study using Student's *t*-test for independent samples. The chi-square test was used to verify the distribution of the different races of the 3 groups. One-way analysis of variance and Tukey's post hoc test were used when necessary to identify statistical differences.

RESULTS

Table 1 shows that the three groups were similar at baseline in terms of biometric characteristics, total calcium, and body composition. The racial distribution (white and no white) did not differ between groups ($p = 0.056$).

After 6 months of study, serum 25(OH)D levels similarly increased in the two groups supplemented with vitamin D3 ($p < 0.001$). The mean value in the CDG group increased by 21% (from 52.9 ± 2.4 to 69.1 ± 2.2; nmol/L, $p < 0.0001$), in the DTG group increased by 23% (from 55.5 ± 3 to 71.5 ± 3 for 3 nmol/L, $p < 0.0001$), and in the CG group did not change significantly (from 50.1 ± 2.6 to 49.82 ± 2.4 nmol/L, $p= 0.4605$) (Figure 2).

Table 1. Clinical features and anthropometric characteristics of the three groups at baseline and study completion

Variable	Control Group (n = 17)			Vitamin D Group (n = 33)			Trained Group (n = 54)		
	Before	After	%	Before	After	%	Before	After	%
Age	59.9 ± 2			58 ± 0.8			59 ± 6		
Weight (kg)	70 ± 3	70 ± 3	0.2 ± 0.4	74 ± 2	75 ± 3	1.3 ± 0.6	73 ± 2	73 ± 2	0.7 ± 0.4
Height (cm)	1.59 ± 2	1.59 ± 2	- 0.01 ± 0.1	1.56 ± 1	1.56 ± 1	0.12 ± 1	1.56 ± 0.1	1.56 ± 0.1	0.22 ± 0.6
BMI (kg/m^2)	27 ± 0.1	27 ± 0.1	0.23 ± 0.40	30 ± 0.7	30 ± 0.8	0.87 ± 0.51	29 ± 0.7	29 ± 0.7	-0.48 ± 0.78
Fat mass (kg)	26 ± 1.7	26 ± 1.8	-7.0 ± 6	29 ± 1.6	29 ± 1.7	-1.3 ± 1.3	28 ± 1.1	28 ± 1.2	-1.0 ± 2
Lean mass (kg)	42 ± 17	42 ± 16	-0.5 ± 1	42 ± 16	44 ± 12	4 ± 3	43 ± 10	43 ± 10	0.8 ± 1
Fat%	37 ± 1.3	36 ± 1.5	- 1 ± 1	38 ± 1.0	38 ± 1.1	-1.5 ± 0.8	38 ± 0.7	38 ± 0.7	-1 ± 0.8
Cirtometry (cm)	2.05 ± 0.3	2.04 ± 0.2	-4 ± 5^a	2.12 ± 0.14	2.45 ± 0.16	4 ± 9^a	2.21 ± 0.13	3.93 ± 0.16*	43 ± 3^b
Ca T (RV: 8.5-10.5 mg/dL)	9.23 ± 0.43	9.14 ± 0.28	-0,9 ± 2	9.50 ± 0.23	9.20 ± 0.31	-3,2 ± 4	9.61 ± 0.33	9.40 ± 0.39	-2,2 ± 3

Values are expressed as the mean ± SE of the biometric measurements and total serum calcium (CaT) levels of the control (CG), control with vitamin D and calcium supplementation (CDG), and training (DTG) groups before and after the intervention. * $p < 0.0001$, indicate differences detected using Student's *t*-test versus before the intervention. Different letters indicate statistically significant differences ($p < 0.05$) on one-way analysis of variance (Tukey's post hoc test) in relation to the percentage change between the groups. BMI, body mass index. RV = Reference values. * $p < 0.05$.

There were similarly significant improvements in PEF (L/m) and FVC (L) in both groups treated with vitamin D3 (CDG and DTG) regardless of physical training, whereas changes were not observed in the CG group (Figure 3). Although FEV_1 values were higher at the end of study than the baseline values in the vitamin D-supplemented groups, this change did not reach statistical significance (Figure 3). The measure of chest expansion (dynamic cirtometry), however, revealed a significant improvement only in the group that underwent physical training (Table 1).

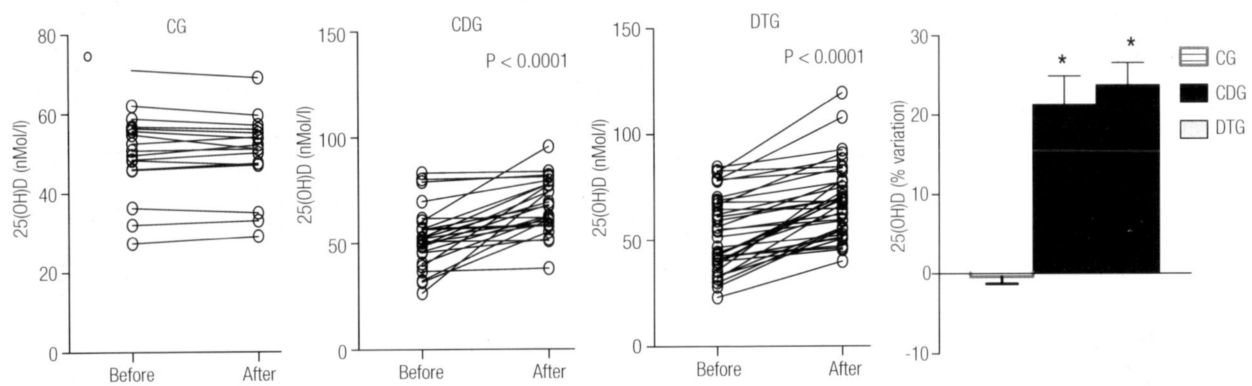

Figure 2. Evolution of serum 25-hydroxyvitamin D (25(OH)D) levels. Values are expressed as the mean ± SE of 25(OH)D levels in the control (CG), control with vitamin D and calcium supplementation (CDG), and training (DTG) groups before and after the intervention. * $p < 0.0001$, indicate differences detected using Student's *t*-test versus before the intervention.

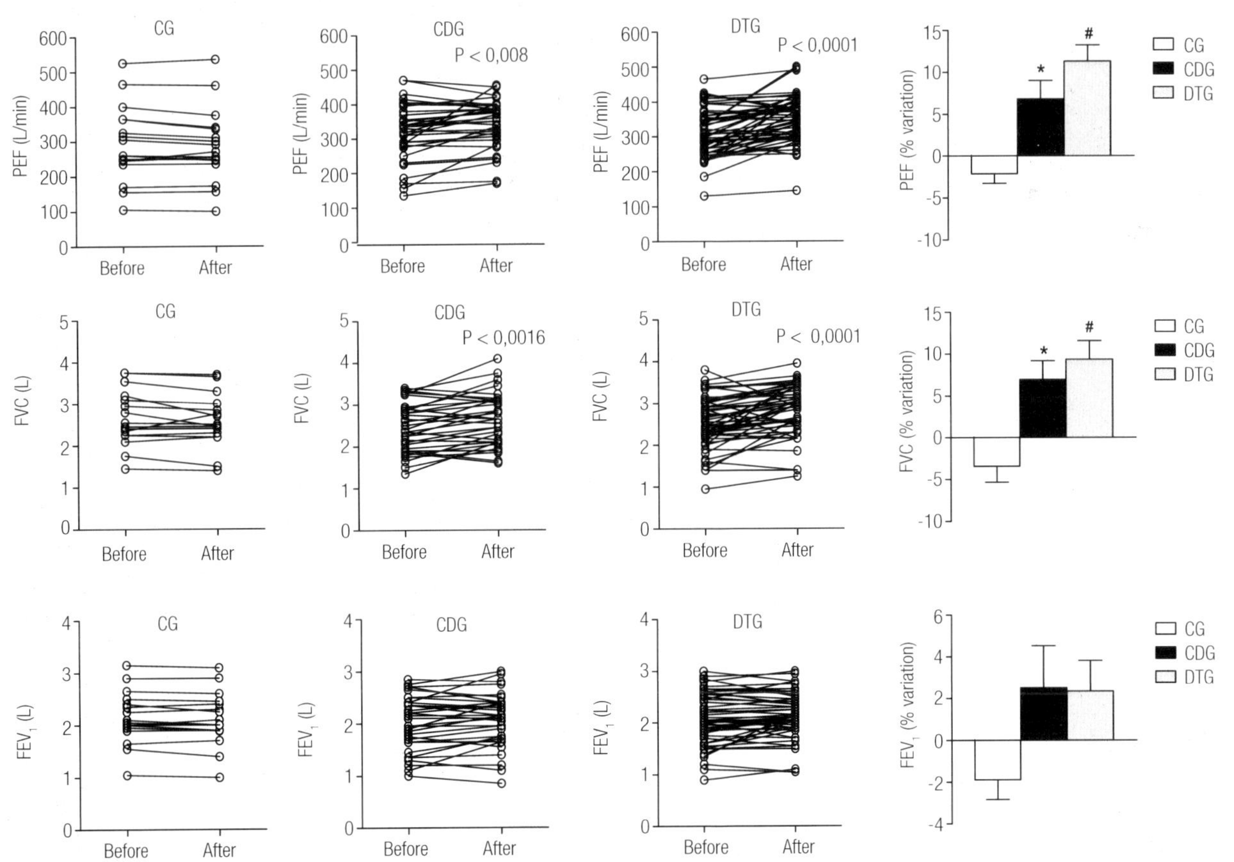

Figure 3. Evolution of pulmonary function test data during the study in the three groups. Values are expressed as the mean ± SE and percentage change for peak expiratory flow (PEF), forced vital capacity (FVC) and forced expiratory volume in 1 s (FEV_1) in the control (CG), control with vitamin D and calcium supplementation (CDG), and training (DTG) groups before and after intervention. * $p < 0.0001$ and # $p < 0.01$, indicate differences detected using Student's *t*-test versus before the intervention.

DISCUSSION

This study is a by-product of a broader protocol that assessed the effects of a high-intensity water aerobics program in postmenopausal women using several physical and laboratory parameters (12,16). Our results demonstrated that daily treatment with 1,000 IU of vitamin D3 for 6 months effectively produced a significant increase in plasma 25(OH)D concentrations in most of the volunteers. In our study, this increase on 25(OH)D levels was associated with an improvement in pulmonary function expiratory parameters (measure by spirometry), even in sedentary women, regardless of no participation in the aquatic exercise program. The trained group, additionally, was the only group to display improvement in the expandability parameter measured by cirtometry, suggesting some effect of water aerobics on this parameter (12). We have to point out that all volunteers had age-related normal values on spirometry at baseline, and both Vitamin D-treated groups improved similarly their expiratory parameters, not seen in the control group (CG). A possible explanation for the similar results on the pulmonary function parameters of DTG and CDG would be related to the increased respiratory muscle mass. The greater dynamic compression (restrictive) of the airways would lead to the fall of the flows measured at nozzle (17). The same dose of supplementation (1,000 IU/day) was used in another study (18) which was able to induce a significant increment on serum levels of 25(OH)D after 3 months (+17,6 nmol/L, in average).

The correlations between vitamin D metabolism and respiratory function have been widely studied in the literature (6). However, the results are not yet conclusive (19); rather, they remain rare in prospective intervention studies, and to our knowledge, no study has examined postmenopausal women without previous lung disease. In a randomized prospective double-blind study, supplementation with vitamin D in asthmatic children reduced the risk of exacerbations triggered by acute respiratory infection and significantly improved FEV_1 values (20). Another prospective study in patients with chronic obstructive pulmonary disease (COPD) and vitamin D deficiency observed increases in respiratory muscle strength, reductions in the degree of dyspnea, and superior physical performance after 1 year of vitamin D supplementation (21).

Several studies observed an increased prevalence of inadequate vitamin D levels in patients with different respiratory diseases such as asthma, COPD, tuberculosis, and a number of infections of the respiratory system (22-24). In observational studies such as the NHANES cohort, a cross-evaluation of 14,000 adults uncovered a significant association between higher 25(OH)D levels and better results for FEV_1 and FVC (5). Similar results were observed by other authors in 1315 Chinese children (25). A Danish longitudinal study that followed 18,507 patients of different age groups for 20 years found that lower serum 25(OH)D concentrations were associated with worse pulmonary function and an accelerated decline in FEV_1 and FVC parameters (6).

Studies have indicated that respiratory epithelial cells express 1α-hydroxylase, which is responsible for the conversion of 25(OH)D to its biologically active form $1,25(OH)_2D_3$, as well as the specific receptor for vitamin D (VDR) (26,27). Cross-sectional and prospective studies uncovered evidence associating the actions of vitamin D with increased surfactant substance levels and reduced inflammation in the respiratory tissues via VDR expressed in the airways (28,29). Besides, there is evidences for the action of vitamin D on the immune system, by increasing levels of LL-37 (cathelicidin), a peptide capable of promoting innate immunity and inducing the destruction of infectious agents, including *Mycobacterium tuberculosis* and influenza virus (19,29,30).

In addition, some studies linked the actions of vitamin D to inhibited proliferation of metalloproteinases of the extracellular matrix (ECM) as well as the balance of type III collagen synthesis by fibroblasts (31). The ECM of lung tissue plays a key role in the structure and mechanical properties of the lungs, thus reflecting pulmonary function (5,32).

Studies in rats evaluated the direct effects of vitamin D on lung growth, and they observed an increased lung volume and improved pulmonary function in these animals. These results were obtained by analyzing the forces generated by the elastic recoil of the lungs in rats with vitamin D deficiency by plethysmography and histological analysis of the lung tissue, respectively (28). Rats born to females not supplemented with vitamin D displayed structural changes, such as a significant increase in airways resistance, and changes in mesenchymal differentiation markers of the trachea compared to rats born to supplemented females (33). The direct effects of active vitamin D on lung tissue observed in these experimental studies could explain our findings in this population of women supplemented with vitamin D, even in the absence of physical training (CDG group).

The improvement observed via cirtometry only in the DTG group suggests that high-intensity aquatic exercises can increase chest expansion, probably by strengthening breathing muscles (17). This improvement may be associated with the influence of the physical properties of water, which increase voluntary breathing. The immersion of a subject in a liquid medium to the level of the xiphoid process promotes an increase of 60-65% in the work of breathing caused by increased resistance to thorax expansion produced by hydrostatic pressure and an increased blood volume in the thorax (34,35). This positive effect of the aquatic environment appears to favor the process of inspiratory force, as demonstrated by some studies in healthy elderly subjects (34).

Despite these findings, this project has limitations such as the discrepancy among the sample sizes, particularly the smaller number of individuals in the control group. A fourth group without vitamin D supplementation subjected exclusively to an aquatic exercise program could be used to evaluate the isolated effects of exercise on pulmonary function. There were no surveys conducted on the time of sun exposure of the study participants. However, the samplings were performed all on the same occasions, therefore, we can suppose that the potential seasonal variations of Vitamin D were similar in the 3 groups, although we have not controlled the individual quantity of exposure to sunlight. Another limiting factor was the lack of an assessment of respiratory muscle strength through measurements of inspiratory and expiratory pressures.

In conclusion, vitamin D supplementation was associated with improved spirometric parameters in postmenopausal women independent of participation in an aquatic exercise program. Aquatic exercises in turn increased chest expansion in the trained group. Based on our findings in addition to related literature, there are strong evidences that Vitamin D can play a role on pulmonary function. The increase of Vitamin D levels could also be a supporting measure for the strategies employed for preventing and treating diseases that impair pulmonary function.

Acknowledgments: this study was supported by Fapesp (*Fundação de Amparo à Pesquisa do Estado de São Paulo*), grant No. 08/50179-9. We are grateful for Yeda Queiroga for their administrative assistance and The Federal Agency for Support and Evaluation of Graduate Education (Higher Education Personnel Improvement Coordination – Capes) for the financial support.

REFERENCES

1. Lunenfeld B, Stratton P. The clinical consequences of an ageing world and preventive strategies. Best Pract Res Clin Obstet Gynaecol. 2013;27(5):643-59.
2. Moazami M, Farahati S. The effects of aerobic training on pulmonary function in postmenopausal women. Int J Sport Std. 2013;3(2):169-74.
3. Maeda SS, Lazaretti-Castro M. Vitamina D. In: Maeda SS, Silva DMW. Guia prático em osteometabolismo. São Paulo: Segmento Farma; 2014. p. 37-51.
4. Gröber U, Spitz J, Reichrath J, Kisters K, Holick MF. Vitamin D: Update 2013: from rickets prophylaxis to general preventive healthcare. Dermato-endocrinology. 2013;5(3):331-47.
5. Black PN, Scragg R. Relationship between serum 25-hydroxyvitamin d and pulmonary function in the third national health and nutrition examination survey. Chest. 2005;128:3792-8.
6. Afzal S, Lange P, Bojesen SE, Freiberg JJ, Nordestgaard BG. Plasma 25-hydroxyvitamin D, lung function and risk of chronic obstructive pulmonary disease. Thorax. 2014;69:24-31.
7. Moreira LD, Oliveira ML, Lirani-Galvão AP, Marin-Mio RV, Santos RN, Lazaretti-Castro M. Physical exercise and osteoporosis: effects of different types of exercises on bone and physical function of postmenopausal women. Arq Bras Endocrinol Metabol. 2014;58(5):514-22.
8. Dawson-Hughes B. Serum 25-hydroxyvitamin D and functional outcomes in the Elderly. Am J Clin Nutr. 2008;88 (suppl):537S-40S.
9. Bischoff-Ferrari HA, Dawson-Hughes B, Staehelin HB, Orav JE, Stuck AE, Theiler R, et al. Fall prevention with supplemental and active forms of vitamin D: a meta-analysis of randomised controlled trials. BMJ. 2009;339:b3692.
10. Takeshima N, Rogers ME, Watanabe E. Water based exercise improves health-related aspects of fitness in older women. Med Sci Sports Exerc. 2002;33:544-51.
11. Vedana TA, Santos RN, Pereira JM, Araujo SP, Portes Júnior MP, Portes LA. Influência da hidroginástica sobre a composição corporal, aspectos cardiovasculares, hematológicos, função pulmonar e aptidão física de adultos e idosos. Braz J Biomotricity. 2011;5(2):65-79.
12. Moreira LDF, Fronza FC, Dos Santos RN, Teixeira LR, Kruel LF, Castro ML. High-intensity aquatic exercises (HydrOS) improve physical function and reduce falls among postmenopausal women. Menopause. 2013;20(10):1012-9.
13. Buzzard M. 24-hours dietary recall and food record methods. In: Willett WC. Nutritional Epidemiology. 2nd.ed. Oxford: Oxford University Press; 1998. p. 50-73.
14. Pardini R, Matsudo S, Matsudo V, Araújo T, Andrade E, Braggion G, et al Validation of the International Physical Activity Questionnaire (IPAQ): Pilot study in Brazilian young adults. Med Sci Sports Exerc. 1997;29(6):s5-9.
15. Miller MR, Hankinson J, Brusasco V, Burgos F, Casaburi R. Standardisation of spirometry. Eur Respir J. 2005;26(2):319-38.
16. Moreira LD, Fronza FC, Dos Santos RN, Zach PL, Kunii IS, Hayashi LF, et al. The benefits of a high-intensity aquatic exercise program (HydrOS) for bone metabolism and bone mass of postmenopausal women. J Bone Miner Metab. 2014;32(4):411-9.
17. Sociedade Brasileira de Pneumologia e Tisiologia. I Consenso Brasileiro de Espirometria. J Pneumol. 1996;22(3):125-9.
18. Canto-Costa MH1, Kunii I, Hauache OM. Body fat and cholecalciferol supplementation in elderly homebound individuals. Braz J Med Biol Res. 2006;39(1):91-8.
19. Persson LJ, Aanerud M, Hiemstra PS, Michelsen AE, Ueland T, Hardie JA, et al. Vitamin D, vitamin D binding protein, and

longitudinal outcomes in COPD. Chalmers JD, ed. PLoS ONE. 2015;10(3):e0121622.

20. Majak P, Olszowiec-Chlebna M, Smejda K, Stelmach I. Vitamin D supplementation in children may prevent asthma exacerbation triggered by acute respiratory infection. J Allergy Clin Immunol. 2011;127(5):1294-6.
21. Rezk NASA, Aly NYA, Hewidy AAH. Effect of vitamin D replacement in chronic obstructive pulmonary disease patients with vitamin D deficiency. Egyptian Journal of Chest Diseases and Tuberculosis. 2015;64(2):353-7.
22. Wacker M, Holick MF. Vitamin D – Effects on skeletal and extraskeletal health and the need for supplementation. Nutrients. 2013;5(1):111-48.
23. Bergman P, Lindh ÅU, Björkhem-Bergman L, Lindh JD. Vitamin D and respiratory tract infections: a systematic review and meta-analysis of randomized controlled trials. PLoS One. 2013;8(6):e65835.
24. Gröber U, Reichrath J, Holick MF. Live Longer with Vitamin D? Nutrients. 2015;7(3):1871-80.
25. Yao TC, Tu YL, Chang SW, Tsai HJ, Gu PW, Ning HC, et al. Serum 25-hydroxyvitamin D levels in relation to lung function and exhaled nitric oxide in children. J Pediatr. 2014;165(6):1098-1103.e1.
26. Hansdottir S, Monick MM, Hinde SL, Lovan N, Look DC, Hunninghake GW. Respiratory epithelial cells convert inactive vitamin D to its active form: potential effects on host defense. J Immunol. 2008;181(10):7090-9.
27. Song Y, Qi H, Wu C. Effect of 1,25-(OH)2D3 (a vitamin D analogue) on passively sensitized human airway smooth muscle cells. Respirology. 2007;12:486-94.
28. Zosky GR, Berry LJ, Elliot JG, James AL, Gorman S, Hart PH. Vitamin D deficiency causes deficits in lung function and alters lung structure. Am J Respir Crit Care Med. 2011;183(10):1336-43.
29. Berry DJ, Hesketh K, Power C, Hyppönen E. Vitamin D status has a linear association with seasonal infections and lung function in British adults. Br J Nutr. 2011;106(9):1433-40.
30. van Schoor NM, de Jongh RT, Daniels JMA, Heymans MW, Deeg DJH, Lips P. Peak expiratory flow rate shows a gender-specific association with vitamin D deficiency. J Clin Endocrinol Metab. 2012;97:2164-71.
31. Finklea JD, Grossmann RE, Tangpricha V. Vitamin D and chronic lung disease: a review of molecular mechanisms and clinical studies. Adv Nutr. 2011;2:244-53; PMID:22332056.
32. Dolhnikoff M, Bernardi FDC, Saldiva PHN. Estrutura morfológica e funcional dos pulmões. In: Carvalho CRR, Rocha e Silva M (Orgs.). Fisiopatologia respiratória. Série Fisiopatologia Clínica. São Paulo: Atheneu, 2005. p. 3-16.
33. Yurt M, Liu J, Sakurai R, Gong M, Husain SM, Siddiqui MA, et al. Vitamin D supplementation blocks pulmonary structural and functional changes in a rat model of perinatal vitamin D deficiency. Am J Physiol Lung Cell Mol Physiol. 2014;307(11):L859-67.
34. Ide MR, Belini MA, Caromano FA. Effects of an aquatic versus non-aquatic respiratory exercise program on the respiratory muscle strength in healthy aged persons. Clinics (Sao Paulo). 2005;60(2):151-8.
35. Pendergast DR, Lundgren CE. The underwater environment: cardiopulmonary, thermal, and energetic demands. J Appl Physiol (1985). 2009;106(1):276-83.

Hounsfield unit value has null effect on thyroid nodules at ^{18}F-FDG PET/CT scans

Filiz Eksi Haydardedeoglu[1], Gulay Simsek Bagir[1], Nese Torun[2], Emrah Kocer[3], Mehmet Reyhan[2], Melek Eda Ertorer[1]

[1] Baskent University Faculty of Medicine Department of Endocrinology and Metabolism, Adana, Turkey
[2] Baskent University Faculty of Medicine Department of Nuclear Medicine, Adana, Turkey
[3] Baskent University Faculty of Medicine Department of Pathology, Adana, Turkey

Correspondence to:
Filiz Eksi Haydardedeoglu,
Baskent University Faculty of Medicine Department of Endocrinology and Metabolism
Dadaloglu mah Serinevler
2591 sk. No: 4/A
01250 – Yüregir, Adana, Turkey
filizeksi@hotmail.com

ABSTRACT

Objectives: Detection rate of thyroid nodules is increasing with the use of new imaging modalities, especially in screening for malignancies. Positron emission tomography/computed tomography (PET/CT)-positive thyroid nodules should be differentiated for malignancy to avoid unnecessary operations and further follow-up. Most trials evaluate the role of SUV_{max}, but there is no definitive information about the utility of Hounsfield unit (HU) values for prediction of malignancy. This study aimed to evaluate the HU values beside SUV_{max} for detecting malignancy risk of PET/CT-positive thyroid nodules. Subjects and methods: Results of 98 cancer patients who had fine needle aspiration biopsy (FNAB) for thyroid nodules detected on PET/CT between January 2011 and December 2015 were assessed. The FNABs and surgical pathological results were recorded. Results: FNABs revealed benign results in 32 patients (32.7%), malignant in 18 (18.4%), non-diagnostic in 20 (20.4%), and indeterminate in 28 (28.5%). Twenty-four patients underwent thyroidectomy. The mean HU values were not significantly different in benign and malignant nodules ($p = 0.73$). However, the mean SUV_{max} was significantly higher ($p < 0.001$) in malignant ones. Area under curve (AUC) was 0.824 for SUV_{max}; the cut-off value was over 5.55 ($p < 0.001$), with 80% sensitivity, 84.5% specificity. Conclusions: Our current study demonstrated that HU value does not add any additional valuable information for discriminating between malignant and benign thyroid nodules. We also defined a SUV_{max} cut-off value of 5.55 for malignant potential of thyroid nodules detected on PET/CT. Arch Endocrinol Metab. 2018;62(4):460-5

Keywords
Thyroid nodules; malignancy; PET-CT, SUV_{max}; Hounsfield Unit

INTRODUCTION

The detection rate of incidental thyroid nodules is increasing steadily due to the use of new radiological imaging modalities, such as ^{18}F-fluorodeoxyglucose (FDG) positron emission tomography/computed tomography (PET/CT). Uptake of ^{18}F-FDG by the thyroid gland can be detected either diffusely or focally. Diffuse ^{18}F-FDG uptake is usually due to benign processes, such as thyroiditis, while focal uptake can be due to either a benign or a malignant nodule. The detection rate of new thyroid nodules by PET/CT has been reported as 1-4% (1).

In the absence of a familial history of thyroid cancer or external beam radiation to the neck, the malignancy rates of thyroid nodules detected on PET/CT ranges between 27.8-74%, whereas it is only 5-13% using ultrasound, CT, or magnetic resonance imaging (MRI) (1-3). Malignant cells tend to have higher glucose metabolism and thus may have positive ^{18}F-FDG PET/CT scans. Although they tend to have higher maximum standardized uptake values (SUV_{max}) than benign nodules, the definitive cut-off SUV_{max} for the prediction of a malignant thyroid nodule has not yet been defined (4).

The Hounsfield unit (HU), which was first introduced by Sir Godfrey Newbold Hounsfield, is used in CT scans and is a quantity proportional to the degree of X-rays that pass through or are absorbed by tissues (5). HU have since been used to evaluate and quantify tissues and fluids. The radiodensity of water is defined as 0, fat has a negative HU, and blood and other tissues have a positive HU, which are measured and reported in a variety of clinical approaches (6). Thus far, there is no clear information about the utility of HU values for the prediction of thyroid malignancy.

^{18}F-FDG PET/CT-positive thyroid nodules tend to have higher rates of malignancy, which should be further investigated by thyroid ultrasonography to enlightment for the features of thyroid nodules. Clinically suspicious features of malignancy on thyroid ultrasonography are hypoechogenicity, taller than wider appearance, irregular margins, hypervascularity, and microcalcifications (7). Many authorities, including the American Thyroid Association (ATA), recommend fine needle aspiration biopsy (FNAB) for exclusion of malignancy in thyroid nodules (8). Although FNAB is a simple, easily performed procedure for the detection of malignancy, in 15-30% of cases the results can be inconclusive. In most cases, repeat FNAB or diagnostic surgery needs to be carried out. More accurate and less invasive diagnostic approaches are required. The aim of this retrospective study is to evaluate the use of SUV_{max} and HU values for detecting the malignancy risk of ^{18}F-FDG PET/CT-positive thyroid nodules.

SUBJECTS AND METHODS

We retrospectively investigated the medical records of 98 patients with various cancers who had FNAB performed following the detection of 18F-FDG PET/CT-positive thyroid nodules between January 2011 and December 2015. None of the patients in our study group were evaluated for thyroid cancer as a primary site. The study was approved by our Institutional Review Board and Ethics Committee (Project number: KA16/23).

Medical records of all cancer patients with ^{18}F-FDG PET/CT-positive thyroid nodules subjected to FNAB were extracted from the hospital database. The ^{18}F-FDG PET/CT procedures were performed for the staging and/or follow-up of a cancer. The ultrasonographic features of these nodules were also noted.

The FNAB examinations were reported according to the Bethesda system for thyroid cytopathology (9). According to the Bethesda system, the cytopathology of thyroid nodules is separated into six groups: 1) nondiagnostic or unsatisfactory, 2) benign, 3) atypia of undetermined significance or follicular lesion of undetermined significance, 4) follicular neoplasm or suspicious for a follicular neoplasm, 5) suspicious for malignancy, and 6) malignant. For this particular study, the FNABs were grouped as: 1) nondiagnostic, 2) benign, 3) malignant and suspicious for malignancy, and 4) indeterminate. The indeterminate group included follicular neoplasm/suspected follicular neoplasm, or Hürthle cell neoplasm and atypia of undetermined significance subgroups. If more than one nodule was detected on a PET/CT scan, FNAB was performed on the nodule that had the higher SUVmax.

Together with SUV_{max}, HU values of the ^{18}F-FDG-positive nodules were also calculated as an additional tool to predict malignancy during non-contrast CT scans taken together with PET imaging. Calculations were performed by the same experienced nuclear medicine physician. The ultrasonographic features and cytological and surgical results were compared with SUV_{max} and HU of ^{18}F-FDG PET/CT-positive nodules.

Whole body ^{18}F-FDG PET/CT imaging

The patients were imaged using a dedicated PET/CT system (General Electric Medical System, Milwaukee, WI, USA). Patients fasted for at least 6 hours before intravenous administration of 2.5 MBq/kg ^{18}F-FDG. Before ^{18}F-FDG injection, blood glucose concentration was measured to confirm that patient levels were below 150 mg/dL. During the distribution phase, the patients were kept in the supine position in a quiet room. Combined image acquisition was performed 60 minutes after ^{18}F-FDG administration. First, an unenhanced CT scan (3.3 mm slice thickness) from the base of the skull to the inferior border of the pelvis was acquired using a standardized protocol (140 kV and 80 mA). The subsequent PET scan was obtained in three-dimensional mode from the base of the skull to the inferior border of the pelvis (6-7 bed positions, 2.5 minutes per bed position) without repositioning the patient on the table. Patients were breathing shallowly while CT and PET images were acquired. Attenuation was corrected by the CT images obtained after ^{18}F-FDG injection.

Thyroid lesions were analyzed semiquantitatively according to SUV_{max} values. The SUV_{max} was calculated automatically by software, as the ratio of the maximum tissue concentration of FDG (kBq/mL) in the structure delineated by the region of interest (ROI) to the activity injected per gram body weight of the patient (kBq/g). An ^{18}F-FDG PET-CT-positive thyroid nodule was defined as a thyroid lesion with a calculated SUV_{max} greater than 2 MBq/kg FDG. The HU value was measured at the region of thyroid nodules marked by a non-contrast CT scan, and calculated as the mean value.

Statistical analysis

The data are expressed as means ± SD or as medians for data that do not fit a normal distribution. The baseline differences between the two groups were analyzed by

Student's *t*-test. Pearson's chi-square test, and Fisher's exact test were used to compare the ratios between groups. The baseline differences between groups were also analyzed by the Kruskal-Wallis test and Mann-Whitney U test. In this study, the cut-off value of SUV_{max} was defined. The sensitivity and specificity of the calculated SUV_{max} and the area under the receiver operating characteristic curve (AUROC) were also measured. A p value < 0.05 was considered statistically significant. All statistical analyses were performed using SPSS for Windows software (ver. 23.0; SPSS Inc., Chicago, IL, USA).

RESULTS

Ninety-eight patients were included in the study. The mean age of the study population (n = 98) was 57.6 ± 13.8 years, and 75 (76.5%) were women. The most common primary malignancy evaluated was breast cancer at 25.5%. Thirty-four patients had solitary nodules (34.7%); the remainder had two or more nodules. Mean maximum diameter of 18F-FDG PET/CT-positive thyroid nodules was 22.5 ± 11.8 mm. The general characteristics and ultrasonographic features of the patients are shown in detail in Table 1.

Cytological examination of FNABs were reported as benign in 32 patients (32.7%), malignant in 18 (18.4%), nondiagnostic in 20 (20.4%), and indeterminate in 28 (28.5%). Thyroidectomy was performed on 24 patients. One of 20 patients in the nondiagnostic FNAB group had surgery, and the nodule was found to be malignant. Two of 32 patients with benign cytology were operated on and were found to have benign nodules. Nine of 18 patients with malignant and suspicious for malignancy FNABs were operated on, and all operation specimens were found to be malignant. The remaining 9 patients with malignant FNABs were not subjected to thyroidectomy because of their accompanying poor general health. Twelve of 28 patients with indeterminate FNABs were subjected to thyroidectomy; 6 of them were diagnosed as malignant, and the remaining were diagnosed as benign. The final pathological examination of 24 cases subjected to thyroidectomy revealed one patient with thyroid metastasis of primary cancer, one with anaplastic thyroid carcinoma, one with follicular carcinoma of thyroid, 13 patients with papillary carcinoma of thyroid, and the remaining eight were diagnosed as benign. These results are summarized in Figure 1.

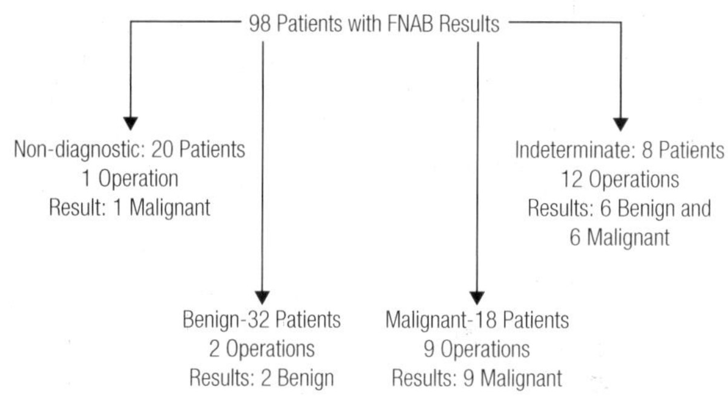

Figure 1. The surgical outcomes of the patients who underwent thyroidectomy.

Table 1. General characteristics of the patients, ultrasonographic features of ^{18}F-FDG PET/CT positive nodules regarding FNAB results

	Benign (n = 32)	Malignant (n = 18)	Indeterminated (n = 28)	Non-diagnostic (n = 20)	*p* value
Age (year)	56.6 ± 14.4	53.55 ± 20.93	57.42 ± 11.61	62.2 ± 10.5	0.15
Female (n, %)	27 (36%)	11 (14.6%)	21 (28%)	16 (21.4%)	NS
Male	5 (21.7%)	7 (30.4%)	7 (30.4%)	4 (17.4%)	NS
Type of nodule					
Solid	24 (33.8%)	8 (11.3%)	21 (29.5%)	18 (25.4%)	0.39
Solid-cystic	4 (44.4%)	1 (11.1%)	2 (22.2 %)	2 (22.2%)	0.29
Size (max diam.mm)	22.03 ± 10.5	21.46 ± 13.73	21.93 ± 11.47	22.5 ± 12.71	0.65
Hypoechogenic	18 (32.7%)	14 (25.5%)	13 (23.6%)	10 (18.2%)	0.52
Hyperechogenic	1 (20%)	1 (20%)	2 (40%)	1 (20%)	0.67
Isoechogenic	10 (50%)	1 (5%)	6 (30%)	3 (15%)	0.27
Microcalcification	2 (25%)	1 (12.5%)	0	5 (62.5%)	**0.034**
Taller than wider	0	1 (33.3%)	2 (66.7%)	0	0.32
Vascularity	3 (30%)	3 (30%)	4 (40%)	0	0.23

NS: not significant.

When we evaluate FNAB and postoperative pathological results of nodules together, 38 of them were considered as benign (32 patients with benign FNAB results and 6 of 12 patients with indeterminate FNAB results who subjected to thyroidectomy) and 25 of them were malignant (18 cases with malignant FNAB results and 6 cases with indeterminate FNAB results who subjected to thyroidectomy) and one with non-diagnostic FNAB result who subjected to thyroidectomy. The mean SUV_{max} was found to be significantly higher ($p < 0.001$) in malignant nodules than benign ones: 17.94 (min = 2.1, max = 82.2, median = 11.3, SD = 19.10) versus 4.68 (min = 2, max = 22.4, median = 3.3, SD = 4.02). The under the curve (AUC) was 0.824 for SUV_{max}; the cut-off value was over 5.55 ($p < 0.001$), with 80% sensitivity and 84.5% specificity (ROC curve) (Figure 2). However, mean HU values of these malignant and benign thyroid nodules were not significantly different ($p = 0.73$), 50.5 (min = 15, max = 91, median = 49, SD = 16.93) and 43.9 (min = 12, max = 67, median = 51, SD = 17.25), respectively (Table 2). We also grouped the patients according to SUV_{max} cut-off level (5.55). We found that SUV_{max} was correlated to HU values in all patients ($p = 0.03$). The nodules that have higher SUV_{max} have higher HU values. However, when only benign and malignant nodules were evaluated, we did not find any correlations between SUV_{max} and HU values.

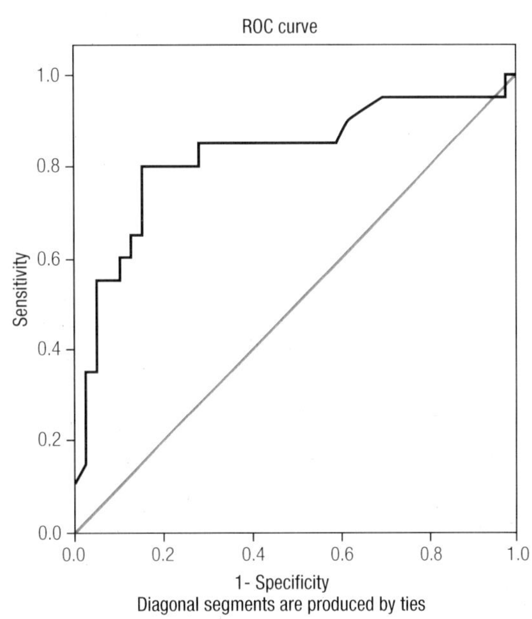

Figure 2. Receiver operating characteristic (ROC) curve of standardized uptake value (SUV max). The sensitivity and specifity in the prediction of malignant thyroid nodules.

Table 2. SUV max and Hounsfield values of ^{18}F-FDG PET/CT positive nodules regarding FNAB and postoperative pathological results

	Benign (n = 38)	Malignant (n = 25)	p value
SUV max	4.68 ± 4.02	17.94 ± 19.10	
	min = 2	min = 2.1	**< 0.001**
	max = 22.4	max = 82.2	
	median = 3.3	median = 11.3	
Hounsfield Unit	43.9 ± 17.25	50.5 ± 16.93	
	min = 12	min = 15	0.73
	max = 67	max = 91	
	median = 51	median = 49	

SUV max: Maximum Standardized Uptake Value.

DISCUSSION

In this study, inquiring the malignancy risk of 18F-FDG PET/CT-positive thyroid nodules via using SUV_{max} and HU values, we found that SUV_{max} values of nodules with malignant pathology were higher. However, the HU values exhibited statistically insignificant difference.

The malignancy risk of thyroid nodules ranges between 5-15% (10), and the risk increases if they are detectable on PET/CT scans 27.8-74% (3). Although the prevalence varies widely, according to a recent meta-analysis, 34.8% of thyroid nodules detected by 18F-FDG PET/CT are malignant (11). Even though, only 24.5% of the cases were subjected to thyroidectomy due to their inconvenient general health conditions, keeping in accordance with the analysis above, the malignancy rate was 25.5% in our cohort. The use of the SUV_{max} as a semiquantitative parameter to discriminate between benign and malignant tumors has been suggested previously (12,13). This measure reflects the metabolic activity of the lesions and, in general, a higher SUV_{max} value may imply malignancy (14). One of the factors affecting SUV_{max} is the expression of glucose transporters, and thyroid cancer cells usually have increased GLUT-1 expression (12). It has also been suggested that the SUV_{max} is influenced by different grades of inflammation, blood flow, and the size of the malignant lesions (15). Because of the high risk of malignancy, it is important to identify malignant 18F-FDG-positive nodules and determine which patients require surgical intervention. However, there is inconsistent information about the diagnostic role of SUV_{max} values for determining malignancy. Some studies have shown no significant difference between the SUV_{max} values of benign and malignant thyroid nodules (16-18), whereas numerous others have suggested its usefulness for identifying malignant lesions (14,19,20). The importance of SUV_{max} and its definitive cut-off value for predicting malignancy have not yet been established among patients with 18F-FDG PET/CT-positive thyroid nodules. The cut-off value for SUV_{max} was found to be 5.55 in the current study, which is corroborated by a previous report (21). The inconsistent results in current medical literature may be due to differences in glucose metabolism among detected lesions and/or differences in tumor size. Accordingly, Kim and cols. reported no significant difference in SUV_{max} between malignant and benign thyroid nodules less than 1 cm in size (22). When the nodules in our study were categorized up to 1 cm size cut-off, there was no significant difference regarding SUV_{max} between malignant and benign nodules, as well.

To avoid unnecessary surgical operations and further investigations, an additional diagnostic tool besides SUV_{max} is required. Recently, Kim and cols. demonstrated that the HU values of thyroid nodules detected on 18F-FDG PET/CT scans were higher in malignant than benign ones, and the sensitivity, specificity, and accuracy of HU values were all higher than those of SUV_{max} (22). This is the only study proposing the use of HU value as a new parameter to classify the risk of malignancy of 18F-FDG PET/CT-positive thyroid nodules. For confirmation, we calculated the HU values of thyroid nodules on non-contrast CT in addition to SUV_{max}. There was no significant difference between mean HU value of benign and malignant thyroid nodules in our study. The HU measurement seems to have no additional value for the identification of malignant and benign thyroid nodules detected on PET/CT scans. Our finding is consistent with the study by Sayman and cols. (23), although conflicting with Kim's study (22). Further studies are required to verify these results.

Our study has some limitations. The retrospective design is one of them. The other is the relatively low number of cases that were subjected to thyroidectomy in indeterminate and non-diagnostic groups. Only one of the 20 patients with nondiagnostic FNAB, and 12 of the 28 patients with indeterminate FNAB, had thyroidectomy. The final pathological examination showed one malignancy in the former group, whereas 6 cases exhibited thyroid malignancy following thyroidectomy in the indeterminate FNAB group. If all of the nondiagnostic and indeterminate results could have been confirmed by repeat FNAB or surgery, the results would have been surely higher. However, this was not possible due to the critical health condition of the patients (most of whom were metastatic). If the cut-off value for SUV_{max} of 5.55 was applied to nondiagnostic thyroid nodules, 9 of 20 patients would have been above that value. If the same cut-off was applied to the indeterminate patients who did not undergo operation, half of them would have been over that value. These probabilities do not necessarily mean that these nodules were malignant, but suggest that the nodules should have been evaluated further.

In conclusion, we defined an SUV_{max} cut-off value of 5.55 and demonstrated its importance in determining the malignant potential of thyroid nodules. Most of the published research on the issue of thyroid incidentaloma detected at 18F-FDG/PET CT focus on the role of SUV_{max} and its potential role in the differentiation of malignant and benign thyroid lesions. Our study deals with the potential role of additional information obtained from the CT part of this imaging modality. The analysis of HUs of metabolically active thyroid nodules does not have any additional valuable information for discriminating between malignant and benign nodules.

Authors' contributions: Dr. Filiz Eksi Haydardedeoglu: Project development, data interpretation/collection, manuscript writing and editing. Gulay Simsek Bagir: Data collection. Nese Torun: Interpretation of PET/CT data and analysis of results. N. Emrah Kocer: Analysis of pathological results. Mehmet Reyhan: Data collection and drafting of manuscript. M. Eda Ertorer: Data interpretation and drafting of manuscript.

Acknowledgment: we do thank Cagla Sariturk for calculating and supporting all statistical analyses.

REFERENCES

1. Chun AR, Jo HM, Lee SH, Chun HW, Park JM, Kim KJ, et al. Risk of Malignancy in Thyroid Incidentalomas Identified by Fluorodeoxyglucose-Positron Emission Tomography. Endocrinol Metab (Seoul). 2015;30(1):71-7.
2. Russ G, Leboulleux S, Leenhardt L, Hegedüs L. Thyroid incidentalomas: epidemiology, risk stratification with ultrasound and workup. Eur Thyroid J. 2014;3(3):154-63.
3. Kao YH, Lim SS, Ong SC, Padhy AK. Thyroid incidentalomas on fluorine-18-fluorodeoxyglucose positron emission tomography-computed tomography: incidence, malignancy risk, and comparison of standardized uptake values. Can Assoc Radiol J. 2012;63(4):289-93.
4. Brindle R, Mullan D, Yap BK, Gandhi A. Thyroid incidentalomas discovered on positron emission tomography CT scanning - Malignancy rate and significance of standardised uptake values. Eur J Surg Oncol. 2014;40(11):1528-32.

5. Lamba R, McGahan JP, Corwin MT, Li CS, Tran T, Seibert JA, et al. CT Hounsfield numbers of soft tissues on unenhanced abdominal CT scans: variability between two different manufacturers' MDCT scanners. AJR Am J Roentgenol. 2014;203(5):1013-20.
6. Kalender WA. Computed tomography: fundamentals, system technology, image quality, applications. 3. Erlangen, Germany: Publicis Publishing; 2011.
7. Yoon JH, Cho A, Lee HS, Kim EK, Moon HJ, Kwak JY. Thyroid incidentalomas detected on 18F-fluorodeoxyglucose-positron emission tomography/computed tomography: Thyroid Imaging Reporting and Data System (TIRADS) in the diagnosis and management of patients. Surgery. 2015;158(5):1314-22.
8. Haugen BR, Alexander EK, Bible KC, Doherty GM, Mandel SJ, Nikiforov YE, et al. 2015 American Thyroid Association Management Guidelines for Adult Patients with Thyroid Nodules and Differentiated Thyroid Cancer: The American Thyroid Association Guidelines Task Force on Thyroid Nodules and Differentiated Thyroid Cancer. Thyroid. 2016;26(1):1-133.
9. Cibas ES, Ali SZ. The Bethesda System for Reporting Thyroid Cytopathology. Thyroid. 2009;19(11):1159-65.
10. Tunbridge WM, Evered DC, Hall R, Appleton D, Brewis M, Clark F, et al. The spectrum of thyroid disease in a community: the Whickham survey. Clin Endocrinol (Oxf). 1977;7(6):481-93.
11. Soelberg KK, Bonnema SJ, Brix TH, Hegedüs L. Risk of malignancy in thyroid incidentalomas detected by 18F-fluorodeoxyglucose positron emission tomography: a systematic review. Thyroid. 2012;22(9):918-25.
12. Chen YK, Ding HJ, Chen KT, Chen YL, Liao AC, Shen YY, et al. Prevalence and risk of cancer of focal thyroid incidentaloma identified by 18F-fluorodeoxyglucose positron emission tomography for cancer screening in healthy subjects. Anticancer Res. 2005;25(2B):1421-6.
13. Yaylalı O, Kirac FS, Yuksel D, Marangoz E. Evaluation of focal thyroid lesions incidentally detected in fluorine-18-fluorodeoxyglucose positron emission tomography/computed tomography images. Indian J Cancer. 2014;51(3):236-40.
14. Stangierski A, Wolinski K, Czepczynski R, Czarnywojtek A, Lodyga M, Wyszomirska A, et al. The usefulness of standardized uptake value in differentiation between benign and malignant thyroid lesions detected incidentally in 18F-FDG PET/CT examination. PLosOne. 2014; 9(10):e109612.
15. Ohba K, Nishizawa S, Matsushita A, Inubushi M, Nagayama K, Iwaki H, et al. High incidence of thyroid cancer in focal thyroid incidentaloma detected by 18F-fluorodeoxyglucose [corrected] positron emission tomography in relatively young healthy subjects: results of 3-year follow-up. Endocr J. 2010;57(5):395-401.
16. Eloy JA, Brett EM, Fatterpekar GM, Kostakoglu L, Som PM, Desai SC, et al. The significance and management of incidental [18F] fluorodeoxyglucose-positron-emission tomography uptake in the thyroid gland in patients with cancer. AJNR Am J Neuroradiol. 2009;30(7):1431-4.
17. Buyukdereli G, Aktar Y, Kara E, Uguz A, Sonmez H. Role of 18F-fluorodeoxyglucose Positron Emission Tomography/Computed Tomography in the Evaluation of Cytologically Indeterminate Thyroid Nodules. Iran J Radiol. 2016;13(1):e21186.
18. Are C, Hsu JF, Schoder JP, Shah JP, Larson SM, Shaha AR. FDG-PET detected thyroid incidentalomas: need for further investigation? Ann Surg Oncol. 2007;14(1):239-47.
19. Wang N, Zhai H, Lu Y. Is fluorine-18 fluorodeoxyglucose positron emission tomography useful for the thyroid nodules with indeterminate fine needle aspiration biopsy? A meta-analysis of the literature. J Otolaryngol Head Neck Surg. 2013;42:38.
20. Kresnik E, Gallowitsch HJ, Mikosch P, Stettner H, Igerc I, Gomez I, et al. Fluorine-18-fluorodeoxyglucose positron emission tomography in the preoperative assessment of thyroid nodules in an endemic goiter area. Surgery. 2003;133(3):294-9.
21. Bertagna F, Treglia G, Piccardo A, Giovannini E, Bosio G, Biasiotto G, et al. F18-FDG-PET/CT thyroid incidentalomas: a wide retrospective analysis in three Italian centres on the significance of focal uptake and SUV value. Endocrine. 2013;43(3):678-85.
22. Kim D, Hwang SH, Cha J, Jo K, Lee N, Yun M. Risk Stratification of Thyroid Incidentalomas Found on PET/CT: The value of Iodine Content on Noncontrast Computed Tomography. Thyroid. 2015;25(11):1249-54.
23. Sayman H, Uslu L, Topuz OV, Sager S, Halac M, Sonmezoglu K. Is adding hounsfield unit measurement on standardized uptake value helpful in differentiating thyroid nodules? J Nucl Med. 2013;54(Suppl 2):1900.

Recent recommendations from ATA guidelines to define the upper reference range for serum TSH in the first trimester match reference ranges for pregnant women in Rio de Janeiro

Nathalie Anne de Oliveira e Silva de Morais[1,2,3], Annie Schtscherbyna Almeida de Assis[1], Carolina Martins Corcino[1,2], Débora Ayres Saraiva[1], Tatiana Martins Benvenuto Louro Berbara[1], Carolina Donner de Drummond Ventura[1], Mario Vaisman[1], Patrícia de Fátima dos Santos Teixeira[1]

[1] Departamento de Medicina Interna e Unidade de Endocrinologia, Faculdade de Medicina e Hospital Universitário Clementino Fraga Filho, Universidade Federal do Rio de Janeiro (HUCFF/UFRJ), Rio de Janeiro, RJ, Brasil
[2] Unidade de Endocrinologia, Instituto Estadual de Diabetes e Endocrinologia Luiz Capriglione (IEDE), Rio de Janeiro, RJ, Brasil
[3] Unidade de Endocrinologia, Instituto Nacional de Câncer José Alencar Gomes da Silva (INCA), Rio de Janeiro, RJ, Brasil

Correspondence to:
Nathalie Anne de Oliveira e Silva de Morais
Hospital Universitário Clementino Fraga Filho, Serviço de Endocrinologia
Rua Rodolpho Paulo Rocco, 255, 9° andar, sala 9E23
21941-913 – Rio de Janeiro, RJ, Brasil
nathalieaos@gmail.com

ABSTRACT

Objectives: American Thyroid Association (ATA)'s new guidelines recommend use of population-based trimester-specific reference range (RR) for thyrotropin (TSH) in pregnancy. The aim of this study was to determine first trimester TSH RR for a population of pregnant women in Rio de Janeiro State. Subjects and methods: Two hundred and seventy pregnant women without thyroid illness, defined by National Academy of Clinical Biochemistry, and normal iodine status were included in this sectional study. This reference group (RG) had normal median urinary iodine concentration (UIC = 219 µg/L) and negative anti-thyroperoxidase antibodies (TPOAb). Twin pregnancy, trophoblastic disease and use of drugs or supplements that influence thyroid function were excluded. In a second step, we defined a more selective reference group (SRG, n = 170) by excluding patients with thyroiditis pattern on thyroid ultrasound and positive anti-thyroglobulin antibodies. This group also had normal median UIC. At a final step, a more selective reference group (MSRG, n = 130) was defined by excluding any pregnant women with UIC < 150 µg/L. Results: In the RG, median, 2.5th and 97.5th percentiles of TSH were 1.3, 0.1, and 4.4 mIU/L, respectively. The mean age was 27.0 ± 5.0 and the mean body mass index was 25.6 ± 5.2 kg/m^2. In the SRG and MSRG, 2.5th and 97.5th percentiles were 0.06 and 4.0 (SRG) and 0.1 and 3.6 mIU/L (MSRG), respectively. Conclusions: In the population studied, TSH upper limit in the first trimester of pregnancy was above 2.5 mIU/L. The value of 3.6 mIU/L, found when iodine deficiency and thyroiditis (defined by antibodies and ultrasound characteristics) were excluded, matches recent ATA guidelines. Arch Endocrinol Metab. 2018;62(4):386-91

Keywords
TSH; pregnancy; reference range

INTRODUCTION

The American Thyroid Association (ATA) has recently published new guidelines for the diagnosis and management of thyroid disease during pregnancy and the postpartum period (1). A substantial difference in these guidelines, compared with the prior version published in 2011 (2), is the question regarding the upper reference limit for serum thyrotropin (TSH) during the first trimester of pregnancy, defined previously as 2.5 mIU/L. ATA's new guidelines recommend the use of population-based trimester-specific reference ranges for serum TSH derived from evaluation of local population data. When local assessments are not available, the panel recommends that lower reference range of TSH should be reduced by approximately 0.4 mIU/L, while the upper reference range should be reduced by approximately 0.5 mIU/L in the first trimester of pregnancy, from the reference values for non-pregnant women (1).

These cutoff changes were based on recent large cohorts from various countries that have published trimester-specific pregnancy reference ranges, demonstrating significantly higher serum TSH concentration in their populations than previously reported in the literature (3-9). Two of these studies showed, by week-to-week evaluation, that TSH reference limits were variable during the first trimester. In their studied populations, median TSH from up to 6 weeks was much higher, similar to the reference range for non-pregnant women, than to the range for 7 to 12 weeks (3,4). This larger analysis also demonstrated substantial population differences in the TSH upper-reference limit that can be explained by differences in ethnicity, geographic location, iodine intake, body mass index (BMI), thyroid peroxidase antibody (TPOAb)-positivity and the TSH assays used for analysis (10).

Recently, there have been published data concerning the normal range of serum TSH for the first trimester of gestation in a non-coastal area of Brazil (11). In the studied population, the TSH value corresponding to the 97.5th percentile was 2.68 mIU/L in the first trimester of gestation, which matches prior guidelines recommendations (2,12,13). In contrast, another smaller Brazilian study, which evaluated pregnant women in the first trimester in a coastal area of the country, found higher TSH levels with a 97.5th percentile of 4.43 mIU/L (14).

The National Academy of Clinical Biochemistry (NACB) states that "TSH reference intervals should be established from 95% confidence limits of the log-transformed values of at least 120 rigorously screened normal euthyroid volunteers who meet the following criteria: no detectable thyroid autoantibodies (TPOAb or thyroglobulin antibody (TgAb), measured by sensitive immunoassay); no personal or family history of thyroid dysfunction; no visible or palpable goiter; and not using any medications (except estrogen)" (15). It is worth mentioning that NACB does not require thyroid ultrasonography to exclude thyroiditis, and that the presence of only one negative thyroid autoantibodies is necessary. The lower and upper limits of TSH are defined by the 2.5th and 97.5th percentile, respectively (16).

In recent years, several studies have shown important additive effects of thyroid autoimmunity on maternal thyroid status with respect to pregnancy outcome. It turns out that women who are antibody positive have a greater risk of adverse events than do antibody-negative women, even when they have identical thyroid function (17,18). There are patients with undetectable thyroid antibodies who may have a thyroiditis pattern on ultrasound (19,20). Furthermore, population studies in non-pregnant women confirm that upper reference range of TSH is reduced after excluding those with ultrasound patterns compatible with thyroiditis (20-22). International guidelines recommend populations with adequate iodine intake to be used to define TSH reference ranges. This is especially important in pregnant populations due to increased iodine demand during pregnancy (1,12,13). Not only iodine deficiency but also high iodine intake is associated with reduced thyroid function (23).

From these data, we proposed this study aiming to establish a serum TSH reference range in the first trimester of gestation for a population that lives in the coastal area of the state of Rio de Janeiro. For this purpose, we assessed a sample of pregnant women without thyroid illness, defined by NACB strict criteria, normal ultrasound patterns, normal iodine status and absence of thyroid autoantibodies (TPOAb and TgAb).

SUBJECTS AND METHODS

This cross-sectional study was performed on a subpopulation from an ongoing prospective cohort, and included pregnant women attending prenatal programs in maternity clinics in the public health system in the State of Rio de Janeiro. Four prenatal outpatient clinics in a coastal area of the state of Rio de Janeiro, Brazil, participated in this study. The study was approved by the local Research Ethics Committee, and all subjects signed consent forms (CAAE: 22546213.0.0000.5275).

A total of 270 pregnant women were enrolled from September 2014 to January 2017. The recruiting criteria included age ≥ 18 and ≤ 35 years old, having a spontaneous pregnancy and gestational age up to 12 weeks (defined by last menstrual period or ultrasound). According to Guideline 22 of the National Academy of Clinical Biochemistry (15), we excluded patients with personal or familiar history of thyroid disease, using drugs or supplements that might influence thyroid function, and with visible or palpable goiter. Women with multiple pregnancies, trophoblastic disease and other chronic diseases history were also excluded.

Specific history and general physical examination were performed. Height and weight were measured with participants barefoot and wearing light clothing. Body mass index (BMI) was calculated as weight (kg) divided by height squared (m^2).

Samples of blood and spot urines were obtained from each participant in the morning, after 10 to 12 hours of fasting, to determine serum TSH, FT4,

TPOAb, TgAb and urinary iodine concentration (UIC). Thyroid ultrasound scan was performed in all participants.

After this analysis, we excluded patients with positive TPOAb to create the reference group.

This final sample, defined as reference group (RG), consisted of 225 pregnant women that filled all NACB criteria and had a normal median UIC.

In a second step, we defined a selective reference group (SRG, n = 170) by excluding those patients with thyroiditis pattern on thyroid ultrasound scan and positive serum TgAb. This group also had normal median UIC.

Ultrasound thyroiditis pattern was defined as the presence of a heterogeneous and/or hypoechoic gland. Classification of iodine status was made according to the World Health Organization (WHO) as follows: severe insufficiency, < 50 µg/L; mild-moderate insufficiency, 50 to 149 µg/L; sufficiency, 150 to 249 µg/L; more than adequate, 250 to 499 µg/L; and excessive, ≥ 500 µg/L.

At a final step, a more selective reference group (MSRG, n = 130) was defined by excluding any pregnant women with UIC < 150 µg/L, which could reflect iodine insufficiency. We emphasize that MSRG meets all NACB criteria, including sample size greater than 120 individuals.

Serum TSH, FT4, TPOAb and TgAb were performed by electrochemiluminescence immunometric assay on the Roche Modular Analytics® E170 (Roche Diagnostics). The Laboratory reference ranges of TSH were 0.4 to 4.3 mIU/L (for non-pregnant women), FT4 0.7 to 1.9 ng/dL, TPOAb < 34 IU/mL and TgAb < 115 IU/mL. The intra-assay coefficients of variation of serum TSH, FT4, TPOAb and TgAb were 7.2%, 2.79%, 6.3% and 4.9%, respectively. The interassay coefficients of variation were 3%, 2.9%, 7.0% and 6.3%, respectively. Urinary iodine concentration was determined by Inductively Coupled Plasma Mass Spectrometry (ICP-MS-Spectroquant® Iodine Test – Merch KGaA, Germany). The manufacturer's reference range was 26 to 705 µg/L.

All thyroid ultrasound scans were performed by a single trained examiner, using a high-frequency SIEMENS-AUSONX 300 transducer (12 MHz). Thyroid volume was calculated by the formula: length x width x thickness x 0.52 of each lobe and the isthmus. Thyroid parenchyma characteristics were described according to their echogenicity and homogeneity.

Statistical analysis was performed using the SPSS for Windows program, version 13.0. Mean, median, 2.5th and 97.5th percentiles were calculated for the TSH and FT4 values. Continuous variables were shown as the mean ± SD (median) and were compared between two groups using the Mann-Whitney test or Student *t*-test, according to the data distribution as evaluated by the Kolmogorov-Smirnov test. Comparisons among three or more groups were assessed by the Kruskal-Wallis test. Categorical variables were expressed as percentages and compared by the chi-squared test (χ^2) or Fisher exact test. The analysis of the correlation between two variables was performed using Spearman's correlation coefficient (rs). A p-value < 0.05 was considered to be significant.

RESULTS

The clinical and biochemical characteristics of the three studied groups are described in Table 1. The RG, SRG and MSRG groups were similar in terms of age, BMI, gestational week at inclusion, frequencies of smoking and iodine status. Although there were no significant differences in UIC among the studied groups, MSRG have a higher median urine iodine, classified as more than adequate status. Our study population presented normal median values of BMI when we use BMI classification tables specific to pregnant women (24).

Table 1. Clinical and biochemical characteristics of the three studied groups of pregnant women, evaluated in the first trimester of gestation, inhabitants a coastal area of Rio de Janeiro State

	RG (n = 225)	SRG (n = 170)	MSRG (n = 130)
Age (years)*	27.0 ± 5.0 (28.0)	27.4 ± 5.2 (28.0)	26.9 ± 5.0 (27.0)
Gestational week at inclusion (weeks)*	9.0 ± 2.0 (9.0)	9.0 ± 2.2 (9.0)	8.9 ± 2.0 (9.0)
BMI (kg/m^2)*	25.6 ± 5.2 (24.6)	25.8 ± 5.0 (25.2)	26.1 ± 5.5 (25.2)
UIC (µg/L)*	234.0 ± 117.0 (219.0)	226.3 ± 103.6 (210.8)	278.6 ± 113.0 (252.8)
Smoking (%)	2.6 (n = 6)	3.5 (n = 6)	3.8 (n = 5)

* Mean ± standard deviation (median); RG: Reference Group; SRG: Selective Reference Group; MSRG: More Selective Reference Group; BMI: body mass index; UIC: urine iodine concentration.

The means, 2.5th percentile, 97.5th percentile and median for serum TSH and FT4 values in the three studied groups are summarized in Table 2. The 97.5th percentile value of TSH decreased from 4.47 mIU/L to 4.00 mIU/L after we excluded pregnant women with positive TgAb or thyroiditis pattern in ultrasound scan. In addition, median TSH and 97.5th percentile value of TSH were lower in the more selective group (MSRG), which excluded any pregnant women with UIC less than 150 μg/L, compared to the other groups. In the reference group (RG), TSH was > 2.5 mIU/L in 19.6%. In the SRG and SSRG this prevalence was 17.1 and 14.6%, respectively.

In the reference group (RG), TSH was slightly negatively correlated with FT4 (r_s -0.142; p = 0.017) but was not correlated with age (r_s -0.052; p = 0.221), BMI (r_s -0.048; p = 0.236), gestational age (r_s -0.025; p = 0.356) or UIC (r_s 0.031; p = 0.323). However, when we evaluated only the group of pregnant women up to 6 weeks of gestation, we found a negative correlation between TSH and gestational age (r_s -0.433; p = 0.025). This correlation was not maintained in the analysis of patients with more than 6 weeks of gestation (r_s 0.065 p = 0.182).

Furthermore, comparing TSH levels in these two subgroups (up to 6 weeks of gestation and > 6 weeks of gestation), we found lower levels of TSH in the group of patients up to 6 weeks of gestation. These data are described in Table 3.

DISCUSSION

This is the first study designed to establish reference limits of serum TSH and FT4 values in a pregnant population that inhabits a coastal Brazilian area, in the state of Rio de Janeiro, that filled all NACB criteria. Additionally, to the best of our knowledge, this is the first study in the literature to apply so strict selection criteria intended to define a rational reference range of serum TSH for pregnant women in the first trimester, considering NACB criteria.

Subclinical hypothyroidism (SCH) is defined as elevated serum TSH concentrations and normal levels of serum FT4. Strategies for the diagnosis of thyroid dysfunction differ in pregnant compared to non-pregnant women.

The definition of a normal reference range of TSH in pregnant women is critical and should ideally be derived from local population data. Substantial variation exists between populations, with many recent investigations confirming a more liberal upper TSH reference range in healthy pregnant women with no thyroid disease (10).

Previously, our group accessed the distribution of serum TSH values in the first trimester of pregnancy in a group of pregnant women with negative TPOAb and iodine sufficiency in Rio de Janeiro (14). This study has also showed a 97.5th percentile value of serum TSH above 2.5 mIU/L (95th percentile:4.43 mIU/L – 95%CI: 3.68 to 5.84). However, the final sample

Table 2. Reference values for serum TSH and FT4 in the first trimester of pregnancy in the three studied subgroups of pregnant women with iodine sufficiency

		TSH (mIU/L)			FT4 (ng/dL)		
	n	**2.5th centile**	**Median**	**97.5th centile**	**2.5th centile**	**Median**	**97.5th centile**
RG	225	0.12	1.33	4.47	0.80	1.10	1.50
SRG	170	0.06	1.26	4.00	0.80	1.20	1.50
MSRG	130	0.14	1.28	3.63	0.80	1.10	1.50

RG: Reference Group; SRG: Selective Reference Group; MSRG: More Selective Reference Group; TSH: thyrotropin; FT4: free thyroxine.

Table 3. Reference values for serum TSH in the first trimester of pregnancy in the three studied subgroups of pregnant women according to gestational age

	TSH		
	Gestational age ≤ 6 weeks	**Gestational age > 6 weeks**	***p* value**
RG*	1.60 ± 1.32 (1.27) n = 21	1.97 ± 0.92 (1.71) n = 204	0.030
SRG*	1.47 ± 1.08 (1.24) n = 18	1.91 ± 0.89 (1.72) n = 152	0.038
MSRG*	1.41 ± 0.97 (1.26) n = 16	1.85 ± 0.93 (1.68) n = 114	0.073

* Mean ± standard deviation (median); RG: Reference Group; SRG: Selective Reference Group; MSRG: More Selective Reference Group; TSH: thyrotropin.

number evaluated in this study, after exclusion of positive TPOAb patients, was below 120, recommended by NACB to define TSH reference range in a given population.

The disagreement between serum TSH reference values found in our study compared to those found by Rosario and cols. (11) may be due to differences between the two populations. Brazil is a continental-sized country with ethnic and geographic characteristics that differ from a region to another. The state of Rio de Janeiro is located in a coastal area, unlike Minas Gerais, which is located in a continental area. In addition, two limitations of that study were absence of iodine status evaluation and absence of ultrasound scan and TgAb measurement to exclude thyroid autoimmunity in their population.

Although some studies have shown that excluding people with thyroid ultrasound abnormalities did not affect TSH reference range (25,26), some authors suggest higher TSH levels in the presence of thyroid autoimmunity detected by both ultrasound and autoantibodies (27). It appears reasonable that, in pregnant women who exhibit immunosuppression of pregnancy, thyroid ultrasound evaluation could add information regarding prediction of autoimmune thyroid disease.

A recent study that evaluated women seeking fertility treatment showed that 5% of patients presented isolated TgAb positivity and 4% isolated TPOAb concentrations. Serum TSH values were significantly higher in the group of women with isolated positive TgAb compared to women without positive thyroid antibodies. This study demonstrated that testing for thyroid autoimmunity using only TPOAb would likely miss a small proportion of women with isolated TgAb (28).

In our study reference population, there were no cases of hypothyroxinemia. Hypothyroxinemia was excluded in the sample of pregnant women studied by the presence of normal FT4 values. We believe that FT4 is a more useful index of thyroid function during early pregnancy than is total T4. Although FT4 immunoassays have been reported to be a less accurate method during pregnancy, this interference occurs mainly in the third trimester of gestation (29,30). In addition, total T4 concentrations are highly dependent on changes in thyroxine-binding globulin (TBG) concentrations, being more variable during early pregnancy than are free T4 concentrations (31).

It should be noted that there are still some concerns about the new reference range suggested by 2017 ATA thyroid and pregnancy guidelines, since it was based on studies that evaluated few women. In the five largest studies cited, only one presented an upper limit of normal TSH above 3.5 mIU/L (32).

Although many studies suggest that subclinical hypothyroidism is associated with obstetric complications and impairment in neurocognitive development of at-risk children (33,34), the recommendations for screening and treatment remain controversial (35). The previously recommended TSH cutoff of 2.5 mIU/L appears to be too low and is likely to leading to overdiagnosis and overtreatment of thyroid disease during pregnancy (1). Additional studies evaluating the safety and benefits of treatment with levothyroxine in pregnant women with subclinical hypothyroidism are needed, especially to assess the differences between TPOAb-positive or negative patients.

In addition, the authors believe that a larger population would be desired to bring more strength to the present study, despite having met the criteria required by NACB.

In conclusion, the upper limit of serum TSH reference in the first trimester was above 2.5 mIU/L in pregnant Brazilian women that live in a coastal area of the country. The value of 3.6 mIU/L, found when iodine deficiency and thyroiditis (defined both by negative TgAb and TPOAb and normal thyroid ultrasound pattern) were excluded, appeared to match the recent ATA guidelines.

Acknowledgments: this study was made possible thanks to grants from the Research Support Foundation of the State of Rio de Janeiro (FAPERJ). The authors are also grateful for the help of Dr. Rosalia Fernandes Cordeiro de Morais, who contributed significantly to this project.

REFERENCES

1. Alexander EK, Pearce EN, Brent GA, Brown RS, Chen H, Dosiou C, et al. 2017 Guidelines of the American Thyroid Association for the Diagnosis and Management of Thyroid Disease During Pregnancy and the Postpartum. Thyroid. 2017;27(3):315-89.
2. Stagnaro-Green A, Abalovich M, Alexander E, Azizi F, Mestman J, Negro R, et al. Guidelines of the American Thyroid Association for the diagnosis and management of thyroid disease during pregnancy and postpartum. Thyroid. 2011;21(10):1081-125.
3. Laurberg P, Andersen SL, Hindersson P, Nohr EA, Olsen J. Dynamics and Predictors of Serum TSH and fT4 Reference Limits

in Early Pregnancy: A Study Within the Danish National Birth Cohort. J Clin Endocrinol Metab. 2016;101(6):2484-92.

4. Li C, Shan Z, Mao J, Wang W, Xie X, Zhou W, et al. Assessment of thyroid function during first-trimester pregnancy: what is the rational upper limit of serum TSH during the first trimester in Chinese pregnant women? J Clin Endocrinol Metab. 2014;99(1):73-9.
5. Lambert-Messerlian G, McClain M, Haddow JE, Palomaki GE, Canick JA, Cleary-Goldman J, et al. First- and second-trimester thyroid hormone reference data in pregnant women: a FaSTER (First- and Second-Trimester Evaluation of Risk for aneuploidy) Research Consortium study. Am J Obstet Gynecol. 2008;199(1):62 e1-6.
6. Mannisto T, Surcel HM, Ruokonen A, Vaarasmaki M, Pouta A, Bloigu A, et al. Early pregnancy reference intervals of thyroid hormone concentrations in a thyroid antibody-negative pregnant population. Thyroid. 2011;21(3):291-8.
7. Springer D, Zima T, Limanova Z. Reference intervals in evaluation of maternal thyroid function during the first trimester of pregnancy. Eur J Endocrinol. 2009;160(5):791-7.
8. Bestwick JP, John R, Maina A, Guaraldo V, Joomun M, Wald NJ, et al. Thyroid stimulating hormone and free thyroxine in pregnancy: expressing concentrations as multiples of the median (MoMs). Clin Chim Acta. 2014;430:33-7.
9. Medici M, de Rijke YB, Peeters RP, Visser W, de Muinck Keizer-Schrama SM, Jaddoe VV, et al. Maternal early pregnancy and newborn thyroid hormone parameters: the Generation R study. J Clin Endocrinol Metab. 2012;97(2):646-52.
10. Medici M, Korevaar TI, Visser WE, Visser TJ, Peeters RP. Thyroid function in pregnancy: what is normal? Clin Chem. 2015;61(5):704-13.
11. Rosario PW, Carvalho M, Calsolari MR. TSH reference values in the first trimester of gestation and correlation between maternal TSH and obstetric and neonatal outcomes: a prospective Brazilian study. Arch Endocrinol Metab. 2016;60(4):314-8.
12. Lazarus J, Brown RS, Daumerie C, Hubalewska-Dydejczyk A, Negro R, Vaidya B. 2014 European thyroid association guidelines for the management of subclinical hypothyroidism in pregnancy and in children. Eur Thyroid J. 2014;3(2):76-94.
13. De Groot L, Abalovich M, Alexander EK, Amino N, Barbour L, Cobin RH, et al. Management of thyroid dysfunction during pregnancy and postpartum: an Endocrine Society clinical practice guideline. J Clin Endocrinol Metab. 2012;97(8):2543-65.
14. Felipe CL, Medina CC, Sieiro NL, Alexandru B, Mario V. Is an upper limit of 2.5 mUI/l for TSH appropriate for the first trimester of pregnancy among young TPO – women? Gynecol Endocrinol. 2010;26(1):54-7.
15. Baloch Z, Carayon P, Conte-Devolx B, Demers LM, Feldt-Rasmussen U, Henry JF, et al. Laboratory medicine practice guidelines. Laboratory support for the diagnosis and monitoring of thyroid disease. Thyroid. 2003;13(1):3-126.
16. Geffre A, Friedrichs K, Harr K, Concordet D, Trumel C, Braun JP. Reference values: a review. Vet Clin Pathol. 2009;38(3):288-98.
17. Chen L, Hu R. Thyroid autoimmunity and miscarriage: a meta-analysis. Clin Endocrinol (Oxf). 2011;74(4):513-9.
18. Thangaratinam S, Tan A, Knox E, Kilby MD, Franklyn J, Coomarasamy A. Association between thyroid autoantibodies and miscarriage and preterm birth: meta-analysis of evidence. BMJ. 2011;342:d2616.
19. Pedersen OM, Aardal NP, Larssen TB, Varhaug JE, Myking O, Vik-Mo H. The value of ultrasonography in predicting autoimmune thyroid disease. Thyroid. 2000;10(3):251-9.
20. Vejbjerg P, Knudsen N, Perrild H, Laurberg P, Pedersen IB, Rasmussen LB, et al. The association between hypoechogenicity or irregular echo pattern at thyroid ultrasonography and thyroid function in the general population. Eur J Endocrinol. 2006;155(4):547-52.
21. Trimboli P, Rossi F, Condorelli E, Laurenti O, Ventura C, Nigri G, et al. Does normal thyroid gland by ultrasonography match with normal serum thyroid hormones and negative thyroid antibodies? Exp Clin Endocrinol Diabetes. 2010;118(9):630-2.
22. Dobert N, Balzer K, Diener J, Wegscheider K, Vaupel R, Grunwald F. Thyroid sonomorphology, thyroid peroxidase antibodies and thyroid function: new epidemiological data in unselected German employees. Nuklearmedizin. 2008;47(5):194-9.
23. Shi X, Han C, Li C, Mao J, Wang W, Xie X, et al. Optimal and safe upper limits of iodine intake for early pregnancy in iodine-sufficient regions: a cross-sectional study of 7190 pregnant women in China. J Clin Endocrinol Metab. 2015;100(4):1630-8.
24. Atalah E, Castillo C, Castro R, Aldea A. [Proposal of a new standard for the nutritional assessment of pregnant women]. Rev Med Chil. 1997;125(12):1429-36.
25. Kratzsch J, Fiedler GM, Leichtle A, Brugel M, Buchbinder S, Otto L, et al. New reference intervals for thyrotropin and thyroid hormones based on National Academy of Clinical Biochemistry criteria and regular ultrasonography of the thyroid. Clin Chem. 2005;51(8):1480-6.
26. Hamilton TE, Davis S, Onstad L, Kopecky KJ. Thyrotropin levels in a population with no clinical, autoantibody, or ultrasonographic evidence of thyroid disease: implications for the diagnosis of subclinical hypothyroidism. J Clin Endocrinol Metab. 2008;93(4):1224-30.
27. Jiskra J, Bartakova J, Holinka S, Limanova Z, Springer D, Fait T, et al. Low concordance between positive antibodies to thyroperoxidase and thyroid ultrasound autoimmune pattern in pregnant women. Endocr J. 2011;58(10):849-59.
28. Unuane D, Velkeniers B, Anckaert E, Schiettecatte J, Tournaye H, Haentjens P, et al. Thyroglobulin autoantibodies: is there any added value in the detection of thyroid autoimmunity in women consulting for fertility treatment? Thyroid. 2013;23(8):1022-8.
29. Anckaert E, Poppe K, Van Uytfanghe K, Schiettecatte J, Foulon W, Thienpont LM. FT4 immunoassays may display a pattern during pregnancy similar to the equilibrium dialysis ID-LC/tandem MS candidate reference measurement procedure in spite of susceptibility towards binding protein alterations. Clin Chim Acta. 2010;411(17-18):1348-53.
30. Berta E, Samson L, Lenkey A, Erdei A, Cseke B, Jenei K, et al. Evaluation of the thyroid function of healthy pregnant women by five different hormone assays. Pharmazie. 2010;65(6):436-9.
31. Korevaar TI, Chaker L, Medici M, de Rijke YB, Jaddoe VW, Steegers EA, et al. Maternal total T4 during the first half of pregnancy: physiologic aspects and the risk of adverse outcomes in comparison with free T4. Clin Endocrinol (Oxf). 2016;85(5):757-63.
32. Stagnaro-Green A. Clinical guidelines: Thyroid and pregnancy – time for universal screening? Nat Rev Endocrinol. 2017;13(4):192-4.
33. Abalovich M, Gutierrez S, Alcaraz G, Maccallini G, Garcia A, Levalle O. Overt and subclinical hypothyroidism complicating pregnancy. Thyroid. 2002;12(1):63-8.
34. Su PY, Huang K, Hao JH, Xu YQ, Yan SQ, Li T, et al. Maternal thyroid function in the first twenty weeks of pregnancy and subsequent fetal and infant development: a prospective population-based cohort study in China. J Clin Endocrinol Metab. 2011;96(10):3234-41.
35. Korevaar TIM, Medici M, Visser TJ, Peeters RP. Thyroid disease in pregnancy: new insights in diagnosis and clinical management. Nat Rev Endocrinol. 2017;13(10):610-22.

Permissions

All chapters in this book were first published in AEM, by The Brazilian Society of Endocrinology and Metabolism; hereby published with permission under the Creative Commons Attribution License or equivalent. Every chapter published in this book has been scrutinized by our experts. Their significance has been extensively debated. The topics covered herein carry significant findings which will fuel the growth of the discipline. They may even be implemented as practical applications or may be referred to as a beginning point for another development.

The contributors of this book come from diverse backgrounds, making this book a truly international effort. This book will bring forth new frontiers with its revolutionizing research information and detailed analysis of the nascent developments around the world.

We would like to thank all the contributing authors for lending their expertise to make the book truly unique. They have played a crucial role in the development of this book. Without their invaluable contributions this book wouldn't have been possible. They have made vital efforts to compile up to date information on the varied aspects of this subject to make this book a valuable addition to the collection of many professionals and students.

This book was conceptualized with the vision of imparting up-to-date information and advanced data in this field. To ensure the same, a matchless editorial board was set up. Every individual on the board went through rigorous rounds of assessment to prove their worth. After which they invested a large part of their time researching and compiling the most relevant data for our readers.

The editorial board has been involved in producing this book since its inception. They have spent rigorous hours researching and exploring the diverse topics which have resulted in the successful publishing of this book. They have passed on their knowledge of decades through this book. To expedite this challenging task, the publisher supported the team at every step. A small team of assistant editors was also appointed to further simplify the editing procedure and attain best results for the readers.

Apart from the editorial board, the designing team has also invested a significant amount of their time in understanding the subject and creating the most relevant covers. They scrutinized every image to scout for the most suitable representation of the subject and create an appropriate cover for the book.

The publishing team has been an ardent support to the editorial, designing and production team. Their endless efforts to recruit the best for this project, has resulted in the accomplishment of this book. They are a veteran in the field of academics and their pool of knowledge is as vast as their experience in printing. Their expertise and guidance has proved useful at every step. Their uncompromising quality standards have made this book an exceptional effort. Their encouragement from time to time has been an inspiration for everyone.

The publisher and the editorial board hope that this book will prove to be a valuable piece of knowledge for researchers, students, practitioners and scholars across the globe.

List of Contributors

José M. Domínguez, Flavia Nilo, María T. Martínez, José M. Massardo, Sueli Muñoz, Tania Contreras, Rocío Carmona and Joaquín Jerez
Department of Endocrinology, Faculty of Medicine, Pontificia Universidad Católica de Chile, Santiago, Región Metropolitana, Chile

Hernán González, Nicolás Droppelmann and Augusto León
Department of Surgery, Faculty of Medicine, Pontificia Universidad Católica de Chile, Santiago, Región Metropolitana, Chile

Fernanda Cristina Carvalho Mattos Magno, Priscila Alves Medeiros de Sousa, José Egídio Paulo de Oliveira, Eliane Lopes Rosado and João Régis Ivar Carneiro
Universidade Federal do Rio de Janeiro (UFRJ), Rio de Janeiro, RJ, Brasil

Marcelo Paiva Rodrigues and Lícia Lopes Pio Pereira
Instituto Fernando Luiz Barroso, Rio de Janeiro, RJ, Brasil

Livia S. Mastella, Letícia S. Weinert and Vanessa Gnielka
Programa de Pós-Graduação em Ciências Médicas: Endocrinologia, Universidade Federal do Rio Grande do Sul (UFRGS), Porto Alegre, RS, Brasil

Sandra P. Silveiro
Programa de Pós-Graduação em Ciências Médicas: Endocrinologia, Universidade Federal do Rio Grande do Sul (UFRGS), Porto Alegre, RS, Brasil
Serviço de Endocrinologia, Hospital de Clínicas de Porto Alegre (HCPA), Porto Alegre, RS, Brasil

Vânia N. Hirakata
Unidade de Bioestatística, Hospital de Clínicas de Porto Alegre (HCPA), Porto Alegre, RS, Brasil

Maria Lúcia R. Oppermann
Serviço de Obstetrícia e Ginecologia, Hospital de Clínicas de Porto Alegre (HCPA), Porto Alegre, RS, Brasil

Angela J. Reichelt
Serviço de Endocrinologia, Hospital de Clínicas de Porto Alegre (HCPA), Porto Alegre, RS, Brasil

Raiane P. Crespo, Tania A. S. S. Bachega, Berenice B. Mendonça and Larissa G. Gomes
Divisão de Endocrinologia e Laboratório de Hormônios e Genética Molecular (LIM-42), Hospital das Clínicas da Faculdade de Medicina da Universidade de São Paulo (HCFMUSP), São Paulo, SP, Brasil

Yang Lin
School of Medicine, Shandong University, Jinan, Shandong 250100, China
Department of Pediatrics, Anhui Provincial Hospital, Hefei, Anhui 230001, China

Shandong Ye
School of Medicine, Shandong University, Jinan, Shandong 250100, China
Department of Endocrinology, Anhui Provincial Hospital, Hefei, Anhui 230001, China

Yuanyuan He and Sumei Li
Department of Endocrinology, Anhui Provincial Hospital, Hefei, Anhui 230001, China

Yan Chen
Endocrinological Laboratory, Anhui Provincial Hospital, Hefei, Anhui 230001, China

Zhimin Zhai
Department of Central lab, Anhui Provincial Hospital, Hefei, Anhui 230001, China

Caroline Pereira Domingueti
Campus Centro Oeste Dona Lindu, Universidade Federal de São João del-Rei (UFSJ), Divinópolis, MG, Brasil

Rodrigo Bastos Fóscolo
Departamento de Clínica Médica, Faculdade de Medicina, Universidade Federal de Minas Gerais (UFMG), Belo Horizonte, MG, Brasil

Luci Maria S Dusse, Maria das Graças Carvalho, Karina Braga Gomes and Ana Paula Fernandes
Departamento de Análises Clínicas e Toxicológicas, Faculdade de Farmácia, Universidade Federal de Minas Gerais (UFMG), Belo Horizonte, MG, Brasil

Janice Sepúlveda Reis
Departamento de Endocrinologia e Metabologia, Instituto de Ensino e Pesquisa da Santa Casa de Belo Horizonte, Belo Horizonte, MG, Brasil

Adriana Cezaretto, Camila Risso de Barros, Bianca de Almeida-Pititto, Antonela Siqueira-Catania, Milena Monfort-Pires, Luciana Gavilan Dias Folchetti and Sandra Roberta Gouvea Ferreira
Departamento de Epidemiologia, Faculdade de Saúde Pública, Universidade de São Paulo
(FSP-USP), São Paulo, SP, Brasil

Abdulzahra Hussain
Doncaster and Bassetlaw Teaching Hospitals, DN2 5LT, Doncaster, UK

Anna Angelousi
Department of Internal Medicine, Laiko General Hospital, National and Kapodistrian
University of Athens, Greece

Evanthia Diamanti-Kandarakis
Department of Internal Medicine, Medical School, National and Kapodistrian University of Athens, Greece

Evangelia Zapanti
Department of Endocrinology and Diabetes, Alexandra Hospital, Athens, Greece

Afroditi Nonni
Department of Pathology, Medical School, Laiko Hospital, National and Kapodistrian
University of Athens, Greece

Eftuxios Ktenas
National School of Public health, National and Kapodistrian University of Athens, Greece

Aimilia Mantzou
Endocrinology laboratory of Evgenidion hospital, Athens, Greece

Konstantinos Kontzoglou
Department of Propaedeutic Surgery, Laiko General Hospital, University of Athens Medical School, Greece

Grigorios Kouraklis
Department of Propaedeutic Surgery, Laiko General Hospital, University of Athens Medical School, Greece

Inés Matia-García, Lorenzo Salgado-Goytia and Luz Elena Ramos-Arellano
Facultad de Ciencias Químico Biológicas, Universidad Autónoma de Guerrero, Chilpancingo, Guerrero, México

José Francisco Muñoz-Valle
Instituto de Investigación en Ciencias Biomédicas, Departamento de Biología Molecular y Genómica, Centro Universitario de Ciencias de la Salud, Universidad de Guadalajara, Jalisco, México

Adakatia Armenta-Solís
Facultad de Medicina, Universidad Autónoma de Guerrero, Acapulco, Guerrero, México

Olga Lilia Garibay-Cerdenares and Mónica Ramírez
Cátedra CONACyT, Facultad de Ciencias Químico Biológicas, Universidad Autónoma de Guerrero, Chilpancingo, Guerrero, México

Isela Parra-Rojas
Laboratorio de Investigación en Obesidad y Diabetes, Facultad de Ciencias Químico Biológicas, Universidad Autónoma de Guerrero, Ciudad Universitaria, Guerrero, México

Inés Califano
Service of Endocrinology, Instituto de Oncología A. H. Roffo, Universidad de Buenos Aires, Ciudad Autónoma de Buenos Aires, Argentina

Susana Deutsch
Endocrine Unit, Hospital General de Agudos J. A. Fernández, Ciudad Autónoma de Buenos Aires, Argentina

Alicia Löwenstein
Division of Endocrinology, Hospital General de Agudos J. M. Ramos Mejía, Ciudad Autónoma de Buenos Aires, Argentina

Carmen Cabezón
Service of Endocrinology and Nuclear Medicine, Hospital Italiano de Buenos Aires, Ciudad Autónoma de Buenos Aires, Argentina

Fabián Pitoia
Division of Endocrinology, Hospital de Clínicas, Universidad de Buenos Aires, Ciudad Autónoma de Buenos Aires, Argentina

Romeu Paulo Martins Silva
Centro de Ciências da Saúde e Desporto, Universidade Federal do Acre (UFAC), Rio Branco, AC, Brasil
Centro Universitário do Planalto de Araxá (Uniaraxá), Araxá, MG, Brasil

Rodrigo Otávio dos Santos, Nelson Eurípedes Matildes Junior and Pâmella Ferreira Rodrigues
Centro Universitário do Planalto de Araxá (Uniaraxá), Araxá, MG, Brasil

Antônio Vicente Mundim, Mario da Silva Garrote-Filho and Nilson Penha-Silva
Instituto de Genética e Bioquímica, Universidade Federal de Uberlândia (UFU), Uberlândia, MG, Brasil

Lucio Vilar and José Luciano Albuquerque
Serviço de Endocrinologia, Hospital das Clínicas, Universidade Federal de Pernambuco (UFPE), Recife, PE, Brasil

Julio Abucham
Unidade de Neuroendócrino, Escola Paulista de Medicina, Universidade Federal de São Paulo (Unifesp/EPM), São Paulo, SP, Brasil

Luiz Antônio Araujo
Centro de Endocrinologia e Diabetes de Joinville (Endoville), Joinville, SC, Brasil

Monalisa F. Azevedo, Luiz Augusto Casulari and Luciana A. Naves
Serviço de Endocrinologia do Hospital Universitário de Brasília, Universidade de Brasília (UnB), Brasília, DF, Brasil

Cesar Luiz Boguszewski
Serviço de Endocrinologia e Metabologia, Hospital de Clínicas, Universidade Federal do Paraná (SEMPR), Curitiba, PR, Brasil

Malebranche B. C. Cunha Neto and Nina R. C. Musolino
Divisão de Neurocirurgia Funcional, Instituto de Psiquiatria do Hospital das Clínicas, Faculdade de Medicina da Universidade de São Paulo (IPq-HC-FMUSP), São Paulo, SP, Brasil

Mauro A. Czepielewski and Camila Viecceli
Serviço de Endocrinologia, Hospital de Clínicas de Porto Alegre, PPG Endocrinologia, Faculdade de Medicina, Universidade Federal do Rio Grande do Sul (UFRGS), Porto Alegre, RS, Brasil

Felipe H. G. Duarte, Andrea Glezer, Raquel S. Jallad and Marcello D. Bronstein
Serviço de Endocrinologia, Hospital das Clínicas, Faculdade de Medicina da Universidade de São Paulo (FMUSP), São Paulo, SP, Brasil

Manuel dos S. Faria
Serviço de Endocrinologia, Hospital Universitário Presidente Dutra, Universidade Federal do Maranhão (UFMA), São Luís, MA, Brasil

Cíntia M. S. Silva
Serviço de Endocrinologia, Hospital Universitário Clementino Fraga Filho, Universidade Federal do Rio de Janeiro (HUCFF-UFRJ), Rio de Janeiro, RJ, Brasil

Monica R. Gadelha
Serviço de Endocrinologia, Hospital Universitário Clementino Fraga Filho, Universidade Federal do Rio de Janeiro (HUCFF-UFRJ), Rio de Janeiro, RJ, Brasil
Unidade de Neuroendocrinologia, Instituto Estadual do Cérebro Paulo Niemeyer, Rio de Janeiro, RJ, Brasil

Heraldo M. Garmes
Departamento de Clínica Médica, Faculdade de Ciências Médicas, Universidade Estadual de Campinas (FCM/Unicamp), Campinas, SP, Brasil

Maria Helane Gurgel, Manoel Martins and Renan M. Montenegro
Serviço de Endocrinologia, Hospital Universitário Walter Cantídio, Universidade Federal do Ceará (UFCE), Fortaleza, CE, Brasil

Paulo A. C. Miranda
Serviço de Endocrinologia e Metabologia, Santa Casa de Belo Horizonte, Belo Horizonte, MG, Brasil

Antônio Ribeiro-Oliveira Júnior
Serviço de Endocrinologia, Hospital das Clínicas, Universidade Federal de Minas Gerais (UFMG), Belo Horizonte, MG, Brasil

Aline Stangherlin Martins, Luiz Oswaldo Carneiro Rodrigues, Camila Maria Matos, Marcio Leandro Ribeiro Souza and Nilton Alves de Rezende
Centro de Referência de Neurofibromatose, Universidade Federal de Minas Gerais (UFMG), Belo Horizonte, MG, Brasil

Ann Kristine Jansen
Departamento de Nutrição, Universidade Federal de Minas Gerais (UFMG), Belo Horizonte, MG, Brasil

Débora Marques Miranda
Departamento de Clínica Médica, Universidade Federal de Minas Gerais (UFMG), Belo Horizonte, MG, Brasil

Pedro Weslley Rosario and Maria Regina Calsolari
Programa de Pós-Graduação e Serviço de Endocrinologia, Santa Casa de Belo Horizonte, Belo Horizonte, MG, Brasil

Luis Fernando Faria Oliveira
Fundação Universidade de Itaúna, Itaúna, MG, Brasil

Fernanda R. Bernaud and Ciglea Nascimento
Divisão de Endocrinologia, Hospital de Clínicas de Porto Alegre (HCPA), Porto Alegre, RS, Brasil

Mileni Vanti Beretta
Divisão de Endocrinologia, Hospital de Clínicas de Porto Alegre (HCPA), Porto Alegre, RS, Brasil
Programa de Pós-graduação em Alimentação, Nutrição e Saúde, Departamento de Nutrição, Universidade Federal do Rio Grande do Sul (UFRGS), Porto Alegre, RS, Brasil

Ticiana C. Rodrigues
Divisão de Endocrinologia, Hospital de Clínicas de Porto Alegre (HCPA), Porto Alegre, RS, Brasil
Departamento de Medicina Interna, Faculdade de Medicina, Universidade Federal do Rio Grande do Sul (UFRGS), Porto Alegre, RS, Brasil

Thais Steemburgo
Programa de Pós-graduação em Alimentação, Nutrição e Saúde, Departamento de Nutrição, Universidade Federal do Rio Grande do Sul (UFRGS), Porto Alegre, RS, Brasil

Monica Marazan and Maria Lesovici
"Louis Turcanu" Emergency Hospital for Children, Timişoara, România

Ramona Stroescu, Teofana Bizerea, Otilia Mãrginean and Gabriela Doroş
"Louis Turcanu" Emergency Hospital for Children, Timişoara, România
"Victor Babes" University of Medicine and Pharmacy, Timişoara, România

Dilek Tuzun, Ayten Oguz, Murat Sahin and Kamile Gul
Kahramanmaras Sutcu Imam University, Faculty of Medicine, Department of Endocrinology and Metabolism, Kahramanmaras, Turkey

Muhammet Naci Aydin, Imran Ceren and Ahmet Akçay
Kahramanmaras Sutcu Imam University, Faculty of Medicine, Department of Cardiology, Kahramanmaras, Turkey

Ergul Belge Kurutas and Velid Ünsal
Kahramanmaras Sutcu Imam University, Faculty of Medicine, Department of Biochemistry, Kahramanmaras, Turkey

Onder Ercan
Kahramanmaras Sutcu Imam University, Faculty of Medicine, Department of Obstetric and Gynecology, Kahramanmaras, Turkey

Valentina Velkoska Nakova
University "Goce Delchev", Faculty of Medical Science, Clinical Hospital, Shtip, R. Macedonia

Brankica Krstevska
University Clinic of Endocrinology, Diabetes and Metabolic Disorders, Medical Faculty, Skopje, R. Macedonia

Elizabeta Srbinovska Kostovska
University Clinic of Cardiology, Medical Faculty, Skopje, R. Macedonia

Olivija Vaskova
Institute of Patophysiology and Nuclear Medicine, Medical Faculty, Skopje, R. Macedonia

Ljubica Georgievska Ismail
University Clinic of Cardiology, Medical Faculty, Skopje, R. Macedonia

Fatemeh Khanizadeh
Obstetrician/Gynecology, Shahid Beheshti University of Medical Science, Tehran, Iran

Asghar Rahmani
Ilam University of Medical Science, Ilam, Iran

Khairollah Asadollahi
Clinical epidemiology, Departament of Social Medicine, Faculty of Medicine, Ilam University of Medical Sciences, Ilam, Iran

Mohammad Reza Hafezi Ahmadi
Department of Pathology, Ilam University of Medical Science, Ilam, Iran

Arunkumar Karthikayan, Sathasivam Sureshkumar, Dharanipragada Kadambari and Chellappa Vijayakumar
Department of Surgery, Jawaharlal Institute of Postgraduate Medical Education and Research (JIPMER), Pondicherry, India

Paulo Eduardo Dietrich Jaworski, Anderson Ramos and Arthur Radaelli Nicoleit
Departamento de Urologia, Hospital Universitário Evangélico de Curitiba, Curitiba, PR, Brasil

Luis Fernando de Almeida Bacarin and Pedro Olivo Neto
Faculdade de Medicina, Faculdade Evangélica do Paraná (Fepar), Curitiba, PR, Brasil

Denise P. Momesso, Rubens Carmo Costa Filho, João Luiz Ferreira Costa, Felipe Saddy, Ayla Mesquita, Marcela Calomeni, Claudia dos Santos Silva, Jacqueline Farret, Mariana Leon Vasques, Aline G. Santos, Ana Paula Vieira Cabral, Dayane Ribeiro, Luciana Reis, Maria de Fátima M. Muino, Roberta Santiago Vitorino, Claudio Amorim Monteiro, Evandro Tinoco and Andre Volschan
Hospital Pró-Cardíaco, Rio de Janeiro, RJ, Brasil

Leila C. B. Zanatta, Cesar L. Boguszewski and Victoria Z. C. Borba
Divisão de Endocrinologia (SEMPR), Departamento de Medicina Interna, Universidade Federal do Paraná (UFPR), Curitiba, PR, Brasil

Carolina A. Moreira
Divisão de Endocrinologia (SEMPR), Departamento de Medicina Interna, Universidade Federal do Paraná (UFPR), Curitiba, PR, Brasil
Laboratório PRO, Seção de Histomorfometria Óssea, Fundação Pró-Renal, Curitiba, PR, Brasil

Francisco Zacaron Werneck and Emerson Filipino Coelho
Universaidade Federal de Ouro Preto (UFOP), Ouro Preto, MG, Brasil

Saulo Peters Almas, Patrícia de Fátima dos Santos Teixeira and Mário Vaisman
Universidade Federal do Rio de Janeiro (UFRJ), Rio de Janeiro, RJ, Brasil

Marília Mendes do Nascimento Garcia and Jorge Roberto Perrout de Lima
Universidade Federal de Juiz de Fora (UFJF), Juiz de Fora, MG, Brasil

Heloina Lamha Machado Bonfante
Faculdade de Ciências Médicas e da Saúde de Juiz de For a (Suprema), Juiz de Fora, MG, Brasil

Patrícia dos Santos Vigário
Centro Universitário Augusto Motta (Unisuam), Rio de Janeiro, RJ, Brasil

Míriam Raquel Meira Mainenti
Escola de Educação Física do Exército (EsEFEx), Rio de Janeiro, RJ, Brasil

Pedro D. Ortolani Jr., João H. Romaldini, Ricardo A. Guerra and Evandro S. Portes
Serviço de Endocrinologia, Hospital do Servidor Público Estadual de São Paulo, Instituto de Assistência Médica ao Servidor Público Estadual (HSPEIAMSPE), São Paulo, SP, Brasil

George C. X. Meireles and João Pimenta
Serviço de Cardiologia, Hospital do Servidor Público Estadual de São Paulo, Instituto de Assistência Médica ao Servidor Público Estadual (HSPE-IAMSPE), São Paulo, SP, Brasil

Gisele Almeida Batista, Aglécio Luiz de Souza, Daniela Miguel Marin, Marina Sider, Vaneska Carvalho Melhado, Arlete Maria Fernandes and Sarah Monte Alegre
Faculdade de Ciências Médicas, Universidade Estadual de Campinas (FCM-Unicamp), Campinas, SP, Brasil

Mariana Veronez Borgo and Rafael de Oliveira Alvim
Programa de Pós-Graduação em Saúde Coletiva, Universidade Federal do Espírito Santo (UFES), Vitória, ES, Brasil

José Geraldo Mill
Programa de Pós-Graduação em Saúde Coletiva, Universidade Federal do Espírito Santo (UFES), Vitória, ES, Brasil
Programa de Pós-Graduação em Ciências Fisiológicas, Universidade Federal do Espírito Santo (UFES), Vitória, ES, Brasil

Marcelo Perim Baldo
Departamento de Fisiopatologia, Universidade Estadual de Montes Claros (Unimontes), Montes Claros, MG, Brasil
Programa de Pós-Graduação em Ciências Fisiológicas, Universidade Federal do Espírito Santo (UFES), Vitória, ES, Brasil

Divanei Zaniqueli and Carmem Luiza Sartório
Programa de Pós-Graduação em Ciências Fisiológicas, Universidade Federal do Espírito Santo (UFES), Vitória, ES, Brasil

Polyana Romano Oliosa
Programa de Pós-Graduação em Nutrição e Saúde, Universidade Federal do Espírito Santo (UFES), Vitória, ES, Brasil

Daniel Pires Capingana, Pedro Magalhães and Amilcar Bernardo da Silva
Departamento de Ciências Fisiológicas, Escola de Medicina, Universidade Agostinho Neto (UAN), Luanda, Angola

Julio Rosenstock
Dallas Diabetes Research Center at Medical City, Dallas, TX, USA

Chantal Mathieu
UZ Leuven, Leuven, Belgium

Hungta Chen, Ricardo Garcia-Sanchez and Gabriela Luporini Saraiva
AstraZeneca, Gaithersburg, MD, USA

Rodrigo Nolasco, Linda D. F. Moreira, Rosangela Villa Marin and Marise Lazaretti-Castro
Departamento de Medicina, Disciplina de Endocrinologia, Faculdade de Medicina, Universidade Federal de São Paulo (Unifesp/EPM), São Paulo, SP, Brasil

Danilo S. Bocalini
Fisiologia Translacional, Programa de Pós-Graduação em Educação Física e Ciências do Envelhecimento, Universidade São Judas Tadeu (USJT), São Paulo, SP, Brasil

Fernanda C. A. O. Fronza
Escola de Educação Física e Esporte da Universidade de São Paulo (EEFE/USP), São Paulo, SP, Brasil

Filiz Eksi Haydardedeoglu, Gulay Simsek Bagir and Melek Eda Ertorer
Baskent University Faculty of Medicine Department of Endocrinology and Metabolism, Adana, Turkey

Nese Torun and Mehmet Reyhan
Baskent University Faculty of Medicine Department of Nuclear Medicine, Adana, Turkey

Emrah Kocer
Baskent University Faculty of Medicine Department of Pathology, Adana, Turkey

Annie Schtscherbyna Almeida de Assis, Débora Ayres Saraiva, Tatiana Martins Benvenuto Louro Berbara, Carolina Donner de Drummond Ventura, Mario Vaisman and Patrícia de Fátima dos Santos Teixeira
Departamento de Medicina Interna e Unidade de Endocrinologia, Faculdade de Medicina e Hospital Universitário Clementino Fraga Filho, Universidade Federal do Rio de Janeiro (HUCFF/UFRJ), Rio de Janeiro, RJ, Brasil

Carolina Martins Corcino
Departamento de Medicina Interna e Unidade de Endocrinologia, Faculdade de Medicina e Hospital Universitário Clementino Fraga Filho, Universidade Federal do Rio de Janeiro (HUCFF/UFRJ), Rio de Janeiro, RJ, Brasil
Unidade de Endocrinologia, Instituto Estadual de Diabetes e Endocrinologia Luiz Capriglione (IEDE), Rio de Janeiro, RJ, Brasil

Nathalie Anne de Oliveira e Silva de Morais
Departamento de Medicina Interna e Unidade de Endocrinologia, Faculdade de Medicina e Hospital Universitário Clementino Fraga Filho, Universidade Federal do Rio de Janeiro (HUCFF/UFRJ), Rio de Janeiro, RJ, Brasil
Unidade de Endocrinologia, Instituto Estadual de Diabetes e Endocrinologia Luiz Capriglione (IEDE), Rio de Janeiro, RJ, Brasil
Unidade de Endocrinologia, Instituto Nacional de Câncer José Alencar Gomes da Silva (INCA), Rio de Janeiro, RJ, Brasil

Index